Psychological Approaches
to Pain Management

Psychological Approaches to Pain Management

A PRACTITIONER'S HANDBOOK

Second Edition

Edited by

Dennis C. Turk
Robert J. Gatchel

THE GUILFORD PRESS
New York   London

© 2002 The Guilford Press
A Division of Guilford Publications, Inc.
72 Spring Street, New York, NY 10012
www.guilford.com

Printed in the United States of America

This book is printed on acid-free paper.

Last digit is print number: 9 8 7 6 5 4 3 2 1

Library of Congress Cataloging-in-Publication Data

Psychological approaches to pain management : a practitioner's handbook
/ edited by Dennis C. Turk, Robert J. Gatchel. — 2nd ed.
    p. cm.
Includes bibliographical references and index.
    ISBN 1-57230-642-4
  1. Pain—Treatment—Handbooks, manuals, etc. 2. Pain—Psychological
aspects—Handbooks, manuals, etc. 3. Psychotherapy—Handbooks, manuals,
etc. I. Turk, Dennis C. II. Gatchel, Robert J., 1947–
RB127 P82 2002
616′.0472—dc21   2002007149

We dedicate this volume to John D. Loeser, MD, for his leadership, wisdom, and commitment to furthering our understanding and treatment of pain sufferers, his outstanding contribution to the field of pain internationally, and especially for his insights regarding the central roles of psychosocial and behavioral factors in the experience of pain and suffering.

About the Editors

Dennis C. Turk, PhD, is the John and Emma Bonica Professor of Anesthesiology and Pain Research at the University of Washington. He was the recipient of the American Psychological Association, Division of Health Psychology, Outstanding Scientific Contribution Award and the American Association of Pain Management's Janet Travell Award. Dr. Turk has over 325 publications and has written and edited 13 volumes. He is currently editor-in-chief of *The Clinical Journal of Pain.*

Robert J. Gatchel, PhD, is the Elizabeth H. Penn Professor of Clinical Psychology and Professor in the Departments of Psychiatry and Rehabilitation Science at the University of Texas Southwestern Medical Center at Dallas, where he is the Director of Graduate Research, Division of Clinical Psychology. He is a Diplomate of the American Board of Professional Psychology and is on the Board of Directors of the American Board of Health Psychology. Dr. Gatchel is also the recipient of consecutive Research Scientist Development Awards from the National Institute of Mental Health. He has published over 190 scientific articles and 60 book chapters, and has authored and edited 20 other books. He is also on the editorial boards of numerous psychological and medical journals. In addition, he is the first psychologist to receive the Henry Farfan Award for Outstanding Contributions to the Field of Spine Care from the North American Spine Society.

Contributors

Janet R. Abrams, PsyD, Department of Psychiatry and Behavioral Sciences, University of Washington School of Medicine, Seattle, Washington

John G. Arena, PhD, Pain Evaluation and Intervention Program, Department of Veterans Affairs Medical Center, Medical College of Georgia, Augusta, Georgia

Ann K. Aspnes, BA, Department of Psychology, Duke University, Durham, North Carolina

Stephen C. Basler, PsyD, Mood Disorders Center, University of Rochester, Rochester, New York

Pat M. Beaupre, PhD, Inland Health Dynamics, San Bernardino, California

Edward B. Blanchard, PhD, Center for Stress and Anxiety Disorders, State University of New York at Albany, Albany, New York

Paul Crichton, MD, MRCPsych, Department of Psychological Medicine, The Royal Marsden Hospital, Surrey, United Kingdom

Geert Crombez, PhD, Department of Psychology, Ghent University, Gent, Belgium

Jeroen de Jong, MSc, Department of Medical, Clinical, and Experimental Psychology, Maastricht University, Maastricht, The Netherlands

Jeffrey Dersch, PhD, PRIDE, Dallas, Texas

Daniel M. Doleys, PhD, Pain and Rehabilitation Institute, Birmingham, Alabama

Robert H. Dworkin, PhD, Department of Anesthesiology, University of Rochester School of Medicine and Dentistry, Rochester, New York

Mark L. Elliott, PhD, Institute for Psychological and Sexual Health, Columbus, Ohio

Noor M. Gajraj, MD, Department of Anesthesia and Pain Management, University of Texas Southwestern Medical Center at Dallas, Dallas, Texas

Robert J. Gatchel, PhD, Department of Psychiatry, University of Texas Southwestern Medical Center at Dallas, Dallas, Texas

Karen M. Gil, PhD, Department of Psychology, University of North Carolina, Chapel Hill, North Carolina

Roy C. Grzesiak, PhD, Department of Psychiatry, University of Medicine and Dentistry of New Jersey, Newark, New Jersey

Loretta M. Hillier, MA, Pain Innovations, Inc., London, Ontario, Canada

Kenneth A. Holroyd, PhD, Psychology Department, Ohio University, Athens, Ohio

Mark P. Jensen, PhD, Department of Rehabilitation Medicine, University of Washington, Seattle, Washington

Francis J. Keefe, PhD, Department of Psychology and Behavioral Science, Duke University Medical Center, Durham, North Carolina

Robert D. Kerns, PhD, Psychology Service, Veterans Affairs Connecticut Healthcare System, West Haven, Connecticut

Steven James Linton, PhD, Department of Occupational and Environmental Medicine, Orebro Medical Center, Orebro, Sweden

Gay L. Lipchik, PhD, St. Vincent Rehabilitation Services, Erie, Pennsylvania

Richard Mayou, BM, FRCPsych, Department of Psychiatry, Warneford Hospital, University of Oxford, Oxford, United Kingdom

Patricia A. McGrath, PhD, Department of Anesthesia, Hospital for Sick Children, and Faculty of Medicine, University of Toronto, Toronto, Ontario, Canada

Kevin McWhorter, PT, MBA, Winnock Reïntegratie, De Bilt, The Netherlands

Susan J. Middaugh, PhD, Department of Anesthesia and Perioperative Medicine, Medical University of South Carolina, Charleston, South Carolina

Elena S. Monarch, PhD, Department of Anesthesiology, University of Washington, Seattle, Washington

Stirling Moorey, MD, FRCPsych, Psychotherapy Department, Maudsley Hospital, London, United Kingdom

Stephen Morley, PhD, Academic Unit of Psychiatry and Behavioral Sciences, School of Medicine, University of Leeds, Leeds, United Kingdom

Justin M. Nash, PhD, Department of Psychiatry and Human Behavior, Centers for Behavioral and Preventive Medicine, Brown Medical School and The Miriam Hospital, Providence, Rhode Island

David V. Nelson, PhD, Department of Anesthesiology, Oregon Health and Science University, Portland, Oregon

John D. Otis, PhD, Psychology Service, Veterans Affairs Connecticut Healthcare System, West Haven, Connecticut

Kim Pawlick, PhD, Department of Anesthesia and Perioperative Medicine, Medical University of South Carolina, Charleston, South Carolina

Peter B. Polatin, MD, Department of Psychiatry, University of Texas Southwestern Medical Center at Dallas, Dallas, Texas

Sheri D. Pruitt, PhD, The Permanente Medical Group, Roseville, California

Meredith E. Rumble, BA, Department of Psychology, Duke University, Durham, North Carolina

Steven H. Sanders, PhD, Siskin Hospital for Physical Rehabilitation, Chattanooga, Tennessee

Michael Sharpe, MD, MRCP, MRCPsych, Department of Psychiatry, University of Edinburgh, Edinburgh, United Kingdom

Jeffrey J. Sherman, PhD, Departments of Oral Medicine and Anesthesiology, University of Washington, Seattle, Washington

Judith Sieben, MSc, Department of General Practice, Maastricht University, Maastricht, The Netherlands

Karen L. Syrjala, PhD, Fred Hutchinson Cancer Research Center and Department of Psychiatry and Behavioral Sciences, University of Washington, Seattle, Washington

Dennis C. Turk, PhD, Department of Anesthesiology, University of Washington, Seattle, Washington

Pieter van Akkerveeken, MD, PhD, Winnock Reïntegratie, De Bilt, The Netherlands

Lex Vendrig, PhD, Winnock Reïntegratie, De Bilt, The Netherlands

Johan W. S. Vlaeyen, PhD, Department of Medical, Clinical, and Experimental Psychology, Maastricht University, Maastricht, The Netherlands

Michael Von Korff, ScD, Center for Health Studies, Group Health Cooperative of Puget Sound, Seattle, Washington

Amanda C. de C. Williams, PhD, INPUT Pain Management Unit, Guys & St. Thomas Hospital, London, United Kingdom

Emily A. Wise, PhD, Psychology Service, Veterans Affairs Connecticut Healthcare System, West Haven, Connecticut

Anna R. Wright, PhD, Departments of Psychiatry and Anesthesiology and Pain Management, University of Texas Southwestern Medical Center at Dallas, Dallas, Texas

Preface

In the Preface to the first edition of this volume, we noted that systematic attempts to treat pain have been closely aligned with how pain is conceptualized and evaluated. Traditionally, the focus in health care has been on the cause of the pain reported, with the assumption that there is a physical basis for the pain and that once it is identified, the source can be either eliminated or blocked by medical, surgical, or other physical interventions. Consequently, assessment was focused on identifying the physical basis—the cause—for the pain. In the absence of "adequate" physical pathology to validate the patient's report, psychological causation was often invoked; hence, the term "psychogenic pain." Thus, the traditional view of persistent pain complaints has been characterized by a simple dichotomy: The pain report had either a physical cause or a psychological one. The psychological causes might be unconscious factors associated with psychopathology, maladaptive personality, or motive in an effort to achieve some type of personal gain.

The dichotomous view of pain has been shown to be incomplete and inadequate. There is no question that physical perturbations contribute to pain symptoms; nor is there any argument anymore that psychological factors may play a part in the symptom reporting of some patients. The weighting or balance between physical and psychological contributors may vary over time and across individuals. These psychosocial factors must be evaluated and treated in conjunction with the physical and predispositional psychological ones in order to ensure therapeutic success. Moreover, research has suggested that the social and familial context in which pain persists can also play a central role in the maintenance of disability.

The observations we outlined underscore the important role of mental health specialists in the assessment and treatment of patients with diverse chronic pain syndromes. A large proliferation of studies, and several meta-analyses, have confirmed the clinical effectiveness and cost-effectiveness of psychological treatments alone and when combined with more traditional methods. In response to the results of this body of research, the role of mental health specialists has been noted in U.S. government publications and initiatives, such as that of the Veterans Administration. Governmental organizations in other countries (e.g., Canada, Australia, United Kingdom, and Sweden), as well as in the United States, have documented the important role of psychological factors and psychologists in the reports of pain and pain management. Private medical certifying agencies such as the Joint Commission on the Accreditation of Healthcare Organizations (JACHO) and the Commission for the Accreditation of Rehabilitation Facilities (CARF), as well as professional organizations that have proposed practice guidelines (e.g., the American Academy of Neurology), also have recognized the importance and complexity of pain and the need to go beyond exclusive reliance on physical modalities to treat pain sufferers. Moreover, the acknowledgment of the importance of psychological factors in pain has resulted in a large number of mental health providers evaluating and treating pain patients in specialized pain clinics, in a variety of medical settings, and in private practices. The American Psychological Association designated psychological treatment of chronic pain patients as one of the 25 areas for which there was empirical validation for psychological intervention.

We have given numerous workshops and presentations on psychological approaches to pain management. What participants are most interested in is going beyond discussions of theory and general principles to more specific details of how to deal with certain patients and common problems raised by individual patients. They raise questions about patient motivation, involvement of families, methods to deal with adherence to treatment recommendations and homework assignments, how to deal with relapses, the role of opioids in treatment of chronic pain patients, can chronicity be predicted, are there ways to prevent long-term problems, and so forth. Essentially, what they are seeking is not only what to do but "how to do it." In response, our emphasis in the first edition and continuing in the present one is on providing details, the "nuts and bolts" of treatment, rather than academic discussions.

Since the publication of the first edition of this volume, there have been tremendous advances in understanding the role and nature of different psychosocial and behavioral factors in acute, recurrent acute, and chronic pain syndromes. Psychological assessment is becoming accepted as essential prior to surgery and implantation of spinal cord stimulators and drug delivery systems. Despite advances in technology, patients who are implanted will likely continue to have some degree of pain. Preparation of these people prior to the procedures may improve outcomes. Predictors of chronicity have received a great deal of attention, and a consistent finding is that psychological variables are better predictors of disability and response to treatment than demographic or physical ones. Identification of psychosocial predictors holds promise for earlier intervention and prevention of chronicity. The interrelationships between physical health and mental health are gaining renewed attention and suggest that traditional psychological approaches are likely to be of importance in the treatment of patients with various pain syndromes. Treatments that combine psychotropic and opioid medications with psychological approaches are gaining renewed interest. More efficient and cost-effective treatment approaches are being driven by changes in health care with concerns about cost containment. In response, psychological approaches are being streamlined and systematically evaluated. Finally, psychological approaches are being extended to patients with many pain syndromes who have previously been treated almost exclusively by physical modalities.

Although patients with diverse chronic pain syndromes have much in common, there are unique characteristics that require attention specific to the problems associated with the syndrome. For example, patients with occupational injuries have concerns about the future and their ability to return to work, those with complex regional pain syndromes must deal with physical limitations, women with chronic pelvic pain must deal with problems associated with sexuality, patients with cancer have to cope with fears of dying, and patients who have sustained injuries in automobile accidents must face their fears of driving and reinjury, all in addition to problems created by persistent pain. In this edition, we have expanded the topics covered to reflect these developments and innovations.

The health care system is changing at a dizzying pace, and there is greater and greater reliance on empirically based outcomes that focus on cost and patient satisfaction, as well as on clinical effectiveness. As a consequence, it is no longer possible to justify treatments based solely on clinicians' beliefs about what is appropriate and likely to be helpful. Reliance on anecdotal reports will not convince third-party payers to invest in such treatment. Clinicians must accept that the plural of anecdote is not evidence. Therefore, outcomes studies are essential as a basis for judging clinical outcomes. In response to this need, we have asked contributors to provide documentation of efficacy of the treatments being described to support their continued use.

To balance the "what to do" and "how to do" of different treatment approaches, with different pain syndromes and the need for a rational theoretical basis and demonstrated evidential base, we have organized this volume in three sections:

Part I, Conceptual, Diagnostic, and Methodological Issues (Chapters 1–3), sets the foundation for the various treatments described. Chapter 1 presents an integrated biopsychosocial perspective that is applicable regardless of the nature of pain or the pain syndrome. The second chapter establishes the interrelationship between psychological disorders and chronic pain, considering the causal relationships between physical health and mental health. Chapter 3 provides important insights into outcomes research and offers suggestions for how to evaluate reports of treatment outcome studies.

Part II, Treatment Approaches and Methods (Chapters 4–13), focuses on important topics and models that transcend specific pain syndromes. There is no question that patient motivation is essential, regardless of the treatment approach adopted. Chapter 4 describes a model for facilitating patient motivation. Chapters 5–7 describe the rationale and methods of three of the most common psychological approaches, namely, insight-oriented psychotherapy, operant conditioning, and the cognitive-behavioral approach to treating chronic pain patients. Chapters 8–10 describe specific techniques—biofeedback, hypnosis, imagery, relaxation, and exposure-based desensitization—that can be used with patients with a number of different pain syndromes. Chapters 11 and 12 address the mode of treatment delivery, group format, and family involvement. There are unique benefits to treating patients in groups, both in efficiency and in the power of group dynamics. Patients, like most people, do not live in isolation but in a social context. Moreover, the vast majority of chronic pain patients (by definition, people with conditions that will extend over long periods) will continue to experience pain long after treatment termination. Consequently, significant others can play an important role in maintaining the benefits derived during formal treatment and generalizing positive results beyond the clinical setting. Involvement of significant others is likely to enhance long-term treatment outcomes.

Part III, Specific Syndromes and Populations (Chapters 14–28), covers secondary prevention, treatment of some of the most common pain syndromes, and pain sufferers at the two extremes of lifespan: children and the elderly. Early interventions in primary care, specialty practice, and in preparing patients for invasive treatments are covered in Chapters 14–16. Chapters 17–26 provide detailed discussions and case examples describing the treatment of patients with specific, prevalent chronic pain syndromes. As we noted earlier, there are commonalities among patients with different pain syndromes, yet there are unique problems that must be addressed in each specific syndrome. These chapters address both the commonalities and the special features that must be targeted to treat successfully patients with this set of pain syndromes. The final two chapters describe the treatment needs of children and the elderly. Although the same psychological principles apply throughout the span of life, the methods used to treat patients at the extremes create unique challenges and require special skills for presentation and delivery. The authors of these two chapters provide insights and make suggestions to increase the likelihood of the best outcomes.

It is our intention for this volume to bridge the gap between laboratory research and direct application to the clinical environment. The National Institutes of Health now emphasize the importance of "transfer of technology" from basic research to clinical populations in the "real world." The contributors, seasoned clinicians who are well-known and respected scholars in the field, were carefully selected. They were given the task of writing chapters for practitioners who desire information about the most effective, empirically documented methods of pain management that can be applied in the clinical arena. We requested that each contributor provide brief overviews of developments, followed by comprehensive recommendations and specific clinical details of how to manage pain most effectively. That is, we asked the contributors to describe, in depth, the details and nuances of their approach to treating their patients.

We believe that this handbook will be of particular relevance and interest to clinicians, whether they see only a small number of pain patients or whether the majority of their practice is devoted to this population. Each chapter provides practical clinical information and guidelines, which can help the practitioner understand the most heuristic ways of managing pain and interfacing with the health care environment. The detailed presentations should facilitate the ability of mental health clinicians and others to treat this diverse population—chronic pain sufferers—more effectively. Moreover, the specific elements of treatment presented should inform clinical investigators about a number of areas in which clinical insights have revealed important issues in need of empirical testing and support.

DENNIS C. TURK
ROBERT J. GATCHEL

Contents

I

CONCEPTUAL, DIAGNOSTIC, AND METHODOLOGICAL ISSUES

1

Biopsychosocial Perspective on Chronic Pain

Dennis C. Turk
Elena S. Monarch

Chronic pain is a demoralizing situation that confronts the sufferer not only with the stress created by pain but with many other ongoing difficulties that compromise all aspects of his or her life. Living with chronic pain requires considerable emotional resilience as it depletes people's emotional reserves. In the presence of chronic pain, the continuing quest for relief often remains elusive, which can lead to feelings of demoralization, helplessness, hopelessness, and outright depression. Moreover, chronic pain taxes not only the sufferer but also the capacity of significant others who provide instrumental and emotional support. Health care providers share patients' and significant others' feelings of frustration as the reports of pain continue, despite the provider's best efforts and, at times, in the absence of pathological signs that can account for the reported pain.

On a societal level, unrelieved pain creates a burden in, health care expenditures, disability benefits, lost productivity, and tax revenue. Third-party payers are confronted with escalating medical costs, compensation payments, and frustration when patients remain disabled despite extensive and expensive treatments.

Despite advances in knowledge of the physical mechanisms, development of sophisticated diagnostic procedures, and development of innovative treatments, currently no treatment is available that consistently and permanently alleviates pain for all those afflicted. This chapter examines how psychological and social factors can be integrated with physical factors to create a biopsychosocial framework that can help us to understand chronic pain patients and their disability. We review research focusing specifically on psychological, behavioral, and social factors, and we discuss the implications of these contributors for treatment and rehabilitation. The factors discussed here underlie many of the treatment approaches described in other chapters of this volume.

The Need for an Alternative to the Disease Model

The biomedical model of pain—which dates back to the ancient Greeks that was inculcated into medical thinking by Descartes in the 17th century—assumes that people's reports result from a specific disease state represented by disordered biology. The diagnosis is confirmed by data from objective tests of physical damage and impairment and medical interventions are specifically directed toward correcting the organic dysfunction or source of pathology. There is general agreement, however, that the presence and extent of physical pathology are not sufficient to account for all reported physical symptoms. Decidedly diverse responses to objectively similar physical perturbations and identical treatments have been noted clinically and have been documented in many empirical investigations. Although they are related, the associations between physical impairments on the one hand and pain report and disability on the other are modest at best (see, e.g., Flor & Turk, 1988; Waddell & Main, 1984). Identified physical pathology does not predict severity of pain or level of disability. Moreover, pain severity does not adequately explain psychological distress or extent of disability observed. The question that remains to be answered is this: What factors can account for the highly varied expression of subjective experience and behavioral responses?

From the perspective of the biomedical model, accompanying features of chronic conditions, such as sleep disturbance, depression, psychosocial disability, and pain, are not viewed as pathognomonic of a particular disease or syndrome. Rather, they are viewed as reactions to the malady and are thus considered of secondary importance. It is assumed that once the disease is "cured," these secondary reactions will evaporate. If they do not, speculations are raised as to possible psychological causation. Thus, traditional medicine has adopted a dichotomous view in which symptoms are either somatogenic or psychogenic. Although evidence to support this dichotomy is lacking, the view remains pervasive.

The biomedical model has been criticized because of its failure to address the roles of psychological and psychosocial variables in health and disease, particularly the dynamic interaction of these variables with pathophysiological factors (Engel, 1977). Specifically, problems arise when patients' symptoms and illnesses are not commensurate with the degree of observable pathology. In these circumstances, common in such chronic pain conditions as back pain,

headache, fibromyalgia syndrome (FMS), and temporomandibular disorders (TMDs), the patient's presentation does not fit neatly within the biomedical model.

Chronic pain is more than a physical symptom. Its continuous presence creates widespread manifestations of suffering, including preoccupation with pain; limitation of personal, social, and work activities; demoralization and affective disturbance; increased use of medications and of health care services; and a generalized adoption of the "sick role" (Parsons, 1958). Although the importance of such factors has been acknowledged for some time, only within the past half century have systematic attempts been made to incorporate these factors within comprehensive models of pain (for a review, see Turk, 2001). Dissatisfaction with the conventional model of pain led to a seminal event: the formulation of the gate control theory of pain by Melzack and his colleagues (Melzack & Casey, 1968; Melzack & Wall, 1965).

The Gate Control Theory of Pain

The first attempt to amalgamate physiological and psychological factors and to develop an integrative model of chronic pain that circumvents shortcomings of unidimensional models was the gate control theory (GCT) (Melzack & Casey, 1968; Melzack & Wall, 1965). Melzack and Casey (1968) differentiated three systems related to the processing of nociceptive stimulation—sensory–discriminative, motivational–affective, and cognitive–evaluative—all of which contribute to the subjective experience of pain. In this way, the GCT specifically includes psychological factors as integral aspects of the pain experience. In addition, by emphasizing central nervous system (CNS) mechanisms, this theory provides a physiological basis for the role of psychological factors in chronic pain.

According to the GCT, peripheral stimuli interact with cortical variables, such as mood and anxiety, in the perception of pain. Pain is not considered either somatic or psychogenic; instead, both factors have either potentiating or moderating effects. From the GCT perspective, the experience of pain is an ongoing sequence of activities, largely reflexive in nature at the outset, but modifiable even in the earliest stages by a variety of excitatory and inhibitory influences, as well as the integration of ascending and descending CNS activity. The process results in overt expressions communicating pain and strategies by the person to terminate the pain. Because the GCT invokes the continuous interaction of multiple systems (sensory–physiological, affect, cognition, and behavior) considerable potential for shaping of the pain experience is implied.

Whereas prior to the GCT formulation psychological processes were largely dismissed as reactions to pain, this new model suggested that cutting or blocking neurological pathways is inadequate because psychological factors are capable of influencing the peripheral input. The emphasis on the modulation of inputs in the dorsal horns and the dynamic role of the brain in pain processes and perception resulted in the integration of psychological variables (e.g., past experience, attention, and other cognitive activities) into current research and therapy on pain. Perhaps the major contribution of the GCT has been its highlighting of the CNS as an essential component in pain processes and perception.

The physiological details of the GCT have been challenged, and it has been suggested that the model is incomplete (see, e.g., Nathan, 1976; Price, 1987). As additional knowledge has been gathered since the original formulation in 1965, specific mechanisms have been disputed and have required revision and reformulation (Nathan, 1976; Wall, 1989). Overall, however, the GCT has proved remarkably resilient and flexible in the face of accumulating scientific data and challenges to these data. It still provides a "powerful summary of the phenomena observed in the spinal cord and brain, and has the capacity to explain many of the most mysterious and puzzling problems encountered in the clinic" (Melzack & Wall, 1982, p. 261). This theory has had enormous heuristic value in stimulating further research in the basic science of pain mechanisms. It has also given rise to new clinical treatments, including neurophysiologically based procedures (e.g., neural stimulation techniques), from peripheral nerves and collateral processes in the dorsal columns of the spinal cord (North, 1989), pharmacological advances (Abram, 1993), behavioral treatments (Fordyce, Roberts, & Sternbach, 1985), and interventions targeting modification of attentional and perceptual processes involved in the pain experience (Turk, Meichenbaum, & Genest, 1983). After the GCT was proposed, no one could continue trying to explain pain exclusively in terms of peripheral factors.

Neuromatrix Theory

Recently, Melzack (1999) extended the GCT and integrated it with Selye's (1950) theory of stress. The neuromatric theory makes a number of assumptions about pain. For example, Melzack proposes that the multidimensional experience of pain produced by characteristic patterns of nerve impulses generated by a widely distributed neural network that comprises a "body–self neuromatrix." The neuromatrix is to some extent genetically determined, but it is modified by sensory experience and learning. Another important feature of the neuromatrix theory is that the patterns of nerve impulses are hypothesized to be triggered either by sensory inputs or centrally, *independent* of any peripheral stimulation.

When an organism receives an injury there is an alteration and disruption of the homeostatic regulation. This deviation from the body's normal state is stressful and initiates a complex of neural, hormonal, and behavioral mechanisms designed to restore homeostasis (Selye, 1950). Melzack (1999) hypothesizes that prolonged stress and ongoing efforts to restore homeostasis can suppress the immune system and activate the limbic system. The limbic system has an important role in emotion, motivation, and cognitive processes. As originally proposed by Selye (1950), prolonged activation of the stress regulation system can lead to a predisposition for the development of different chronic pain states (e.g., FMS, cumulative trauma disorders, whiplash-associated disorders).

According to Melzack (1999), a person's unique body–self neuromatrix is the *primary* determinant of whether the organism experiences pain and is the basis for the individual differences observed. Building on the

GCT, pain suppression can be produced by sensory and evaluative processes, as well as activation of the endogenous opioid system.

The cumulative effects of stresses that preceded or are concomitant with the current stress may account for the large variation in individual responses to what might appear to be objectively the same degree of physical pathology. In this way, the theory incorporates the pain sufferer's prior learning history to shape the neuromatrix by influencing interpretive processes and individual physiological and behavioral response patterns. A new stressor may amplify baseline stress and related efforts of homeostatic regulation. Prolonged stress augments tissue breakdown as the body continues to attempt to return to its "normal" state. In a sense, the neuromatix theory proposes a diathesis–stress model in which predispositional factors interact with an acute stressor (Okifuji & Turk, in press; Turk, 2002). Once pain is established, however, it becomes a stressor in and of itself, as the body continues to attempt return to homeostasis and the presence of pain is a continual threat that creates demands on the body. Fear, worry about the future, and the meaning of the nociceptive stimulation contribute to the ongoing stress producing additional deviations from homeostasis.

Nociception involves activation of energy impinging on specialized nerve endings. The nerve(s) involved conveys information about tissue damage to the CNS. A growing body of animal research suggests that repetitive or ongoing nociceptive input can lead to structural and functional changes that may cause altered perceptual processing and contribute to pain chronicity (Woolf & Mannion, 1999). These structural and functional changes, demonstrate plasticity in the nervous system and may explain why a person experiences a gradual increase in the perceived magnitude of pain referred to as neural (peripheral and central) sensitization. Moreover, once these changes have occurred, they may contribute to nociception even after the initial cause has resolved. These changes in the CNS offer an explanation for the reports of pain in many chronic pain syndromes (e.g., FMS, whiplash-associated disorders and back pain) even when no physical pathology is identified. According to Melzack, these CNS changes can be accounted for by modification of the body–self neuromatrix.

The neuromatrix theory poses intriguing hypotheses and integrates a great deal of physiological and psychological knowledge. However, components of the theory and the theory itself await systematic investigation. As was the case with the GCT, the neuromatrix theory offers a heuristic way of thinking that should stimulate research.

The Biopsychosocial Perspective: A Basic Description

People differ markedly in how frequently they report physical symptoms, in their propensity to visit physicians when experiencing identical symptoms, and, as noted, in their response to the same treatments (Desroches, Kaimen, & Ballard, 1967; Zborowski, 1969). Often the nature of patients' responses to treatment has little to do with their objective physical condition (Mechanic, 1962). For example, White, Williams, and Greenberg (1961) noted that less than one-third of people with clinically significant symptoms consult a physician. Conversely, from 30 to 50% of patients who seek treatment in primary care do not have specific diagnosable disorders (Dworkin & Massoth, 1994), and for up to 80% of people with back pain (Deyo, 1986) and the majority of chronic headache suffers, no physical basis for the pain can be identified.

The distinction between "disease" and "illness" is crucial to understanding chronic pain. Disease is generally defined as an "objective biological event" that involves disruption of specific body structures or organ systems caused by pathological, anatomical, or physiological changes (Mechanic, 1986). In contrast to this customary view of physical disease, illness is defined as a "subjective experience or self-attribution" that a disease is present; it yields physical discomfort, emotional distress, behavioral limitations, and psychosocial disruption. In other words, illness refers to how the sick person and members of his or her family and wider social network perceive, live with, and respond to symptoms and disability.

The distinction between disease and illness is analogous to the distinction between "pain" and "nociception." Nociception entails stimulation of nerves that convey information *about* tissue damage to the brain. Pain is a subjective perception that results from the transduction, transmission, and modulation of sensory input filtered through a person's genetic composition and prior learning history and modulated further by the person's current physiological status, idiosyncratic appraisals, expectations, current mood state, and sociocultural environment (body–self neuromatix). This is why we emphasize assessment of the person, as we cannot assess pain removed from the person who is being exposed to the nociception.

In contrast to the biomedical model's emphasis on disease, the biopsychosocial model focuses on both disease and illness, a complex interaction of biological, psychological, and social variables. From this perspective, diversity in illness expression (which includes its severity, duration, and consequences for the individual) is accounted for by the interrelationships among biological changes, psychological status, and the social and cultural contexts. All these variables shape the person's perception and response to illness.

The biopsychosocial way of thinking about the differing responses of people to symptoms and the presence of chronic conditions is based on an understanding of the dynamic nature of these conditions. That is, by definition, chronic syndromes extend over time. Therefore, these conditions need to be viewed longitudinally as ongoing, multifactorial processes in which there is a vibrant reciprocal interplay among biological, psychological, and social factors that shape the experience and responses of patients. Biological factors may initiate, maintain, and modulate physical perturbations, whereas psychological variables influence appraisals and perception of internal physiological signs and social factors shape patients' behavioral responses to the perceptions of their physical perturbations.

Conversely, psychological factors may influence biology by affecting hormone production (see, e.g., Bandura, O'Leary, Taylor, Gauthier, & Gossard, 1987), brain structure and processes (see, e.g., Flor et al., 1998; Knost, Flor, Braun, & Birbaumer, 1997), and the autonomic nervous system (see, e.g., Bansevicius, Westgaard, & Jensen, 1997;

Flor, Turk, & Birbaumer, 1985). Behavioral responses may also affect biological contributors, as when a person avoids engaging in certain activities in order to reduce his or her symptoms. Although avoidance may initially reduce symptoms, in the long run it will lead to further physical deconditioning, which can exacerbate nociceptive stimulation.

The picture is not complete unless we consider the direct effects of disease factors and treatment on cognitive and behavioral factors. Biological influences and medications (e.g., steroids and opioids) may affect the ability to concentrate, induce fatigue, and modulate peoples' interpretation of their state as well as of their ability to engage in certain activities.

At different points during the evolution of a disease or impairment, the relative weighting of physical, psychological, and social factors may shift. For example, during the acute phase of a disease biological factors may predominate, but over time psychological and social factors may assume a disproportionate role in accounting for symptoms and disability. Moreover, there is considerable variability in behavioral and psychological manifestations of dysfunction, both across persons with comparable symptoms and within the same person over time (Crook, Weir, & Tunks, 1989).

To understand the variable responses of people to chronic conditions, it is essential that biological, psychological, and social factors each be considered. Moreover, a longitudinal perspective is essential. A cross-sectional approach will only permit consideration of these factors at a specific point in time, and chronic conditions continually evolve. What is observed at any one time is a person's adaptation to interacting biological, personal, and environmental factors. In sum, the hallmarks of the biopsychosocial perspective are (1) integrated action, (2) reciprocal determinism, and (3) development and evolution. This perspective can be contrasted with the traditional biomedical model, whose emphasis on the somatogenic–psychogenic dichotomy is too narrow in scope to accommodate the complexity of chronic pain.

According to the biopsychosocial model, elements of symptom reporting and disability are common to all pain conditions. Research supporting the role of a common set of psychological and social factors across diagnoses has been reported by several investigators. For example, Turk and Rudy (1988) used cluster analyses of patients' responses to the West Haven–Yale Multidimensional Pain Inventory (MPI; Kerns, Turk, & Rudy, 1985) to discover empirically three subgroups of a heterogeneous sample of chronic pain patients based on psychosocial and behavioral factors. In subsequent studies, covariance structures of MPI scores were similar for back pain, headache, TMD patients (Turk & Rudy, 1990), FMS patients (Turk, Okifuji, Starz, & Sinclair, 1996), and cancer patients (Turk et al., 1998) resulting in similar profiles regardless of the anatomical site of pain. The percentages of patients with the different diagnoses varied; however, regardless of physical diagnosis, significant numbers of patients were classified within one of these three subgroups. These results have been replicated in several additional studies of different pain samples (e.g., Bergstrom, Bodin, Jensen, Linton, & Nygren, 2001; Johansson & Lindberg, 2000; Lousberg, Groenman, & Schmidt, 1996).

Consistent with the Turk and Rudy (1988, 1990) studies, Von Korff, Dworkin, and LeResche (1990) demonstrated that different measures of pain experience (e.g., intensity, interference, duration) showed similar intercorrelations across back, abdominal, chest, TMD pain, and headache. They also found that it was useful to employ consistent criteria for classifying chronic pain patients, regardless of the anatomical site. These results suggest that a standard set of criteria for grading chronic pain and dysfunction can be applied to diverse pain patients, and that such a classification yields groups that are similar in terms of unemployment rates, depression, use of opioids, and use of pain-related health care (Von Korff, Ormel, Keefe, & Dworkin, 1992). As noted, in the traditional disease model emotional and behavioral responses are viewed as reactions to disease and trauma and thus have been considered of secondary importance. However, a large number of studies published since the 1960s support the significant role of psychological, behavioral, and social factors in the severity, maintenance, and exacerbation of pain. Despite the proliferation of research,

these factors often are not incorporated within the treatment of chronic pain patients. In the remainder of this chapter, we discuss some of the psychological and social factors involved in pain and disability along with treatment implications.

Support for the Importance of Nonphysiological Factors

The history of medicine is replete with descriptions of interventions believed to be appropriate for alleviating pain, many of which are now known to have little therapeutic merit and some of which may actually have been harmful to patients (Turk et al., 1983). Prior to the second half of the 19th century and the advent of research on sensory physiology, much of the pain treatment arsenal consisted of interventions that had no direct mode of action upon organic mechanisms associated with the source of the pain. Despite the absence of an adequate physiological basis, these treatments proved to have some therapeutic merit, at least for some patients. The effects were desparagingly referred to as "placebo effects" or "psychological cures," with the implicit message being that alleviated symptoms must be psychological (i.e., imaginary) (Turner, Deyo, Loeser, VonKorff, & Fordyce, 1994).

Although some treatment regimens are based on specific knowledge of physiology, the mode of action may be unrelated to modification of physiological processes. For example, in a study of headache patients treated with pharmacological preparations, Fitzpatrick, Hopkins, and Harvard-Watts (1983) concluded that although a large number of patients benefited from drug treatment, most improvements appeared to be unrelated to the pharmacological action per se. Similarly, although biofeedback is beneficial for a several disorders (e.g., headache and back pain), the actual effects of biofeedback may be unrelated to modification of physiological activity (Blanchard, 1987; Holroyd et al., 1984; see also Arena & Blanchard, Chapter 8, this volume).

Deyo, Walsh, and Martin (1990) studied patients who suffered with intractable low back pain for a mean duration of over 4 years. Given the long duration of symptoms, few improvements would be expected in the absence of an efficacious treatment. Following treatment, however, patients experienced statistically significant and substantial improvements in overall functioning, physical functioning, and pain severity. Remarkably, however, the same results were produced with *sham* transcutaneous electrical nerve stimulation (TENS), suggesting that the treatment effects were not related to the physiological mechanism on which treatment was based.

Some pain syndromes seem responsive to almost any treatment. For example, Greene and Laskin (1974) followed TMD patients treated with a diverse set of treatments (e.g., analgesic medication, tranquilizers, physical exercises, intraoral appliances, injections into muscles and nerves, physical therapy, and psychological counseling), including various "placebo" treatments (inert drugs, nonoccluding bite plates, mock equilibration of the bite, and nonfunctional biofeedback) from 6 months to 8 years. These treatments were all given in combination with reassurances, explanation for self-management, and sympathetic understanding. Remarkably, 92% of the patients had no or only minor recurrences of symptoms. The common factors for the diverse set of successful treatments appear to be nonspecific features. Should this be taken as an indication that TMDs are psychological and have no physical basis? Absolutely not; rather, they highlight the important role of non-physiological factors in the maintenance of these symptoms and responses to treatment.

Sociocultural Factors

Commonsense beliefs about illness and health care providers are based both on prior experience and on social and cultural transmission of beliefs and expectations. Ethnic group membership influences how one perceives, labels, responds to, and communicates various symptoms, as well as from whom one elects to obtain care when it is sought, and the types of treatments received (Mechanic, 1978). Several authors have specifically noted the importance of sociocultural factors (e.g., Lipton & Marbach, 1984; Nerenz & Leventhal, 1983; Zborowski, 1969) and sex differences (e.g., Unruh, 1996) in beliefs about and responses to pain. Social factors influence how families and local groups respond to and interact with patients (see discussion of operant conditioning later). Furthermore, ethnic expectations and sex and age stereotypes may influence the practitioner–patient relationship (see, e.g., Turk, Okifuji, & Scharff, 1994, 1995; Unruh, 1996).

Social Learning Mechanisms

The role of social learning has received some attention in the development and maintenance of chronic pain states. From this perspective, pain behaviors (i.e., overt expressions of pain, distress, and suffering) may be acquired through observational learning and modeling processes. That is, people can learn responses that were not previously in their behavioral repertoire by observing others who respond in these ways (Bandura, 1969).

Children acquire attitudes about health and health care, perceptions and interpretations of symptoms, and appropriate responses to injury and disease from their parents, cultural stereotypes, and the social environment (see, e.g., Bachanas & Roberts, 1995; see McGrath & Hillier, Chapter 27, this volume). Based on their experiences, children develop strategies to help them avoid pain and learn "appropriate" (acceptable) ways to react. Children are exposed to numerous minor injuries throughout the day (Fearon, McGrath, & Achat, 1996). How adults address these experiences provides ample learning opportunities. Children's learning influences whether they will ignore or how they will respond or overrespond to symptoms. The observation of others in pain is an event that captivates attention. There is a large amount of experimental evidence of the role of social learning from controlled studies in the laboratory (Craig, 1986, 1988) and observations of patients' behavior in clinical settings (e.g., Schanberg, Keefe, Lefebvre, Kredich, & Gil, 1998). For example, Vaughan and Lanzetta (1980, 1981) demonstrated that physiological responses to pain stimuli may be conditioned simply by observation of others in pain. Richard (1988) found that children whose parents had chronic pain chose more pain-related responses to scenarios presented to them and were more external in their health locus of control than were children with healthy or diabetic parents. Moreover, teachers rated the pain patients' children as displaying more illness behaviors (e.g., complaining, days absent, and visits to school nurse) than the children of the diabetics and healthy controls.

Operant Learning Mechanisms

Early in the last century, Collie (1913) discussed the effects of environmental factors in shaping the experience of people suffering with pain. However, a new era in thinking about pain was initiated with Fordyce's (1976) description of the role of operant factors in chronic pain. The operant approach stands in marked contrast to the disease model of pain described earlier (see Sanders, Chapter 6, this volume).

In the operant formulation, behavioral manifestations of pain rather than pain per se are central. When people are exposed to a stimulus that causes tissue damage, their immediate response is withdrawal or an attempt to escape from the noxious sensations. Their behaviors are observable and consequently are subject to the principles of reinforcement. Behaviors that are positively reinforced will increase and persist, whereas behaviors that receive no positive response will decrease and be diminished. Those behaviors that permit avoidance of aversive events (negatively reinforced) will also increase.

The operant view proposes that through external contingencies of reinforcement, acute pain behaviors, such as limping to protect a wounded limb from producing additional nociceptive input, can evolve into chronic pain problems. Pain behaviors may be positively reinforced directly, for example, by attention from a spouse or health care provider. They may also be maintained by the escape from noxious stimulation through the use of drugs or rest or avoidance of undesirable activities such as work.

In addition, "well behaviors" (e.g., activity and working) may not be sufficiently positively reinforced and will be extinguished. Pain behaviors originally elicited by organic factors may thus occur totally or in part in response to reinforcing environmental events. Because of the consequences of specific behavioral responses, Fordyce (1976) proposed that pain behaviors might persist long after the initial cause of the pain is resolved or greatly reduced. The operant conditioning model does not concern itself with the initial cause of pain. Rather, it considers pain an internal subjective experience that may be maintained even after its initial physical basis is resolved.

Several studies have provided evidence that supports the underlying assumptions of the operant conditioning model. For example, Cairns and Pasino (1977) and Doleys, Crocker, and Patton (1982) showed that pain behaviors (specifically, inactivity) could be decreased and well behaviors (specifically, activity) could be increased by verbal reinforcement and by setting exercise quotas. Interestingly, Block, Kremer, and Gaylor (1980) demonstrated that pain patients reported differential levels of pain in an experimental situation, depending on whether they knew they were being observed by their spouses or by ward clerks. Pain patients with nonsolicitous spouses reported more pain when neutral observers were present than when the spouses were present and patients with solicitous spouses reported more pain when their spouses were present than when neutral observers were present. On the other hand, patients with solicitous spouses reported more pain when their spouses were present than when more neutral ward clerks were present.

Romano and colleagues (1992) videotaped patients and their spouses engaged in a series of cooperative household activities and recorded patients' pain behaviors and spouses' responses. Sequential analyses revealed that spouses' solicitous behaviors were more likely to precede and follow pain behaviors in pain patients than in healthy controls. Two additional studies (Flor, Kerns, & Turk, 1987; Turk, Kerns, & Rosenberg, 1992) observed that chronic pain patients reported more intense pain and less activity when they indicated that their spouses were solicitous. Taken together, these studies suggest that spouses can serve as important discriminative stimuli for the display of pain behaviors, including their reports of pain severity.

Treatment from the operant perspective focuses on extinction of pain behaviors and increasing well behaviors by positive reinforcement. This treatment has proven to be effective for select samples of chronic pain patients (see, e.g., Nicholas, Wilson, & Goyen, 1991; Vlaeyen, Haazen, Schuerman, Kole-Snijders, & Van Eek, 1995; see also Sanders, Chapter 6, this volume). Although operant factors undoubtedly play a role in the maintenance of pain and disability, the operant conditioning model of pain has been criticized for its exclusive focus on motor pain behaviors, failure to consider the emotional and cognitive aspects of pain (Schmidt, 1985a, 1985b; Schmidt, Gierlings, & Peters, 1989; Turk & Flor, 1987), and failure to treat the subjective experience of pain (Kotarba, 1983). Moreover, Turk and Okifuji (1997) demonstrated that patients' appraisals were better predictors of pain behavior than environmental factors, including responses from significant others.

Respondent Learning Mechanisms

Factors contributing to chronicity that have previously been conceptualized in terms of operant learning may also be initiated and maintained by respondent conditioning (Gentry & Bernal, 1977). Fordyce, Shelton, and Dundore (1982) hypothesized that intermittent sensory stimulation from the site of bodily damage, environmental reinforcement, or successful avoidance of aversive social activity are not necessarily required to account for the maintenance of avoidance behavior or protective movements; anticipation of pain may be sufficient to maintain avoidance behavior. Linton (1985), among others showed, that avoidance of activities was elated more to anxiety about pain than to actual pain.

Once an acute pain problem is established; fear of motor activities that the patient *expects* to result in pain may develop and motivate avoidance of activity (Lenthem, Slade, Troup, & Bentley, 1983; Linton, Melin, & Götestam, 1984; Vlaeyen, Kole-Snijders, Boeren, & van Eek, 1995). Nonoccurrence of pain is a powerful reinforcer for future reduction of activity. In this way, the original respondent conditioning may be followed by an operant learning process whereby the nociceptive stimuli and the associated responses need no longer be present for the avoidance behavior to occur.

In acute pain states it may be useful to reduce movement, and consequently to avoid pain, in order to accelerate the healing process. Over time, however, anticipatory anxiety related to activity may develop and act as a conditioned stimulus for sympathetic activation (the conditioned response), which may be maintained after the original unconditioned stimulus (injury) and unconditioned response (pain and sympathetic activation) have subsided (Lenthem et al., 1983; Linton et al., 1984; Philips, 1987a).

Sympathetic activation and increases in muscle tension may be viewed as unconditioned responses that can elicit more pain. Even when no injury is present, pain related to sustained muscle contractions may also be conceptualized as an unconditioned stimulus, and conditioning may proceed in the same fashion as outlined previously. Although an original association between pain and pain-related stimuli may result in anxiety regarding these stimuli, with time the expectation of pain related to activity may lead to avoidance of adaptive behaviors even if the nociceptive stimuli and the related sympathetic activation are no longer present.

In acute pain, many activities that are otherwise neutral or pleasurable may elicit or exacerbate pain and are thus experienced as aversive and avoided. Over time, more and more activities may be seen as eliciting or exacerbating pain and thus are feared and avoided (stimulus generalization). Avoided activities may involve simple motor behaviors as well as work, leisure, and sexual activity (Philips, 1987a). In addition to the avoidance learning, pain may be exacerbated and maintained in an expanding number of situations because anxiety-related sympathetic activation and accompanying muscle tension may occur both in anticipation and also as a consequence of pain (cf. Flor, Birbaumer, & Turk, 1990). Thus, psychological factors may directly affect nociceptive stimulation and need not be viewed merely as reactions to pain. We return to this point later in this chapter.

Persistent avoidance of specific activities prevents disconfirmations that are followed by corrected predictions (Rachman & Arntz, 1991). Prediction of pain promotes pain avoidance behavior and overprediction of pain promotes excessive avoidance behavior (Schmidt, 1985a, 1985b). Insofar as pain avoidance succeeds in preserving the overpredictions from repeated disconfirmation, they will continue unchanged (Rachman & Lopatka, 1988). By contrast, people who repeatedly engage in behavior that produces significantly less pain than they *predicted* will likely make adjustments in subsequent expectations, which will eventually become more accurate. Increasingly accurate predictions will be followed by reduction of avoidance behavior (Vlaeyen, de Jong, Geilen, Heuts, & van Breukelen, 2001). These observations support the importance of physical therapy and exercise quota, with patients progressively increasing their activity levels despite their fears of injury and discomfort associated with renewed use of deconditioned muscles.

From the respondent conditioning perspective, the pain sufferers may have learned to associate increases in pain with all kinds of stimuli that were originally associated with nociceptive stimulation (i.e., stimulus generalization). As the pain symptoms persist, more and more situations may elicit anxiety and anticipatory pain and depression because of the low rate of reinforcement obtained when behavior is greatly reduced (cf. Lenthem et al., 1983). Sitting, walking, cognitively demanding work or social interaction, sexual activity, or even thoughts about these activities may increase anticipatory anxiety and concomitant physiological and biochemical changes (Philips, 1987a). Subsequently, patients may respond inappropriately to many stimuli, reducing the frequency of numerous activities in addition to those that initially induced nociception. Physical abnormalities often observed in chronic pain patients (e.g., distorted gait, decreased range of motion, and muscular fatigue) may actually result from secondary changes initiated in behavior through learning rather than continuing nociception. In short, the anticipation of suffering or prevention of suffering may be sufficient for the long-term maintenance of avoidance behaviors.

Cognitive Factors

As noted earlier, people are not passive responders to physical sensation. Rather, they actively seek to make sense of their experience. They appraise their conditions by matching sensations to some preexisting implicit model and determine whether a particular sensation is a symptom of a particular physical disorder that requires attention or can be ignored. In this way, to some extent, each person functions with a uniquely constructed reality (i.e., a body–self neuromatrix). When information is ambiguous, people rely on general attitudes and beliefs based on experience and prior learning history. These beliefs determine the meaning and significance of the problems, as well as the perceptions of appropriate treatment. If we accept the premise that pain is a complex, subjective phenomenon that is uniquely experienced by each person, then knowledge about idiosyncratic beliefs, appraisals, and coping repertoires becomes critical for optimal treatment planning and for accurately evaluating treatment outcome (Reesor & Craig, 1988; Turk & Okifuji, 1996).

A great deal of research has been directed toward identifying cognitive factors that contribute to pain and disability (e.g., De-Good & Tait, 2001; Jensen, Turner, Romano, & Karoly, 1991; Turk & Rudy, 1992). These studies have consistently demonstrated that patients' attitudes, beliefs, and expectancies about their plight, themselves, their coping resources, and the health care system affect their reports of pain, activity, disability, and response to treatment (e.g., Flor & Turk, 1988; Jensen, Turner, Romano, & Lawler, 1994; Tota-Faucette, Gil, Williams, & Goli, 1993).

Beliefs about Pain

Clinicians working with chronic pain patients are aware that patients who have similar pain histories may differ greatly in their beliefs about their pain. Certain beliefs may lead to maladaptive coping, exacerbation of pain, increased suffering, and greater disability. For example, if pain is interpreted as signifying ongoing tissue damage rather than viewed as being the result of a stable problem that may improve, it is likely to produce considerably more suffering and behavioral dysfunction even though the amount of nociceptive input in the two cases may be equivalent (see, e.g., Spiegel &

Bloom, 1983). People who believe that their pain is likely to persist may be quite passive in their coping efforts and may fail to make use of cognitive or behavioral strategies to cope with pain. Pain sufferers who consider their pain to be an unexplainable mystery may minimize their own abilities to control or decrease pain and may be less likely to rate their coping strategies as effective in controlling and decreasing pain (Williams & Keefe, 1991; Williams & Thorn, 1989).

Moreover, pain sufferers' beliefs about the implications of a disease can affect their perception of symptoms (Turk & Okifuji, 1996; Turk et al., 1996). For example, Cassell (1982) cited the case of a patient whose pain could easily be controlled with codeine when he attributed it to sciatica but required significantly greater amounts of opioids to achieve the same degree of relief when he attributed it to metastatic cancer. Cassell's observation was confirmed in a study published by Spiegel and Bloom (1983) who found that the pain severity ratings of cancer patients could be predicted by the use of analgesics and by the patients' affective state as well as by their *interpretations of pain*. Patients who attributed their pain to a worsening of their underlying disease experienced more pain than did patients with more benign interpretations, despite the same level of disease progression.

A person's cognitions (beliefs, appraisals, expectancies) regarding the consequences of an event and his or her ability to deal with it are hypothesized to affect functioning in two ways—by directly influencing mood and indirectly influencing coping efforts. Both influences may affect physiological activity associated with pain such as muscle tension (see, e.g., Flor et al., 1985) and production of endogenous opioids (see, e.g., Bandura et al., 1987).

The presence of pain may change the way people process pain-related and other information. For example, chronic pain may focus attention on all types of bodily signals. Arntz and Schmidt (1989) have suggested that the processing of internal information may become disturbed in chronic pain patients. It is possible that pain patients become preoccupied with and over emphasize physical symptoms and interpret them as painful stimulation. In fact, studies of patients with diverse conditions (e.g., irritable

bowel syndrome [Whitehead, 1980]; FMS [Tunks, Crook, Norman, & Kalasher, 1988]; angina pectoris [Droste & Roskamm, 1983]; headaches [Borgeat, Hade, Elie, & Larouche, 1984]; see also Mayou, Chapter 24, and Turk and Sherman, Chapter 19, this volume) support the presence of what appears to be a hypersensitivity characterized by a lowered threshold for labeling stimuli as noxious. Patients may interpret pain symptoms as indicative of an underlying disease, and they may do everything to avoid pain exacerbation, most often by resorting to inactivity (Okifuji & Turk, 1999; Vlaeyen, Kole-Snijders, Boeren, & van Eek, 1995). For example, in acute pain states, bed rest is often prescribed to relieve pressure on the spine. These pain sufferers may subsequently ascribe to a belief that any movement of the back may worsen their condition, and they may still maintain this belief in the chronic state, when inaction is not only unnecessary but also detrimental.

In a set of studies, Schmidt (1985a, 1985b) found that people with low back pain demonstrated poor behavioral persistence in various exercise tasks, and that their performance on these tasks was independent of physical exertion or actual self-reports of pain. Instead, these patients' exercise behaviors were related to their previous pain reports, suggesting that having a negative view of their abilities and expecting increased pain influenced their behavior more than did actual events or sensations. In another study, Council, Ahern, Follick, and Cline (1988) noted that 83% of patients with low back pain reported that they were unable to complete a movement sequence, including leg lifts and lateral bends because of *anticipated* pain; yet, only 5% were unable to perform the activities because of actual lack of ability. Thus, the rationale for their avoidance of exercise was not the presence of pain but their *learned expectation* of heightened pain and accompanying physical arousal, factors which might further aggravate pain and reinforce the patients' beliefs regarding the pervasiveness of their disability (Turk & Okifuji, 1996; Turk et al., 1996). These results are consistent with the respondent learning factors described previously. Patients' negative perceptions of their capabilities for physical performance form a vicious circle, with the failure to perform activities reinforcing the perception of helplessness and incapacity (Schmidt, 1985a, 1985b).

Jensen and colleagues (1994) demonstrated that patients' beliefs that emotions affected their pain, that others should be solicitous when they experienced pain, and that they were disabled by pain were positively associated with psychosocial dysfunction. For example, patients who believed that they were disabled by pain and should avoid activity because pain signified damage were more likely to reveal physical disability than were patients who did not hold these beliefs.

Once cognitive structures (based on memories and meaning) about a disease are formed, they become stable and difficult to modify. Patients tend to avoid experiences that could invalidate their beliefs, and they guide their behavior in accordance with these beliefs even in situations in which the beliefs are no longer valid. Consequently, as noted previously in describing respondent conditioning, they do not receive corrective feedback.

In addition to beliefs about the ability to function despite pain, beliefs about pain per se appear to be important in understanding patients' compliance with treatment, response to treatment, and disability. For example, Schwartz, DeGood, and Shutty (1985) presented patients with information about the role of cognitive, affective, and behavioral factors and their own role in the rehabilitation process. Following treatment, patients who had rated the information as applicable to their pain condition had much better outcomes. Those who disagreed with the concepts presented were found at follow-up to have higher levels of pain, lower levels of activity, and a high degree of dissatisfaction.

The results of several studies suggest that when successful rehabilitation occurs, there appears to be an important cognitive shift— a shift from beliefs about helplessness and passivity to resourcefulness and ability to function regardless of pain. For example, Williams and Thorn (1989) found that chronic pain patients who believed that their pain was an "unexplained mystery" reported high levels of psychological distress and pain and also showed poorer

treatment compliance than did patients who believed that they understood their pain.

In a process study designed to evaluate the direct association between patients' beliefs symptoms, a thought-sampling procedure was used to evaluate the nature of patients' cognitions during and immediately following headache, both prior to, and following treatment (Newton & Barbaree, 1987). Results indicated that there were significant changes in certain aspects of headache-related thinking in treated groups compared to a control group. Treated participants made significantly fewer negative appraisal (e.g., "It's getting worse" and "There is nothing I can do") and significantly more positive appraisals than did untreated participants. Treated participants learned to evaluate headaches in a more positive fashion. Importantly, patients who had the largest positive shifts in appraisal reported the greatest reduction in headache intensity, significantly fewer headache days per week, and lower intensity of pain than did untreated controls.

The results of Newton and Barbaree's (1987) study support the argument that changes in cognitive reactions to headache may underlie headache improvement (see also Arena and Blanchard, Chapter 8, this volume). Many additional pain treatment outcome studies support the idea that reducing negative appraisals is one way to reduce pain and associated suffering. In considering the efficacy of biofeedback for back pain patients, Nouwen and Solinger (1979) concluded that "simultaneous accomplishment of muscle tension reduction and lowering reported pain convinced patients that muscle tension, and subsequently pain, could be controlled. As self-control could not be demonstrated in most patients, it seems plausible that the feeling of self-control, rather than actual control of physiological functions or events is crucial for further reductions" (p. 110). In other words, it appears that the extent to which patients believe that voluntary control over muscles has been achieved dictates the outcome, even when their beliefs are not accompanied by lasting reductions in muscular reactivity.

Similar to Nouwen and Solinger's (1979) interpretation, Blanchard (1987) speculated that for headache patients the maintenance of treatment effects endures in spite of almost universal cessation of regular home practice of biofeedback, because the self-perpetuating cycle of chronic headache has been broken. The experience of headache serves as a stressor, which can contribute to future headaches. By the end of biofeedback treatment, when patients have experienced noticeable headache relief, it is as if they have redefined themselves as able to cope with headaches. Removing one source of stress appears to help patient to cope with recurrences more adaptively.

Clearly, it appears essential for people with chronic pain to develop adaptive beliefs about the relation among impairment, pain, suffering, and disability and to deemphasize the role of experienced pain in their regulation of functioning. In fact, results from numerous treatment outcome studies have shown that changes in pain level do not parallel changes in other variables of interest, including activity level, medication use, return to work, rated ability to cope with pain, and pursuit of further treatment (see Flor, Fydrich, & Turk, 1992).

Beliefs about Controllability

Many laboratory studies demonstrate that controllability of aversive stimulation reduces its impact (e.g., Jensen & Karoly, 1991; Wells, 1994). Conversely, there is evidence that the explicit expectation of uncontrollable pain stimulation may cause subsequent nociceptive input to be perceived as more intense (Leventhal & Everhart, 1979). Because people who have associated activity with pain may expect heightened levels of pain when they attempt to get involved in activity, they may actually perceive higher levels of pain or avoid activity altogether.

Chronic pain sufferers typically perceive a lack of personal control, which probably relates to their ongoing but unsuccessful efforts to influence the pain they experience. A large proportion of chronic pain patients appear to believe that they have limited ability to exert control over their pain (Turk & Rudy, 1988). Such negative, maladaptive appraisals about the situation and their personal efficacy may reinforce the experience of demoralization, inactivity, and overreaction to nociceptive stimulation commonly observed in chronic pain sufferers (Biedermann, McGhie, Monga, & Shanks, 1987).

The relationship between perceived controllability and pain has been demonstrated in a variety of chronic pain syndromes. Mizener, Thomas, and Billings (1988) demonstrated that among successfully treated migraine headache patients, increases in perceived control over physiological activity and general health were significantly correlated with reduction in headache activity. Flor and Turk (1988) examined the relationship among general and situation-specific pain-related thoughts, conceptions of personal control, pain severity, and disability levels in people with low back pain and rheumatoid arthritis (RA). General and situation-specific convictions of uncontrollability and helplessness were more highly related to pain and disability than were disease-related variables for both samples. The combination of both situation-specific and general cognitive variables explained 32% and 60% of the variance in pain and disability, respectively. The addition of disease-related variables improved the predictions only marginally. Peoples' beliefs about the extent to which they can control their pain are associated with various other outcome variables including medication use, activity levels, and psychological functioning (see, e.g., Jensen & Karoly, 1991).

Self-Efficacy

Closely related to the sense of control over aversive stimulation is the concept of "self-efficacy." A self-efficacy expectation is defined as a personal conviction that one can successfully execute a course of action (i.e., perform required behaviors) to produce a desired outcome in a given situation. This construct appears to be a major mediator of therapeutic change.

Bandura (1997) suggested that if a person has sufficient motivation to engage in a behavior, the person's self-efficacy beliefs are what determine which activities to initiate, the amount of effort expended, and the extent of persistence in the face of obstacles and aversive experiences. Efficacy judgments are based on the following four sources of information regarding one's capabilities, in descending order of impact:

1. One's own past performance at the task or similar tasks.

2. The performance accomplishments of others who are perceived to be similar to oneself.
3. Verbal persuasion by others that one is capable.
4. Perception of one's own state of physiological arousal, which is in turn partly determined by prior efficacy estimation.

Encouraging patients to undertake subtasks that are increasingly difficult or close to the desired behavioral repertoire can create performance mastery experience. From this perspective, the occurrence of coping behaviors is conceptualized as being mediated by the person's beliefs that situational demands do not exceed his or her coping resources.

Dolce, Crocker, Moletteire, and Doleys (1986) and Litt (1988) reported that low self-efficacy ratings regarding pain control are related to low pain tolerance, and that they are better predictors of tolerance than are objective levels of noxious stimuli. The relationship between pain sufferers' self-efficacy ratings of perceived ability to control pain has been confirmed in disparate samples. For example, Manning and Wright (1983) obtained self-efficacy ratings from women expecting their first child concerning their ability to have a medication-free childbirth. These ratings were good predictors of medication use and time in labor without medication. Similarly, Council and colleagues (1988) had patients rate their self-efficacy as well as expectancy of pain related to the performance of movement tasks. Patients' performance levels were highly related to their self-efficacy expectations, which in turn appeared to be determined by their expectancy of pain levels.

Converging lines of evidence from investigations of both laboratory and clinical pain indicate that perceived self-efficacy operates as an important cognitive factor in pain control (e.g., Bandura et al., 1987; Lorig, Chastain, Ung, Shoor, & Holman, 1989), adaptive psychological functioning (e.g., Lorig et al., 1989; Spinhoven, Ter Kuile, Linssen, & Gazendam, 1989), disability (e.g., Dolce, Crocker, & Doleys, 1986; Lorig et al., 1989), impairment (e.g., Lorig et al., 1989), and treatment outcome (e.g., O'Leary, Shoor, Lorig, & Holman, 1988; Philips, 1987b). What are the mechanisms that account for the association between

self-efficacy and behavioral outcome? Cioffi (1991) has suggested that at least four psychological processes may be responsible:

1. As perceived self-efficacy decreases anxiety and its concomitant physiological arousal, the person may approach the task with less potentially distressing physical information to begin with.
2. The efficacious person is able to willfully distract attention from potentially threatening physiological sensations.
3. The efficacious person perceives and is distressed by physical sensations, but simply persists in the face of them (stoicism).
4. Physical sensations are neither ignored nor necessarily distressing, but rather are relatively free to take on a broad distribution of meanings (change interpretations).

Bandura (1997) suggested that those techniques that most enhance mastery experiences would be the most powerful tools for bringing about behavioral change. He proposed that cognitive variables are the primary determinants of behavior but that these variables are most affected by performance accomplishments. The studies on headache, back pain, and RA cited earlier appear to support Bandura's proposal.

Cognitive Errors

In addition to specific self-efficacy beliefs, a number of investigators have suggested that a common set of "cognitive errors" affect perceptions of pain, affective distress, and disability (Smith, Aberger, Follick, & Ahern, 1986; Smith, Follick, Ahern, & Adams, 1986; Smith, Peck, Milano, & Ward, 1990). A cognitive error is a negatively distorted belief about oneself or one's situation.

Lefebvre (1981) developed a Cognitive Errors Questionnaire to assess cognitive distortions. He found that patients with chronic low back pain were particularly prone to such cognitive errors as "catastrophizing" (self-statements, thoughts, and images anticipating negative outcomes or aversive aspects of an experience, or misinterpreting the outcome of an event as extremely negative); "overgeneralization" (assuming that the outcome of one event necessarily applies to the outcome of future or similar events); "personalization" (interpreting negative events as reflecting personal meaning or responsibility); and "selective abstraction" (selectively attending to negative aspects of experience). Dufton (1989) reported that persons experiencing chronic pain had a tendency to make cognitive errors related to the emotional difficulties associated with living with pain, rather than to the pain intensity alone; moreover, those who made such errors were more depressed.

As is the case with self-efficacy, specific cognitive errors and distortions have been linked consistently to depression (see, e.g., Gil, Williams, Keefe, & Beckham, 1990), self-reported pain severity (see, e.g., Gil et al., 1990), and disability (see, e.g., Flor & Turk, 1988; Smith, Follick, et al., 1986) in chronic pain patients. Such negative thoughts (1) appear to predict long-term adjustment to chronic pain; (2) may mediate a portion of the relationship between disease severity and adjustment; and (3) uniquely contribute (over and above other cognitive factors) to the prediction of adjustment (Smith et al., 1990).

Catastrophizing appears to be a particularly potent cognitive error that greatly influences pain and disability (Keefe et al., 1990a, 1990b). Several lines of research, including experimental laboratory studies of acute pain with normal volunteers and field studies with patients suffering clinical pain, show that catastrophizing and adaptive coping strategies (see later) are important in determining the reaction to pain. People who spontaneously used fewer catastrophizing self-statements and more adaptive coping strategies rated experimentally induced pain as lower and tolerated painful stimuli longer than did those who reported more catastrophizing thoughts (Heyneman, Fremouw, Gano, Kirkland, & Heiden, 1990; Spanos, Horton, & Chaves, 1975). People who spontaneously use more catastrophizing self-statements reported more pain, distress, and disability in several acute and chronic pain studies (e.g., Main & Waddell, 1991; Wells, 1994).

Butler, Damarin, Beaulieu, Schwebel, and Thorn (1989) demonstrated that in the case of postsurgical pain, cognitive coping strategies and catastrophizing thoughts correlated significantly with medication use, pain reports, and nurses' judgments of people's pain tolerance. Turner and Clancy (1986) showed that during cognitive-behavioral treatment, reductions in catastrophizing were significantly related to increases in pain tolerance and reductions in physical and psychosocial impairment. Conversely, following treatment, reductions in catastrophizing were related to reduction in pain intensity and physical impairment. As noted earlier, Flor and Turk (1988) found that in low back pain sufferers and people with RA, significant percentages of the variance in pain and disability were accounted for by cognitive factors that were labeled catastrophizing, helplessness, adaptive coping, and resourcefulness. In both the low back pain and the RA groups, the cognitive variables of catastrophizing and adaptive coping had substantially more explanatory power than did disease-related variables or impairment. Finally, Keefe, Brown, Wallston, and Caldwell (1989) found that RA patients who reported high levels of pain, physical disability, and depression had reported excessive catastrophizing ideation on questionnaires administered 6 months earlier (for detailed discussions of catastrophizing, see Sullivan et al., 2001; Turner & Aaron, 2001).

Coping

Self-regulation of pain and its impact depend on people's specific ways of dealing with pain, adjusting to pain, and reducing or minimizing distress caused by pain—in other words, their coping strategies. Coping is assumed to be involve spontaneously employed purposeful and intentional acts, and it can be assessed in terms of overt and covert behaviors. Overt behavioral coping strategies include rest, use of relaxation techniques, or medication. Covert coping strategies include various means of distracting oneself from pain, reassuring oneself that the pain will diminish, seeking information, and problem solving. Coping strategies are thought to act to alter both the perception of pain intensity and the ability to manage or tolerate pain and to continue everyday activities (DeGood & Tait, 2001; Turk et al., 1983).

Studies have found active coping strategies (efforts to function in spite of pain or to distract oneself from pain, such as engaging in activity or ignoring pain) to be associated with adaptive functioning and passive coping strategies (such as depending on others for help in pain control and restricting one's activities) to be related to greater pain and depression (e.g., Lawson, Reesor, Keefe, & Turner, 1990; Tota-Faucette et al., 1993). However, beyond this, there is no evidence supporting the greater effectiveness of any one active coping strategy compared to any other (Fernandez & Turk, 1989). It seems more likely that different strategies will be more effective than others for some people at some times, but not necessarily for all people all the time.

A number of studies have demonstrated that if people are instructed in the use of adaptive coping strategies, their ratings of pain intensity decrease and tolerance for pain increases (for a review, see Fernandez & Turk, 1989). The most important factor in poor coping appears to be the presence of catastrophizing rather than differences in the nature of specific adaptive coping strategies (see, e.g., Heyneman et al., 1990; Martin, Nathan, Milech, & van Keppel, 1989). Turk and colleagues (1983) concluded that "what appears to distinguish low from high pain tolerant individuals are their cognitive processing, catastrophizing thoughts and feelings that precede, accompany, and follow aversive stimulation" (p. 197).

Affective Factors

Pain is ultimately a subjective, private experience, but it is invariably described in terms of sensory and affective properties. As defined by the International Association for the Study of Pain: "[Pain] is unquestionably a sensation in a part or parts of the body but it is also always unpleasant and therefore also an emotional experience" (Merskey & Bogduk, 1986, p. S217). The central and interactive roles of sensory information and affective state are supported by an overwhelming amount of evidence (Fernandez & Turk, 1992).

The affective components of pain include many different emotions, but they are primarily negative in quality. Anxiety and depression have received the greatest amount of attention in chronic pain patients. The importance of anxiety in maintaining chronic pain was described previously.

Depression

After reviewing a large body of literature, Romano and Turner (1985) concluded that from 40% to 50% of chronic pain patients suffer from depression. In the majority of cases, depression appears to be patients' reaction to their plight. Some have suggested that chronic pain is a form of masked depression. Although this may be true in a small number of cases, there is no empirical support for the hypothesis that depression precedes the development of chronic pain (Turk & Salovey, 1984).

Given our description of the plight of the chronic pain sufferer, it is not surprising that a large number of chronic pain patients are depressed. It is interesting to ponder the other side of the coin. How is it that all people with chronic pain disorders are *not* depressed? Turk and colleagues (Okifuji, Turk, & Sherman, 2000; Rudy, Kerns, & Turk, 1988; Turk et al., 1994, 1995) examined this question and determined that patients' appraisals of the impact of the pain on their lives and of their ability to exert any control over their pain and lives mediated the pain–depression relationship. That is, those patients who believed that they could continue to function despite their pain, and that they could maintain some control despite their pain, did not become depressed.

Anxiety

Anxiety is commonplace in chronic pain. Pain-related fear and concerns about harm–avoidance appear to exacerbate symptoms (Vlaeyen, Kole-Snijders, Boeren, & van Eek, 1995). Anxiety is an affective state that is influenced by appraisal processes, to cite Hamlet, "There is nothing either bad or good but thinking makes it so." There is a reciprocal relationship between affective state and cognitive–interpretive processes whereby thinking affects mood and mood influences appraisals and ultimately the experience of pain.

Threat of intense pain captures attention and is difficult to disengage. Continual vigilance and monitoring of noxious stimulation and the belief that they signify disease progression may render even low intensity nociception less bearable. As we noted in our discussion of respondent conditioning, the experience of pain may initiate a set of extremely negative thoughts and arouse fears—fears of inciting more pain, injury, and the future impact (see Vlaeyen & Linton, 2000, and Vlaeyen, de Jong, Sieben, & Crombez, Chapter 10, this volume). Fear of pain and anticipation of pain are cognitive–perceptual processes that are not driven exclusively by the actual sensory experience of pain and can exert a significant impact on the level of function and pain tolerance (Feuerstein & Beattie, 1995; Vlaeyen et al., 1999). As noted earlier (see, e.g., Lenthem et al., 1983; Vlaeyen, Kole-Snijders, Rooteveel, Ruesink, & Heuts, 1995), fear of pain, driven by the anticipation of pain and not by the sensory experience of pain, is a strong negative reinforcement for the persistence of avoidance behavior and the functional disability.

Avoidance behavior is reinforced in the short term, through the reduction of suffering associated with nociception (McCracken, Gross, Sorg, & Edmands, 1993). Avoidance, however, can be a maladaptive response if it persists and leads to increased fear, limited activity, and other physical and psychological consequences that contribute to disability and persistence of pain. Studies have demonstrated that fear of movement and fears of (re)injury are better predictors of functional limitations than are biomedical parameters (e.g., McCracken et al., 1993; Vlaeyen, Kole-Snijders, Rooteveel, et al., 1995). For example, Crombez, Vlaeyen, and Heuts (1999) showed that pain-related fear was the best predictor of behavioral performance in trunk extension, flexion, and weight-lifting tasks, even after partialing out the effects of pain intensity. Moreover, Vlaeyen, Kole-Snijders, Rooteveel, and colleagues (1995) found that fear of movement/(re)injury was the best predictor of the patient's self-reported disability among chronic back pain patients and that physiological sensory perception of pain and biomedical findings did not add any predictive value. Approximately two-thirds of chronic nonspecific low back pain sufferers avoid back-straining activities because of fear of (re)injury (Crombez, Vervaet, Lysens, Eelen, & Baeyerns, 1998). Interestingly, reduction in pain-related anxiety predicts improvement in functioning, affective distress, pain, and pain-related interference with activity (McCracken & Gross, 1998). Clearly, pain-related anxiety and concerns about harm–avoidance all play an important role in chronic pain and need to be assessed and addressed in treatment.

Enduring psychological and functional limitation following a traumatic event is frequently indicative of posttraumatic stress disorder (PTSD). Traumatic events have been associated with a set of symptoms including nightmares, recurrent and intrusive recollections about the trauma, avoidance of thoughts or activities associated with the traumatic event, and symptoms of increased arousal such as insomnia and hyperarousal. When this set of symptoms closely follows a known traumatic event over an extended period of time, they are labeled PTSD. Significant minorities of chronic pain sufferers attribute the onset of their symptoms to a specific trauma such as a motor vehicle accident. Results of research suggest an exceedingly high prevalence of PTSD in patients presenting to chronic pain clinics (Aghabeigi, Feinmann, & Harris, 1992; Sherman et al., 1988).

In a preliminary study, Sherman, Turk, and Okifuji (2000) found that more than 50% of a sample of 93 treatment-seeking FMS patients reported symptoms of PTSD. Those who experienced these anxiety-related symptoms reported significantly greater levels of pain, life interference, emotional distress, and greater inactivity than did the patients who did not report PTSD-like symptoms. Over 85% of the sample with significant PTSD symptoms compared to 50% of the patients without significant PTSD symptoms demonstrated significant disability. Geisser, Roth, Bachman, & Eckert (1996) reported similar results for a heterogeneous sample of chronic pain patients. Sherman and colleagues suggest that based on these results, clinicians should assess the presence of these symptoms as the failure to attend to them in treatment may undermine successful outcomes.

Anger

Anger has been widely observed in patients with chronic pain (see, e.g., Fernandez &

Turk, 1995; Schwartz, Slater, Birchler, & Atkinson, 1991). Summers, Rapoff, Varghese, Porter, and Palmer (1992) examined patients with spinal cord injuries and found that anger and hostility explained 33% of the variance in pain severity. Kerns, Rosenberg, and Jacobs (1994) found that the internalization of angry feelings accounted for a significant proportion of variances in measures of pain intensity, perceived interference, and reported frequency of pain behaviors.

Frustrations related to persistence of symptoms, limited information on etiology, and repeated treatment failures, along with anger toward employers, insurance companies, the health care system, family members, and themselves, contributes to the general dysphoric mood of patients (Okifuji, Turk, & Curran, 1999).

The precise mechanisms by which anger and frustration exacerbate pain are not known. One reasonable possibility is that anger exacerbates pain by increasing autonomic arousal. Anger may also block motivation for and acceptance of treatments oriented toward rehabilitation and disability management rather than cure. Yet rehabilitation and disability management are often the only treatments available for these patients.

It is important to be aware of the role of negative mood in pain sufferers because it is likely to affect treatment motivation and compliance with treatment recommendations. For example, patients who are depressed and who feel helpless may have little initiative to comply, patients who are anxious may fear engaging in what they perceive as physically demanding activities, and patients who are angry at the health care system are not likely to be motivated to respond to recommendations from yet another health care professional.

It is reasonable to suggest that anger serves as a complicating factor, by increasing autonomic arousal and blocking motivation and acceptance of treatments oriented toward rehabilitation and disability management rather than cure, which are often the only treatments available for chronic pain (Fernandez & Turk, 1995). Suppression of anger has been found to predict worse outcome following pain rehabilitation (Burns, Johnson, Devine, Mahoney, & Pawl, 1998).

Personality Factors

The search for specific personality factors that predisposes people to develop chronic pain has been a major emphasis of psychosomatic medicine. Studies have attempted to identify a specific "migraine personality," a "rheumatoid arthritis personality," and a more general "pain-prone personality" (Blumer & Heilbronn, 1982). By and large, these efforts have received little support and have been challenged (Turk & Salovey, 1984). However, on the basis of their prior experiences, people develop idiosyncratic ways of interpreting information and coping with stress. Avoidance and the resulting failure to experience disconfirmation prevent the extinction or modification of these interpretations and expectations. There is no question that these unique patterns will have an effect on their perceptions of and responses to the presence of pain (Weisberg & Keefe, 1999; see also Gatchel, Chapter 21, this volume).

Anxiety sensitivity refers to the fear of anxiety symptoms based on the belief that they will have harmful consequence (Reiss & McNally, 1985). Anxiety sensitivity appears to be a vulnerability factor (i.e., diathesis) that may condition specific fears that contribute to the development and maintenance of distress.

Pain is essential for survival. Thus, attention may be primed to process painful stimuli ahead of other attentional demands. People with high levels of anxiety sensitivity may be especially hypervigilant to pain as well as to other noxious sensations. Selective attention directed toward threatening information such as bodily sensations leads to greater arousal. Because of this attentional process, those with high anxiety sensitivity may be primed such that minor painful stimuli may be amplified (Okifuji & Turk, 1999; Turk, 2002).

Asmundson, Norton, and Norton (1999) have demonstrated that anxiety sensitivity is correlated with exaggerated fear responses. The unpleasantness of this exaggerated fear response can lead people with high anxiety sensitivity to behave in ways that reduce fear and anxiety-related bodily sensations. Such behavior often takes the form of avoidance to prevent exacerbation of symptoms and further injury.

Preliminary studies that demonstrate the importance of anxiety sensitivity as a predispositional factor in chronic pain have been reported. Asmundson and Norton (1995) found a positive association between anxiety sensitivity and pain-related anxiety, escape/avoidant behaviors, fear of negative consequences of pain, and negative affect. Not only were patients with high anxiety sensitivity more likely to experience greater cognitive disturbance as a result of their pain, they were likely to use greater amounts of analgesic medication to control equal amounts of pain compared to those with low or medium anxiety sensitivity. Furthermore, Asmundson and Taylor (1995) demonstrated that anxiety sensitivity directly exacerbates fear of pain and indirectly exacerbates pain-specific avoidance behavior even after controlling for the direct influences of pain severity on these variables. For a more extensive review, see Asmundson and colleagues (1999).

General fearful appraisals of bodily sensations may sensitize predisposed people and cause high awareness of bodily sensations. Thus, anxiety sensitivity is only one individual difference characteristics that might predispose people to develop and maintain chronic pain and disability. For example, somatization, negative affectivity, bodily preoccupation, and catastrophic thinking also may be involved (Linton, Buer, Vlaeyen, & Hellsing, 2000; Turk, 2002). Vlaeyen, Kole-Snijders, Boeren, and van Eek (1995) argue that a style of catastrophic thinking about pain may be a risk factor for the emergence of pain-related fear.

Many studies have attempted to use different measures of psychopathology to predict pain patients' responses to conservative and surgical interventions, but discussion of this topic is beyond the scope of this chapter. Several papers have reviewed this extensive literature (e.g., Bradley & McKendree-Smith, 2001; see also Gatchel, Chapter 21, this volume).

The Effect of Psychological and Social Factors on Pain

Psychological and social factors may act indirectly on pain and disability by reducing physical activity, and consequently reducing muscle flexibility, muscle tone, strength, and physical endurance. Fear of reinjury, fear of loss of disability compensation, and job dissatisfaction can also influence the return to work. Several studies have suggested that psychological factors may also have a direct effect on physiological parameters associated more directly with the production or exacerbation of nociception. Cognitive interpretations and affective arousal may directly affect physiology by increasing sympathetic nervous system arousal (Bandura, Taylor, Williams, Mefford, & Barchas, 1985), endogenous opioid (endorphin) production (Bandura et al., 1987), and elevated levels of muscle tension (Flor et al., 1985; Flor, Birbaumer, Schugens, & Lutzenberger, 1992).

Effect of Thoughts on Sympathetic Arousal and Muscle Tension

Circumstances that are appraised as potentially threatening to safety or comfort are likely to generate strong physiological reactions. For example, Rimm and Litvak (1969) demonstrated that subjects exhibited physiological arousal by simply thinking about a painful stimulus. In an early study, Barber and Hahn (1962) showed that subjects' self-reported discomfort and physiological responses (frontalis electromyographic activity, heart rate, skin conductance) were similar whether they imagined taking part in a cold-pressor test or actually participated in it. In patients suffering from recurrent migraine headaches simply processing words describing migraine headaches can increase skin conductance (Jamner & Tursky, 1987).

Chronic increases in sympathetic nervous system activation, known as increased skeletal muscle tone, may set the stage for hyperactive muscle contraction and possibly for the persistence of a contraction following conscious muscle activation. Excessive sympathetic arousal and maladaptive behaviors can be immediate precursors of muscle hypertonicity, hyperactivity, and persistence. These in turn may be the proximate causes of chronic muscle spasm and pain. It is common for persons in pain to exaggerate or amplify the significance of their problem and needlessly "turn on" their sympathetic nervous systems (Ciccone & Grzesiak, 1984). In this way, cognitive processes may influence sympathetic arousal and thereby predispose individuals to further injury or otherwise complicate the process of recovery.

Several studies support the direct effect of cognitive factors on muscle tension. For example, Flor and colleagues (1985) demonstrated that discussing stressful events and pain produced elevated levels of EMG activity localized to the site of back pain patients' pain. The extent of abnormal muscular reactivity was better predicted by depression and cognitive coping style than by pain demographic variables (e.g., number of surgeries or duration of pain). Flor, Birbaumer, and colleagues (1992) replicated these results and extended them to patients with TMDs. For this group, imagery reconstruction of pain episodes produced elevated tension in facial muscles.

The natural evolution and course of many chronic pain syndromes are unknown. At the present time, it is probably more appropriate to refer to abnormal psychophysiological patterns as antecedents of chronic pain states or to view them as consequences of chronic pain that subsequently maintain or exacerbate the symptoms, rather than to assign them any direct etiological significance (Hatch et al., 1991).

Implications for Treatment

We have emphasized that pain is a subjective perceptual event that is not solely dependent on the extent of tissue damage or organic dysfunction. The intensity of pain reported and the responses to the perception of pain are influenced by a wide range of factors, such as meaning of the situation, attentional focus, mood, prior learning history, cultural background, environmental contingencies, social supports, and financial resources, among others. The research we reviewed supports the importance of these factors in the etiology, severity, exacerbation, and maintenance of pain, suffering, and disability.

Treatment based on the biopsychosocial perspective not only must address the biological basis of symptoms, but must incorporate the full range of social and psychological factors that have been shown to affect pain, distress, and disability. Therefore, treatment should be designed not only to alter physical contributors but also to change the patient's behaviors regardless of the patient's specific pathophysiology and without necessarily controlling pain per se (Fordyce, 1976; Turk et al., 1983).

Treatment from the biopsychosocial perspective focuses on providing the patient with techniques to gain a sense of control over the effects of pain on his or her life, by modifying the affective, behavioral, cognitive, and sensory facets of the experience. Behavioral experiences help to show patients that they are capable of more than they assumed they were, thus increasing their sense of personal competence. Cognitive techniques help to place affective, behavioral, cognitive, and sensory responses under a patient's control. The assumption is that long-term maintenance of behavioral changes will occur only if the patient has learned to attribute success to his or her own efforts. There are suggestions that these treatments can result in changes in beliefs about pain, coping style, and reported pain severity, as well as in direct behavioral changes (Jensen, Romano, Turner, Good, & Wald, 1999; Turner & Clancy, 1986, 1988). Treatment that results in increased perceived control over pain and decreases in catastrophizing has also been associated with decreased pain severity ratings and functional disability (Jensen et al., 1991; Turner, 1991).

An important implication of the biopsychosocial perspective is the need first to identify the relevant physical, psychological, and social characteristics of patients and then to develop treatments matched to patients' characteristics and to evaluate their efficacy. The ultimate aim is the prescription of treatment components that have been shown to maximize outcome for different subsets of patients (Turk, 1990).

Summary and Conclusions

The variability of patients' responses to nociceptive stimuli and treatment is somewhat more understandable when we consider that pain is a personal experience influenced by attention, meaning of the situation, and prior learning history as well as physical pathology. In the majority of cases, biomedical factors appear to instigate the initial report of pain. Over time, however, secondary problems associated with deconditioning may exacerbate and maintain the problem. Inactivity leads to increased focus on and preoccupation with the body and pain, and these cognitive–attentional changes increase the likelihood of misinterpreting symptoms, the overemphasis on symptoms, and the patient's self-perception as disabled. Reduction of activity, anger, fear of reinjury, pain, loss of compensation, and an environment that perhaps unwittingly supports the *pain patient role* can impede alleviation of pain, successful rehabilitation, reduction of disability, and improvement in adjustment.

Pain that persists over time should not be viewed as either solely physical or solely psychological. Rather, the experience of pain is a complex amalgam maintained by an interdependent set of biomedical, psychosocial, and behavioral factors, whose relationships are not static but evolve and change over time. The various interacting factors that affect a person with chronic pain suggest that the phenomenon is quite complex and requires a biopsychosocial perspective.

From the biopsychosocial perspective, each of these factors contributes to the experience of pain and the response to treatment. The interaction among the various factors is what produces the subjective experience of pain. There is a synergistic relationship whereby psychological and socioenviromental factors can modulate nociceptive stimulation and the response to treatment. In turn, nociceptive stimulation can influence patients' appraisals of their situation and the treatment, their mood states, and the ways they interact with significant others, including medical practitioners. An integrative, biopsychosocial model of chronic pain needs to incorporate the mutual interrelationships among physical, psychological, and social factors and the changes that occur among these relationships over time (Flor et al., 1990; Turk & Rudy, 1991). A model and treatment approach that focuses on only one of these three core sets of factors is inevitably incomplete.

Acknowledgments

Preparation of this chapter was supported in part by grants from the National Institute of Arthritis and Musculoskeletal and Skin Diseases (AR/AI44724, AR47298) and the National Institute of Child Health and Human Development/National Center for Medical Rehabilitation Research (HD33989).

References

Abram, S. E. (1993). Advances in chronic pain management since gate control. *Regional Anesthesia, 18*, 66–81.

Aghabeigi, B., Feinmann, C., & Harris, M. (1992). Prevalence of post-traumatic stress disorder in patients with chronic idiopathic facial pain. *British Journal of Oral and Maxillofacial Surgery, 30*, 360–364.

Arntz, A., & Schmidt, A. J. M. (1989). Perceived control and the experience of pain. In A. Steptoe & A. Appels (Eds.), *Stress, personal control and health* (pp. 131–162). Brussels-Luxembourg: Wiley.

Asmundson, G. J. G, & Norton, G. R. (1995). Anxiety sensitivity in patients with physically unexplained chronic back pain: a preliminary report. *Behaviour Research and Therapy, 33*, 771–777.

Asmundson, G. J. G., Norton, P. J., & Norton, G. R. (1999). Beyond pain: The role of fear and avoidance in chronicity. *Clinical Psychology Review, 19*, 97–119.

Bachanas, P. J., & Roberts, M. D. (1995). Factors affecting children's attitudes toward health care and responses to stressful medical procedures. *Journal of Pediatric Psychology, 20*, 261–2175.

Bandura, A. (1969). *Principles of behavior modification*. New York: Holt, Rinehart & Winston.

Bandura, A. (1997). *Self-efficacy: The exercise of control*. New York: Freeman.

Bandura, A., O'Leary, A., Taylor, C. B., Gauthier, J., & Gossard, D. (1987). Perceived self-efficacy and pain control: Opioid and nonopioid mechanisms. *Journal of Personality and Social Psychology, 53*, 563–571.

Bandura, A., Taylor, C. B., Williams, S. L., Mefford, I. N., & Barchas, J. D. (1985). Catecholamine secretion as a function of perceived coping self-efficacy. *Journal of Consulting and Clinical Psychology, 53*, 406–414.

Bansevicius, D., Westgaard, R. H., & Jensen, C.

(1997). Mental stress of long duration: EMG activity, perceived tension, fatigue, and pain development in pain-free subjects. *Headache, 37,* 499–510.

Barber, T., & Hahn, K. W. (1962). Physiological and subjective responses to pain producing stimulation under hypnotically-suggested and waking-imagined "analgesia. " *Journal of Abnormal and Social Psychology, 65,* 411–418.

Bergstrom, G., Bodin, L., Jensen, I. B., Linton, S. J., & Nygren, A. L. (2001). Long-term, non-specific spinal pain: Reliable and valid subgroups of patients. *Behaviour Research and Therapy, 39,* 75–87.

Biedermann, H. J., McGhie, A., Monga, T. N., & Shanks, G. L. (1987). Perceived and actual control in EMG treatment of back pain. *Behaviour Research and Therapy, 25,* 137–147.

Blanchard, E. B. (1987). Long-term effects of behavioral treatment of chronic headache. *Behavior Therapy, 18,* 375–385.

Block, A. R., Kremer, E. F., & Gaylor, M. (1980). Behavioral treatment of chronic pain: Variables affecting treatment efficacy. *Pain, 8,* 367–375.

Blumer, D., & Heilbronn, M. (1982). Chronic pain as a variant of depressive disease: The pain-prone disorder. *Journal of Nervous and Mental Disease, 170,* 381–406.

Borgeat, F., Hade, B., Elie, R., & Larouche L. M. (1984). Effects of voluntary muscle tension increases in tension headache. *Headache, 24,* 199–202.

Bradley, L. A., & McKendree-Smith, N. L. (2001). Assessment of psychological status using interviews and self-report instruments. In D. C. Turk & R. Melzack (Eds.), *Handbook of pain assessment* (2nd ed., pp. 292–319). New York: Guilford Press.

Burns, J. W., Johnson, B. J., Devine, J., Mahoney, N., & Pawl, R. (1998). Anger management style and the prediction of treatment outcome among male and female chronic pain patients. *Behaviour Research and Therapy, 36,* 1051–1062.

Butler, R., Damarin, F., Beaulieu, C., Schwebel, A., & Thorn, B. E. (1989). Assessing cognitive coping strategies for acute post-surgical pain. *Psychological Assessment: A Journal of Consulting and Clinical Psychology, 1,* 41–45.

Cairns, D., & Pasino, J. (1977). Comparison of verbal reinforcement and feedback in the operant treatment of disability of chronic low back pain. *Behavior Therapy, 8,* 621–630.

Cassell, E. J. (1982). The nature of suffering and the goals of medicine. *New England Journal of Medicine, 396,* 639–645.

Ciccone, D. S., & Grzesiak, R. C. (1984). Cognitive dimensions of chronic pain. *Social Science and Medicine, 19,* 1339–1345.

Cioffi, D. (1991). Beyond attentional strategies: A cognitive-perceptual model of somatic interpretation. *Psychological Bulletin, 109,* 25–41.

Collie, J. (1913). *Malingering and feigned sickness.* London: Edward Arnold.

Council, J. R., Ahern, D. K., Follick, M. J., & Kline,

C. L. (1988). Expectancies and functional impairment in chronic low back pain. *Pain, 33,* 323–331.

Craig, K. D. (1986). Social modeling influences: Pain in context. In R. A. Sternbach (Ed.), *The psychology of pain* (2nd ed., pp. 67–95). New York: Raven Press.

Craig, K. D. (1988). Consequences of caring: Pain in human context. *Canadian Psychologist, 28,* 311–321.

Crombez, G., Vervaet, L., Lysens, R., Eelen, P., & Baeyerns F. (1998). Avoidance and confrontation of painful, back straining movements in chronic back pain patients. *Behavior Modification, 22,* 62–77.

Crombez, G., Vlaeyen, J. W., & Heuts, P. H. (1999). Pain-related fear is more disabling than pain itself: Evidence on the role of pain-related fear in chronic back pain disability. *Pain, 80,* 329–339.

Crook, J., Weir, R., Tunks, E. (1989). An epidemiologic follow-up survey of persistent pain sufferers in a group family practice and specialty pain clinic. *Pain, 36,* 49–61.

DeGood, D. E., & Tait, R. C. (2001). Assessment of pain beliefs and pain coping. In D. C. Turk & R. Melzack (Eds.), *Handbook of pain assessment* (2nd ed., pp. 320–345). New York: Guilford Press.

Desroches, H. F., Kaiman, B. D., & Ballard, H. T. (1967). Factors influencing reporting of physical symptoms by aged patients. *Geriatrics, 22,* 169–175.

Deyo, R. A. (1986). The early diagnostic evaluation of patients with low back pain. *Journal of General Internal Medicine, 1,* 328–338.

Deyo, R. A., Walsh, N. E., Martin, D., Schoenfeld, L. S., & Ramamurthy, S. (1990). A controlled trial of transcutaneous electrical nerve stimulation (TENS) and exercise for chronic low back pain. *New England Journal of Medicine, 322,* 1627–1634.

Dolce, J. J., Crocker, M. F., & Doleys, D. M. (1986). Prediction of outcome among chronic pain patients. *Behaviour Research and Therapy, 24,* 313–319.

Dolce, J. J., Crocker, M. F., Moletteire, C., & Doleys, D. M. (1986). Exercise quotas, anticipatory concern and self-efficacy expectancies in chronic pain: A preliminary report. *Pain, 24,* 365–375.

Doleys, D. M., Crocker, M., & Patton, D. (1982). Response of patients with chronic pain to exercise quotas. *Physical Therapy, 62,* 1112–1115.

Droste, C., & Roskamm, H. (1983). Experimental pain measurement inpatients with asymptomatic myocardial ischemia. *Journal of the American College of Cardiology, 1,* 940–945.

Dufton, B. D. (1989). Cognitive failure and chronic pain. *International Journal of Psychiatry in Medicine, 19,* 291–297.

Dworkin, S. F., & Massoth, D. L. (1994). Temporomandibular disorders and chronic pain: Disease or illness. *Journal of Prosthetic Dentistry, 7,*

29–38.

Engel, G. L. (1977). The need for a new medical model: A challenge for biomedical science. *Science, 196,* 129–136.

Fearon, I., McGrath, P. J., & Achat, H. (1996). "Booboos": The study of everyday pain among young children. *Pain, 68,* 55–62.

Fernandez, E., & Turk, D. C. (1989). The utility of cognitive coping strategies for altering perception of pain: A meta-analysis. *Pain, 38,* 123–135.

Fernandez, E., & Turk, D. C. (1992). Sensory and affective components of pain: Separation and synthesis. *Psychological Bulletin, 112,* 205–217.

Fernandez, E., & Turk, D. C. (1995). The scope and significance of anger in the experience of chronic pain. *Pain, 61,* 165–175.

Feuerstein, M., & Beattie, P. (1995). Biobehavioral factors affecting pain and disability in low back pain: Mechanisms and assessment. *Physical Therapy, 75,* 267–269.

Fitzpatrick, R. M., Hopkins, A. P., & Harvard-Watts, O. (1983). Social dimensions of healing: A longitudinal study of outcomes of medical management of headaches. *Social Science and Medicine, 17,* 501–510.

Flor, H., Birbaumer, N., Schugens, M. M., & Lutzenberger, W. (1992). Symptom-specific psychophysiological responses in chronic pain patients. *Psychophysiology, 29,* 452–460.

Flor, H., Birbaumer, N., & Turk, D. C. (1990). The psychobiology of chronic pain. *Advances in Behaviour Research and Therapy, 12,* 47–84.

Flor, H., Elbert, T., Muhlnickel, W., Pantev, C., Wienbruch, C., & Taub, E. (1998). Cortical reorganization and phantom phenomena in congenital and traumatic upper extremity amputees. *Experimental Brain Research, 119,* 205–212.

Flor, H., Fydrich, T., & Turk, D. C. (1992). Efficacy of multidisciplinary pain treatment centers: A meta-analytic review. *Pain, 49,* 221–230.

Flor, H., Kerns, R. D., & Turk, D. C. (1987). The role of spouse reinforcement, perceived pain, and activity levels of chronic pain patients. *Journal of Psychosomatic Research, 31,* 251–259.

Flor, H., & Turk, D. C. (1988). Chronic back pain and rheumatoid arthritis: Predicting pain and disability from cognitive variables. *Journal of Behavioral Medicine, 11,* 251–265.

Flor, H., Turk, D. C., & Birbaumer, N. (1985). Assessment of stress-related psychophysiological responses in chronic pain patients. *Journal of Consulting and Clinical Psychology, 35,* 354–364.

Fordyce, W. E. (1976). *Behavioral methods for chronic pain and illness.* St. Louis, MO: Mosby.

Fordyce, W. E., Roberts, A. H., & Sternbach, R. A. (1985). The behavioral management of chronic pain: A response to critics. *Pain, 22,* 113–125.

Fordyce, W. E., Shelton, J., & Dundore, D. (1982). The modification of avoidance learning pain behaviors. *Journal of Behavioral Medicine, 4,* 405–414.

Geisser, M. E., Roth, R. S., Bachman, J. E., & Eckert, T. A. (1996). The relationship between symptoms of post-traumatic stress disorder and pain, affective disturbance and disability among patients with accident and non-accident related pain *Pain, 66,* 207–214.

Gentry, W. D., & Bernal, G. A. A. (1977). Chronic pain. In R. Williams & W. D. Gentry (Eds.), *Behavioral approaches to medical treatment* (pp. 171–182). Cambridge, MA: Ballinger.

Gil, K. M., Williams, D. A., Keefe, F. J., & Beckham, J. C. (1990). The relationship of negative thoughts to pain and psychological distress. *Behavior Therapy, 21,* 349–352.

Greene, C. S., & Laskin, D. M. (1974). Long-term evaluation of conservative treatments for myofascial pain dysfunction syndrome. *Journal of the American Dental Association, 89,* 1365–1368.

Hatch, J. P., Prihoda, T. J., Moore, P. J., Cyr-Provost, M., Borcherding, S., Boutros, N. N., & Seleshi, E. (1991). A naturalistic study of the relationship among electromyographic activity, psychological stress, and pain in ambulatory tension-type headache patients and headache-free controls. *Psychosomatic Medicine, 53,* 576–584.

Heyneman, N. E., Fremouw, W. J., Gano, D., Kirkland, F., & Heiden, L. (1990). Individual differences in the effectiveness of different coping strategies. *Cognitive Therapy and Research, 14,* 63–77.

Holroyd, K. A., Penzien, D. B., Hursey, K. G., Tobin, D. L., Rogers, L., & Holm, J. E. (1984). Change mechanisms in EMG biofeedback training: Cognitive changes underlying improvements in tension headache. *Journal of Consulting and Clinical Psychology, 52,* 1039–1053.

Jamner, L. D., & Tursky, B. (1987). Syndrome-specific descriptor profiling: A psychophysiological and psychophysical approach. *Health Psychology, 6,* 417–430.

Jensen, M. P., & Karoly, P. (1991). Control beliefs, coping effort, and adjustment to chronic pain. *Journal of Consulting and Clinical Psychology, 59,* 431–438.

Jensen, M. P., Romano, J. M., Turner, J. A., Good, A. B., & Wald, L. H. (1999). Patient beliefs predict patient functioning: Further support for a cognitive-behavioral model of chronic pain. *Pain, 81,* 95–104.

Jensen, M. P., Turner, J. A., Romano, J. M., & Karoly, P. (1991). Coping with chronic pain: A critical review of the literature. *Pain, 47,* 249–283.

Jensen, M. P., Turner, J. A., Romano, J. M., & Lawler, B. K. (1994). Relationship of pain-specific beliefs to chronic pain adjustment. *Pain, 57,* 301–309.

Johansson, E., & Lindberg, P. (2000). Low back pain patients in primary care: Subgroups based on the Multidimensional Pain Inventory. *International Journal of Behavioral Medicine, 7,* 340–352.

Keefe, F. J., Brown, G. K., Wallston, K. S., & Caldwell, D. S. (1989). Coping with rheumatoid arthritis pain. Catastrophizing as a maladaptive strategy. *Pain, 37,* 51–56.

Keefe, F. J., Caldwell, D. S., Williams, D. A., Gil, K. M., Mitchell, D., Robertson, C., Martinez, S.,

Nunley, J., Beckham, J. C., Crisson, J. E., & Helms, M. (1990a). Pain coping skills training in the management of osteoarthritis knee pain: A comparative approach. *Behavior Therapy, 21,* 49–62.

Keefe, R. J., Caldwell, D. S., Williams, D. A., Gil, K. M., Mitchell, D., Robertson, C., Martinez, S., Nunley, J., Beckham, J. C., Crisson, J. E., & Helms, M. (1990b). Pain coping skills training in the management of osteoarthritis knee pain II. Follow-up results. *Behavior Therapy, 21,* 435–447.

Kerns, R. D., Rosenberg, R., & Jacob, M. C. (1994). Anger expression and chronic pain. *Journal of Behavioral Medicine, 17,* 57–68.

Kerns, R. D., Turk, D. C., & Rudy, T. E. (1985). The West Haven–Yale Multidimensional Pain Inventory (WHYMPI). *Pain, 23,* 345–356.

Knost, B., Flor, H., Braun, C., & Birbaumer, N. (1997). Cerebral processing of words and the development of chronic pain. *Psychophysiology, 34,* 474–481.

Kotarba, J. A. (1983). *Chronic pain: Its social dimensions.* Beverly Hills, CA: Sage.

Lawson, K., Reesor, K. A., Keefe, F. J., & Turner, J. A. (1990). Dimensions of pain-related cognitive coping: Cross validation of the factor structure of the Coping Strategies Questionnaire. *Pain, 43,* 195–204.

Lefebvre, M. F. (1981). Cognitive distortion and cognitive errors in depressed psychiatric low back pain patients. *Journal of Consulting and Clinical Psychology, 49,* 517–525.

Lenthem, J., Slade, P. O., Troup, J. P. G., & Bentley, G. (1983). Outline of a fear-avoidance model of exaggerated pain perception. *Behaviour Research and Therapy, 21,* 401–408.

Leventhal, H., & Everhart, D. (1979). Emotion, pain and physical Illness. In C. E. Izard (Ed.), *Emotion and psychopathology* (pp. 263–299). New York: Plenum Press.

Linton, S. (1985). The relationship between activity and chronic back pain. *Pain, 21,* 289–294.

Linton, S. J., Buer, N., Vlaeyen, J. W. S., & Hellsing, A.-L. (2000). Are fear-avoidance beliefs related to the inception of an episode of back pain: A prospective study. *Psychology and Health, 14,* 1051–1059.

Linton, S. J., Melin, L., & Götestam, K. G. (1984). Behavioral analysis of chronic pain and its management. In M. Hersen, R. Eisler, & P. Miller (Eds.), *Progress in behavior modification* (Vol. 7, pp. 1–38). New York: Academic Press.

Lipton, J. A., & Marbach, J. J. (1984). Ethnicity and the pain experience. *Social Science and Medicine, 19,* 1279–1298.

Litt, M. D. (1988). Self-efficacy and perceived control: Cognitive mediators of pain tolerance. *Journal of Personality and Social Psychology, 54,* 149–160.

Lorig, K., Chastain, R. L., Ung, E., Shoor, S., & Holman, H. R. (1989). Development and evaluation of a scale to measure perceived self-efficacy in people with arthritis. *Arthritis and Rheumatism, 32,* 37–44.

Lousberg, R., Groenman, N., & Schmidt, A. (1996). Profile characteristics of the MPI-DVL clusters of pain patients. *Journal of Clinical Psychology, 52,* 161–167.

Main, C. J., & Waddell, G. (1991). A comparison of cognitive measures in low back pain: Statistical structure and clinical validity of initial assessment. *Pain, 46,* 287–298.

Manning, M. M., & Wright, T. L. (1983). Self-efficacy expectancies, outcome expectancies, and the persistence of pain control in childbirth. *Journal of Personality and Social Psychology, 45,* 421–431.

Martin, P. R., Nathan, P., Milech, D., & Van Keppel, M. (1989). Cognitive therapy vs. self-management training in the treatment of chronic headaches. *British Journal of Clinical Psychology, 28,* 347–361.

McCracken, L. M., & Gross R T. (1998). The role of pain-related anxiety reduction in the outcome of multidisciplinary treatment for chronic low back pain: Preliminary results. *Journal of Occupational Rehabilitation, 8,* 179–189.

McCracken, L. M., Gross, R. T., Sorg, P. J., & Edmands, T. A. (1993). Prediction of pain in patients with chronic low back pain: Effects of inaccurate prediction and pain-related anxiety. *Behavior Research and Therapy, 31,* 647–652.

Mechanic, D. (1962). The concept of illness behavior. *Journal of Chronic Disease, 15,* 189–194.

Mechanic, D. (1978). Effects of psychological distress on perceptions of physical health and use of medical and psychiatric facilities. *Journal of Human Stress, 4,* 26–32.

Mechanic, D. (1986). Illness behavior: An overview. In S. McHugh & T. M. Vallis (Eds.), *Illness behavior: A multidisciplinary model* (pp. 101–110). New York: Plenum Press.

Melzack, R. (1999). Pain and stress: A new perspective. In R. J. Gatchel & D. C. Turk (Eds.), *Psychosocial factors in pain: Critical perspectives* (pp. 89–106). New York: Guilford Press.

Melzack, R., & Casey, K. L. (1968). Sensory, motivational and central control determinants of pain: A new conceptual model. In D. Kenshalo (Ed.), *The skin senses* (pp. 423–443). Springfield, IL: Thomas.

Melzack, R., & Wall, P. D. (1965). Pain mechanisms: A new theory. *Science, 50,* 971–979.

Melzack, R., & Wall, P. D. (1982). *The challenge of pain.* New York: Basic Books.

Merskey, H., & Bogduk, N. (1986). Classification of chronic pain. Description of chronic pain syndromes and definitions of pain terms. *Pain* (Suppl. 3), S1–S225.

Mizener, D., Thomas, M., & Billings, R. (1988). Cognitive changes of migraineurs receiving biofeedback training. *Headache, 28,* 339–343.

Nathan, P. W. (1976). The gate control theory of pain: A critical review. *Brain, 99,* 123–158.

Nerenz, D. R., & Leventhal H. (1983). Self regulation theory in chronic illness. In T. Burish & L. A. Bradley (Eds.), *Coping with chronic illness* (pp.

13–37). Orlando, FL: Academic Press.

Newton, C. R., & Barbaree, H. E. (1987). Cognitive changes accompanying headache treatment: The use of a thought-sampling procedure. *Cognitive Therapy and Research, 11,* 635–652.

Nicholas, M. K., Wilson, P. H., & Goyen, J. (1991). Operant-behavioural and cognitive-behavioral and cognitive-behavioral treatment for chronic back pain. *Behaviour Research and Therapy, 29,* 225–238.

North, R. B. (1989). Neural stimulation techniques. In C. D. Tollison (Ed.), *Handbook of chronic pain management* (pp. 136–146). Baltimore: Williams & Wilkins.

Nouwen, A., & Solinger, J. W. (1979). The effectiveness of EMG biofeedback training in low back pain. *Biofeedback and Self-Regulation, 4,* 103–111.

Okifuji, A., & Turk, D. C. (1999). Fibromyalgia: Search for mechanisms and effective treatments. In R. J. Gatchel & D. C. Turk (Eds.), *Psychosocial factors in pain: Critical perspectives* (pp. 227–246). New York: Guilford Press.

Okifuji, A., & Turk, D. C. (in press). Stress and psychophysiological dysregulation in patients with fibromyalgia syndrome. *Biofeedback and Applied Psychophysiology.*

Okifuji, A., Turk, D. C., & Curran, S. L. (1999). Anger in chronic pain: Investigation of anger targets and intensity. *Journal of Psychosomatic Research, 61,* 771–780.

Okifuji, A., Turk, D. C., & Sherman, J. J. (2000). Evaluation of the relationship between depression and fibromyalgia syndrome: Why aren't all patients depressed? *Journal of Rheumatology, 27,* 212–219.

O'Leary, A., Shoor, S., Lorig, K., & Holman, H. R. (1988). A cognitive-behavioral treatment for rheumatoid arthritis. *Health Psychology, 7,* 527–544.

Parsons, T. (1958). Definitions of health and illness in the light of American values and social structure. In E. G. Jaco (Ed.), *Patients, physicians, and illness* (pp. 3–29). New York: Free Press.

Pennebaker, J. W. (1982). *The psychology of physical symptoms.* New York: Springer-Verlag.

Philips, H. C. (1987a). Avoidance behaviour and its role in sustaining chronic pain. *Behaviour Research and Therapy, 25,* 273–279.

Philips, H. C. (1987b). The effects of behavioural treatment on chronic pain. *Behaviour Research and Therapy, 25,* 365–377.

Price, D. D. (1987). *Psychological and neural mechanisms of pain.* New York: Raven Press.

Rachman, S., & Arntz, A. (1991). The overprediction and underprediction of pain. *Clinical Psychology Review, 11,* 339–356.

Rachman, S., & Lopatka, C. (1988). Accurate and inaccurate predictions of pain. *Behaviour Research and Therapy, 26,* 291–296.

Reesor, K. A., & Craig, K. (1988). Medically incongruent chronic pain: Physical limitations, suffering and ineffective coping. *Pain, 32,* 35–45.

Reiss, S., & McNally, R. J. (1985). The expectancy model of fear. In S. Reiss & R. R. Bootzin (Eds.), *Theoretical issues in behavior therapy* (pp. 107–121). New York: Academic Press.

Richard, K. (1988). The occurrence of maladaptive health-related behaviors and teacher-related conduct problems in children of chronic low back pain patients. *Journal of Behavioral Medicine, 11,* 107–116.

Rimm, D. C., & Litvak, S. B. (1969). Self-verbalizations and emotional arousal. *Journal of Abnormal Psychology, 74,* 181–187.

Romano, J., & Turner, J. A. (1985). Chronic pain and depression: Does the evidence support a relationship? *Psychological Bulletin, 97,* 18–34.

Romano, J. M., Turner, J. A., Friedman, L. S., Bulcroft, R. A., Jensen, M. K., & Hops, H. (1992). Sequential analysis of chronic pain behaviors and spouse responses. *Journal of Consulting and Clinical Psychology, 60,* 777–782.

Rudy, T. E., Kerns, R. J., & Turk, D. C. (1988). Chronic pain and depression: Toward a cognitive-behavioral mediation model. *Pain, 35,* 179–183.

Schanberg, L. E., Keefe, F. J., Lefebvre, J. C., Kredich, D. W., & Gil, K. M. (1998). Social context of pain in children with juvenile primary fibromyalgia syndrome: Parental pain history and family environment. *Clinical Journal of Pain, 14,* 107–115.

Schmidt, A. J. M. (1985a). Cognitive factors in the performance of chronic low back pain patients. *Journal of Psychosomatic Research, 29,* 183–189.

Schmidt, A. J. M. (1985b). Performance level of chronic low back pain patients in different treadmill test conditions. *Journal of Psychosomatic Research, 29,* 639–646.

Schmidt, A. J. M., Gierlings, R. E. H., & Peters, M. L. (1989). Environment and interoceptive influences on chronic low back pain behavior. *Pain, 38,* 137–143.

Schwartz, D. P., DeGood, D. E., & Shutty, M. S. (1985). Direct assessment of beliefs and attitudes of chronic pain patients. *Archives of Physical Medicine and Rehabilitation, 66,* 806–809.

Schwartz, L., Slater, M., Birchler, G., & Atkinson, J. H. (1991). Depression in spouses of chronic pain patients: The role of pain and anger, and marital satisfaction. *Pain, 44,* 61–67.

Selye, H. (1950). *Stress.* Montreal: Acta Medical.

Sherman, J., Carlson, C., Cordova, M., Mager, W., Studts, J., Moesko, M., & Okeson, J. (1988). Identification of posttraumatic stress disorder in orofacial pain patients. *Journal of Dental Research, 77,* 111–117.

Sherman, J. J., Turk, D. C., & Okifuji, A. (2000). Prevalence and impact of posttraumatic stress disorder (PTSD) symptoms on patients with fibromyalgia syndrome. *Clinical Journal of Pain, 16,* 212–219.

Smith, T. W., Aberger, E. W., Follick, M. J., & Ahern, D. L. (1986). Cognitive distortion and psychological distress in chronic low back pain. *Journal of Consulting and Clinical Psychology,*

54, 573–575.

Smith, T. W., Follick, M. J., Ahern, D. L., & Adams, A. (1986). Cognitive distortion and disability in chronic low back pain. *Cognitive Therapy and Research, 10*, 201–210.

Smith, T. W., Peck, J. R., Milano, R. A., & Ward, J. R. (1990). Helplessness and depression in rheumatoid arthritis. *Health Psychology, 9*, 377–389.

Spanos, N. P., Horton, C., & Chaves, J. F. (1975). The effect of two cognitive strategies on pain threshold. *Journal of Abnormal Psychology, 84*, 677–681.

Spiegel, D., & Bloom, J. R. (1983). Pain in metastatic breast cancer. *Cancer, 52*, 341–345.

Spinhoven, P., Ter Kuile, M. M. Linssen, A. C. G., & Gazendam, B. (1989). Pain coping strategies in a Dutch population of chronic low back pain patients. *Pain, 37*, 77–83.

Sullivan, M. J. L., Thorn, B., Hatyhornthwaite, J. A., Keefe, F., Martin, M., Bradley, L. A., & Lefebvre, J. C. (2001). Theoretical perspectives on the relationship between catastrophizing and pain. *Clinical Journal of Pain, 17*, 52–64.

Summers. J. D., Rapoff, M. A., Varghese, G., Porter, K., & Palmer, K. (1992). Psychological factors in chronic spinal cord injury pain. *Pain, 47*, 183–189.

Tota-Faucette, M. E., Gil, K. M., Williams. F. J., & Goli, V. (1993). Predictors of response to pain management treatment. The role of family environment and changes in cognitive processes. *Clinical Journal of Pain, 9*, 115–123.

Tunks, E., Crook, J., Norman, G., & Kalasher, S. (1988). Tender-points in fibromyalgia. *Pain, 34*, 11–19.

Turk, D. C. (1990). Customizing treatment for chronic pain patients. Who, what and why. *Clinical Journal of Pain, 6*, 255–270.

Turk, D. C. (2001). Physiological and psychological bases of pain. In A. Baum, T. Revenson, & J. Singer (Eds.), *Handbook of health psychology* (pp. 117–138). Hillsdale, NJ: Erlbaum.

Turk, D. C. (2002). A diathesis-stress model of chronic pain and disability following traumatic injury. *Pain Research and Management, 7*, 10–19.

Turk, D. C., & Flor, H. (1987). Pain > pain behaviors: The utility and limitations of the pain behavior construct. *Pain, 31*, 277–295.

Turk, D. C., Kerns, R. D., & Rosenberg, R. (1992). Effects of marital interaction on chronic pain and disability: Examining the down-side of social support. *Rehabilitation Psychology, 37*, 259–274.

Turk, D. C., Meichenbaum, D., & Genest, M. (1983). *Pain and behavioral medicine: A cognitive-behavioral perspective.* New York: Guilford Press.

Turk, D. C., & Okifuji, A. (1996). Perception of traumatic onset and compensation status: Impact on pain severity, emotional distress, and disability in chronic pain patients. *Journal of Behavioral Medicine, 9*, 435–453.

Turk, D. C., & Okifuji, A. (1997). Evaluating the role of physical, operant, cognitive, and affective factors in pain behavior in chronic pain patients. *Behavior Modification, 21*, 259–280.

Turk, D. C., Okifuji, A., & Scharff, L. (1994). Assessment of older women with chronic pain. *Journal of Women and Aging, 6*, 25–42.

Turk, D. C., Okifuji, A., & Scharff, L. (1995). Chronic pain an depression: Role of perceived impact and perceived control in different age cohorts. *Pain, 61*, 93–102.

Turk, D. C., Okifuji, A., Starz, T. W., & Sinclair, J. D. (1996). Effects of type of symptom onset on psychological distress and disability in fibromyalgia syndrome patients. *Pain, 68*, 423–430.

Turk, D. C., & Rudy, T. E. (1988). Toward an empirically derived taxonomy of chronic pain patients: Integration of psychological assessment data. *Journal of Consulting and Clinical Psychology, 56*, 233–238.

Turk, D. C., & Rudy, T. E. (1990). Robustness of an empirically derived taxonomy of chronic pain patients. *Pain, 43*, 27–36.

Turk, D. C., & Rudy, T. E. (1991). Persistent pain and the injured worker: Integrating biomedical, psychosocial, and behavioral factors. *Journal of Occupational Rehabilitation, 1*, 159–179.

Turk, D. C., & Rudy, T. E. (1992). Cognitive factors and persistent pain: A glimpse into Pandora's box. *Cognitive Therapy and Research, 16*, 99–112.

Turk, D. C., & Salovey, P. (1984). "Chronic pain as a variant of depressive disease": A critical reappraisal. *Journal of Nervous and Mental Disease, 172*, 398–404.

Turk, D. C., Sist, T. C., Okifuji, A., Miner, M. F., Florio, G., Harrison, P., Massey, J., Lema, M. L., & Zevon, M. A. (1998). Adaptation to metastatic cancer pain, regional/local cancer pain and non-cancer pain: Role of psychological and behavioral factors. *Pain, 74*, 247–256.

Turner, J. A. (1991). Coping and chronic pain. In M. R. Bond, J. E. Charlton, & C. J. Woolf (Eds.), *Proceedings of the VIth World Congress on Pain* (pp. 219–227). Amsterdam: Elsevier.

Turner, J. A., & Aaron, L. A. (2001). Pain-related catastrophizing: What is it? *Clinical Journal of Pain, 17*, 65–71.

Turner, J. A., & Clancy, S. (1986). Strategies for coping with chronic low back pain: Relationship to pain and disability. *Pain, 24*, 355–363.

Turner, J. A., & Clancy, S. (1988). Comparison of operant behavioral and cognitive-behavioral group treatment for chronic low back pain. *Journal of Consulting and Clinical Psychology, 56*, 261–266.

Turner, J., Deyo, R. A., Loeser, J. D., Von Korff, M., & Fordyce, W. E. (1994). The importance of placebo effects in pain treatment and research. *Journal of the American Medical Association, 271*, 1609–1614.

Unruh, A. M. (1996). Gender variations in clinical pain experience. *Pain, 65*, 123–167.

Vaughan, K. B., & Lanzetta, J. T. (1980). Vicarious instigation and conditioning of facial expressive and autonomic responses to a model's expressive display of pain. *Journal of Personality and Social Psychology, 38*, 909–923.

Vaughan, K. B., & Lanzetta, J. T. (1981). The effect of modification of expressive displays on vicarious emotional arousal. *Journal of Experimental Social Psychology, 17*, 16–30.

Vlaeyen, J. W. S., de Jong, J., Geilen, M., Heuts, P. H. T. G., & van Breukelen, G. (2001). Graded exposure in vivo in the treatment of pain-related fear: A replicated single-case experimental design in four patients with chronic low back pain. *Behaviour Research and Therapy, 39*, 151–166.

Vlaeyen, J. W. S., Haazen, I. W. C. J., Schuerman, J. A., Kole-Snijders, A. M. J., & van Eek, H. (1995). Behavioral rehabilitation of chronic low back pain—comparison of an operant, and operant cognitive treatment and an operant respondent treatment. *British Journal of Clinical Psychology, 34*, 95–118.

Vlaeyen, J,W. S., Kole-Snijders, A. M., Boeren, R. G. B., & van Eek, H. (1995). Fear of movement/(re)injury in chronic low back pain and its relation to behavioral performance. *Pain, 62*, 363–372.

Vlaeyen, J. W. S., Kole-Snijders, A., Rooteveel, A., Ruesink, R., & Heuts, P. (1995). The role of fear of movement/(re)injury in pain disability. *Journal of Occupational Rehabilitation, 5*, 235–252.

Vlaeyen, J. W. S., & Linton, S. J. (2000). Fear-avoidance and its consequences in chronic muculoskeletal pain: A state of the art. *Pain, 85*, 317–332.

Vlaeyen, J. W. S., Seelen, H. A. M., Peters, M., de Jong, P., Aretz, E., Beisiegel, E., & Weber, W. E. J. (1999). Fear of movement/(re)injury and muscular reactivity in chronic low back pain patients: An experimental investigation. *Pain, 82*, 297– 304.

Von Korff, M., Dworkin, S., & LeResche, L. (1990). Graded chronic pain status: An epidemiologic evaluation. *Pain, 40*, 279–291.

Von Korff, M., Ormel, J., Keefe, F. J., & Dworkin, S. F. (1992). Grading severity of chronic pain: Concepts, use, and validity. *Pain, 50*, 133–149.

Waddell, G., & Main, C. J. (1984). Assessment of severity in low back disorders. *Spine, 9*, 204–208.

Wall, P. D. (1989). The dorsal horn. In P. D. Wall & R. Melzack (Eds.), *Textbook of pain* (2nd ed., pp. 102–111). New York: Churchill Livingstone.

Weisberg, J. N., & Keefe, F. J. (1999). Personality, individual differences, and psychopthology in chronic pain. In R. J. Gatchel & D. C. Turk (Eds.), *Psychosocial factors in pain: Critical perspectives* (pp. 56–73). New York: Guilford Press.

Wells, N. (1994). Perceived control over pain: Relation to distress and disability. *Research in Nursing and Health, 17*, 295–302.

White, K. L., Williams, F., & Greenberg, B. G. (1961). The ecology of medical care. *New England Journal of Medicine, 265*, 885–886.

Whitehead, W. E. (1980). Interoception, In R. Holzl & W. E. Whitehead (Eds.), *Psychophysiology of the gastrointestinal tract* (pp. 145–161). New York: Plenum Press.

Williams, D. A., & Keefe, F. J. (1991). Pain beliefs and the use of cognitive-behavioral coping strategies. *Pain, 46*, 185–190.

Williams, D. A., & Thorn, B. E. (1989). An empirical assessment of pain beliefs. *Pain, 36*, 251–258.

Woolf, C. J., & Mannion, R. J. (1999). Neuropathic pain: Aetiology, symptoms, mechanisms, and management. *Lancet, 353*, 1959–1964.

Zborowski, M. (1969). *People in pain*. San Francisco: Jossey-Bass.

2

Psychological Disorders and Chronic Pain: Are There Cause-and-Effect Relationships?

Robert J. Gatchel
Jeffrey Dersh

With the introduction of the *gate control theory* of pain by Melzack and Wall (1965), the scientific community came to accept the importance of central, psychological factors in the pain perception process. As a result, a great deal of research has attempted to isolate the psychological characteristics associated with chronic pain patients. For example, the Minnesota Multiphasic Personality Inventory (MMPI) has been widely used to delineate these psychological characteristics. This early work attempted to differentiate "functional" pain from "organic" pain. However, Sternbach (1974) challenged the utility and validity of attempting to make a functional–organic dichotomy when dealing with chronic pain. Chronic pain is a complex psychophysiological behavior pattern that cannot be broken down into distinct, psychological and physical components.

The *biopsychosocial model* of pain, which includes physical, psychological, and social elements, moves away from an overly simplistic biomedical disease model of pain and replaces it with an alternative multidimensional perspective. In this model, psychosocial factors are viewed as intricately related to the pain perception process. As pain becomes more chronic, the psychosocial vari-

ables play an increasingly dominant role in the maintenance of pain behaviors and suffering (see Turk & Monarch, Chapter 1, this volume.

In this chapter, we discuss the issue of one of the important concomitants that clinicians must be prepared to deal with when treating chronic pain patients—psychopathology. Relatedly, the complex "chicken or egg" question of what occurs first—the chronic pain or psychopathology—is addressed.

Psychological Concomitants of Pain

There is evidence to suggest that chronic pain patients develop specific psychological problems because of the failure to alleviate their pain, which distinguishes them from acute pain patients. For example, in an early study, Sternbach, Wolf, Murphy, and Akeson (1973) compared the MMPI profiles of a group of acute low back pain patients (pain present for less than 6 months) to those of a group of chronic low back pain patients (more than 6 months). Results indicated significant differences between the two groups on the first three clinical scales

(Hypochondriasis, Depression, and Hysteria). The combined elevation of these three scales is often referred to as the *neurotic triad* because it is commonly found in neurotic individuals who are experiencing a great deal of anxiety (another typical pattern often found is the Conversion V, in which Scales 1 and 3 are more elevated than Scale 2). These results indicate that during the early stages of pain, no major psychological problems are produced by it. However, as the pain becomes chronic in nature, psychological changes begin to occur. These changes are most likely due to the constant discomfort, despair, and preoccupation with the pain that comes to dominate the lives of these patients, as well as their inability to fulfill customary familial, vocational, and recreational roles. This may produce a "layer" of behavioral and psychological problems over the original nociception or pain experience itself.

We have found a similar pattern of results from research conducted with chronic low back pain patients participating in an intensive 3-week rehabilitation program (Barnes, Gatchel, Mayer, & Barnett, 1990). In this study, patients were administered the MMPI before the start of the program. Results clearly showed that the first three clinical scales were significantly elevated in these chronic patients before the start of the treatment program, as would be expected on the basis of past clinical research. However, at a 6-month follow-up after successful completion of this program (which produced successful rehabilitation and return to work in the great majority of these patients), the three scales were significantly *decreased* to normal levels. Thus, these results again suggest that elevations of scores are related to the trauma and stress associated with the chronic pain condition. When successfully treated, these clinically significant elevations disappear.

The foregoing findings indicate that one of the consequences of dealing with chronic pain is the development of emotional reactions such as anxiety and dysphoria produced by the long-term "wearing down" effects and drain of psychological resources. Again, such data suggest that this may produce a layer of behavioral and psychological problems over the original nociception or pain experience itself. Indeed, it is generally accepted that chronic low back pain is a complex behavior that does not merely result from some specific structural cause. When the chronic pain is effectively treated, many of the problematic psychosocial symptoms tend also to be alleviated.

A Conceptual Model of the Transition from Acute to Chronic Pain

Gatchel (1991, 1996) has proposed a broad conceptual model that hypothesizes three stages that may be involved in the transition of acute low back pain into chronic low back pain disability and accompanying psychosocial distress. To summarize, and as presented in Figure 2.1, Stage 1 is associated with emotional reactions such as fear, anxiety, worry, and so forth, as a consequence of the perception of pain during the acute phase. Pain or hurt is usually associated with harm, and thus there is a natural emotional reaction to the potential for physical harm. If the pain persists past a reasonable acute period of time (2–4 months), this leads to the progression into Stage 2. Stage 2 is associated with a wider array of behavioral–psychological reactions and problems, such as learned helplessness–depression, distress–anger, and somatization, that are the result of suffering with the now more chronic nature of the pain.

Gatchel (1991, 1996) hypothesized that the form these problems take primarily depends on the *premorbid* or preexisting personality/psychological characteristics of the individual, as well as current socioeconomic–environmental conditions. Thus, for a person with a premorbid problem with depression who is seriously affected economically by loss of a job due to the pain and disability, depressive symptomatology is greatly exacerbated during this stage. Similarly, a person who had premorbid hypochondriacal characteristics, and who receives a large amount of secondary gain for remaining disabled, will most likely display a great deal of somatization and symptom magnification.

This model does *not* propose that there is one primary preexisting "pain personality." It is assumed that there is a general *nonspecificity* in terms of the relationship between personality or psychological problems and

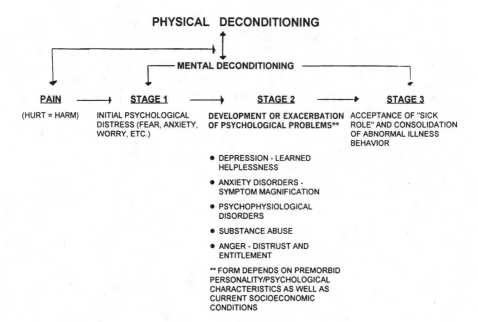

FIGURE 2.1. A conceptual model of the transition from acute to chronic pain. From Gatchel (1991). Copyright 1991 by Lea & Febiger. Adapted by permission.

pain. This is in keeping with a great deal of research that has not found any such consistent personality syndrome (Gatchel, 1996). Moreover, even though there is a relationship usually found between pain and certain psychological problems such as depression (Romano & Turner, 1985), the nature of the relationship between the two variables remains inconclusive.

In a study initially evaluating one aspect of this "chicken and/or egg" question, Polatin, Kinney, Gatchel, Lillo, and Mayer (1993) assessed 200 chronic low back pain patients (pain disability present an average of well over 1 year) for current and lifetime psychiatric syndromes using a structured psychiatric interview to make diagnoses according to Axis I and Axis II of the revised third edition of *Diagnostic and Statistical Manual of Mental Disorders* (DSM-III-R; American Psychiatric Association, 1987). Results showed that, even when the somewhat controversial category of somatoform pain disorder was excluded, 77% of patients met lifetime diagnostic criteria and 59% demonstrated current symptoms for at least one psychiatric diagnosis. In comparison, lifetime and current rates of mental disorders in the general population were estimated to be 29–38% and 15%, respectively

(American Psychiatric Association, 1987; Regier et al., 1988; Robins et al., 1984). The most common diagnoses in the Polatin and colleagues (1993) study were major depression, substance use disorders, and anxiety disorders. In addition, 51% met criteria for at least one personality disorder. All the rates were significantly greater than the base rates of the general population. These were strikingly high rates of psychopathology in this chronic pain population (an issue we return to later in this chapter). More important, however, was the finding that of those patients with a positive lifetime history for psychiatric syndromes, 54% of those with major depression, 94% of those with substance use disorders, and 95% of those with anxiety disorders had experienced these syndromes *before* the onset of their back pain. These were the first results to suggest that certain psychiatric syndromes appear to precede chronic low back pain (substance use disorders and anxiety disorders), whereas others (specifically, major depression) develop either before or after the onset of their low back pain. The interesting aspect of these findings was that depression was demonstrably high in chronic low back pain patients, and patients appear to be divided *equally* between those who were depressed before the onset of low back pain and those in whom depression developed after the onset of low back pain. Clearly, a prospective study is needed to more clearly substantiate these retrospective-recall results as the findings cannot definitively answer the question whether psychopathological disorders in chronic pain patients are a consequence of experiencing the chronic pain or whether preexisting disorders act as a "predisposition" to develop chronicity.

Returning to Gatchel's (1991, 1996) conceptual model, it is assumed that patients "bring with them" certain predisposing personalities/psychological characteristics that differ from one patient to the next, and that may be exacerbated by the stress of attempting to cope with the chronic pain. Indeed, the relationship between stress and exacerbation of mental health problems has long been documented in the scientific literature (e.g., Barrett, Rose, & Klerman, 1979). This conceptual model proposes that as the "layer" of behavioral and psychological problems persists, it leads to the progression into Stage 3 that can be viewed as the acceptance or adoption of a "sick role" during which patients are excused from their normal responsibilities and social obligations. This may become a potent reinforcer for not becoming "healthy." The medical and psychological "disabilities" or "abnormal illness behaviors" (Pilowsky, 1978) are consolidated during this phase. Moreover, if compensation issues are present, they can also serve as disincentives for becoming well again because compensation is a critical factor in the persistence of disabilities (Beals, 1984; Gatchel, Polatin, & Mayer, 1995; Robinson, Rondinelli, Scheer, & Weinstein, 1997).

This conceptual model also proposes that superimposed on these three stages is what is known as the physical "deconditioning syndrome" (Mayer & Gatchel, 1988). This syndrome refers to a significant decrease in physical capacity (strength, flexibility, and endurance) due to disuse and resultant atrophy of the injured area. There is usually a two-way pathway between the physical deconditioning and the foregoing stages. For example, research has clearly demonstrated that physical deconditioning can "feed back" and have a negative effect on the emotional well-being and self-esteem of people (Gatchel, Baum, & Krantz, 1989). This two-way path can lead to further psychological sequelae. Conversely, negative emotional reactions such as depression can significantly "feed back" to physical functioning by, for example, decreasing the motivation to get involved in work or recreational activities and thereby further contributing to physical deconditioning.

Data Supporting the Conceptual Model

Over the past decade, a great deal of research data supportive of the conceptual model just described have accumulated. Studies have documented elevated rates of psychopathology in various types of chronic pain conditions, higher rates of psychopathology in chronic versus acute pain patients, and decreased rates of psychopathology after successful treatment of chronic pain. Further, psychosocial variables have been found to be better predictors of pain and disability chronicity than physical variables (see Linton, Chapter 15, this volume). These findings, which lend indirect support to the model, are discussed in more detail later.

The Polatin and colleagues (1993) study previously reviewed documented high rates of psychopathology in chronic pain patients compared to the general population. These results were consistent with previous research, conducted mostly on chronic low back pain (CLBP) patients who showed increased prevalence of depressive disorders, anxiety disorders, substance use disorders, "somatization," and personality disorders in this population (e.g., Fishbain, Goldberg, Meagher, Steele, & Rosomoff, 1986; Magni, Caldieron, Rigatti-Luchini, & Merskey, 1990). For example, rates of major depressive disorder (MDD) ranged from 34% to 57% in these studies, compared to rates of 5% to 26% in the general population (American Psychiatric Association, 1987). More recent research has documented elevated rates of psychopathology in other types of chronic pain conditions, including headaches (Okasha et al., 1999), temporomandibular disorders (Dohrenwend, Raphael, Marbach, & Gallagher, 1999), pelvic pain (Savidge & Slade, 1997), and fibromyalgia syndrome (Epstein et al., 1999).

Another relevant issue that has been investigated is the prevalence of psychiatric disorders in acute versus chronic pain. Kinney, Gatchel, Polatin, Fogarty, and Mayer (1993) examined this issue in acute versus CLBP patients. They found higher rates of psychopathology in the CLBP group. In particular, the CLBP patients had higher rates of MDD, substance use disorders, and personality disorders than did the acute low back pain patients. In contrast, the acute patients were diagnosed with more anxiety disorders. This pattern of results, which was also found in a study of acute and chronic pain patients with temporomandibular disorder (Gatchel, Garofalo, Ellis, & Holt, 1996; see also Gatchel, Chapter 21, this volume), indicates that higher rates of psychiatric disorders are not solely related to the onset of pain per se, but are linked to the development of chronicity. Furthermore, these results lend support to Gatchel's (1991, 1996) model of the progression from acute pain to chronic pain disability, in which anxiety is considered to be a common reaction to acute pain, with more disabling and varied psychopathology associated with chronic pain. It should be noted that anger is a common, and perhaps the most prominent, affective response to chronic pain (Fernandez, Clark, & Rudick-Davis, 1999; Fernandez & Turk, 1995). However, the current version of DSM (DSM-IV; American Psychiatric Association, 1994) fails to address anger as a mental disorder. As future versions of DSM begin to address this issue, anger disorders are expected to be frequent diagnoses in this population.

Recent studies also lend support to Gatchel's (1991, 1996) conceptual model, showing that elevated rates of psychopathology significantly decrease following intensive rehabilitation of CLBP patients (e.g., Owen-Salters, Gatchel, Polatin, & Mayer, 1996; Vittengl, Clark, Owen-Salters, & Gatchel, 1999). Owen-Salters and colleagues (1996) used the Structured Clinical Interview for DSM (SCID; Spitzer, Williams, Gibbon, & First, 1988) to evaluate patients for current psychiatric disorders on admission to a comprehensive 3-week rehabilitation program and again at 6 months following completion of the treatment program. The results documented significant decreases in the prevalence of psychiatric disorders, particularly somatoform pain dis-

order and MDD. In a methodologically similar study, Vittengl and colleagues (1999) found decreased prevalence of Axis II personality disorders 6 months after completion of the treatment program in a sample of CLBP patients. These two studies demonstrate that effective rehabilitation can significantly decrease the high rates of psychiatric disorders found in CLBP patients, which is consistent with earlier research showing normalization of MMPI scores after successful treatment (Barnes et al., 1990).

Support for Gatchel's model (1991, 1996) is also drawn from studies that demonstrated that psychosocial variables are potent predictors of pain and disability chronicity. In fact, attempts to predict which individuals with an acute back pain injury will go on to develop chronic difficulties, including a poor response to rehabilitation treatment, have demonstrated that psychosocial factors, more than physical factors, are instrumental in failure to return to work after a spinal injury (see Gatchel & Gardea, 1999, for a review of relevant studies; see also Linton, Chapter 15, this volume). For example, Gatchel, Polatin, and Mayer (1995) evaluated whether a comprehensive assessment of psychosocial characteristics is useful in characterizing those acute low back pain patients who subsequently develop chronic pain disability problems (as measured by job work status at 1-year postevaluation). In this study, patients were administered a standard battery of psychological assessment tests (SCID, MMPI, and Million Visual Pain Analog Scale) within 6 weeks of acute lumbar spine pain onset. A structured telephone interview was conducted 1 year after the psychological assessment in order to evaluate return-to-work status. Logistic regression analyses, conducted to differentiate between those patients who were back at work at 1 year versus those who were not, revealed the importance of two psychosocial measures: level of self-reported pain and disability and scores on Scale 3 (Hysteria) of the MMPI. In addition, two other variables were found to be significant: gender of the patient (female) and workers' compensation/personal injury cases at 1 year. The model generated correctly identified 90.7% of the cases. There were no differences between the two groups for the physician-related severity of the initial back injury or the physical demands of the job to which patients had to return.

One of the notable findings of the Gatchel, Polatin, and Kinney (1995) study was that SCID-diagnosed psychopathology was not predictive of the development of chronic pain disability, as one might expect on the basis of Gatchel's model. However, it must be kept in mind that this model does not propose that psychopathology causes chronic pain. Rather, if psychopathology is present in the chronic pain patient, then the form displayed depends on the premorbid characteristics of the particular patient. During the evaluation of the early acute stage, many symptoms of psychopathology may have still been relatively "dormant" and may not express themselves until the stress of more chronic experiences with pain and disability begin to dominate the lives of these patients.

Additional related research has focused on determining whether psychiatric disorders are a limiting factor in the successful rehabilitation of patients with CLBP. Gatchel, Polatin, Mayer, and Garcy (1994) used the SCID to assess the prevalence of current and lifetime DSM diagnoses in a sample of CLBP patients beginning an intensive 3-week rehabilitation program. These patients were then followed over time, with treatment outcome being defined as return-to-work status 1 year after program completion. Despite high rates of Axis I and Axis II psychiatric disorders in this sample, neither type nor degree of psychopathology was found to be predictive of a patient's ability to successfully return to work. In a methodologically similar study involving chronic pain patients with work-related upper extremity disorders, a different set of results were obtained. Burton, Polatin, and Gatchel (1997) found that several factors, including the number of Axis I disorders, a past diagnosis of substance abuse, a past and/or current diagnosis of an anxiety disorder, a diagnosis of borderline personality disorder, and a variety of other demographic and psychosocial variables, were associated with lower return-to-work rates 1 year after completion of the rehabilitation program. The contradictory findings of this study and the Gatchel and colleagues (1994) study may be the result of differences in the two treatment programs, although both

were based on a similar rehabilitation model. A more interesting possible explanation is that the nature of the relationship between psychopathology and long-term disability is different for various musculoskeletal conditions.

The "Psychosocial Disability Factor"

The results of the Gatchel and colleagues (1995) study clearly demonstrate the presence of a robust "psychosocial disability factor" that is associated with those injured workers who are likely to develop CLBP disability problems. Such results again highlight the fact that chronic pain disability reflects more than just the presence of some physical symptomatology or a single psychosocial characteristic; it is a complex psychosocioeconomic phenomenon. In fact, some investigators have argued that only a small amount of the total disability phenomenon in someone complaining of chronic back pain can be attributed to physical impairment (e.g., Waddell, Main, & Morris, 1984). Indeed, physical findings, such as radiographic results, have not been found to be reliable indices of low back pain (Mayer & Gatchel, 1988). Even recent improvements in diagnostic imaging instrumentation, such as computed tomography (CT) and magnetic resonance imaging (MRI) have not produced reliable indices of pain (Deyo, 1998). Most cases of low back pain are ill defined and physically unverifiable and are often classified as "soft tissue injuries" that cannot be visualized or verified on physical examination. The correlation between radiographic-documented disc space narrowing and disc rupture level in proven disc herniation is less than 50% (Pope, Frymoyer, & Andersson, 1984). Moreover, even when MRI studies reveal identifiable lesions, the presence of such lesions in asymptomatic populations raises doubts about their significance in a given patient (Boden et al., 1994; Jensen et al., 1994). A similar dissociation between self-report of pain and actual physical abnormalities has also been found in other chronic pain conditions such as temporomandibular disorders.

Emotional or psychological characteristics make a significant contribution in characterizing which injured workers will develop CLBP disability. This is *not* to suggest that these patients are "malingerers." Psychosocial factors can interact with physical symptoms to contribute to disability. Such psychosocial factors will need to receive additional careful attention in the primary care setting. Medical evaluation will be required to take into account more than pure biomechanical factors in assessing low back pain. Indeed, today it is generally accepted that the phenomenon of pain is more than a straight-through physical process.

Chronic Pain and Specific Psychological Disorders

As discussed previously, elevated rates of depressive, anxiety, substance use, somatoform, and personality disorders have been documented in chronic pain patients. In the next sections, we examine the relationship between chronic pain and each of these types of psychopathology separately. Although there are unique aspects to the relationship between chronic pain and each specific type of psychopathology, a *diathesis–stress model* consistent with Gatchel's (1991, 1996) model is emerging as the dominant overarching theoretical perspective. In this model, diatheses are conceptualized as preexisting semidormant characteristics of the individual prior to the onset of chronic pain, which are then activated by the stress of this chronic condition, eventually resulting in diagnosable psychopathology.

Chronic Pain and Depression

Beginning with the influential article of Romano and Turner (1985), the association between chronic pain and depression has generated more research and theoretical interest than any other area of the chronic pain psychopathology literature. Much of this interest can be attributed to the frequency with which chronic pain patients suffer from depression (Polatin, 1991). A number of the studies reviewed earlier (i.e., Burton et al., 1997; Kinney et al., 1993; Polatin et al., 1993) identified extremely high rates of MDD in chronic pain patients, with current and lifetime rates of this disorder of about 45% and 65%, respectively, in the CLBP population, and both current and

lifetime rates of about 80% in the chronic upper extremity pain population. However, most studies report prevalences in the moderately high range. For example, Banks and Kerns (1996) reviewed 14 studies that used DSM criteria for diagnosing depression in chronic pain patients, and found that nine of these studies reported current prevalence rates of MDD 30% and 54%. In contrast, recent estimates of current and lifetime major depression for the entire U.S. population are 5% and 17%, respectively (Blazer, Kessler, McGonagle, & Swartz, 1994).

Despite wide agreement that depression is frequently associated with chronic pain conditions, several problematic issues have proven to be barriers to research in this area (Polatin, 1991b). The first is the definition of depression itself. The term "depression" has been used to refer to a mood, a symptom, and a syndrome (Banks & Kerns, 1996; Polatin, 1991b). As a result, depression has been assessed in a variety of ways, including self-report instruments, projective tests, chart reviews, and structured and unstructured clinical interviews. The definitional and assessment variability have made it difficult to compare the results of different studies.

One additional problem in studying the relationship between depression and chronic pain is "criterion contamination" (Pincus & Callahan, 1993; Williams, 1998). This term refers to the overlapping symptomatology of chronic pain and depression. Because the diagnostic criteria for MDD include several somatic symptoms that can also be attributed to chronic pain (e.g., sleep disturbance, motor retardation, loss of energy, and change in appetite and weight), diagnosing depression in this population is not always straightforward. This problem may not be limited to diagnosing depression in chronic pain patients but may extend to the medically ill in general (Rodin & Voshart, 1986). Criterion contamination may be particularly problematic with psychological instruments assessing depression, such as the Beck Depression Inventory, which were standardized on psychiatric populations from which those with significant physical illness and disability were excluded (see, e.g., Wesley, Gatchel, Garofalo, & Polatin, 1999; Williams, 1998). Banks and Kerns (1996) suggest that until future research determines appropriate diagnostic criteria and measures of depression among chronic pain patients (see Aronoff, 1999, for a proposal about such criteria) and the medically ill, standardized diagnostic systems such as the DSM are the most reliable means of producing valid diagnoses of MDD.

Despite significant barriers to answering research questions, recent progress has been made, particularly in terms of understanding the causal nature of the relationship between chronic pain and depression. In terms of the temporal relationship between these disorders, depression has been shown to be an antecedent to chronic pain (Polatin, 1991a), a consequence of chronic pain (see, e.g., Brown, 1990; Dohrenwend et al., 1999; Magni, Moreschi, Rigatti-Luchini, & Merskey, 1994), and a concomitant biological relative of chronic pain (Roy, Thomas, & Matas, 1984). Fishbain, Cutler, Rosomoff, and Rosomoff (1997) reviewed these and other studies and found that five major hypotheses have been proposed concerning the timing and causal relationship of depression to chronic pain. These have been termed the (1) *antecedent hypothesis*—depression precedes the development of chronic pain; (2) *consequence hypothesis*—depression is a consequence and follows the development of pain; (3) *scar hypothesis*—episodes of depression occurring before the onset of pain predispose an individual to a depressive episode after pain onset; (4) *cognitive-behavioral mediation model*—cognitions mediate the relationship between chronic pain and the development of depression; and (5) *common pathogenic mechanisms model*.

Fishbain and colleagues (1997) reviewed 40 studies either directly or indirectly addressing the foregoing hypotheses. Overall, these authors concluded that the consequence model is most strongly supported, with additional support for the cognitive-behavioral mediation and scar models. A recent theoretical proposal by Banks and Kerns (1996), when placed within the framework of Fishbain and colleagues' study, may help to further clarify the relationship between chronic pain and depression. After demonstrating that rates of depression appear to be higher in chronic pain versus other chronic medical populations, Banks and Kerns proposed a diathesis–stress model of the development of depression in chronic pain patients that is consistent with the consequence, scar, and cognitive-behavioral mediation hypotheses. In their model, the diathesis is psychological in nature and could include negative psychological schemas (Beck, 1967, 1976); internal, stable, and global attributions leading to learned helplessness (Abramson, Seligman, & Teasdale, 1978); or deficits in instrumental skills (Fordyce, 1976). These diatheses are conceptualized as preexisting, semidormant characteristics of the person prior to the onset of chronic pain, which are then activated by the stress of this chronic condition.

The stress component of the model proposed by Banks and Kerns (1996) refers to the nature of the chronic pain experience. They suggest that chronic pain is more likely to result in depression than are other chronic medical conditions because of the uniquely challenging nature of stressors associated with chronic pain, including the aversive sensory and distressful emotional aspects of the pain symptom, impairment and disability, secondary losses that occur across various domains (e.g., work and social relationships), and perceived invalidating responses from the medical system. May, Doyle, and Chew-Graham (1999) have recently discussed the last stressor in some detail, noting that the disparity between expressed symptoms, pathological signs, and perceived disability in CLBP has led to the moral character of the sufferer forming a constant subtext to medical discourse about the condition.

The model proposed by Banks and Kerns (1996) is obviously consistent with the consequence hypothesis. It is also consistent with the cognitive-behavioral mediation hypothesis in that cognitions (negative schemas, attributions) and behaviors (instrumental skills) mediate the relationship between pain and depression. Finally, if the scar hypothesis could be broadened to include not only a genetic predisposition to recurrent major depression but also psychological predispositions such as negative schemas or a depressive attributional style, then the diathesis–stress model would also be consistent with this hypothesis. Empirical support for the diathesis–stress model was recently obtained by Maxwell, Gatchel, and Mayer (1998), who found that each of the three cognitive and behavioral variables outlined by Banks and Kerns (1996) emerged as unique predictors of self-reported depression in CLBP patients. Moreover, consistent with the cognitive-behavioral mediation hypothesis, when theses three variables were held constant, pain and disability did not have a significant association with self-reported depression.

The similarities between the models proposed by Banks and Kerns (1996) and, earlier, by Gatchel (1991, 1996) are striking. Gatchel stated "many patients whose pain later becomes chronic may 'bring with them' certain pre-morbid or predisposing psychological/personality characteristics or disorders (a diathesis) that are exacerbated by the stress of attempting to cope with pain" (Gatchel, 1996, p. 40). With a diathesis–stress theoretical framework emerging, future research will focus on identifying additional psychological diatheses, further understanding the stressful nature of the chronic pain experience, and, most important, on clarifying the factors that mediate the relationship between diathesis–stress and the development of MDD and other forms of diagnosable psychopathology.

Chronic Pain and Substance Use Disorders

Numerous studies have identified high prevalence rates of substance use disorders in chronic pain patients (e.g., Hoffman, Olofsson, Salem, & Wickstrom, 1995; Katon, Egan, & Miller, 1985; Polatin et al., 1993; for a review, see Brown, Patterson, Rounds, & Papasouliotis, 1996). Of the studies using standard measures for diagnostic assessment, including the SCID, these reviewers found that prevalences of *current* substance use disorders ranged from 15% to 28%, whereas *lifetime* rates ranged from 23% to 41%. Lifetime prevalences are clearly higher than the 16.7% found in the general population (National Institute on Drug Abuse, 1991), while current rates are "probably" higher (Fishbain, Steele-Rosomoff, & Rosomoff, 1992). Substance use disorders are more prevalent for males than females, both in the general population (National Institute on Drug Abuse, 1991) and

in the chronic pain population (Brown et al., 1996).

Turning to the issue of the relationship between chronic pain and substance use disorders, the research literature suggests that a variety of temporal and causal pathways are likely. Polatin and colleagues (1993) found that 94% of the chronic pain patients with lifetime substance use disorders experienced the onset of these disorders before the onset of their chronic pain. They suggested that chronic pain may not precipitate substance use disorders as often as many clinicians believe. Others (e.g., Compton, Darakjian, & Miotto, 1998) have speculated that premorbid substance use disorders may increase the risk for traumatic illness and work-related accidents, a certain proportion of which will develop into chronic pain conditions. As mentioned earlier, rates of current substance use disorders are "probably" higher in chronic pain patients than in the general population. However, Brown and colleagues (1996) found that chronic pain patients were no more likely to have a current substance use disorder than were other patients in a primary care setting, suggesting that chronic pain is not associated with a unique risk for substance abuse.

Despite findings on prior substance use, Brown and colleagues (1996) found that chronic pain patients are at an increased risk for new substance use disorders during the 5 years following the onset of chronic pain, as compared with other 5-year periods in their lives. The risk may be related to iatrogenic factors, with estimates of current addiction to opiod analgesics ranging from 3% to 16% (Miotto, Compton, Ling, & Conolly, 1996). This risk appears to be greatest in people with a previous history of substance abuse/dependence, and in those with a childhood history of physical or sexual abuse, suggesting that these factors are premorbid (i.e., prechronic pain) diatheses for new or recurrent substance dependence. In addition, Fishbain, Cutler, and Rosomoff (1998) examined the comorbidity of substance use disorders with other DSM disorders. They found that patients with a substance diagnosis had higher rates of depression, anxiety disorders, and personality disorders than did patients with no substance diagnosis, suggesting that these patients may be self-medicating psychiatric symptoms with drugs or alcohol.

Before proceeding further, it should be noted that substance use disorders are typically broken down into the categories of abuse and dependence. Substance abuse is defined in DSM-IV as a maladaptive pattern of substance use leading to clinically significant impairment or distress, as manifested by at least one of several criteria (e.g., recurrent substance use in situations in which it physically hazardous). The diagnostic criteria for substance dependence involve both behavioral (or "psychological") dependence and physiological dependence. The criteria for behavioral dependence emphasize the substance-seeking activities and related evidence of pathological use patterns, whereas the criteria for physiological dependence emphasize the body's reaction to heavy and prolonged use of a substance (i.e., tolerance and withdrawal; Kaplan, Sadock, & Grebb, 1994).

The most commonly abused substances in chronic pain patients appear to be alcohol (current and lifetime) and opiods (current). However, a controversy exists in the chronic pain literature about how to classify patients who are maintained on narcotic analgesic medications (Aronoff, 1999; Compton et al., 1998; Miotto et al., 1996). Most of these patients will meet the criteria for tolerance and withdrawal, almost ensuring them a DSM-IV diagnosis of substance dependence. However, the overwhelming majority of these patients are not actually behaviorally or psychologically "addicted" to opiod medications (Miotto et al., 1996). In light of the unique issues relating to this patient population, the American Society for Addiction Medicine (ASAM) developed separate criteria for defining addiction in chronic pain patients treated with opiods (unpublished, as cited in Compton et al., 1998). These criteria are focused on symptoms of behavioral dependence, including the presence of adverse consequences associated with the use of narcotics, loss of control over the use of narcotics, and preoccupation with obtaining narcotics despite the presence of adequate analgesia.

The best method to identify substance use disorders in chronic pain patients has also been an ongoing issue. With substance-abusing individuals in general, there is always the potential for denial, social desirability bias, and memory lapse (Brown et al., 1996). With chronic pain patients, there may also be fears that pain-relieving medications will be reduced or discontinued, that they will not be considered good candidates for pain rehabilitation treatment if the physician finds out about their patterns of medication and other substance use (Miotto et al., 1996), or that this information will work against them in potential future workers' compensation litigation (Fishbain, Cutler, Rosomoff, & Rosomoff, 1999).

Fishbain and colleagues (1999) investigated the concordance of self-reported substance use and urine toxicology indicators of substance use in a sample of chronic pain patients. They found that 9% of the patients provided incorrect self-report information about current substance use, mostly about illicit substances (cocaine and cannabis). Chronic pain patients who incorrectly denied substance use were more likely to be younger, to have a workers' compensation case, and to have been assigned a DSM diagnosis of polysubstance dependence in remission. The authors suggest that this last variable may be attributable to chronic pain patients feeling comfortable in disclosing a past history of substance abuse, knowing that such disclosure would in no way affect their current situation. Fishbain and colleagues indicate that young age, workers' compensation status, and a diagnosis of polysbstance abuse in remission may indicate a need for urine toxicology for a chronic pain patient who denies illicit drug use but who is suspected of such. Despite the concerns and factors outlined by Fishbain and colleagues and others, there is widespread agreement that self-report is the most accurate method currently available for assessing substance use disorders (see, e.g., Babor, Kranzler, & Lauerman, 1989; Keso & Salaspuro, 1990).

Chronic Pain and Anxiety Disorders

Several studies have documented high rates of anxiety disorders among chronic pain patients (e.g., Burton et al., 1997; Polatin et al., 1993). Anxiety disorders include panic disorder, agoraphobia, specific phobia, social phobia, posttraumatic stress disorder, obsessive–compulsive disorder, and generalized anxiety disorder. Although there is little consistency in the chronic pain research literature regarding specific anxiety disorder diagnoses (Fishbain, 1999), panic disorder and generalized anxiety disorder appear to be the most commonly diagnosed (Asmundson, Jacobson, Allerdings, & Norton, 1996). The non-anxiety disorder diagnosis of adjustment disorder with anxious mood has also been frequently used (e.g., Fishbain et al., 1986). In studies that used a structured DSM clinical interview, such as the SCID, overall prevalences for anxiety disorders ranged from 16.5% to 28.8% (Asmundson et al., 1996). Although overall prevalences are close to those estimated for the general population, Fishbain (1999) has recently presented evidence suggesting that anxiety disorders are more often associated with chronic pain than has been reported in the research literature. Finally, studies that have made a distinction between lifetime and current anxiety disorders (e.g., Burton et al., 1997; Polatin et al., 1993) have found that lifetime prevalences rates are close to those estimated for the general population, while current prevalences rates are significantly higher in chronic pain patients.

In several studies described earlier (Gatchel, Garofalo, Ellis, & Holt, 1996; Kinney et al., 1993), investigators found that although chronic pain patients had much higher rates of overall psychopathology than did acute pain patients, anxiety disorders were diagnosed frequently in both groups. These data support Gatchel's (1991, 1996) model of the progression from acute pain to chronic pain disability, in which anxiety is considered to be a common reaction to acute pain, with more disabling and varied psychopathology associated with chronic pain. The diathesis–stress model, described in the earlier section on depression, may also be applicable to the relationship between chronic pain and anxiety disorders. Polatin and colleagues (1993) found that 95% of those diagnosed with anxiety disorders in their sample of work-disabled CLBP patients had experienced these disorders before the onset of pain, suggesting that a premorbid physiological or psychological diathesis exists, which is then exacerbated by the stress of the chronic pain experience. One diathesis may be a genetic predisposition to panic disorder or one of the other anxiety disorders. Another diathesis may be anxiety sensitivity, which is considered to be one of three fundamental trait sensitivities that amplify an array of fear reactions and phobias, according to the expectancy model of fear (Reiss, 1991; Reiss & McNally, 1985).

Once an anxiety response is in place, chronic pain may be maintained or exacerbated through direct physiological mechanisms (Flor & Turk, 1989). Fear of pain and fear of movement/reinjury, both of which lead to further physical deconditioning through avoidance of activities that have potential for long-term pain reduction, may also contribute to the maintenance of pain (Asmundson, Norton, & Norton, 1999). Avoidance, in turn, may be reinforced through operant learning mechanisms. For example, unwanted responsibilities may be avoided or anxiety associated with the anticipation of further pain-related experiences may be reduced (McCracken, Zayfert, & Gross, 1993). Cognitive factors may also be involved, with avoidance leading to decreased self-efficacy and increased expectations that stimulation will increase pain, which, in turn, leads to increased avoidance. The result is a self-defeating cycle between cognition and behavior (Phillips, 1987). Supporting evidence for these ideas has come from Waddell, Newton, Henderson, Sommerville, and Main (1993), who found that pain-related fear-avoidance beliefs about work are the most specific and powerful factors accounting for disability and work loss associated with CLBP. One additional cognitive factor that may be important in maintaining chronic pain is the tendency of anxiety-sensitive patients to catastrophically misinterpret sensations of arousal that are associated with pain (Asmundson et al., 1999).

Chronic Pain and Somatoform Disorders

Perhaps the most common psychiatric disorder diagnosis that chronic pain patients receive is pain disorder, which is one of the somatoform disorders listed in DSM-IV (American Psychiatric Association, 1994). According to DSM-IV, "The common feature of the Somatoform Disorders is the presence of physical symptoms that suggest a general medical condition and are not fully explained by a general medical condition, by the direct effects of a substance, or by another mental disorder" (American Psychiatric Association, 1994, p. 445). Other somatoform disorders, including somatization disorder, conversion disorder, and hypochondriasis, are not frequently diagnosed in chronic pain populations.

Pain disorder is diagnosed when pain is the predominant focus of clinical presentation, when the pain causes significant distress or functional impairment, and when psychological factors are judged to have an important role in the onset, severity, exacerbation, or maintenance of the pain (American Psychiatric Association, 1994). The names and diagnostic criteria for pain disorder have evolved from the two most recent versions of the DSM. In DSM-III (American Psychiatric Association, 1980), psychogenic pain disorder was diagnosed when psychological factors were judged to play an etiological role in the development of pain and when organic factors were absent or not severe enough to explain the pain complaint. The diagnostic criteria for somatoform pain disorder in DSM-III-R (American Psychiatric Association, 1987) no longer specified that psychological factors had to play an etiological role. In addition, the primary criterion was changed from pain to a "preoccupation" with pain for at least 6 months. The criterion of absent/insufficient organic findings was removed from DSM-IV for several reasons, including the lack of clear correlation between physical findings and the level of pain, and the realization that failure to detect organic factors does not mean that such factors are absent (King, 1995). The clinician can now diagnose pain disorder in both acute and chronic pain conditions. Current criteria also allow for the clinician to choose between pain disorder associated with psychological factors and pain disorder associated with *both* psychological factors and a general medical condition (American Psychiatric Association, 1994).

The current and previous DSM pain disorder(s) have been widely criticized over the years. In the past, controversy existed as to what constituted an adequate organic find-

a.
in
for
spec.

Th
vious pain
tic criteria, and
make these diagnose
ly disparate findings reg
rates in chronic pain popula.
ample, Polatin and colleagues (19
that 97% of a sample of CLBP patien
an intensive rehabilitation setting had current somatoform pain disorder. In all cases, the disorder developed after the onset of pain associated with an injury. In contrast, only 0.3% of chronic pain patients (73% with CLBP) were diagnosed with psychogenic pain disorder in a study conducted by Fishbain and colleagues (1986). To our knowledge, no studies have addressed the prevalence of pain disorder using DSM-IV criteria. However, prevalences are expected to be higher in light of the research and theory described in earlier sections of this chapter, which draw a clear connection between chronic pain and various psychological factors. It appears that pain disorder, by definition, will apply to most or all chronic pain patients. In light of the controversy regarding pain disorder, and the unreliability of this diagnostic category, many researchers (e.g., Burton et al., 1997; Polatin et al., 1993) have reported the prevalence of psychogenic and/or somatoform pain disorder but have excluded them from discussions of overall prevalence of psychopathology, as well as from the majority of other analyses.

The nature of the causal relationship between chronic pain and DSM pain disorders currently receives minimal attention in the research literature. Engel (1959) first described "the pain-prone" patient, a concept that was later revived by Blumer and Heilbronn (1982). Aronoff (1999) recently pro-

sorder" be includ-
of DSM. Although
that there are "pain-
es" that precede devel-
pain, most research has
there is a general non-
ms of the relationship be-
lity/psychological problems
chel, 1996; Mayer & Gatchel,
hat significant psychopathology
develops (or recurs) only after
of experiencing disabling pain
l, 1996). However, there appears to
subset of chronic pain patients who
onstrate a consistent tendency to expe-
nce and communicate emotional distress
s somatic symptoms (Fishbain, 1999). This
syndrome, which may or may not approach
the severity of a somatoform disorder, has
been called somatization.

The construct of somatization has received a great deal of attention in the psychological, medical, and, more specifically,
chronic pain literature. As currently conceptualized, somatization involves the focusing
of attention on internal stimuli ("somatosensory amplification"; Barsky, 1992)
and the denial of psychological or interpersonal difficulties (Sternbach, 1974), resulting in an increased tendency to report somatic symptoms, many of which cannot be
medically explained (Barsky, 1992; see also
Mayou, Chapter 24, this volume). Main
and colleagues (Main, 1983; Main, Wood,
Hollis, Spanswick, & Waddell, 1992) use
the term "somatic distress" to bring attention to the function of somatization as an
alternate means of communicating emotional distress. Although somatization is a widespread phenomenon in the chronic pain
population (Main et al., 1992), perhaps because the reporting of somatic symptoms is
viewed as a more appropriate route for
seeking help from a physician (Simon, Von
Korff, Piccinelli, Fullerton, & Ormel,
1999), there appears to be a subset of this
population in which this process is amplified (Fishbain, 1999). For these patients,
somatization is conceptualized as a stable
trait (diathesis) that becomes activated in response to situations and events the individual finds stressful, such as a painful injury.
Although not necessarily meeting the DSM
criteria for a somatoform pain disorder,

somatization has been found to be associated with increased risk for developing chronic pain and greater health utilization in
acute pain patients (Dworkin, 1995;
Dworkin, Wilson, & Massoth, 1994), and
poorer treatment outcomes in chronic pain
patients (Dionne et al., 1997; Vassend,
Krogstad, & Dahl, 1995).

Chronic Pain and Personality Disorders

According to DSM-IV, "Personality traits
are enduring patterns of perceiving, relating
to, and thinking about the environment and
oneself that are exhibited in a wide range of
social and personal contexts. Only when
personality traits are inflexible and maladaptive and cause significant functional
impairment or subjective distress do they
constitute personality disorders" (American
Psychiatric Association, 1994, p. 630). Personality disorders (PDs) are thought to develop during childhood or adolescence and
must be evident by late adolescence or early
adulthood. As long-term patterns, these disorders, by definition, precede the development of pain episodes. DSM-IV recognizes
10 distinct PDs, including paranoid,
schizoid, schizotypal, borderline, histrionic,
narcissistic, antisocial, dependent, obsessive–compulsive, and avoidant PDs, which
are coded on Axis II. Research indicates
that patients with codiagnoses on Axis I and
Axis II have a poor psychiatric prognosis
and higher relapse rate than do comparable
patients without an Axis II diagnosis (e.g.,
Fyer, Frances, Sullivan, Hurt, & Clarkin,
1988; Joffe & Regan, 1988).

Several studies have documented high
rates of PDs among chronic pain patients
(e.g., Burton et al., 1997; Gatchel et al.,
1996; Weisberg, Gallagher, & Gorin,
1996). Prevalence ranged from 31% (Weisberg et al., 1996) to 81% (Burton et al.,
1997) in these studies. Although no firm
statistics are available regarding overall
rates of PDs in the general population, examination of the prevalence of specific PDs
indicates that these disorders are more common in the chronic pain population (Fishbain et al., 1999; Weisberg & Keefe, 1999).
In terms of specific PDs among chronic
pain patients, little consistency has been

found among different research groups. For example, histrionic (Reich et al., 1983), dependent (Fishbain et al., 1986), paranoid (Polatin et al., 1993), and borderline (Weisberg et al., 1996) PDs have been identified as the most common specific Axis II disorders in different studies. Discrepancies in patient samples and diagnostic methods (semistructured vs. unstructured interview) may be partially responsible for this lack of consistency, as well as the lack of consistency in overall rates of PDs between different studies. The overlap between various DSM-IV PD categories (Widiger, Trull, Hurt, Clarkin, & Frances, 1987) may also play a part in these findings.

Additional important findings related to chronic pain and personality disorders have also been discussed in the research literature. Prevalence of PDs was found to be much higher in a sample of CLBP patients (60%) compared to samples of acute low back pain patients (21%; Kinney et al., 1993) and acute carpal tunnel syndrome patients (Mathis, Gatchel, Polatin, Boulas, & Kinney, 1994), further supporting Gatchel's (1991, 1996) model of the progression from acute to chronic pain. Gatchel, Polatin, and Kinney (1995) found that the presence of any SCID-diagnosed PD, along with several other psychosocial variables, was predictive of which acute low back pain patients had not returned to work 6 months later. The authors noted that no specific type of PD was found to predict chronicity, leading them to suggest that an Axis II diagnosis of any type may reflect a general deficit in coping skills that is linked to chronic disability. However, in a follow-up to their study, Gatchel, Polatin, and Mayer (1995) did not find PDs to be predictive of return-to-work status 1 year later.

Finally, Weisberg and Keefe (1997, 1999) suggest that there is a great deal of support for a *diathesis–stress* model of the relationship between chronic pain and PDs. According to these authors, personality patterns that are associated with marginally adaptive coping styles commonly decompensate under the stress of injury, disability, and pain, resulting in the expression of a personality disorder. Following treatment that has improved function as a primary goal, stress is likely to decrease. In these cases, individuals who met the criteria for PDs prior to treatment may still possess the criterion traits but to a lesser extent than required for a categorical diagnosis. Weisberg and Keefe's (1997, 1999) model is intuitively appealing and is also consistent with other diathesis–stress models (e.g., Banks & Kerns, 1996; Gatchel, 1991, 1996) of the relationship between psychopathology and chronic pain.

Treatment Implications: Acute Stage

What implications do the foregoing reviewed results of the relationship between psychological disorders and chronic pain have for the treatment of pain? There can be little doubt that such psychosocial variables are important in not only pain perception but also the subsequent development of pain-related disability. As in other areas of the growing field of health psychology–behavioral medicine, medical personnel will need to be concerned with the psychological characteristics of their patients in order to prevent costly effects (both economic and human productivity losses) of prolonged bouts of pain disability. Many patients, who later become chronic, may "bring with them" certain premorbid or predisposing psychological and personality characteristics (a *diathesis*) that are exacerbated by the *stress* of attempting to cope with pain. Thus, early intervention may be important for more effective management of these patients, (see also Linton, Chapter 15, this volume). Within this diathesis–stress model, though, there are also other factors that can lead to chronicity. A number of important socioeconomic and environmental variables can significantly contribute to it (e.g., secondary gain such as workers' compensation). These predisposed patients, however, are the ones who have the greater likelihood of subsequently becoming the difficult-to-treat chronic patients. Finally, this is not to say that these predisposing factors make chronic pain cases "functional" disorders and that it is "all in the patient's head." The chronic problem represents a complex interaction between physical and psychosocioeconomic variables (i.e., a biopsychosocial phenomenon; see also Turk & Monarch, Chapter 1, this volume).

Types of Treatment

At this point, it will be useful to differentiate among primary, secondary, and tertiary care because the type of psychological treatment required for each type of care will be substantially different. Primary care is applied generally to acute cases of pain of very limited severity and generally consists of "passive modalities" (i.e., treatments done *to* a person in hopes of palliating pain during a normal early healing period from an injury). Traction, heat, ice, and manipulation fall into this pattern. Instruction and education may be included, and merely some effective psychological reassurance that the acute pain episode will soon be resolved is all that is needed (however, see Pruitt & Von Korff, Chapter 14, this volume).

Secondary care represents reactivation treatment intended for those people who have not been able to return to productivity simply through the normal healing process. It occurs during the transition from acute (primary) care to return to work and is designed to facilitate return to productivity before chronic disability supervenes (see Pruitt & Von Korff, Chapter 14, this volume). It is designed to prevent chronic disability, advanced deconditioning, and the development of psychosocial barriers to work return. "Work hardening" and "work conditioning" approaches fall into this category and are designed to be used toward the end of a normal soft tissue healing period. During this phase, more active psychological intervention may be needed for those patients who may not be progressing.

Finally, tertiary care is an interdisciplinary, individualized, and intensive treatment designed for patients already demonstrating changes consistent with chronic disability. In general, differentiation from secondary treatment includes medical direction, intensity of service, severity of injury, universal application of psychological and disability management services, and specificity of physical/psychosocial assessment.

In terms of primary and secondary care, the clinician must be aware of many psychological factors that can contribute to an acute pain episode becoming subacute and then chronic. As Gatchel (1991, 1996) suggests, a patient may progress through a number of stages as his or her pain and disability becomes more chronic. These psychological factors may create formidable barriers to recovery if they are not effectively dealt with. These barriers to recovery include the psychosocial variables discussed earlier, as well as functional, legal, social, and work-related issues that can significantly interfere with the patient's return to full functioning and a productive lifestyle. Treatment personnel must also be alert to potential secondary gains of continued disability, whether legal, financial, job-related, or familial. It is important that members of the treatment team be knowledgeable of all psychosocial issues while the patient is in rehabilitation. This knowledge allows staff members not only to better understand and serve the patient but also to be more effective in problem solving when the patient is not physically progressing as expected. At other times, real interfering circumstances may be used as a "smoke screens" or excuses for suboptimal performance and failure to adhere to the treatment regimen. Indeed, failure to progress physically generally represents psychosocial barriers to recovery. These barriers to recovery issues must be effectively assessed and brought to the attention of the entire treatment team. Steps can then be taken to understand their origins and avoid their interference with treatment goals.

In a recent review of epidemiological studies, Gatchel and Epker (1999) delineated a number of risk factors or barriers to recovery that have been found to be associated with an increased likelihood of an acute pain episode developing into chronic disability (Table 2.1). As can be seen, there are a number of risk factors or barriers that have been consistently found across a number of epidemiological studies to be important. These may provide important "flags" for clinicians to be aware of in order to anticipate important barriers to recovery in the treatment setting, (see also Linton, Chapter 14, this volume).

The transition from the acute to more subacute stage at about 3 months is a point where psychopathology may begin to emerge as a potentially significant barrier to recovery. Of course, it must be emphasized

TABLE 2.1. Summary of Psychosocioeconomic Risk Factors That May Predict the Development of Chronic Pain Disability

- High self-reported pain and disability
- Elevation of MMPI Scale 3 (Hysteria)
- Depression
- Somatization
- Poor coping skills/strategies
- Poor quality of social support
- Unresolved workers' compensation/personal injury cases
- Gender
- Reinforcement of pain behaviors
- Job dissatisfaction
- Maladaptive attitudes and beliefs about pain
- History of childhood sexual abuse

Note. From Gatchel and Epker (1999). Copyright 1999 by The Guilford Press. Reprinted by permission.

to the patient that psychological and emotional factors are invariably involved in the pain syndrome in such a manner as not to alienate the patient into assuming that the clinician thinks that the pain "is all in his or her head." Figure 2.2 presents a diagram that can be shown to patients to explain this relationship. Physical changes due to injury and their aftereffects (e.g., disruption in ac-tivities of daily living such as work and play) can lead to emotional changes. Such emotional changes, due to the forced decrease in everyday activities, can produce significant emotional distress such as increased anxiety, depression, and anger. This emotional distress, in turn, can lead to increased psychophysiological tension and stress. Such stress and tension can substantially affect pain threshold and exacerbation, ultimately feeding back and affecting physical functioning and changes. The cycle can also work in the opposite direction, with physical changes affecting pain threshold and exacerbation, leading to increased psychophysiological stress and tension, producing additional emotional distress and changes that can, in turn, produce disruptions in activities of daily living (e.g., depression may decrease interest in getting involved in work or social activities). Once the cycle is completed, it can begin at any new point in the interrelated process and start the whole vicious cycle over gain. If this process is explained in an appropriate and clinically sensitive manner, the patient will become more receptive to the role that psychosocial stress factors can play in contributing to (*not* causing) the pain and disability process. Patients can also be shown a diagram depicting the many factors that can affect the stress/tension-pain cycle (see Figure 2.3).

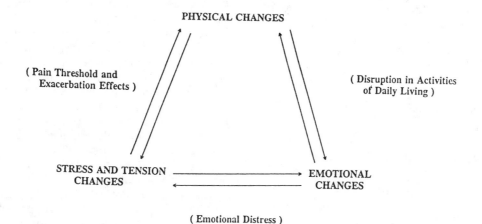

FIGURE 2.2. The cycle of physical changes, emotional changes, and psychophysiological stress and tension changes in the chronic pain process. From Mayer and Gatchel (1988). Copyright 1988 by Lea & Febiger. Adapted by permission.

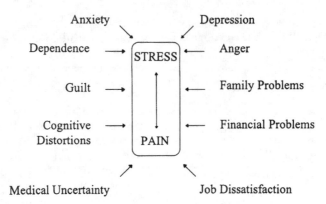

FIGURE 2.3. Factors magnifying the stress–pain cycle. From Mayer and Gatchel (1988). Copyright 1988 by Lea & Febiger. Adapted by permission.

Treatment Implications: Chronic Stage

Table 2.2 summarizes psychosocioeconomic factors that appear to be important for treatment outcome with chronic pain patients, based on a review of epidemiological studies. Psychopathology is included in the list. Indeed, as we have seen, when patients reach the more chronic stages of pain, usually some significant psychopathology needs to be dealt with that may impede the rehabilitation process. As discussed earlier, not all studies (e.g., Gatchel et al., 1994) have demonstrated a relationship between psy-

chopathology and treatment outcome. However, in a study we are currently undertaking with a large and heterogeneous sample of chronic musculoskeletal pain patients, Axis I psychopathology is linked to poorer socioeconomic outcomes at 1-year postevaluation, and Axis II psychopathology is associated with noncompletion of an intensive rehabilitation program.

These results again indicate that one of the important factors that makes the treatment of chronic pain patients traditionally so challenging is the high prevalence of emotional distress and psychopathology commonly displayed. This comorbidity clearly highlights the fact that pain treatment staff must be sensitive to high rates of psychopathology and must be prepared to use mental health professionals to assist them in stabilizing these patients. One of the major factors that makes a functional restoration program or other tertiary multidisciplinary programs so time-intensive and professional staff-intensive is the need to carefully address such psychopathology in order to effectively manage these patients during the program. Programs that do not have an adequate mental health component may well be doomed to failure in the treatment of chronic pain patients. Not that such rehabilitation programs should be developed to try to "cure" such psychopathology, but, rather, the philosophy of a tertiary treatment program, such as functional restoration, is that many of these patients were likely to have been functioning adequately before the onset of their pain dis-

---

TABLE 2.2. Summary of Potential Psychosocioeconomic Predictors of Response to Treatment

- Depression
- Somatization
- History of childhood abuse
- Psychiatric disturbance (presence of Axis I clinical disorders)
- Multidimensional Pain Inventory subgroup categories
- Elevation of the Emotional Vulnerability scale of the Millon Behavioral Health Inventory
- Poor coping skills/strategies
- Unresolved workers' compensation/personal injury cases
- Positive attitudes and expectations about pain and disability

Note. From Gatchel and Epker (1999). Copyright 1999 by The Guilford Press. Reprinted by permission.

abilities in spite of any overt or subthreshold psychopathology. The aim of the program is to provide a multidisciplinary disability management approach to use in a crisis intervention manner in order to better manage these patients. Indeed, there has been an increase in the development of effective brief or short-term therapeutic approaches to replace the traditional long-term therapies that have been used in the past (see, e.g., Budman & Gurman, 1988; Dattilio & Freeman, 1994; Puryear, 1988). Moreover, the recent development of brief cognitive-behavioral techniques for pain management also fits this philosophy well (see Linton, Chapter 14, this volume). Many of these chronic patients still might have some signs of psychopathology after finishing the program (as they may also have had before their injury or pain episode), but they no longer have the chronic low back pain disability that seriously interfered with their working and social lives.

Finally, related to the aforementioned treatment issues, one question often asked by clinicians is: "What is the best battery of assessment tests to use in evaluating patients with pain and disability?" However, there is no single answer to this question because the question itself needs to be prefaced by a number of more specific questions, such as: "For what purpose is the assessment being performed (e.g., patient management and treatment planning; disability determination; surgical pre-screening purposes, etc.)?" "Is the assessment purely for clinical purposes or for research outcome purposes?" The first of these more specific questions is most often asked in terms of answering the question: "What's the best battery of assessment tests to use for patient management/treatment planning?" Gatchel (2000) has recommended a "step-wise" approach" in which one chooses the most time- and cost-efficient biopsychosocial assessment of patients. Of course, one must not assume that there is a single instrument than can serve as the best assessment method. For most patients, several assessment methods are needed.

Summary and Conclusions

As pain becomes more chronic, psychosocial variables play an increasingly dominant role in the maintenance of pain behavior and suffering. A conceptual model of the transition from acute to chronic pain was presented in which it is assumed that the type of psychological distress displayed by patients who become subacute or chronic depends on the premorbid or preexisting personality/psychological characteristics of that individual. One of the major psychosocial concomitants or sources of distress clinicians must be prepared to deal with when treating chronic pain patients is psychopathology. Elevated rates of depressive, somatoform, anxiety, substance use, and personality disorders have been identified as the most common diagnostic categories. Although there are unique aspects to the relationship between chronic pain and each specific type of psychopathology, a diathesis–stress model is emerging as the dominant overarching theoretical perspective. In this model, diatheses are conceptualized as preexisting semidormant characteristics of the person prior to the onset of chronic pain, which are then activated by the stress of this chronic condition, eventually resulting in diagnosable psychopathology.

Regardless of the type of psychopathology, however, clinicians need to evaluate the presence of psychopathology and be prepared to effectively manage it during the course of rehabilitation. The increase in recent years in the development of effective brief or short-term therapeutic approaches nicely coincides with the philosophy of effective management of psychopathology while rehabilitation of the chronic pain disability occurs. By embracing such a philosophy, the probability of rehabilitation success is greatly increased, even in the presence of psychopathology.

Acknowledgments

Much of the research by the authors reported in this chapter was supported by grants from the National Institutes of Health (MH46452, MH01107, and DE10713).

References

Abramson, L. Y., Seligman, M. E. P., & Teasdale, J. D. (1978). Learned helplessness in humans: Critique and reformulation. *Journal of Abnormal Psychology, 87*, 49–74.

American Psychiatric Association. (1980). *Diagnostic and statistical manual of mental disorders* (3rd ed.). Washington, DC: Author.

American Psychiatric Association. (1987). *Diagnostic and statistical manual of mental disorders* (3rd ed., rev.). Washington, DC: Author.

American Psychiatric Association. (1994). *Diagnostic and statistical manual of mental disorders* (4th ed.). Washington, DC: Author.

Aronoff, G. M. (1999). Psychiatric aspects of nonmalignant chronic pain: A new nosology. In G. Aronoff (Ed.), *Evaluation and treatment of chronic pain* (3rd ed., pp. 4–31). Baltimore: Williams & Wilkins.

Asmundson, G. J., Jacobson, S. J., Allerdings, M. D., & Norton, G. R. (1996). Social phobia in disabled workers with chronic musculoskeletal pain. *Behavior Research and Therapy, 34,* 939–943.

Asmundson, G. J. G., Norton, P. J., & Norton G. R. (1999). Beyond pain: The role of fear and avoidance in chronicity. *Clinical Psychology Review, 19,* 97–119.

Babor, T. F., Kranzler, H. R., & Lauerman, R. J. (1989). Early detection of harmful alcohol consumption: Comparison of clinical, laboratory, and self-report screening procedures. *Addictive Behavior, 14,* 139–157.

Banks, S. M., & Kerns, R. D. (1996). Explaining high rates of depression in chronic pain: A diathesis–stress framework. *Psychological Bulletin, 119,* 95–110.

Barsky, J. C. (1992). Amplification, somatization, and the somatoform disorders. *Psychosomatics, 33,* 28–34.

Barnes, D., Gatchel, R. J., Mayer, T. G., & Barnett, J. (1990). Changes in MMPI profiles of chronic low back pain patients following successful treatment. *Journal of Spinal Disorders, 3,* 353–355.

Barrett, J. F., Rose, R. M., & Klerman, G. L. (Eds.). (1979). *Stress and mental disorder.* New York: Raven Press.

Beals, R. K. (1984). Compensation and recovery from injury. *Western Journal of Medicine, 40,* 276–283.

Beck, A. T. (1967). *Depression: Clinical, experimental, and theoretical aspects.* New York: Harper & Row.

Beck, A. T. (1976). *Cognitive therapy and the emotional disorders.* New York: International Universities Press.

Biering-Sorensen, F. (1983). A prospective study of LBP in a general population, II, location, character, aggravating and relieving factors. *Scandinavian Journal of Rehabilitation Medicine, 14,* 15–81.

Bigos, S. J., Battie, M. C., & Spengler, D. M. (1991). A prospective study of work perceptors and psychosocial factors affecting the report of back injury. *Spine, 16,* 1–6.

Blazer, D. G., Kessler, R. C., McGonagle, K. A., & Swartz, M. S. (1994). The prevalence and distribution of major depression in a national community sample: The national comorbidity survey. *American Journal of Psychiatry, 151,* 979–986.

Blumer, D., & Heilbronn, M. (1982). Chronic pain as a variant of depressive disease. *Journal of Nervous and Mental Disease, 170,* 381–406.

Boden, S. D., McCowin, S. R., Davis, D. O., Dina, T. S., Mark, A. S., & Wiesel, S. (1994). Abnormal magnetic-resonance scans of the cervical spine in asymptomatic subjects. *Journal of Bone and Joint Surgery, 72,* 1178–1184.

Brown, G. K. (1990). A causal analysis of chronic pain and depression. *Journal of Abnormal Psychology, 99,* 127–137.

Brown, R. L., Patterson, J. J., Rounds, L. A., & Papasouliotis, O. (1996). Substance use among patients with chronic back pain. *Journal of Family Practice, 43,* 152–160.

Budman, S. H., & Gurman, A. V. (1988). *Theory and practice of brief therapy.* New York: Guilford Press.

Burton, K., Polatin, P. B., & Gatchel, R. J. (1997). Psychosocial factors and the rehabilitation of patients with chronic work-related upper extremity disorders. *Journal of Occupational Rehabilitation, 7,* 139–153.

Compton, P., Darakjian, J., & Miotto, K. (1998). Screening for addiction in patients with chronic pain and "problematic" substance use: Evaluation of a pilot assessment tool. *Journal of Pain and Symptom Management, 16,* 355–363.

Dattilio, F. M., & Freeman, A. (Eds.). (1994). *Cognitive-behavioral strategies in crisis intervention.* New York: Guilford Press.

Deyo, R. A. (1998). Low-back pain. *Scientific American, 279,* 48–53.

Dionne, C. E., Koepsell, T. D., Von Korff, M., Deyo, R. A., Barlow, W. E., & Checkoway, H. (1997). Predicting long-term functional limitations among back pain patients in primary care settings. *Journal of Clinical Epidemiology, 50,* 31–43.

Dohrenwend, B. P., Raphael, K. G., Marbach, J. J., & Gallagher, R. M. (1999). Why is depression comorbid with chronic myofascial face pain? A family study of alternative hypotheses. *Pain, 83,* 183–192.

Dworkin, S. F. (1995). Personal and societal impact of orofacial pain. In J. R. Fricton & R. B. Dubner (Eds.), *Orofacial pain and temporomandibular disorders* (pp. 15–32). New York: Raven Press.

Dworkin, S. F., Wilson, L., & Massoth, D. L. (1994). Somatizing as a risk factor for chronic pain. In R. C. Grzesiak & D. S. Ciccone (Eds.), *Psychological vulnerability to chronic pain* (pp. 28–54). New York: Springer-Verlag.

Engel, G. L. (1959). "Psychogenic" pain and the pain-prone patient. *American Journal of Medicine, 26,* 899–918.

Epstein, S. A., Kay, G., Clauw, D., Heaton, R., Klein, D., Krupp, L., Kuck, J., Leslie, V., Masur, D., Wagner, M., Waid, R., & Zisook, S. (1999). Psychiatric disorders in patients with fibromyalgia: A multicenter investigation. *Psychosomatics, 40,* 57–63.

Fernandez, E., Clark, T. S., & Rudick-Davis, D. (1999). A framework for conceptualization and assessment of affective disturbance in pain. In A. R. Block, E. F. Kremer, & E. Fernandez (Eds.), *Handbook of pain syndromes* (pp. 90–112). Mahwah, NJ: Erlbaum.

Fernandez, E., & Turk, D. C. (1995). The scope and significance of anger in the experience of chronic pain. *Pain, 61,* 165–175.

Fishbain, D. A. (1995). DSM-IV: Implications and issues for the pain clinician. *American Pain Society Bulletin, 5,* 6–18.

Fishbain, D. A. (1996). Where have two DSM revisions taken us for the diagnosis of pain disorder in chronic pain patients? *American Journal of Psychiatry, 153,* 137–138.

Fishbain, D. A. (1999). Approaches to treatment decisions for psychiatric comorbidity in the management of the chronic pain patient. *Medical Clinics of North America, 83,* 737–763.

Fishbain, D. A., Cutler, R., & Rosomoff, H. L. (1998). Comorbid psychiatric disorders in chronic pain patients. *Pain Clinic, 11,* 79–87.

Fishbain, D. A., Cutler, R., Rosomoff, H. L., & Rosomoff, R. S. (1997). Chronic pain-associated depression: Antecedent or consequence of chronic pain? A review. *Clinical Journal of Pain, 13,* 116–137.

Fishbain, D. A., Cutler, R., Rosomoff, H. L., & Rosomoff, R. S. (1999). Validity of self-reported drug use in chronic pain patients. *Clinical Journal of Pain, 15,* 184–191.

Fishbain, D. A., Goldberg, M., Meagher, B. R., Steele, R., & Rosomoff, H. (1986). Male and female chronic pain patients categorized by DSM-III psychiatric diagnostic criteria. *Pain, 26,* 181–197.

Fishbain, D. A., Steele-Rosomoff, R., & Rosomoff, H. (1992). Drug abuse, dependence, and addiction in chronic pain patients. *Clinical Journal of Pain, 8,* 77–85.

Flor, H., & Turk, D. C. (1989). Psychophysiology of chronic pain: Do chronic pain patients exhibit symptom-specific physiological responses? *Psychological Bulletin, 105,* 215–259.

Fordyce, W. (1976). *Behavioral methods of control of chronic pain and illness.* St. Louis, MO: Mosby.

Fyer, M. R., Frances, A. J., Sullivan, T., Hurt, S. W., & Clarkin, J. (1988). Comorbidity of borderline personality disorder. *Archives of General Psychiatry, 45,* 348–352.

Gatchel, R. J. (1991). Early development of physical and mental deconditioning in painful spinal disorders. In T. G. Mayer, V. Mooney & R. J. Gatchel (Eds.), *Contemporary conservative care for painful spinal disorders* (pp. 278–289). Philadelphia: Lea & Febiger.

Gatchel, R. J. (1996). Psychological disorders and chronic pain: Cause-and-effect relationships. In R. J. Gatchel & D. C. Turk (Eds.), *Psychological approaches to pain management: A practitioner's handbook* (pp. 33–52). New York: Guilford Press.

Gatchel, R. J. (2000). How practitioners should evaluate personality to help manage patients with chronic pain. In R. J. Gatchel & J. N. Wesberg (Eds.), *Personality characteristics of patients with pain.* Washington, DC: American Psychological Association Press.

Gatchel, R. J., Baum, A., & Krantz, D. S. (1989). *An introduction to health psychology* (2nd ed.). New York: Random House.

Gatchel, R. J., & Epker, J. (1999). Psychosocial predictors of chronic pain and response to treatment. In R. J. Gatchel & D. C. Turk (Eds.), *Psychosocial factors in pain: Critical perspectives* (pp. 412–434). New York: Guilford Press.

Gatchel, R. J., & Gardea, M. A. (1999). Psychosocial issues: Their importance in predicting disability, response to treatment, and search for compensation. *Neurologic Clinics, 17*(1), 149–166.

Gatchel, R. J., Garofalo, J. P., Ellis, E., & Holt, C. (1996). Major psychological disorders in acute and chronic TMD: An initial examination. *Journal of the American Dental Association, 127,* 1365–1374.

Gatchel, R. J., Polatin, P. B., & Kinney, R. K. (1995). Predicting outcome of chronic back pain using clinical predictors of psychopathology: A prospective analysis. *Health Psychology,14,* 415–420.

Gatchel. R. J., Polatin, P. B., & Mayer, T. G. (1995). The dominant role of psychosocial risk factors in the development of chronic low back pain disability. *Spine, 20,* 2702–2709.

Gatchel, R. J., Polatin, P. B., Mayer, T. G., & Garcy, P. D. (1994). Psychopathology and the rehabilitation of patients with low back pain disability. *Archives of Physical Medicine and Rehabilitation, 75,* 666–670.

Hodgkiss, A. (1997). Rediscovering the psychopathology of chronic pain. *Journal of Psychosomatic Research, 42,* 221–224.

Hoffman, N., Olofsson, O., Salem, B., & Wickstrom, L. (1995). Prevalence of abuse and dependency in chronic pain patients. *International Journal of Addiction, 30,* 919–927.

Jensen, M. C., Brant-Zawadzki, M. N., Obuchowski, N., Modic, M. T., Malkasian, D., & Ross, J. S. (1994). Magnetic resonance imaging of the lumbar spine in people without back pain. *New England Journal of Medicine, 331,* 69–73.

Joffe, R. T., & Regan, J. J. (1988). Personality and depression. *Journal of Psychiatric Research, 22,* 279–286.

Kaplan, H. I., Sadock, B. J., & Grebb, J. A. (1994). *Synopsis of psychiatry* (7th ed.). Baltimore: Williams & Wilkins.

Katon, W., Egan, K., & Miller, D. (1985). Chronic pain: Lifetime psychiatric diagnoses and family history. *American Journal of Psychiatry, 142,* 1156–1160.

Keso, L., & Salaspuro, M. (1990). Comparative value of self-report and blood tests in assessing outcome amongst alcoholics. *British Journal of Addiction, 85,* 209–215.

King, S. A. (1995). Review: DSM-IV and beyond. *Clinical Journal of Pain, 11,* 171–176.

Kinney, R. K., Gatchel, R. J., Polatin, P. B., Fogarty, W. J., & Mayer, T. G. (1993). Prevalence of psychopathology in acute and chronic low back pain patients. *Journal of Occupational Rehabilitation, 3*, 95–103.

Magni, G., Caldieron, C., Rigatti-Luchini, S., & Merskey, H. (1990). Chronic musculoskeletal pain and depressive symptoms in the general population: An analysis of the first national and nutrition examination survey data. *Pain, 43*, 299–307.

Magni, G., Moreschi, C., Rigatti-Luchini, S., & Merskey, H. (1994). Prospective study on the relationship between depressive symptoms and chronic musculoskeletal pain. *Pain, 56*, 289–297.

Main, C. J. (1983). The Modified Somatic Perception Questionnaire (MSPQ). *Journal of Psychosomatic Research, 27*, 503–514.

Main, C. J., Wood, P. L., Hollis, S., Spanswick, C. C., & Waddell, G. (1992). The distress and risk assessment method: A simple patient classification to identify distress and evaluate the risk of poor outcome. *Spine, 17*, 42–52.

Mathis, L. B., Gatchel, R. J., Polatin, P. B., Boulas, H. J., & Kinney, R. K. (1994). Prevalence of psychopathology in carpal tunnel syndrome patients. *Journal of Occupational Rehabilitation, 4*, 199–209.

Maxwell, T. D., Gatchel, R. J., & Mayer, T. G. (1998). Cognitive predictors of depression in chronic low back pain: Toward an inclusive model. *Journal of Behavioral Medicine, 21*, 131–143.

May, C., Doyle, H., & Chew-Graham, C. (1999). Medical knowledge and the intractable patient: The case of chronic low back pain. *Social Science and Medicine, 48*, 523–534.

Mayer, T. G., & Gatchel, R. J. (1988). *Functional restoration for spinal disorders: The sports medicine approach*. Philadelphia: Lea & Febiger.

McCracken, I. M., Zayfert, C., & Gross, R. T. (1993). The pain anxiety symptom scale (PASS): A multimodal measure of pain-specific anxiety symptoms. *Behavior Therapist, 16*, 183–184.

Melzack, R., & Wall, P. (1965). Pain mechanisms: A new theory. *Science, 50*, 971–979.

Miotto, K., Compton, P., Ling, W., & Conolly, M. (1996). Diagnosing addictive disease in chronic pain patients. *Psychosomatics, 37*, 223–235.

National Institute on Drug Abuse (1991). *National Household Survey on Drug Abuse: Highlights 1991*. Washington, DC: U.S. Government Printing Office.

Okasha, A., Ismail M. K., Khalil, A. H., El Fiki, R., Soliman, A., & Okasha, T. (1999). A psychiatric study of nonorganic chronic headache patients. *Psychosomatics, 40*, 233–238.

Owen-Salters, E., Gatchel, R. J., Polatin, P. B., & Mayer, T. G. (1996). Changes in psychopathology following functional restoration of chronic low back pain patients: A prospective study. *Journal of Occupational Rehabilitation, 6*, 215–223.

Phillips, H. (1987). Avoidance behavior and its role in sustaining chronic pain. *Behaviour Research and Therapy, 25*, 273–279.

Pilowsky, I. (1978). A general classification of abnormal illness behavior. *British Journal of Medical Psychiatry, 51*, 131–137.

Pincus, T., & Callahan, L. F. (1993). Depression scales in rheumatoid arthritis: Criterion contamination in interpretation of patient responses. *Patient Education and Counseling, 20*, 133–143.

Polatin P. (1991a). Affective disorders in back pain. In T. G. Mayer, V. Mooney, & R. J. Gatchel (Eds.), *Contemporary conservative care for painful spinal disorders* (pp. 149–154). Philadelphia: Lea and Febiger.

Polatin, P. (1991b). Predictors of low back pain. In A. White & R. Anderson (Eds.), *Conservative care of low back pain* (pp. 265–273). Baltimore: Williams & Wilkins.

Polatin, P. B., Kinney, R. K., Gatchel, R. J., Lillo, E., & Mayer, T. G. (1993). Psychiatric illness and chronic low back pain. *Spine, 18*, 66–71.

Pope, M. H., Frymoyer, J. W., & Andersson, G. (1984). *Occupational low back pain*. New York: Praeger.

Puryear, D. A. (1988). *Helping people in crisis*. San Francisco: Jossey-Bass.

Regier, D. A., Boyd, J. H., Burke, J. D., Rae, D. S., Myers, J. K., Kramer, M., Robins, L. N., George, L. K., Karno, M., & Locke, B. Z. (1988). One-month prevalence of mental disorders in the United States. *Archives of General Psychiatry, 45*, 977–986.

Reiss, S. (1991). Expectancy theory of fear, anxiety, and panic. *Clinical Psychology Review, 11*, 141–153.

Reiss, S., & McNally, R. J. (1985). The expectancy model of fear. In S. Reiss & R. R. Bootzin (Eds.), *Theoretical issues in behavior therapy* (pp. 107–121). New York: Academic Press.

Robins, L. N., Helzer, J. E., Weissman, M. M., Orvaschel, D. A., Gruenberg, E., Burke, J. D., & Regier, D. A. (1984). Lifetime prevalence of specific psychiatric disorders in three sites. *Archives of General Psychiatry, 41*, 949–958.

Robinson, J. P., Rondinelli, R. D., Scheer, S. J., & Weinstein, S. M. (1997). Industrial rehabilitation medicine. 1. Why is industrial rehabilitation medicine unique? *Archives of Physical Medicine and Rehabilitation, 78*(Suppl.), S3–S9.

Rodin, G., & Voshart, K. (1986). Depression in the medically ill: An overview. *American Journal of Psychiatry, 143*, 696–705.

Romano, J. M., & Turner, J. A. (1985). Chronic pain and depression: Does the evidence support a relationship? *Psychological Bulletin, 97*, 18–34.

Roy, R., Thomas, M., & Matas, M. (1984). Chronic pain and depression: A review. *Comphrehensive Psychiatry, 25*, 96–105.

Savidge, C. J., & Slade, P. (1997). Psychological aspects of chronic pelvic pain. *Journal of Psychosomatic Research, 42*, 433–444.

Simon, G. E., Von Korff, M., Piccinelli, M., Fullerton, C., & Ormel, J. (1999). An international study of the relation between somatic symptoms and depression. *New England Journal of Medicine, 341*, 1329–1335.

Spitzer, R. L., Williams, J. B. W., Gibbon, M., &

First, M. (1988). *Structured Clinical Interview for DSM-III-R*. New York: New York State Psychiatric Institute.

Sternbach, R. A. (1974). *Pain patients: Traits and treatments*. New York: Academic Press.

Sternbach, R. A., Wolf, S. R., Murphy, R. W., & Akeson, W. H. (1973). Traits of pain patients: The low-back "loser." *Psychosomatics, 14,* 226–229.

Vassend, O., Krogstad, B. S., & Dahl, B. L. (1995). Negative affectivity, somatic complaints, and symptoms of temporamandibular disorders. *Journal of Psychosomatic Research, 39,* 889–899.

Vittengl, J. R., Clark, L. A., Owen-Salters, E., & Gatchel, R. J. (1999). Diagnostic change and personality stability following functional restoration treatment in chronic low back pain patients. *Psychological Assessment, 6,* 79–91.

Waddell, G., Main, C. J., & Morris, E. W. (1984). Chronic low back pain, psychologic distress, and illness behavior. *Spine, 5,* 117–125.

Waddell, G., Newton, M., Henderson, I., Sommerville, D., & Main, C. J. (1993). A fear-avoidance beliefs questionnaire (FABQ) and the role of fear-avoidance beliefs in chronic low back pain and disability. *Pain, 52,* 157–168.

Weisberg, J. N., Gallagher, R. M., & Gorin, A. (1996, November). *Personality disorder in chronic pain: A longitudinal approach to validation of diagnosis*. Poster presented at the 15th annual Scientific Meeting of the American Pain Society, Washington, DC.

Weisberg, J. N., & Keefe, F. J. (1997). Personality disorders in the chronic pain population: Basic concepts, empirical findings, and clinical implications. *Pain Forum, 6,* 1–9.

Weisberg, J. N., & Keefe, F. J. (1999). Personality, individual differences, and psychopathology in chronic pain. In R. J. Gatchel & D. C. Turk (Eds)., *Psychosocial factors in pain* (pp. 56–73). New York: Guilford Press.

Wesley, A. L., Gatchel, R. J., Garofalo, J. P., & Polatin, P. B. (1999). Toward more accurate use of the Beck Depression Inventory with chronic back pain patients. *Clinical Journal of Pain, 15,* 117–121.

Widiger, T. A., Trull, T. J., Hurt, S. W., Clarkin, J., & Frances, A. (1987). A multidimensional scaling of the DSM-III personality disorders. *Archives of General Psychiatry, 44,* 557–563.

Williams, A. (1998). Depression in chronic pain: Mistaken models, missed opportunities. *Scandinavian Journal of Behavior Therapy, 27,* 61–80.

3

Conducting and Evaluating Treatment Outcome Studies

Stephen Morley
Amanda C. de C. Williams

Most readers will never be responsible for conducting an outcome trial, but some may consider evaluating a clinical service and most will want to know what to look for when they examine reports of treatment trials and service evaluations and they will want to appraise the emerging literature against the background of what is known and what is accepted as competent. To achieve these ends, we begin with an overview of development of psychological treatments for chronic pain and the current evidence for the efficacy and effectiveness of psychological treatments for chronic pain. We highlight what we perceive as issues that need further conceptual development and research.

Overview

Contemporary psychological treatments for chronic pain have their origins in several distinct formulations. The earliest is Fordyce's operant analysis (Fordyce, 1976; Fordyce, Fowler, Lehmann, & DeLateur, 1968) in which publicly observable responses such as medication consumption, limping, and other motor activities are governed by their contingent consequences. The focus of treatment is the manipulation of the contingencies and their reinforcer value. The operant approach to treatment presupposes a precise behavioral analysis of people and individually tailored interventions. Single-case methodology (Hersen & Barlow, 1984; Morley, 1996) has been used to demonstrate the influence of reinforcement and contingencies on behavior associated with pain (Block, Kremer, & Gaylor, 1980; Fordyce, Shelton, & Dunmore, 1982; see also Sanders, Chapter 6, this volume).

The respondent formulation of pain identifies the pain–tension cycle as a focus of treatment (Gessel & Alderman, 1971)[1]: Pain elicits a response of increased muscle tension which itself produces more pain as well as contributing directly to secondary problems such as sleep disturbance and immobilization. The simple generic intervention of relaxation aims to break the pain–tension cycle. The primary outcome target is reduction in subjective pain experience, and treatment validity can be assessed by reductions in electromyographic levels.

By the early 1980s, the third element of contemporary treatment was established (Turk, Meichenbaum, & Genest, 1983).

The experience and behavioral consequences of pain were conceptualized as a function of the person's cognitive appraisals of the pain and the person's ability to manage and control the pain and its consequences. The formulation implies that successful manipulation of the key cognitive elements will alter not only the patient's subjective experience of pain but also his or her behavioral and emotional state. Turk and Rudy (1992) encapsulated the general cognitive-behavioral formulation, describing patients as

> active processors of information. They have negative expectations about their own ability and responsibility to exert any control over their pain. Moreover they often view themselves as helpless. Such negative, maladaptive appraisals about their situation and their personal efficacy may reinforce the experience of demoralization, inactivity, and overreaction to nociceptive stimulation. Such cognitive appraisals and expectations are postulated as having an effect on behavior, leading to reduced effort and activity and increased psychological distress. (Turk & Rudy, 1992, p. 103; see also Turk, Chapter 7, this volume)

Within a short time the three elements were being combined in varying quantities within a generic cognitive-behavioral approach to which additional elements drawn from cognitive therapy for depression were added.

As clinicians and researchers recognized the complexity of pain, treatment programs developed pragmatically within the cognitive-behavioral framework outlined by Turk and his colleagues (Turk & Meichenbaum, 1994; Turk et al., 1983) and therapeutic procedures were added to the treatment of pain without prior evaluation of their impact. The specificity that in earlier behavioral studies linked treatment to outcome has largely been lost. In a review of treatment efficacy, Morley, Eccleston, and Williams (1999) conducted a content analysis of treatments used in 30 trials retrieved in a systematic review of the literature. More than 40 different specific[2] therapeutic procedures were identified and grouped into the following components: education, exercise, relaxation, goal setting, graded increase in activity, problem solving, attention diversion, cognitive therapy, and maintenance. At present, not only is pain treatment multicomponent, but it is frequently delivered in a multidisciplinary format to groups of patients and assessed with multiple outcome measures.

Efficacy and Effectiveness

In evaluating the impact of health care technologies, the distinction between efficacy and effectiveness studies is important (Nathan, Stuart, & Dolan, 2000). Efficacy studies seek to determine the impact of a specified intervention. The primary concern is to maximize the internal validity of the study by controlling as many sources of variability as possible so that any differences in the outcomes between the intervention and control condition(s) may confidently be attributed to the intervention. By common consent, the best form of efficacy study is the randomized controlled trial (RCT).[3] Critics of the RCT emphasize its inability to generalize to the everyday clinical environment. Effectiveness research is therefore required to determine whether treatments are both feasible and have clinical and social benefits in other environments. Table 3.1 contrasts some of the differences between efficacy and effectiveness research.

The catholic approach to pain treatment has generated a significant number of controlled trials and program evaluations spanning the range of the efficacy and effectiveness dimension. Recent narrative reviews (Chambless & Ollendick, 2001; Compas, Haaga, Keefe, Leitenberg, & Williams, 1998) and systematic reviews and meta-analyses (Flor, Fydrich, & Turk, 1992; Guzmán, Esmail, Karjalainen, Irvin, & Bombadier, 2001; Morley et al., 1999; Turner, 1996; van Tulder et al., 2000) have concluded that the available published data demonstrate that therapy is effective when compared with minimal control conditions (waiting list and treatment as usual) and at least as good as other active treatments.

Although the value of psychological treatments is now broadly established there is a need to conduct further evaluations. Demands from governments, health service managers and employers, funding sources (payers), and ethical considerations about best use of resources all require that redun-

TABLE 3.1. Efficacy and Effectiveness

	Efficacy	Effectiveness
Aims	Are there measurable effects of specific interventions?	Is the treatment feasible and does it have benefits in the real world?
Design	Treatment versus control (standard treatment/placebo/waiting list)—to control for "nonspecifics" of treatment.	Treatment versus treatment as usual or no control group.
	Patients randomly allocated to treatment.	Random allocation useful but not necessary
Patient selection	Restrictive inclusion/exclusion criteria. Specific diagnostic categories. Comorbidity excluded.	Unrestricted selection of patients in need regardless of diagnosis and comorbidity.
	Often selected from referrals to university-based clinics.	Broader sampling frame. Often evaluations of particular service.
	Treatment free at point of delivery in private health care systems (United States).	Treatment costs incurred by patient (United States) but not necessarily in social health care systems (e.g., U.K. National Health Service).
Treatment protocols	Tightly defined, manualized, adherence checks of therapists to ensure purity of treatment, therapists specially trained in the protocol.	Clinicians not trained to specific protocol, adherence checks not mandatory.
Outcomes	Theoretically important, predominantly symptom focused.	Broader measures of disability, quality of life.

dant or ineffective components of the program be cut and that the effectiveness and efficiency of the treatments be improved (see Pruitt & Von Korff, Chapter 14, and Linton, Chapter 15, this volume). In addition to these practical considerations, research and clinical curiosity drive us to ask further questions about therapy and the processes of therapeutic change.

Improving effectiveness and identifying procedures essential for therapeutic change are challenging tasks. Trials are characterized by marked heterogeneity, and the pragmatic development of pain management has made for relatively little theorizing and research on the process of change. We suggest that the key tasks of researchers and clinicians are to understand the impact and nature of the sources of variability outlined in Table 3.2 and to integrate them in theoretically productive ways. The remainder of this chapter highlights some of the issues that deserve consideration when thinking about conducting and evaluating treatments.

Patients: The Patient Uniformity Myth

It is now 35 years since Keisler (1966) described the myth of patient uniformity—that is, the unspoken assumption that patients with a disorder are psychologically homogeneous and will respond identically to treatment. Once heterogeneity is recognized, the issues of targeting treatments for subsets of patients and aptitude–treatment interactions must be considered.

Heterogeneity between studies is readily apparent in the variation in their sampling frames, sociodemographic characteristics, and the diagnostic groups used. Some investigators have recruited specific diagnostic groups with correspondingly intensive medical workups to ensure homogeneity, but others studied chronic pain patients with a mix of diagnoses. Although this information is important, because it helps to contextualize the samples, it rarely contributes to understanding the impact of patient heterogeneity on treatment outcome. We cautiously interpret the current evidence as sup-

TABLE 3.2. Sources of Heterogeneity in Trials

Patients
Demographics: age, socioeconomic status; diagnostic status; biomedical status; psychological status

Therapies
Type of therapy: content, number, duration, and frequency of sessions; manualization; group or individual

Therapist
Training, experience, and level of qualification; competence; adherence to protocol; supervision

Outcomes
See Table 3.3 for details.

---

port for the conclusion that cognitive-behavioral therapy (CBT) is equally effective regardless of diagnostic group (Morley et al., 1999). Indeed, this should not be too surprising as the treatments are designed to attack the problem of chronic pain rather than a specific diagnosis or aspects of gender or socioeconomic status.

The possibility that treatments may be tailored to fit patients is enticing because of the presumed increase in treatment efficiency, cost savings, expected improvement in treatment outcome, and patient satisfaction. The issue has been debated for many years in the wider literature on psychotherapy and behavioral change. Despite its desirability commentators have noted that progress has been remarkably slow (Dance & Neufeld, 1988; Garfield, 1994; Smith & Sechrest, 1991), but the same commentators "remain optimistic about the future of . . . research" (Dance & Neufeld, 1988, p. 209). We give two examples of approaches to tailoring treatments: profiling and aptitude–treatment interaction.

Profiling: Patient Typologies

This approach disaggregates patients into subsets each with a set of treatment needs and outcomes and also indicates which treatment procedures "fit" each subset of patients. There is a subsidiary issue concerned with using criteria to select patients

most likely to benefit from a treatment. This issue will occur when there are limited and costly treatment resources and when it is known that a significant proportion of patients will not respond. The pragmatic and ethical issue of selecting patients for treatment should not overshadow the need for research into ways in which putative nonresponders might be moved to a state in which they are likely to respond.

Within pain there are several emerging approaches to disaggregating patients. Turk and Rudy (1988; Rudy, Turk, Zaki, & Curtin, 1989) have cluster analyzed the Multidimensional Pain Inventory (MPI) and identified three groups of patients (dysfunctional, interpersonally distressed, and adaptive copers). There is some evidence for the robustness of this solution from several other studies (Bergstrom, Bodin, Jensen, Linton, & Nygren, 2001; Hellstrom, Jansson, & Carlsson, 2000; Jamison, Rudy, Penzien, & Mosley, 1994). The profiles suggest that patients have different treatment needs that might be met by distinct treatment packages. The strongest test of this would be to randomly assign patients within each profile to treatments that have been optimally designed for each profile: patients assigned to their optimal therapy should show greatest therapeutic change on the target outcomes, whereas patients allocated to the nonoptimal group should show a poorer response.

Preliminary work provides support for some aspects of the model. Two studies (Rudy, Turk, Kubinski, & Zaki, 1995; Turk, Okifuji, Sinclair, & Starz, 1998) have treated patients (temporomandibular disorders and fibromyalgia syndrome) from each profile with a standard protocol that included biofeedback and stress management and was hypothesized to best "fit" the dysfunctional group. As predicted, patients classified as dysfunctional demonstrated greater improvements in pain intensity, perceived impact of pain, depression, and negative thoughts, compared with those classified as interpersonally distressed or adaptive copers. In a third study, Turk, Rudy, Kubinski, Zaki, and Greco (1996) selected only dysfunctional patients with temporomandibular disorder (TMD) and randomly allocated them to a standardized treatment package with or without the addition of a cognitive therapy (CT) component aimed at changing the maladaptive cognitions presumed to underpin their dysfunction or to nondirective supportive counseling. As predicted, the group receiving CT showed greater reductions in pain, depression, and medication use and continued improvement at the 6-month follow-up assessment.

A second example of disaggregating patients demonstrates the potential for defining a precise link between clearly defined psychological process and a relevant pain outcome. Vlaeyen and Linton (2000) have recently drawn the literature together and formulated a model in which the relationship between fear of pain, behavioral avoidance, and the establishment and maintenance of low activity levels has been made explicit (see also Vlaeyen, de Jong, Sieben, & Crombez, Chapter 10, this volume). Their model implies that there is a distinct group of patients who have a strong fear that physical activity will cause injury. Consistent avoidance of feared activity underpins these patients' accumulated deficits, but this behavior can be modified by the application of a well-specified protocol with an established track record in the wider field of anxiety and phobia. The initial test of the treatment used an experimental single-case approach with sophisticated time-series analysis (Vlaeyen, de Jong, Geilen, Heuts, & van Breukelen, 2001) to demonstrate that therapeutic reduction in fear of movement and fear of pain, and in catastrophizing, is associated with introduction of graded exposure to the feared activity rather than graded activity.

Aptitude–Treatment Interactions

Aptitude–treatment interactions (ATI) relate individual differences to variation in outcomes when different treatments are offered for the same outcome or set of outcomes. In the prototypical study, a critical aptitude is identified and it is predicted that patients who possess more of this characteristic will profit from a particular treatment. In contrast, patients with less of the characteristic will be more likely to profit from another treatment. The study of ATI raises a number of important issues and although the complexity of the topic is beyond detailed discussion, we highlight three of them. More detailed discussions can be found in Dance

and Neufeld (1988), Snow (1991), and Shoham-Saloman and Hannah (1991).

• *Which aptitudes are important?* Given the number of possible variables, the challenge is to determine which, individually or in combination, are important. Investigators may select variables with little psychological meaning simply because they are measurable (e.g., demographic variables), often only weak proxy measures of meaningful psychological ones (Beutler, Brown, Crothers, Booker, & Seabrook, 1996). Identification of a single critical variable would indicate the development of specific treatment. If multiple variables are implicated, we need to know how they interrelate to produce coherent models of chronic pain that lead to different treatments. In each case the goal is the psychological equivalent of mechanism based classification and treatment (Woolf et al., 1998)

• *How can we identify aptitudes?* A frequently used strategy has been to conduct post hoc analyses of trials and patient series. This is generally unsatisfactory for a number of reasons. First, although individual studies may generate "predictors," they are usually derived from an atheoretical analysis of the data. Second, the data bases typically comprise relatively small groups of patients who are selected on unknown or restricted criteria and subjected to therapeutic conditions that are poorly controlled and understood. However competently these studies are conducted, it is likely that they will produce only local solutions dependent on the context of the study (Vlaeyen et al., 1997).

Shoham-Salomon and Hannah (1991) describe the pervasive approach to identifying attribute–treatment interaction as *pragmatic* with the primary aim of establishing predictive validity. In contrast, a *heuristically* directed approach tries to establish construct validity in which the key aim is to articulate and understand the relationship between "change mechanisms that underlie therapeutic processes and the aptitudes that are hypothesized to thrive on such processes" (Shoham-Salomon & Hannah, 1991, p. 211).

• *How does one conduct an ATI study?* Several issues arise with respect to the statistical treatment of ATIs and readers are referred to Snow (1991) for detailed guidance. Among the most important is the representation of the key aptitude. The approach that is generally not advised is to form groups by a median split of a variable. There are serious problems with this strategy. First, the median is a function of sample size and entirely dependent on that particular sample. Second, persons on either side of the median will psychologically resemble one another more than they will resemble the extremes. For these reasons, and also for considerations of statistical power, analysis should be based on regression rather than analysis of variance (ANOVA). Even when groups are formed by other means (e.g., cluster analysis), continuity between members in different groups is still likely.

The ATI is often considered in the simplified context of a single outcome. Given the multidimensional nature of chronic pain, this view seems inappropriate. When multidimensionality is taken into account, we need to consider the possibility that while possession of one aptitude may confer an advantage for one outcome, it may be disadvantageous for another. On the other hand, a second aptitude may confer the reverse ordering of advantages.

Our final consideration concerns the content and delivery of therapy. The implicit assumption is that therapy is constant and in some sense fixed. Although manuals, therapist training, and supervision (see below) strive to maintain the quality of specific components of therapy, variation in the nonspecific components of therapy (e.g., therapeutic alliance), and cohort effects for patients treated in groups may provide the source of the ATI. The assessment of the nonspecific effects of therapy is necessary to determine the relative contribution of the specific and nonspecific aspects of treatment.

Summary

A significant challenge is to understand why patients vary in their response to treatment and to develop interventions that are sensitive to individual needs. The examples we have highlighted give some indication of the current state of the art. It is important to note that the approaches to tailoring treatment are not independent. For example, it is possible to develop procedures for targeting possible outcomes, as in the work of Turk and his colleagues, and also to consider

variations in the degree to which patients in one typology may respond to a particular treatment.

Identifying variation in treatment need does not necessarily tell us a great deal about possible variation in response to a treatment protocol. For example, patients categorized as interpersonally distressed may show marked variation in their interpersonal styles that have implications for the way in which they will respond to treatment (Safran & Segal, 1990). Second, a degree of caution is warranted when considering profiling systems. Such systems frequently produce a group of unclassifiable patients who will vary in study to study. For example, Okifuji, Turk, and Eveleigh (1999) report that the MPI clusters produce between 3% and 30% "unclassifiable." In addition, one must bear in mind the fact that even when clusters are identified there is often substantial overlap between groups on several key variables and that members of clusters may have similar expressed needs (see later discussion on stakeholder definitions of outcome). As Snow (1991) points out, profiles do not necessarily contain information about likely response to treatment and we must be aware of confusing treatment need with the capacity to respond to treatment.

Therapies

Critical Ingredients or Essential Processes?

Interpreting evaluations of complex packages of treatment is further confounded by the apparent equivalence of different treatments, or of the same treatment for different populations: The picture is of moderate outcome almost whatever the treatment content and patient population (Morley et al., 1999; Turk 2000a). Some hypotheses proposed to explain this focus not on the designated content of treatment but on nonspecific effects common to most therapies inherent in the trial design and assessment materials (e.g., therapist attention to patients' concerns, the generation of hope and positive expectancies, and education in the model of chronic pain). Certainly, these process issues deserve more attention and quantification.

When patients are selected for treatment

close to the time of referral, it may be that the timing of treatment coincides with the nadir of their problems, and that spontaneous recovery and regression to a healthier mean produce good outcome results. However, when the mean is that of a chronically disabled population and the wait for treatment is prolonged, regression to the mean is not a likely explanation for change. But whatever the variance attributable to any or all of these processes, it is worth also examining the evidence for the efficacy and effectiveness of each of the components involved in treatment.

One approach to this is the component analysis (dismantling) study in which the complete treatment is contrasted with the treatment minus one component that is presumed to be critical to effect a particular change. There are, however, logical problems with this design: Only if the relationship between component and outcome is specific and *independent* of other component-outcome relationships can the difference in outcomes between the complete and dismantled treatments be attributed to the subtracted component. But the relationship between component and outcome is designed not to be independent: treatment is given as a package in order to benefit from synergistic interactions between components. Not only does complexity arise from the combined effects of components, which may be synergistic or antagonistic (components may be effective, ineffective, or harmful, individually or by interaction), but also from the interaction of therapy and therapist in producing the outcome of interest (Grimshaw, Freemantle, Langhorne, & Song, 1995). Without an adequate theoretical basis, the most sophisticated statistical analysis cannot disentangle these effects.

Furthermore the component-outcome relationship may not be specific. For example, four patients who substantially increase their activity may do so for different reasons: One may have been sufficiently reassured by education to restart avoided activities; another may increase activity through graded exposure to feared movements and exertion; a third may benefit from cognitive therapy and with improved mood will see increased activity as a source of pleasure and satisfaction instead of failure and discouragement; a fourth may find that on re-

ducing large doses of opioid analgesics and sedating psychotropic drugs, she has energy and enthusiasm whose loss she had attributed to pain. Careful examination of the various dismantling studies bears out the nonspecificity of outcome to component, producing apparently disappointing results in terms of the contribution of any single component, despite substantial improvement across outcomes in treated groups compared with untreated controls (e.g., Newton-John, Spence, & Schotte, 1995; Nicholas, Wilson, & Goyen, 1991).

A further practical consideration against extensive use of dismantling studies is that the required study size is comparatively large in a field in which the average size of treatment and control groups is 21.[4] Ethical considerations encourage the design of control groups with best standard care, requiring large sample sizes to provide the power to show differences between treatment and control (Kopta, Lueger, Saunders, & Howard, 1999). For example, Turner and Jensen (1993) compared cognitive therapy versus cognitive therapy plus relaxation versus a wait-list control in a study that had adequate power to detect an effect size of 1 ($n = 34$ per group). To detect effect size differences of 0.5 with 80% power, they calculated they would need 64 subjects per group, almost doubling the demands of the study. When we consider that the median effect size of differences between active treatments and wait-list control is about 0.5 (Morley et al., 1999), the magnitude of difference between two active treatments is likely to be significantly smaller. Although large trials might be feasible with brief and economical interventions with minimal follow-up, this clearly does not describe the sort of trials needed to answer current questions in pain management. In addition to this constraint, Stiles, Shapiro, and Elliott (1986) argued that the number of permutations of treatments, settings, outcomes, and patients was simply too large be a realistic basis for progress by the brute empiricism of factorial designed trials (Jones, Jarvis, Lewis, & Ebutt, 1996).

Although it arises from a wish to make best use of resources, the "critical ingredients" model may be neither appropriate nor achievable. What are the alternatives to dismantling studies? Campbell and colleagues

(2000), Stiles and colleagues (1986), and others emphasize the importance of the first step of defining and modeling each mechanism in the complex treatment, and relating it to particular outcomes. This is equivalent to Phase I of pharmaceutical studies, for which intensive qualitative and single-case methods should be considered (Vlaeyen et al., 2001). Process of change remains underaddressed in many areas of the pain field and establishing relationships between therapeutic events and outcome would enable more useful Phase 2, 3, and 4 studies in which the new treatment is sequentially tested against standard treatments and in effectiveness settings (Schwartz, Chesney, Irvine, & Keefe, 1997).

Process Variables

Exploring the relationships between process and outcome is complex: Radically different conclusions are drawn from findings in the psychotherapy field. One extreme is to disregard process variables and address only the intended content of treatment and argue that treatment outcome is attributable to the specific content of therapy. The broad equivalence of therapies renders this position untenable.

The other extreme is represented by Frank and Frank (1991), who identified the therapeutic content of specific therapies such as cognitive-behavioral therapy (CBT) with the processes common to therapy: reduced alienation and isolation for patients as they were accepted by a normative group, the generation of the expectation of help, direct and vicarious learning of new behaviors, enhancing self-efficacy, and modifying unrealistic expectations of outcome. The components of therapy and its rationale needed only to be plausible, not correct, to bring about the changes. Therapeutic techniques work by "giving the patient and therapist something to do together, the ritual sustains mutual interest" (Frank & Frank 1991, p. 44).

What methods are appropriate for resolving this question? Searching for correlations between the quantity of a process (such as rated empathy) and the extent of outcome may fail to demonstrate any connection when there is insufficient variability, for instance, when there is a generally low or high level across therapists of empathy. Finding

associations also requires that processes be identified and that adequate measures are available, not always the case, as in, for instance, group processes in psychoeducational groups.

Some processes themselves constitute subgoals of therapy, complicating the model: for instance, the establishment of a therapeutic alliance or treatment credibility. Process research comparing different psychotherapies with similar outcomes for the same patients produces conclusions largely consistent with Rogerian tenets of the importance of empathy, support, and nonjudgmental acceptance in bringing about change. Ablon and Jones (1999) point out the difficulty of dismantling therapeutic effects that are summed across patients and therapists when "specific interventions do not have fixed meanings independent of context and cannot be assumed to contribute discretely and uniquely to outcome" (p. 73). Turner, Deyo, Loeser, Von Korff, and Fordyce (1994) make similar points about the extent to which patients' positive expectancies of change can be attached to treatment staff.

Setting and Delivery Variables

Most published studies of pain management involve group-based treatment, although some also contain individual treatment, and individual treatment is common in clinical practice. Because the group format is used to teach common principles and to promote self-management and vicarious learning, it is more psychoeducation than group psychotherapy. However, group dynamics are relevant, promoting, inhibiting, or undermining patient progress. They depend in part on the skills of therapists, largely trained in individual therapy, being effectively applied to group settings, with which the principles of CBT are entirely compatible (see Keefe, Beaupre, Gil, Rumble, & Aspnes, Chapter 11, this volume).

The intensity and length of treatment programs are little investigated, and one meta-analysis reported no association between program length (number of hours) and outcome (Flor et al., 1992). However, when differences between inpatient and outpatient delivery are considered, in which length is confounded with intensiveness of treatment (there are further confounds such as environmental support for rehearsing new behaviors, and process variables such as the extent of group cohesion) results support a dose–response effect (Peters & Large, 1990; Williams, Nicholas, Richardson, Pither, & Fernandes, 1999). Although the argument in favor of outpatient or more extensive programs is the opportunity for patients to establish and generalize new behaviors in their own environments, for some patients and some behaviors, an inpatient setting provides safety and protection from external pressures and may therefore be a more effective way to make major changes. As in other areas, the separate factors of overall length, number of hours per week, and dose–response effects require further investigation.

Comment

Given the surprising gaps in theoretical and empirical support for aspects of the content and delivery of pain management, and the heterogeneity of patients treated within the same group, the package approach is both a practical and probably economical way for clinical work to proceed. While often referred to as a "blunderbuss"[5] approach, the notion of passive (and mortally threatened!) patients is perhaps less appropriate than that of a supermarket, from which the patient selects specifically and according to his or her needs and plans, although what she or he takes home may not match the shopping list made at the outset. Greater specificity of treatment is desirable, but we doubt if this can be achieved using a "critical ingredients" model for the theoretical and practical reasons stated. Similarly, there are severe limits to the extensive testing of all the parameters of treatment such as length and intensity.

We suggest that the way forward must include the careful articulation of theories of change, both specific and process components, and testing for efficacy and effectiveness. We also observe that despite the presence of several high-quality outcome trials, there is an almost complete lack of secondary analyses of the process of change. This contrasts markedly with the research in change on affective disorders where both the NIMH Treatment of Depression Collab-orative Research Program (Elkin, 1999; Shaw et al., 1999) and the Sheffield psychotherapy trials (Raue, Goldfried, & Barkham, 1997; Stiles, Agnew-Davies, Hardy, Barkham, & Shapiro, 1998) have produced extensive secondary analyses relating to process.

Therapists: Manualization, Treatment Integrity, and Accountability

Studies of treatment efficacy need to demonstrate precise control of the independent variable (the treatment). In practice, this demonstration requires the control of content of treatment and ensuring that it is administered within agreed parameters in a competent manner. The accepted methods of controlling treatment content are to manualize the treatment and to ensure that therapists adhere to the manual during treatment.[6] The purpose of a manual is to prescribe the essential elements of the treatment and to proscribe other elements that are deemed to be extraneous to the treatment. Well-specified manuals also facilitate the training of therapists to a common standard and the replication of treatment across therapists, both within and between different trials. Ideally, investigators should demonstrate that therapists have been trained to the treatment protocol and that they adhere to it throughout the period of the trial.

An additional problem of therapist variance occurs when there are two or more possible treatments. If different therapists are assigned to the treatments, differences in outcome at the end of treatment could be ascribed to differences in the therapists' characteristics (therapeutic allegiance, motivation, inherent competence). This is particularly likely when a treatment trial uses "treatment as usual" as the comparator treatment as it is unlikely that the trial therapists will also provide treatment for the control group. In the ideal trial, therapists should deliver each of the treatments equally competently and without bias to avoid therapist–treatment confounding.

In their review of trials, Morley and his colleagues (1999) observed a marked discrepancy between the published trials and the ideal features. For example, only one-third of the trials reported using fully manualized protocols and about one-half reported no manualization or that the treatment was conducted in line with other published accounts. The remaining authors stated that at least one component of the treatment was conducted to a manualized standard. Similarly, only 40% of authors reported that they had made adherence checks on the therapists' performance and even fewer (32%) reported that therapists had received supervision during the trial. There was also marked variance between trials in the level of therapists used, with 20% using unqualified graduate students. There is clearly room for significant improvement in this component of trial design and execution.

Although manuals and assessment of therapist adherence are mandatory in randomized trials of therapeutic efficacy, they have been subject to criticism on a number of grounds. Some concerns are raised by the proposal that only manualized therapies validated in RCTs should be sanctioned for use. Significant concerns are that manuals prepared for efficacy trials may be too narrow and too rigid for application in effectiveness settings; that they infringe on the capacity of the skilled clinician to exercise clinical judgment; that they fix therapy so that it stagnates and prevents innovation; and that they are too cumbersome, time-consuming, expensive, and difficult to train and supervise (Kazdin, 1998; Parloff, 1998; Strosahl, 1998; Wilson, 1998). Some of these issues are practical; for example, a manual need not be written as a set of instructions for assembling a kit, but in a more strategic, problem-solving style (Beutler, 1999).

Within the context of psychological treatment of pain, we are persuaded that manuals are not only necessary in efficacy trials but need to be developed for effectiveness settings and use in everyday clinical settings. They offer considerable advantages in settings in which teams of therapists from different disciplines manage difficult clinical problems and team membership is variable. Manuals can provide guidance on how the separate parts of a program interrelate, set minimal standards of therapeutic activity, facilitate training and supervision, and expedite clinical audit. Manuals need not stifle

therapeutic innovation, and we suggest that it is only when programs have established a solid baseline of performance that an innovation can be truly implemented and assessed against the expected outcome (Beiber, Wroblewski, & Barber, 1999).

Although there are a number of unpublished manuals and some excellent accounts of psychological treatments (Gatchel & Turk, 1996; Main & Spanswick, 2000; Nicholas, Molloy, Tonkin, & Beeston, 2000; Philips & Rachman, 1996), the extent to which they have been adopted by programs is unknown but we regard their use as essential in studies evaluating treatments. Finally, we note that manuals and the associated monitoring of therapist adherence can only guarantee that the relevant input has been delivered. The extent to which the input has been taken up by patients is a different question and we note that there appears to be an almost complete lack of studies on patient's compliance with therapy and the process of therapy.

Outcomes

"Whose Outcome Is It Anyway?": A Stakeholder Analysis

Although there is at first glance a consensus on the broad domains of outcome of pain management, a closer look reveals a less satisfactory picture. There is often a rather tenuous relationship between the outcomes measured (pain, mood, disability) and the reasons given by authors for attempting to mitigate the effects of chronic pain on the person (suffering, limitations on activity, high consumption of health care resources, loss of work and other meaningful activity, poor quality of life), on those close to the person (suffering, limitation of social activity), and on society as a whole (substantial costs in health care, welfare, and lost workdays). Behavioral outcomes (Kaplan, 1990) are surprisingly rare given that pain management aims to change a range of behaviors. Moreover, the modality of measurement is predominantly self-report, even when external sources of information are in principle available; even observations made within the treatment program (such as progress in exercises) are rarely reported.

At present, researchers and clinicians select most outcomes and there is little recognition of the various "stakeholders" in patients' recovery or rehabilitation (Howard, Moras, Brill, & Martinovich, 1996). The priorities of various stakeholders are unlikely to coincide and at times they will conflict. An employer may want full return to work and minimal sickness absence or special-needs provision or complete cessation of employment. In contrast, the patient's quality of life (with which his or her family's quality of life is often associated) may improve with adjusted or assisted work demands. The patient's doctor may wish to reduce the frequency of consultation, the prescription of drugs, and referrals for investigation and treatment, but these are rarely high priorities for patients or their families. The family may wish to retain disability-linked welfare assistance, while the therapeutic team holds its withdrawal as a high-priority goal.

Further problems arise within various domains of outcome. Although there is a proliferation of overlapping measures in areas such as cognitive content and process or disability, there is a regrettable neglect of measurement of work or meaningful activity, even less of health care and drug use, and (common to many RCTs) a relative neglect of quality of life (Sanders, Egger, Tallon, & Frankel, 1998).

There are various sources to guide selection of measures (McDowell & Newell, 1996; Turk & Melzack, 1992; Williams, 1999). Measure selection is best considered a compromise between several features: the underlying theoretical constructs, the content (included and omitted), psychometric properties (which depend on the context of testing), previous performance in the field; the type of scores produced (dichotomous, categorical, continuous), and their susceptibility to the planned statistical analysis. Although at one level this is obvious, it is alarming to read simple claims in accounts of trials that each measure represents, with excellent reliability and validity, the construct of interest when reading the questionnaire and the account of its development would lead to substantial modification of these claims. There is also a continuing tendency to develop new scales, for the purpose of a single trial or for others to use, with little consideration of measurement theory. Michell (1977) questions whether some psychological constructs and their relationships can properly be represented by linear scales rather than, for instance, tree structure).

Although the outcomes to be measured should be indicated by the aims and methods of treatment under investigation, their choice often seems less well grounded, and we would recommend reference to a checklist of domains (see Table 3.3)—whatever the treatment—at least to arrive at the initial list of possible measures. Changes in domains may be only loosely coupled; for example, improved physical performance in terms of walking, lifting, and standing does not necessarily imply a return to work or other activities. The mode of measurement also requires consideration: Too many outcomes are assessed only by self-report, using measures which in turn have been validated by cross correlation with other self-report measures; the relationship to any desired behavior can be remote. More independence of measures, and more direct behavioral measurement, would considerably improve the overall credibility of outcome.

Analyzing Outcomes

Statistical and Clinical Significance

Readers cannot but be familiar with the statement that clinical significance and statistical significance are not the same, but the implications of this statement are rarely addressed in the design of trials. This is not least because defining clinical significance is complex and appears to lack the scientific certainty offered by the chosen p value by which findings are judged to be "significant." Traditional methods in psychology and behavioral sciences involve evaluating outcomes using the language of inferential statistics on differences between groups. Although an effective tool, such evaluation does not provide an obvious way of determining how much better or worse a treatment is, and the results are dependent on the sample size.

Before exploring the alternatives, a little further elaboration of what statistical significance does tell us may be useful. As Cohen (1994) pointed out, the common interpreta-

TABLE 3.3. Measurement Domains and Example Measures

Domain	Comments
Pain experience. Measures of subjective pain experience captured by ratings of intensity, sensory qualities and unpleasantness, and frequency and duration.	Good multidimensional measures available. Still frequently treated as a single dimension.
Mood/affect. Primary measure of mood or affective state, but not a trait assessment.	General psychopathology measures less applicable; recent specific pain-related ones most relevant.
Cognitive and coping. Content and process of cognitive and behavioral coping strategies	Catastrophizing has emerged as a significant feature of coping. Perception of control of pain and self-efficacy in behavioral coping attempts are also important.
Pain-related behavior. Overt behavioral acts associated with pain.	Good systems available for quantifying behaviors (e.g., guarding and bracing); interpretation is more difficult when they are not the target of treatment.
Biology/physical fitness. Assessment of biological function and physical fitness, but not including measures of behavioral activity as in previous category.	Clinical measures (e.g., straight leg raise) lack external validity except where they are the target of treatment (e.g., joint stiffness in rheumatoid arthritis).
Social role functioning. Assessments of the impact of pain on the ability of the person to function in a variety of social roles: work; leisure; marital and family.	Inventories vary in breadth and depth of coverage and congruence with patient and treatment goals.
Use of health care system. Use of health care facilities, including clinic visits and drug use.	A major target of treatment: aspects easily assessed but need clear rationale and norms.

tion of p as the probability that the null hypothesis (of no change with treatment, or no difference between treatments or groups) is false, and therefore that the cherished hypothesis is true, is incorrect. p gives the probability, if the null hypothesis were true, of the data in question occurring, so if the value of p is small, and if the null hypothesis were true, the data are unlikely. This is not the same as saying that given these data, the probability of the null hypothesis being true is small. He recommends careful exploration of data before analysis, the use of the standardized difference or effect sizes with its confidence limits to describe differences or change, and replications to establish the actual likelihood of the data occurring.

One of the questions raised by the focus on clinical significance is who is to define what amount of change or threshold achieved is clinically significant given the diverse opinions on which outcomes matter. Turk (2000b) suggests that whoever has the most stake in the outcome should define what is clinically meaningful: the patient for pain relief, the clinician for opioid reduction, and so on. The definition is reasonably straightforward when this is a measurable event, such as return to or abstinence from analgesic drugs. Only recently have researchers begun to ask whether the almost universal 50% pain relief as outcome coincides with patients' definition of meaningful change.

The Reliable Change Index

Jacobson and his colleagues (Jacobson, Roberts, Berns, & McGlinchey, 1999; Jacobson & Truax, 1991) described and discussed the Reliable Change Index (RCI). The RCI is a statistical technique for defining clinically significant change. It has two separate but interrelated functions. First, it takes into account the reliability properties of a measure to test the hypothesis that the observed change is not merely attributable to the unreliability of the measure. The second function is to determine whether the change corresponds to what might be regarded as a clinically significant change. The criterion for this is dependent on the availability of normative data for the measure.

Assuming that the scores of the healthy population and untreated population both approximate to normal distributions and do not overlap greatly, significant clinical change is deemed to have taken place if a posttreatment score falls within one of three bands: (1) within two standard deviations of the healthy mean, (2) beyond two standard deviations from the untreated mean toward the healthy mean, or (3) on the healthy side of the intersection of the two distributions. These three criteria may coincide, but they can be usefully contrasted and compared. The RCI has one marked advantage over other statistical methods for data analysis because it can be applied to pre–posttreatment differences without the need for a control group and is recommended as the preferred statistic for uncontrolled program evaluations. However, the assumption of a healthy norm may not always be applicable to the chronic pain population and the subject urgently requires debate that would arise from more attention to defining and reporting clinically significant change.

Odds Ratio and Number Needed to Treat

These two statistics are not widely used in analyzing data from psychological treatment trials, but they are applicable to categorical outcomes (e.g., the proportion of patients in each group making a clinically significant change). In the field of headache research, there is consensus that a 50% reduction in scores on the Headache Index is clinically meaningful. It is therefore possible to represent outcomes from trials in terms of the proportion of patients who make clinically significant gains. An odds ratio (OR) of 1 implies that the two conditions are equivalent. Deviations to either side of 1 indicate that one or other of the treatments is more or less effective.

The number needed to treat (NNT) is simply interpreted as the as the number of patients one needs to treat in order to obtain an effect. An NNT of 1 would mean that every patient treated meets the posttreatment criterion, however it is defined, and none in the control group. NNTs approaching 2 to 3 are observed in pharmacological treatment of acute pain. Where NNTs have been used with psychological data, the results may be comparable with those achieved in medical treatments (Eccleston, Morley, Williams, Yorke, & Mastroyannopoulou, in press). The disadvantage is that there is no indication of the fate of those who did not attain the outcome in question: They may have fallen slightly below the cut point, worsened, or dropped out of treatment (for more detail, see McQuay & Moore, 1997; Sackett & Cook, 1994). Computation of the OR is simple, but the computation of its confidence interval and NNT are more complex. Appropriate software is readily available.

The Effect Size

There is a family of effect size (ES) statistics with a large technical literature (Rosenthal, 1994). A commonly used effect size is the difference between two sets of scores represented as a ratio of standard deviation of the difference. The resulting statistic is a z score from a normal distribution. The advantages of this statistic are that measurement on different scales can be compared on a standard metric and that differences between two groups can be represented in percentage point. For example, a difference between a treatment group and control group of 1 can be expressed as the average member of the treatment group being at the 84th percentile of the untreated group. The ES does not, of course, offer any inherent guide to what constitutes clinically significant change, but its applicability to clinical populations makes it easier to translate into clinical significance terms. The ES is also used as a measurement statistic when one combines studies as in a meta-analysis.

Conclusion

There is solid evidence from several rigorous trials and evaluations of programs to indicate that psychological treatments conducted within the broad framework of CBT are both efficacious and effective. In reflecting on the current state of play in this chapter, we identified several issues that need to be addressed in future evaluations of outcomes for pain treatment. Despite the current success, our knowledge is still limited and there is a substantial gap between where we are now and Gordon Paul's expression of the ideal "What treatment, by whom, is most effective for (this) individual, with that specific problem, under which set of circumstances?" (Paul, 1967, p. 111).

We suggest that the next stage of research should refine the formulation of pain and attempt to make explicit links between the process of therapy and outcomes and to attack the problems of heterogeneity. In the selection and development of outcome measures we need to look both at our own theoretical concerns and at the needs of the various stakeholders. Finally we suggest that no one method will suffice. Although quantitative randomized control trials will remain the bedrock of research, well-planned single-case designs and program evaluations will be equally important. There should also be a place for developing process research and for the use of qualitative methods to understand the processes of change.

Notes

1. Relaxation was also introduced as a direct treatment of the presumed pathophysiology in tension headache.
2. We use the term "specific" to refer to procedures prescribed by the therapeutic model that are presumed to have an impact on an outcome measure. In contrast, there are nonspecific components of treatment that are often common to many treatments and are not a central component of the therapeutic rationale (e.g., therapeutic alliance).
3. In evaluating many medical technologies, the preferred RCT is double blinded so that neither the patient nor the therapist is aware of which treatment is being administered. This is clearly not feasible in most studies of psychological treatments.
4. This figure is derived from Table 3 in Morley and colleagues (1999). In 25 trials there were 1,626 patients allocated to 78 treatment and control groups
5. A blunderbuss is a 16th-century gun with a large bore and flared muzzle. It was loaded with shot and was inaccurate even at a short range.

6. There is a critical distinction to make between adherence and competence. Adherence refers to the extent to which a therapist uses the prescribed interventions and abjures from proscribed interventions. Competence refers to the level of skill demonstrated by the therapist in delivering the treatment. Waltz, Addis, Koerner, and Jacobson (1993) have discussed this in detail. In general, it is both easier and economically cheaper to conduct adherence checks. In the trials reviewed by Morley and colleagues (1999), none gave details of competence checks.

References

Ablon, J. S., & Jones, E. E. (1999). Psychotherapy process in the National Institute of Mental Health Treatment of Depression Collaborative Research Program. *Journal of Consulting and Clinical Psychology, 67,* 64–75.

Beiber, J., Wroblewski, J. M., & Barber, C. M. (1999). Design and implementation of an outcomes management system within inpatient and outpatient behavioral health settings. In M. E. Marhuish (Ed.), *The use of psychological testing for treatment planning and outcomes assessment* (2nd ed., pp. 171–210). Mahwah, NJ: Erlbaum.

Bergstrom, G., Bodin, L., Jensen, I. B., Linton, S. J., & Nygren, A. L. (2001). Long- term, non-specific spinal pain: Reliable and valid subgroups of patients. *Behaviour Research and Therapy, 39,* 75–87.

Beutler, L. E. (1999). Manualizing flexibility: The training of eclectic therapists. *Journal of Clinical Psychology, 55,* 399–404.

Beutler, L. E., Brown, M. T., Crothers, L., Booker, K., & Seabrook, M. K. (1996). The dilemma of factitious demographic distinctions in psychological research. *Journal of Consulting and Clinical Psychology, 64,* 892–902.

Block, A. R., Kremer, E. F., & Gaylor, M. (1980). Behavioral treatment of chronic pain: The spouse as a discriminative cue for pain behavior. *Pain, 9,* 243–252.

Campbell, M., Fitzpatrick, R., Haines, A., Kinmonth, A. L., Sandercock, P., Spiegelhalter, D., & Tyrer, P. (2000). Framework for design and evaluation of complex interventions to improve health. *British Medical Journal, 321,* 694–696.

Chambless, D. L., & Ollendick, T., H. (2001). Empirically supported psychological interventions. *Annual Review of Psychology, 52,* 685–716.

Cohen, J. (1994). The earth is round (p < .05). *American Psychologist, 49,* 997–1003.

Compas, B. E., Haaga, D. A. F., Keefe, F. J., Leitenberg, H., & Williams, D. A. (1998). Sampling of empirically supported psychological treatments from health psychology: Smoking, chronic pain, cancer, and bulimia nervosa. *Journal of Consulting and Clinical Psychology, 66,* 89–112.

Dance, K. A., & Neufeld, R. W. J. (1988). Aptitude-treatment interaction research in the clinical setting: A review of attempts to dispel the "patient-uniformity" myth. *Psychological Bulletin, 104,* 192–213.

Eccleston, C., Morley, S., Williams, A. C., Yorke, L., & Mastroyannopoulou, K. (in press). Systematic review and meta-analysis of randomised controlled trials of psychological therapy for chronic pain in children and adolescents. *Pain.*

Elkin, I. (1999). A major dilemma in psychotherapy outcome research: Disentangling therapists from therapies. *Clinical Psychology-Science and Practice, 6,* 10–32.

Flor, H., Fydrich, T., & Turk, D. C. (1992). Efficacy of multidisciplinary pain treatment centers: A meta-analytic review. *Pain, 49,* 221–230.

Fordyce, W. E. (1976). *Behavioral methods for chronic pain and illness.* St. Louis, MO: Mosby.

Fordyce, W. E., Fowler, R., Lehmann, J., & DeLateur, B. (1968). Some implications of learning in problems of chronic pain. *Journal of Chronic Disease, 21,* 179–190.

Fordyce, W. E., Shelton, J. L., & Dundore, D. E. (1982). The modification of avoidance learning pain behaviors. *Journal of Behavioral Medicine, 5,* 405–414.

Frank, J. D., & Frank, J. B. (1991). *Persuasion and healing: A comparative study of psychotherapy* (3rd ed.). Baltimore: Johns Hopkins University Press.

Garfield, S. L. (1994). Research on client variables in psychotherapy. In A. E. Bergin & S. L. Garfield (Eds.), *Handbook of psychotherapy and behavior change* (4th ed., pp. 190–228). New York: Wiley.

Gatchel, R. J., & Turk, D. C. (Eds.). (1996). *Psychological approaches to pain management: A practitioner's handbook.* New York: Guilford Press.

Gessel, A., & Alderman, M. (1971). Management of myofascial pain dysfunction syndrome of the temporomandibular joint by tension control. *Psychosomatics, 12,* 302–309.

Grimshaw, J., Freemantle, N., Langhorne, P., & Song, F. (1995). *Complexity and systematic reviews: Report to the US Congress, Office of Technology Assessment.* Aberdeen, UK: University of Aberdeen.

Guzmán, J., Esmail, R., Karjalainen, K., Irvin, E., & Bombadier, C. (2001). Multidisciplinary rehabilitation for chronic low back pain: Systematic review. *British Medical Journal, 322,* 511–516.

Hellstrom, C., Jansson, B., & Carlsson, S. G. (2000). Perceived future in chronic pain: the relationship between outlook on future and empirically derived psychological patient profiles. *European Journal of Pain, 4,* 283–290.

Hersen, M., & Barlow, D. H. (1984). *Single case experimental designs: Strategies for studying behavior change* (2nd ed.). New York: Pergamon Press.

Howard, K. I., Moras, K., Brill, P. L., & Martinovich, Z. (1996). Evaluation of psychotherapy: Efficacy, effectiveness, and patient progress. *American Psychologist, 51,* 1059–1064.

Jacobson, N. S., Roberts, L. J., Berns, S., B., & McGlinchey, J. B. (1999). Methods for defining and determining the clinical significance of treatment effects: Description, application, and alternatives. *Journal of Consulting and Clinical Psychology, 67,* 300–307.

Jacobson, N. S., & Truax, P. (1991). Clinical significance: A statistical approach to defining meaningful change in psychotherapy research. *Journal of Consulting and Clinical Psychology, 59,* 12–19.

Jamison, R. N., Rudy, T. E., Penzien, D. B., & Mosley, T. H., Jr. (1994). Cognitive-behavioral classifications of chronic pain: Replication and extension of empirically derived patient profiles. *Pain, 57,* 277–292.

Jones, B., Jarvis, P., Lewis, J. A., & Ebbutt, A. F. (1996). Trials to assess equivalence: The importance of rigorous methods. *British Medical Journal, 313,* 36–39.

Kaplan, R. M. (1990). Behavior as the central outcome in health care. *American Psychologist, 45,* 1211–1220.

Kazdin, A. E. (1998). Treatment manuals in clinical practice: Introduction to the series. *Clinical Psychology Science and Practice, 5,* 361–632.

Keisler, D. J. (1966). Some myths of psychotherapy research and the search for a paradigm. *Psychological Bulletin, 65,* 110–136.

Kopta, S. M., Lueger, R. J., Saunders, S. M., & Howard, K. I. (1999). Individual psychotherapy outcome and process research: Challenges to greater turmoil or a positive transition? *Annual Review of Psychology, 50,* 441–469.

Main, C. J., & Spanswick, C. C. (2000). *Pain management: An interdisciplinary approach.* Edinburgh, UK: Churchill Livingstone.

McDowell, I., & Newell, C. (1996). *Measuring health: A guide to rating scales and questionnaires* (2nd ed.). New York: Oxford University Press.

McQuay, H. J., & Moore, R. A. (1997). Using numerical results from systematic reviews in clinical practice. *Annals of Internal Medicine, 126,* 712–720.

Michell, J. (1977). Quantitative science and the definition of measurement in psychology. *British Journal of Psychology, 88,* 355–383.

Morley, S. (1996). Single case research. In G. Parry & F. N. Watts (Eds.), *Behavioural and mental health research: A handbook of skills and methods* (2nd ed., pp. 277–314). Hove, UK: Erlbaum.

Morley, S., Eccleston, C., & Williams, A. (1999). Systematic review and meta-analysis of randomized controlled trials of cognitive behaviour therapy and behaviour therapy for chronic pain in adults, excluding headache. *Pain, 80,* 1–13.

Nathan, P. E., Stuart, S. P., & Dolan, S. L. (2000). Research on psychotherapy efficacy and effectiveness: Between Scylla and Charybdis? *Psychological Bulletin, 126,* 964–981.

Newton-John, T. O., Spence, S. H., & Schotte, D. (1995). Cognitive-behavioural therapy versus EMG biofeedback in the treatment of chronic low back pain. *Behaviour Research and Therapy, 33,* 691–697.

Nicholas, M., Molloy, A., Tonkin, L., & Beeston, L. (2000). *Manage your pain.* Sydney, Australia: ABC Books.

Nicholas, M. K., Wilson, P. H., & Goyen, J. (1991). Operant-behavioural and cognitive-behavioural treatment for chronic low back pain. *Behaviour Research and Therapy, 29,* 225–238.

Okifuji, A., Turk, D. C., & Eveleigh, D. J. (1999). Improving the rate of classification of patients with the multidimensional pain inventory (MPI): Clarifying the meaning of "significant other." *Clinical Journal of Pain, 15,* 290–296.

Parloff, M. B. (1998). Is psychotherapy more than manual labor? *Clinical Psychology-Science and Practice, 5,* 376–381.

Paul, G. L. (1967). Strategy of outcome research in psychotherapy. *Journal of Consulting Psychology, 31,* 109–118.

Peters, J. L., & Large, R. G. (1990). A randomised control trial evaluating in- and outpatient pain management programmes. *Pain, 41,* 283–293.

Philips, H. C., & Rachman, S. (1996). *The psychological management of chronic pain: A treatment manual* (2nd ed.). New York: Springer.

Raue, P. J., Goldfried, M. R., & Barkham, M. (1997). The therapeutic alliance in psychodynamic-interpersonal and cognitive-behavioral therapy. *Journal of Consulting and Clinical Psychology, 65,* 582–587.

Rosenthal, R. (1994). Parametric measures of effect size. In H. Cooper & L. V. Hedges (Eds.), *The handbook of research synthesis* (pp. 231–244). New York: Russell Sage Foundation.

Rudy, T. E., Turk, D. C., Kubinski, J. A., & Zaki, H. S. (1995). Differential treatment responses of TMD patients as a function of psychological characteristics. *Pain, 61,* 103–112.

Rudy, T. E., Turk, D. C., Zaki, H. S., & Curtin, H. D. (1989). An empirical taxometric alternative to traditional classification of temporomandibular disorders. *Pain, 36,* 311–320.

Sackett, D. L., & Cook, R. J. (1994). Understanding clinical trials. *British Medical Journal, 309,* 755–756.

Safran, J. D., & Segal, Z. V. (1990). *Interpersonal processes in cognitive therapy.* New York: Basic Books.

Sanders, C., Egger, M., Donovan, J., Tallon, D., & Frankel, S. (1998). Reporting on quality of life in randomised controlled trials: Bibliographic study. *British Medical Journal, 317,* 1191–1194.

Schwartz, C. E., Chesney, M. A., Irvine, J., & Keefe, F. J. (1997). The control group dilemma in clinical research: Applications for psychosocial and behavioral medicine trials. *Psychosomatic Medicine, 59,* 362–371.

Shaw, B. F., Elkin, I., Yamaguchi, J., Olmsted, M., Vallis, T. M., Dobson, K. S., Lowery, A., Sotsky, S. M., Watkins, J. T., & Imber, S. D. (1999). Therapist competence ratings in relation to clinical outcome in cognitive therapy of depression. *Journal of Consulting and Clinical Psychology, 67,* 837–846.

Shoham-Salomon, V., & Hannah, M. T. (1991). Client-treatment interaction in the study of differential change processes. *Journal of Consulting and Clinical Psychology, 59,* 217–225.

Smith, B., & Sechrest, L. (1991). Treatment of aptitude-treatment interactions. *Journal of Consulting and Clinical Psychology, 59,* 233–244.

Snow, R. E. (1991). Aptitude-treatment interaction as a framework for research on individual differences in psychotherapy. *Journal of Consulting and Clinical Psychology, 59,* 205–216.

Stiles, W. B., Agnew-Davies, R., Hardy, G. E., Barkham, M., & Shapiro, D. A. (1998). Relations of the alliance with psychotherapy outcome: Findings in the second Sheffield Psychotherapy Project. *Journal of Consulting and Clinical Psychology, 66,* 791–802.

Stiles, W. B., Shapiro, D. A., & Elliott, R. (1986). Are all psychotherapies equivalent? *American Psychologist, 41,* 165–180.

Strosahl, K. (1998). The dissemination of manual-based psychotherapies in managed care: Promises, problems, and prospects. *Clinical Psychology-Science and Practice, 5,* 382–386.

Turk, D. C. (2000a). Everyone has won and all must have prizes. [Editorial]. *Clinical Journal of Pain, 16,* 93–94.

Turk, D. C. (2000b). Statistical significance and clinical significance are not synonyms! [Editorial]. *Clinical Journal of Pain, 16,* 185–187.

Turk, D. C., & Meichenbaum, D. (1994). A cognitive-behavioral approach to pain management. In P. D. Wall & R. Melzack (Eds.), *Textbook of pain* (3rd ed., pp. 1337–1348). Edinburgh, UK: Churchill Livingstone.

Turk, D. C., Meichenbaum, D., & Genest, M. (1983). *Pain and behavioral medicine: A cognitive-behavioral perspective.* New York: Guilford Press.

Turk, D. C., & Melzack, R. (Eds.). (1992). *Handbook of pain assessment.* New York: Guilford Press.

Turk, D. C., Okifuji, A., Sinclair, J. D., & Starz, T. W. (1998). Differential responses by psychosocial subgroups of fibromyalgia syndrome patients to an interdisciplinary treatment. *Arthritis Care and Research, 11,* 397–404.

Turk, D. C., & Rudy, T. E. (1988). Toward an empirically derived taxonomy of chronic pain patients: Integration of psychological assessment data. *Journal of Consulting and Clinical Psychology, 56,* 233–238.

Turk, D. C., & Rudy, T. E. (1992). Cognitive factors and persistent pain: A glimpse into Pandora's box. *Cognitive Therapy and Research, 16,* 99–122.

Turk, D. C., Rudy, T. E., Kubinski, J. A., Zaki, H. S., & Greco, C. M. (1996). Dysfunctional patients with temporomandibular disorders: Evaluating the efficacy of a tailored treatment protocol. *Journal of Consulting and Clinical Psychology, 64,* 139–146.

Turner, J. A. (1996). Educational and behavioral interventions for back pain in primary care. *Spine, 21,* 2851–2857.

Turner, J. A., Deyo, R. A., Loeser, J. D., Von Korff, M., & Fordyce, W. E. (1994). The importance of placebo effects in pain treatment and research. *Journal of the American Medical Association, 271,* 1609–1614.

Turner, J. A., & Jensen, M. P. (1993). Efficacy of cognitive therapy for chronic low back pain. *Pain, 52,* 169–177.

van Tulder, M. W., Ostelo, R. W., Vlaeyen, J., Linton, S., Morley, S., & Assendelft, W. J. (2000). Behavioral treatment for chronic low back pain: a systematic review within the framework of the Cochrane Back Review Group. *Spine, 25,* 2688–2699.

Vlaeyen, J. W., de Jong, J., Geilen, M., Heuts, P. H., & van Breukelen, G. (2001). Graded exposure *in vivo* in the treatment of pain-related fear: A replicated single-case experimental design in four patients with chronic low back pain. *Behaviour Research and Therapy, 39,* 151–166.

Vlaeyen, J. W., & Linton, S. J. (2000). Fear-avoidance and its consequences in chronic musculoskeletal pain: A state of the art. *Pain, 85,* 317–332.

Vlaeyen, J. W. S., Nooyen-Haazen, I. W. C. J., Goossens, M. E. J. B., van Breukelen, G., Heuts, P. H., & The, H. G. (1997). The role of fear in the cognitive-educational treatment of fibromyalgia. In T. S. Jensen, J. A. Turner, & Z. Wiesenfeld-Hallin (Eds.), *Proceedings of the 8th World Congress on Pain* (Vol. 8, pp. 693–704). Seattle, WA: IASP Press.

Waltz, J., Addis, M. E., Koerner, K., & Jacobson, N. S. (1993). Testing the integrity of a psychotherapy protocol: Assessment of adherence and competence. *Journal of Consulting and Clinical Psychology, 61,* 620–630.

Williams, A. C. de C. (1999). Measures of function and psychology. In R. Melzack & P. D. Wall (Eds.), *Textbook of pain* (4th ed., pp. 427–444). Edinburgh: Churchill Livingstone.

Williams, A. C. de C., Nicholas, M. K., Richardson, P. H., Pither, C. E., & Fernandes, J. (1999). Generalizing from a controlled trial: the effects of patient preference versus randomization on the outcome of inpatient versus outpatient chronic pain management. *Pain, 83,* 57–65.

Wilson, G. T. (1998). Manual-based treatment and clinical practice. *Clinical Psychology-Science and Practice, 5,* 363–375.

Woolf, C. J., Bennett, G. J., Doherty, M., Dubner, R., Kidd, B., Koltzenburg, M., Lipton, R., Loeser, J. D., Payne, R., & Torebjork, E. (1998). Towards a mechanism-based classification of pain? *Pain, 77,* 227–229.

II

TREATMENT APPROACHES AND METHODS

4

Enhancing Motivation to Change in Pain Treatment

Mark P. Jensen

Pain clinicians and researchers have many reasons to be proud. They have eased the pain and suffering of countless individuals through the development, refinement, and provision of a great variety of pain treatments. Most of these treatments, such as relaxation training, coping skills training, and multidisciplinary treatment, have all been shown to be effective in controlled studies (see, e.g., Becker, Sjorgren, Bech, Olsen, & Eriksen, 2000; Keefe & Caldwell, 1997; Moore, Von Korff, Cherkin, Saunders, & Lorig, 2000; Vlaeyen et al., 1996). That is, *on average*, individuals who received these treatments have done significantly better than those who did not receive treatment.

Unfortunately, despite the growing research base that supports the effectiveness of current pain treatments on average, many people remain who do not improve or who relapse (Turk, 1990; Turk & Rudy, 1991). There are numerous possible explanations for treatment failure, including the likelihood that some treatments are effective only for subgroups of pain sufferers (Turk, 1990). Another possible explanation concerns *motivation* for treatment (Karoly, 1980). To the extent that an intervention requires a patient to be an active participant, treatment should

be effective only for those individuals who demonstrate a willingness to participate. If this is true, then assessing and enhancing patient motivation prior to treatment should help to reduce treatment failure.

On the assumption that client motivation is an important component of behavior change, William Miller and his colleagues (Miller, 1983; Miller & Rollnick, 1991; Miller, Zweben, DiClemente, & Rychtarik, 1992; Rollnick & Miller, 1995) have been developing an approach to clinician–client interactions that focuses on enhancing client's motivation to change. This approach, called motivational interviewing (MI), was initially developed to help problem drinkers cut down on or abstain from drinking alcohol (see, e.g., Bien, Miller, & Boroughs, 1993; Brown & Miller, 1993: Miller, Benefield, & Tongigan, 1993). However, MI has also been used to help individuals change a number of other problem behaviors (e.g., smoking, heroin dependency, HIV risk behaviors, and child sexual abuse; see Miller, 1996).

My purpose in this chapter is to review, for pain clinicians, the principles and strategies of MI, and to examine how this approach may be used to facilitate changes in health behaviors thought to influence the long-term adaptation to pain conditions. Because MI focuses on patient motivation, it may be used in a variety of settings and in conjunction with a variety of interventions. For the purposes of this chapter, *motivation* refers to "the probability that a person will enter into, continue, and adhere to a specific change strategy" (Miller & Rollnick, 1991, p. 19). Motivation is demonstrated by what a patient *does*, not by what he or she *says*.

An assumption of MI is that people generally have the skills necessary to be able to engage in adaptive behaviors. Concerning adaptive responses to pain, for example, nearly everyone with a pain problem knows how to exercise (e.g., walk), to relax, or to refuse suggestions that they take analgesic medications on a pain-contingent basis. A lack of skill or knowledge, then, may not explain people's choice to display maladaptive responses to pain. Some of these individuals may lack motivation to engage in adaptive coping strategies. MI strategies, as applied to chronic pain problems, are designed primarily to address this motivational problem. In MI, the role of the clinician is to provide an environment that will lead to a greater probability that the patient will respond in an adaptive way—that is, an environment that increases motivation.

My primary hope is that this chapter will interest pain clinicians in incorporating MI strategies into their practice to increase the chances that their patients will follow through with recommendations for those changes deemed necessary for treatment success. I also hope that the ideas expressed here will encourage continued empirical investigations into the application of these strategies with chronic pain patients. I begin the chapter with an outline of the stages-of-change model and a review of the assumptions on which MI is based. In the remainder (and bulk) of the chapter, I present the principles and therapeutic strategies of MI. Throughout, my discussion focuses on how these strategies can be applied to the treatment of pain problems.

Stages of Change

MI is based on the assumption that people vary in the degree to which they are ready to engage in new adaptive behaviors. This assumption has been supported in the research of DiClemente and Prochaska (1982), who have identified specific stages through which people move as they change from maladaptive to adaptive behaviors (graphically presented in Figure 4.1). According to this model, each stage poses different challenges for the individual that need to be addressed before that person can move on to the next stage (Prochaska, DiClemente, & Norcross, 1992). People who are not considering any changes in their behavior are in the *precontemplation* stage. Precontemplators will show active resistance to change when and if they feel coerced into changing some behavior that other people, not they themselves, view as a problem. *Contemplation* is a stage in which a person sees the need to change and is seriously considering making some change in the near future but has yet to commit to that change. Contemplators are in a state of weighing the pros and cons of changing their behavior. *Preparation* (also known as the *decision making* or *determination* stage) involves both an intention to make changes and initial behavioral steps in the direction of change. The fourth stage, *action*, is evidenced by concrete activities that will lead to the desired change. Individuals in the fifth stage, called *maintenance,* are making active efforts to sustain the changes made in the action stage. Those unable to sustain the changes they have made are said to be in the stage of *relapse.* From there, they may reenter the change cycle at any point (e.g., give up and become precontemplators or start right back in again at the action stage).

Some important characteristics of the stages-of-change model influence how a clinician might think about and intervene with individuals engaging in problem behaviors. First, the model predicts who is most likely to benefit from interventions that require a patient to take action. People in different change stages should evidence different treatment success rates, with those in the action stage more likely to benefit than those in the precontemplation stage. Treatment outcome research supports this prediction for a number of treatments and conditions (e.g., Beitman et al., 1994; Prochaska & DiClemente, 1992; Treasure et al., 1999; Wells-Parker, Kenne, Spratke, &

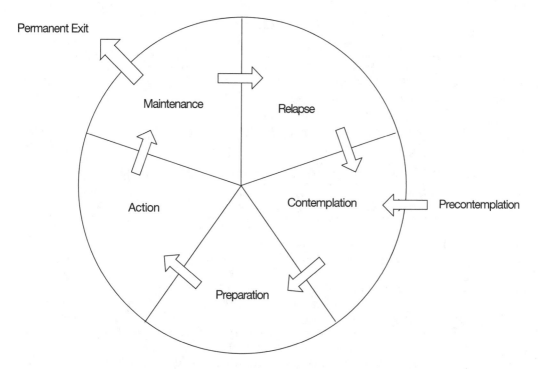

FIGURE 4.1. Prochaska and DiClemente's stage model of the process of change. Adapted from Miller and Rollnick (1991). Copyright 1991 by The Guilford Press. Adapted by permission.

Williams, 2000). Moreover, in two separate studies, pretreatment scores on the Precontemplation subscale of a recently developed measure of readiness to adopt a self-management approach to chronic pain (the Pain Stages of Change Questionnaire, or PSOCQ; Kerns, Rosenberg, Jamison, Caudill, & Haythornthwaite, 1997) predicted lack of completion of pain self-management treatment programs (Biller, Arnstein, Caudill, Federman, & Guberman, 2000; Kerns & Rosenberg, 2000).

The implication of these findings is that the same treatment should not be provided to everyone who is engaging in a problem behavior. Rather, treatment should be tailored to each patient's readiness stage. Those in the preparation or action stage should be provided with specific advice, recommendations, and encouragement on how to make behavioral changes. However, those in the precontemplation or contemplation stage should first be provided with therapeutic responses that will facilitate their moving into the preparation and action stages. In support of this idea, Prochaska, DiClemente, and Norcross (1992) note that merely helping patients move from one change stage to the next *doubles* their chances of taking action to quit smoking within the next 6 months. Table 4.1 lists the specific clinician tasks associated with each change stage, according to MI principles (Miller & Rollnick, 1991).

Another important implication of the stages-of-change model is its recognition that relapse is a part of the change process. For example, in their initial research, Prochaska and DiClemente (1982) found that smokers tended to move through the various stages from three to seven times (on average, four) before finally quitting smoking for good. For many patients, relapse can be predicted, prepared for, and (perhaps most important) learned from, so that relapse is less likely to occur next time.

Basic Assumptions of Motivational Interviewing

The MI clinician has a single major purpose: to provide a patient with a response,

TABLE 4.1. **Stages of Change and Therapist Tasks**

Patient's stage	Clinician's motivational tasks
Precontemplation	Raise doubt—increase the patient's perception of the risks and problems associated with the current behavior.
Contemplation	Tip the balance—evoke reasons to change, risks of not changing; strengthen the patient's self-efficacy for change of current behavior.
Preparation	Help the patient to determine the best course of action to take in seeking change.
Action	Help the patient to take steps toward change.
Maintenance	Review progress; renew motivation and commitment as needed.
Relapse	Help the patient review the processes of contemplation, determination, and action, without becoming stuck or demoralized because of relapse.

appropriate to his or her stage of readiness to change, that will facilitate movement through the stages toward maintenance of some adaptive behavior. This requires an ongoing assessment of each patient's readiness to change, as well as flexible and timely application of therapeutic strategies chosen specifically for that patient to enhance movement through the change cycle. However, MI has some assumptions that should be explicitly acknowledged. First the clinician assumes that the behavior change being encouraged is beneficial for the patient. There is little controversy regarding the need to change most of the problem behaviors to which MI approaches have already been applied (e.g., smoking, problem drinking, and heroin abuse). However, some controversy remains concerning the relative adaptiveness of specific behaviors related to pain management. For example, although opioid medication use is strongly discouraged in some treatment programs (Loeser & Turk, 2001), some clinicians believe that there is a place for opioid medications for the management of chronic nonmalignant pain (Portenoy, 1996; Schofferman, 1993; see also McCarberg & Barkin, 2001). Even exercise, which may be considered an essential component of multidisciplinary pain treatment (Loeser & Turk, 2001), has not necessarily been shown to be important to short-term treatment effectiveness (Jensen, Turner, & Romano, 1994, 2001). There is a strong need in the pain treatment literature for well-designed research that will identify which patient behaviors are most adaptive and most maladaptive for which individuals suffering from pain problems. This research may then be used as a guide for clinicians who are in a position to encourage or discourage specific responses to pain.

In the absence of clear empirical guidelines concerning which pain-related behaviors to encourage or discourage in the individuals we serve, perhaps the role of the clinician should be to help motivate the patient to try *something different* from what he or she is currently doing or has tried in the past and then to monitor the effects of this on the functioning of this particular patient. The clinician may thus assist the patient to determine which behaviors seem to be most adaptive for him or her. In fact, given the fact that it is unlikely that specific coping responses are necessarily adaptive or maladaptive for all individuals at all times, such an individualized empirical approach may be useful even after more knowledge is obtained concerning the relative adaptiveness of specific pain responses. In any case, the clinician is in a position to provide specific treatments, and to ensure that the patient gives the intervention an adequate trial, MI strategies may be used to prepare the patient for and maximize adherence to a particular treatment regimen.

Although an assumption of MI is that clinician behavior plays a key role in the development and maintenance of patient motivation, the approach paradoxically argues that the ultimate responsibility for change lies within the patient. In short, the clinician's task is to enhance motivation; the patient's task is to take action. MI clinicians actively avoid doing anything "for" patients or strongly advocate for any one particular action. Interestingly, it appears that placing more responsibility on the patient for action actually increases rather than decreases the probability of behavior change (Miller et al., 1993).

In the remainder of this chapter I outline the five basic principles of MI and then describe motivational enhancement therapy, an approach that may be used to apply MI in persons with chronic pain. In the examples that follow, the "adaptive" pain responses to which the MI strategies are applied include exercise, relaxation, and avoidance of pain-contingent rest and medication use. However, it is important to acknowledge that these responses may not be adaptive for all individuals at all times. To provide examples of the MI approach, it has been necessary to select *some* behaviors to encourage and discourage. However, MI principles and strategies may be applied to *any* behavior.

Five Principles of Motivational Interviewing

Miller and Rollnick (1991) list five principles or tasks that guide the MI clinician. The MI clinician should (1) express empathy, (2) develop discrepancy, (3) avoid argumentation, (4) roll with resistance, and (5) support self-efficacy.

Expressing Empathy

Accurate empathy has been described in detail by Carl Rogers (1957, 1959). It involves efforts to communicate respect for the patient and includes active support for the patient's right to self-determination and direction. The important attitude underlying accurate empathy is acceptance without judgment, criticism, or blame. Such acceptance is not the same thing as agreement. It reflects a desire to understand the patient's perspective and a willingness to reflect that understanding back to the patient. Interestingly, as Miller and Rollnick (1991) point out, this approach seems to have a paradoxical effect of freeing people to change, whereas a more judgmental approach, by forcing resistance, can actually inhibit change.

Developing Discrepancy

The second principle of MI is to develop discrepancy between the patient's current behavior and important goals in his or her life. *How* the clinician helps the patient develop this discrepancy is crucial. So-called confrontational approaches are to be avoided, as they often result in defensive patient responses. Rather, the MI clinician encourages the patient to talk about the problem, listens specifically for discrepancies between patient goals and patient problem behaviors, reflects back discrepancies that are verbalized, and encourages the patient to elaborate these discrepancies. In this process, the patient becomes increasingly aware of how his or her current behavior conflicts with important personal goals.

Avoiding Argumentation

The MI clinician avoids argumentation at all costs—especially that which might involve the clinician's arguing *for* a specific behavior change, resulting in the patient's arguing *against* an adaptive change. Argumentation often gives the patient the opportunity to list reasons to avoid change and may thus inhibit rather than promote change. MI assumes that patient resistance is influenced by clinician behavior. For example, resistance is likely when a clinician tries to pressure a patient to make some change before that patient feels ready to change. If a clinician finds that the patient begins to argue against adaptive behavior change, that is a signal for the clinician to switch strategies.

Rolling with Resistance

Related to the principle of avoiding argumentation is the fourth MI principle—rolling with resistance. The MI clinician avoids argumentation by switching strategies. But what should the clinician switch strategies to? There are several responses to patient resistance other than direct disagreement or arguing. These are described in more detail later, but they generally involve reframing or restating the patient's comment(s) in such a way as to demonstrate the clinician's understanding of the patient's ambivalence about change. Sometimes, when the clinician reflects back the patient's resistant statement, the patient may actually respond by taking on the other side of the argument that he or she just started and come up with arguments for behavior change.

Supporting Self-Efficacy

The fifth principle important to MI is self-efficacy. *Self-efficacy* may be defined as the belief in one's ability to perform a specific behavior (Bandura, 1977). It includes beliefs in one's capabilities and optimism about being successful in behavior change efforts. All efforts to express empathy, develop discrepancy, avoid argumentation, and roll with resistance may prove ineffective if the patient does not believe he or she is capable of making the needed changes. Thus, an important aspect of MI is to make statements and ask questions that promote the patient's hope that change is possible.

Specific Motivational Strategies

The five principles of MI, outlined earlier, may be seen as the overriding tasks or goals of the MI clinician. Next I review specific intervention strategies that are consistent with these principles. What makes these strategies "motivational" is that they have empirical support for influencing patient behavior change. In one application of MI principles, Miller and his colleagues developed a three-phase intervention, called motivational enhancement therapy (MET), to decrease alcohol abuse and dependence (Miller et al., 1992). Phase 1 strategies generally are best used with precontemplators and contemplators and are designed to encourage patients to consider change. Phase 2 strategies may be used with contemplators who appear almost ready to make a commitment for change and are designed to "tip the balance" from ambivalence about change to preparation. Phase 3 strategies are used in follow-up sessions, after the patient has made a commitment to change and has had an opportunity to take action.

Phase 1: Strategies That Enhance Motivation for Behavior Change

Miller and colleagues (1992) describe eight specific therapeutic strategies that encourage motivation to change. These strategies can be used with patients in the precontemplation stage but are especially helpful for contemplators to move them toward preparation and action. In Phase 1, the clinician (l) elicits self-motivational statements, (2) listens with empathy, (3) questions, (4) presents personal feedback, (5) affirms the patient, (6) handles resistance, (7) reframes, and (8) summarizes. Each of these strategies is described here and is illustrated by examples involving encouragement of adaptive pain coping.

ELICITING SELF-MOTIVATIONAL STATEMENTS

Perhaps the skill that distinguishes a MI therapist most clearly from other clinicians is the extent to which he or she asks questions and listens to the patient in such a way as to elicit self-motivational statements. *Self-motivational statements* may be defined simply as arguments for behavior change (e.g., "It's time I did something about this," "OK, I'm ready to try something new," and "I can't go on like this any more").

A number of psychological theories provide a strong rationale for the importance of patients', not clinicians', arguing for change. For example, cognitive dissonance theory (Festinger, 1957) asserts that when people are enticed to make public statements that differ from their previous statements, their beliefs and values shift in the direction of the new statements. Similarly, self-perception theory (Bem, 1967) argues that people learn about themselves through their actions. People know what they believe by what they hear themselves say and see themselves do.

For the purposes of building patient motivation to alter pain-related behaviors, the clinician's task is to elicit from the patient statements that support the following: (1) the patient's recognition of the full nature and extent of the problem, (2) the patient's concern about how he or she is currently managing the problem, (3) the patient's intention of changing in the direction of adaptive pain management, and (4) the patient's optimism that change is possible.

There are two ways to begin to elicit such statements (Miller & Rollnick, 1991). First, the clinician can simply ask for self-motivational statements from the patient. For example, a clinician might ask, "Tell me, what is it that you would like to change about what you are doing now to manage your pain problem?" A second strategy is to ask the patient to express the positive aspects of some maladaptive behavior before asking about the costs of that behavior. Most of us engage in maladaptive behaviors for specific reasons. If nothing else, behaviors such as smoking, eating a high-calorie meal, and inactivity can feel good, at least in the short run. Asking patients to discuss their reasons for maladaptive behaviors, prior to discussing the costs, indicates an acceptance of the ambivalence that most contemplators feel about such behaviors. Moreover, if the major arguments for a maladaptive behavior are reviewed first, the patient will probably feel less of a need to bring up these arguments later; it frees him or her to discuss the "downside" at length. Table 4.2 presents some specific questions that may elicit self-motivational statements among individuals with pain problems. Examples of possible dialogues between a clinician and a patient [with comments in square brackets] in which these questions are used to elicit motivational self-statements follow.

Problem Recognition. The clinician can ask questions to determine whether the problem, as identified by the patient, is getting worse over time rather than better. Frequently, patients report that their pain problem is getting worse, and this information can be used to begin to build a case for making some changes in how the problem is being addressed.

CLINICIAN: During the past several months, do you see your pain problem getting worse, getting better, or staying the same?

PATIENT: Oh, things are much worse.

CLINICIAN: What exactly—

PATIENT: Well, the pain has been getting worse and worse, and I am getting at the end of my rope. I just can't seem to handle it any more.

CLINICIAN: So the pain is getting worse? How much worse?

PATIENT: Well, not a lot, but my bad days seem to be happening a lot more often.

CLINICIAN: What is a bad day like for you?

TABLE 4.2. Examples of Questions That May Evoke Self-Motivational Statements in Individuals with Pain Problems

1. *Problem recognition*
   "Have things gotten better or worse in the past 6 months?" [Follow up with questions about current coping strategies].
   "What are you now doing to cope with your pain problem? Is this working?"
   "What do you miss most about your life before the pain problem?"

2. *Concern*
   "What concerns you the most about your pain problem?"
   "What scares you about what might happen if you don't try a new approach to this problem?"

3. *Intention to change*
   "The fact that you are here suggests to me that you are interested in seeing things change. How would you like your life to be different?"
   "If you received treatment here, how would you know whether treatment was successful? What would be different in your life?"
   "Of the things that you have control over, what would you like to see change the most?"

4. *Optimism*
   "Have you tried _____ in the past? What was easy and what was difficult about this?"
   "What area of your life has not yet been touched by the pain problem?"
   "What evidence do you have in your life that you could succeed here?"
   "What will make [decreasing your medication use, engaging in an exercise program, etc.] easier for you?"
   "What aspect of your life do you feel the most control over?"
   "What things in your life have you absolutely refused to let the pain control?"

Note. Adapted from Miller and Rollnick (1991). Copyright 1991 by The Guilford Press. Adapted by permission.

Nearly every patient uses *some* strategies to manage pain; some of these may be adaptive and some may be maladaptive. The clinician can use responses to questions about coping to reflect and emphasize (1) the usefulness of adaptive strategies and (2) problems with and concerns about maladaptive ones. By asking about both the benefits and costs, the clinician can get a more balanced picture of the patient's beliefs.

CLINICIAN: What do you do now to cope with your pain problem? Is this working?

PATIENT: Nothing seems to help.

CLINICIAN: I noticed on your diaries that you take an analgesic every day. Is this for pain?

PATIENT: Well, it sometimes takes the edge off the pain, but it doesn't really help much.

CLINICIAN: So the medication helps a little, but it has not taken your pain away. [The clinician hears ambivalence and reflects this to emphasize ambivalence about medication use.]

PATIENT: Yes, and I've had to take more and more to have any effect.

CLINICIAN: That must be very frustrating, to have the drug lose its effectiveness. [The clinician reflects a possible negative emotion and consequence associated with the use of the medication.] Are there any other problems with this medication?

PATIENT: Well, my doctor keeps telling me she does not want to prescribe it, and my husband does not like me using drugs. Sometimes I take many more than I am supposed to, just to try and get some relief. [The patient is providing a number of motivational statements, each of which, as they are emphasized and elaborated, should lead him or her closer to making a decision to try something new.]

Concern. Presumably, the patient is concerned about the problem; otherwise, he or she would not be seeking assistance. Discussing how the patient's life is different, and especially how it is worse, since the pain problem began can be one way to focus on reasons the patient has for managing the pain better.

CLINICIAN: What concerns you most about your pain problem?

PATIENT: It's taken over my life. I can't play with my kids, and I'm no longer working.

CLINICIAN: Which of these has been harder on you? [In order to help the patient develop discrepancies, the clinician should always try to be aware of which problems are of primary concern to the patient.]

PATIENT: I really miss playing with my kids. I can't pick them up or run with them—it's like they don't have a mother any more.

CLINICIAN: You really want to be a good parent. [The clinician reflects a potentially deeply held value to better understand what is important to the patient, as well as to enhance the patient's awareness of this value. Later, the patient may identify maladaptive responses to pain (using excessive opioid or sedative medications, becoming increasingly inactive) that are inconsistent with this value.]

Chances are that if a patient does nothing to change how he or she is managing the problem, or continues to seek invasive medical procedures that have not been recommended or have already been tried without success, the patient will continue to have difficulties managing the pain problem. It is not usually difficult for patients to reach this conclusion, but some direct questions can help emphasize this fact.

CLINICIAN: What scares you about what might happen if you don't try a new approach?

PATIENT: I suppose things will continue to get worse.

CLINICIAN: In what ways? [The clinician asks the patient to elaborate on the self-motivational statement indicating concern about inaction.]

Intention to Change. Asking patients to envision a life in which they are managing the pain problem better can help to begin to establish treatment goals that have meaning to the patient, and can also help to shift the patient in the direction of working toward those goals. Several simple questions may be used to elicit such statements, and the clinician can ask for elaboration or use reflective listening to obtain more detailed information.

CLINICIAN: How would you like your life to be different?

PATIENT: I would like to be pain-free. [The patient begins by setting an unlikely goal, and also a goal that may be incompatible with an active lifestyle.]

CLINICIAN: I can certainly understand wanting to be free of pain. How would your life be different if your pain were to go away? [Rather than pointing out that total pain relief is unlikely—a point better made by the patient than by the clinician—the clinician gives an empathetic response that shows an understanding of the patient's stated wish, while still trying to elicit what a "better life" might look like.]

Optimism. It is not uncommon for people with pain problems to have tried adaptive strategies at some time previously, and to have had at least some success with these strategies. For example, some individuals naturally use distraction and report that they feel better when they are actively engaged in an interesting task. Others report that they experience less pain when they are calm or relaxed. Still others may have tried and experienced an increase in confidence and strength as a result of exercise. Information concerning these past successes is important, and their empathic reflection can help to build optimism for success in the future.

CLINICIAN: I'm interested in hearing about your experience with exercise. Have you tried an exercise program since the onset of the pain problem? If you have, what was easy and what was difficult about this? [As is frequently the case, the clinician is interested in hearing "both sides of the story" about efforts to manage the problem in the past.]

PATIENT: Right after the surgery, my doctor wanted me to walk every day. I was able to do it at first—for about 3 months. But then I fell and had to stay in bed for several weeks. After that, I couldn't walk without a lot of pain.

CLINICIAN: So you were able to maintain a walking program for 3 months [The clinician reflects past success]. During this time, did your tolerance for walking change? [The clinician wants to know about the patient's perceptions of the effects of the walking program. The clinician may reflect and/or ask for elaboration on perceived benefits and improvements. A lack of perceived benefit may be responded to with an affirmation (see below) that the patient's ability to maintain the exercise program, despite immediate benefits, suggests a lot of determination.]

Given the potential importance that perceptions of control may have on the well-being of people with pain problems (see, e.g., Jensen et al., 1994: Lorig, Chastain, Ung, Shoor, & Holman, 1989), as well as the established connection between self-efficacy beliefs and adaptive pain-related behaviors (see, e.g., Jensen, Turner, & Romano, 1991), patients are likely to benefit from increases in self-efficacy and perceived control over pain. Discussions that focus on those times when, or those activities in which, self-control and self-efficacy were maximized should help to enhance patients' self-efficacy.

CLINICIAN: Sometimes people feel like their activities are controlled by their pain; at other times they feel like they are controlling what they do despite the pain. What areas of your life have not yet been touched by the pain problem?

PATIENT: Well, I haven't been able to work because of pain, but I still insist on doing a lot of yardwork. I can't let my husband do *all* the work.

CLINICIAN: I'd like to hear more about how you've managed to do the yardwork despite pain. [And then after discussion of the yardwork, eliciting and praising the patient's efforts to maintain some degree of functioning, the clinician can seek to identify other times when the patient is able to function despite pain. This should remind the patient of her abilities and resources for pain management.] Are there other areas of your life that you feel you've managed to keep on top of, despite the pain problem?

Some patients may feel that they are almost completely controlled by their pain problems, and it may therefore be difficult to elicit self-motivational statements that indicate self-efficacy. Nevertheless, it is true that patients, at least at some level, make choices about control. Emphasizing and reflecting statements that show an understanding of this type of control should also enhance self-efficacy.

CLINICIAN: Sometimes people feel like their activities are controlled by their pain; at other times they feel like they are controlling what they do despite the pain. What areas of your life have not yet been touched by the pain problem?

PATIENT: Everything has been affected by pain. My pain controls everything I do.

CLINICIAN: Have you ever just decided to go ahead and do something despite the pain?

PATIENT: Oh yeah, I used to try and get my work done no matter what. Then the pain would get me, and I've had to learn to tone down my activities quite a bit.

CLINICIAN: So in the past, when you've tried to control over your activities, you've experienced increases in pain. At this point, if I am hearing you right, you maintain a low profile as one way to manage pain. [The clinician reflects the patient's current pattern of decreased activity because of pain. However, by framing this as something the patient does "at this point," the clinician hints at the possibility that the patient may choose another way to handle activities in the future.]

In summary, the goal of the questions listed in Table 4.2 and discussed earlier is to elicit statements indicating problem recognition, concern about how things are going, intention to change, and optimism that change is possible. The goal here is to ask questions and listen carefully to the patient's responses so as to get to the most important reasons for change *from the perspective of the patient*. To the extent that a high number of self-motivational statements are elicited and resistance is minimized (Miller et al., 1993), the patient should be more motivated to try something new.

LISTENING WITH EMPATHY

According to MI principles, empathic listening provides an environment that is extremely important if not essential for helping people take on difficult behavior changes (Miller & Rollnick, 1991; Miller et al., 1992). This therapeutic strategy involves listening carefully to the patient and then reflecting accurately what the patient has said. Empathic listening also acts to minimize patient resistance. It is more difficult for patients to argue with someone who is seeking to understand them than with someone who is challenging them.

Given the high volume of both verbal and nonverbal communication that can occur with every patient phrase, the clinician cannot hope to accurately reflect *everything* a patient says. Through careful selection of

what to reflect back to the patient, reflective listening also may be used to emphasize and reinforce self-motivational statements. The following example illustrates how a clinician might use reflective listening to help a patient clarify the costs of maladaptive pacing (periods of high activity followed by increases in pain and periods of inactivity).

CLINICIAN: Do you ever find that on some days when you are feeling better, you try and get a lot of things done that you have been unable to do, only to find you pay for this later by an increase in pain?

PATIENT: (*Nods vigorously and smiles.*)

CLINICIAN: I seem to have touched a chord. Tell me about that.

PATIENT: Sometimes I just get sick of not being able to do the dishes, so I do them anyway. Then I feel excruciating pain for the next few days and I can't get anything done.

CLINICIAN: There is a lot you would like to be able to do.

PATIENT: I would love to be able to just hold my children again. And I really miss . . .

The clinician in this example is seeking to discover what is important to the patient that the pain problem interferes with. The fact that the patient misses certain activities will become important information to summarize back to the patient as he or she begins to consider trying alternative, adaptive coping strategies. Because it is more patient-directed than direct questioning, empathic listening tends to elicit information that may be more relevant to the patient's perceived needs and desires.

QUESTIONING

There are at least two situations that call for direct questioning. First, direct questions can be used to elicit initial patient responses, which can then be responded to with empathic listening. Many of the interactions presented earlier begin with such questions. A second way to use direct questioning is to ask a series of planned questions (an interview protocol) as a means of efficiently obtaining a great deal of specific information in a short time. In this case, the clinician needs to be aware that the patient has less control over the interaction, so the information obtained may not seem as relevant to the patient concerning his or her pain problem. Therefore, a long series of direct questions without empathic listening may result in increasing patient resistance and should be avoided during most interactions. If the clinician chooses to ask a number of such questions in a series, he or she should watch carefully for signs of resistance and interject empathic listening to minimize any resistance as the session progresses.

"What Seems to Increase Your Pain?" Given the likelihood that patients find pain punishing, knowledge concerning activities that are associated with increased pain gives the clinician knowledge about activities that are perhaps being consistently punished. A patient's report indicating that specific activities are decreasing over time provides further evidence that these activities are being punished, perhaps by the increase in pain associated with them. Often these activities include standing, bending, and lifting. It is unfortunate when such behaviors are punished in the short run because they are often beneficial in moderate amounts for the patient in the long run. A challenge for the clinician is therefore to help the patient develop rewards for these activities, as well as methods for short-circuiting the punishing qualities of pain experience. Rewards may include affirmations from a spouse and self-affirmations for engaging in the activity despite pain. Coping self-statements may decrease the punishing qualities of pain by reframing the pain experience (e.g., "Pain means that the activity is challenging the muscles that need to be challenged; it is a *good* pain," "Despite the pain, I am increasing my tolerance for standing; this will make it easier for me to return to work").

"What Decreases Your Pain?" It is possible that activities associated with decreased pain are negatively reinforced by this pain decrease. Such activities may include medication use and rest. If these activities are increasing over time, it could be construed as further evidence that something, perhaps a decrease in pain, is reinforcing the behavior. To the extent that such activities are maladaptive in the long run, the challenge for the patient and clinician is to develop motivation

for stopping or decreasing these activities, despite the presence of the reinforcement. This development may include contingency management, the use of appropriate coping self-statements, and/or changes in beliefs about the meaning of the pain relief associated with these activities.

"What Is the Effect of Deep Relaxation on Your Pain Experience?" Patients who report a decrease in pain experience with relaxation may be in a good position to seriously consider relaxation training. To the extent that relaxation training may be a treatment option, knowledge concerning the patient's experience and beliefs about relaxation is important.

"How Has the Pain Problem Affected Your Spouse?" MI assumes that clinician behavior influences patient motivation to engage in new, adaptive pain management strategies. Consistent with the MI approach, and with models of chronic pain that focus on the importance of environmental influences on adaptation (Fordyce, 1976; Romano et al., 1992), information concerning the responses of other people to the person in pain is important in developing a viable treatment plan. For example, what, if anything, would a spouse gain or lose as the patient begins to feel better? What could the patient gain or lose from his or her spouse as the patient starts to feel better?

"What Do You Think Is Causing Your Pain?" Patients often have strong beliefs about what is wrong with their bodies that is causing the pain (e.g., "a pinched nerve," "a bulging disk," and "nerve damage"). These beliefs may or may not be consistent with what they have been told by physicians. Concerns and fears about the meaning of pain, unless understood and dealt with, can interfere with progress. This is especially important if progress is initially associated with greater pain, as is often the case with reactivation programs. The answers to questions concerning a patient's beliefs about the cause of pain provide important clues to the frequency and amount of reassurance the patient may need as treatment progresses.

Direct questioning, especially if it can be done with sensitivity and willingness to hear the patient's full response, is an important aspect of assessing motivation to change. Questions can be used to elicit information that can later be summarized to encourage patients to consider approaching their problem in a new way.

PRESENTING PERSONAL FEEDBACK

An additional Phase 1 strategy is providing feedback concerning the effects of the problem behavior on the patient's life. When MET is used with problem drinking, for example, patients are given feedback (based on a pretreatment assessment) on their level of drinking relative to that of same-gender peers, level of intoxication, risk factors for problem drinking, negative consequences of drinking, blood test results, and neuropsychological test results (Miller et al., 1992). Feedback information concerning the effects of maladaptive pain responses would obviously differ from this. However, the primary goal of feedback is the same: to bring into better focus discrepancies between what the patient is doing now to manage the problem and his or her personal goals and core values.

For the purposes of adaptive pain management, feedback given to patients may include (but is not necessarily limited to) the following:

Level of physical functioning relative to same-age, same-gender, and same-level-of-pain-report peers (according to a standardized measure of physical functioning such as the Sickness Impact Profile [SIP]; Bergner, Bobbitt, Carter, & Gilson, 1981).
Use of opioid medications as a risk factor for increased pain over time.
Presence of sleep disturbance (including sleep onset insomnia, early morning awakening, and nocturnal awakenings).
Impact of pain problem on social role functioning, including family and work responsibilities.

Of course, for the clinician to provide feedback, information concerning each of the components of the feedback needs to be obtained prior to the feedback session. Much of this information may be obtained by administering standardized tests (e.g.,

the Sickness Impact Profile) or specific items on questionnaires. Other information may be obtained in a prior interview. The key is to consolidate this information and then to present it in such a way as to encourage the patient's motivation to change in the direction of more effective pain management, as well as to build hope that such efforts will be beneficial.

Once the feedback information to be provided has been consolidated, the clinician is ready to present it to the patient. The most important, and most challenging, aspect of this portion of the session is the way feedback is presented. Each important piece of information is reviewed with the patient. Patients are given time to ask questions about and respond to the information provided. The clinician's task is to adapt the timing of feedback to fit each patient's ability to process the information. Self-motivational statements that patients make during the feedback session should be accurately reflected as they occur. In addition, as the data are discussed, questions may be asked to elicit such motivational statements (e.g., What do you think of this? and Does it make sense to you?). Patient responses that reflect resistance to the information may be responded to with reflection or reframing (see below). Here are some examples of feedback that is likely to support greater patient motivation to change:

CLINICIAN: [presenting feedback] First, my reading of your medical record indicates that your physicians see you as medically stable. That is, although you continue to experience significant pain, they have not yet found a specific disease process that is causing the pain or that will seriously harm you, over and above the effect of pain on your life. People have a lot of different responses to this type of information, from relief that they do not have some deteriorating disease to frustration that they do not have a specific diagnosis. What is your response to it? Does it make sense to you?

PATIENT: I'd rather have a diagnosis, but if my doctors don't know, they don't know. I know that something is wrong. [This response suggests something in between the belief in the traditional biomedical approach to pain (if it hurts, there must be a physical cause that can be found and fixed) and acceptance that the problem may not have a single specific treatable cause.]

CLINICIAN: Given all this, what are your thoughts and feelings about a new approach? I mean an approach where you stop looking to doctors for a diagnosis or a treatment that will cure pain, and begin to think about ways to manage the pain so you can get on with your life—like working to be the parent you'd like to be? [Here the clinician presents the option of pain management, and raises one of the patient's core values that emerged in earlier discussions.]

CLINICIAN: [presenting feedback] From what you have said to me and your responses to the Sickness Impact Profile, it appears that your pain has had a profound impact on your life. Your percentile score of 75% indicates that you are more disabled than 75 out of 100 of the people we see here who have the same level of pain intensity.

PATIENT: I am more disabled than other people with the same pain level?

CLINICIAN: Yes. Does it make sense to you that different people can be affected differently by the same amount of pain? [The clinician here suggests the possibility that people can vary in their adaptation to pain, implicitly indicating that the patient may be able to function better even with the same amount of pain. As always, making this suggestion and then asking the patient whether the idea makes sense to him or her should make the idea easier to accept than lecturing would.]

PATIENT: I guess some people can handle pain more than others. I have a real hard time with pain. [The patient seems to view pain tolerance as a trait rather than a learned skill—an idea inconsistent with his or her learning how to tolerate pain well.]

CLINICIAN: I'm curious, in yourself, do you find that there are days when you seem to be better able to manage the pain? [This question is designed to encourage the patient to consider the possibility that pain tolerance may not be consistent from day to day, and therefore may be changeable through purposeful efforts.]

A defensive response to feedback, that the patient is having a difficult time managing the pain's impact on his or her life, relative to other individuals reporting the same pain level, should be met with reflection rather than argumentation. Perhaps such a patient needs additional reassurance that the clinician understands how difficult the pain problem is for the patient:

PATIENT: I think I am doing as good as I can.

CLINICIAN: I actually think you've done very well, considering how difficult pain can be to deal with. You've kept up on a lot of yardwork, and you've made a lot of effort to continue to be as good a parent as you can for your children.

Some patients may also have a difficult time understanding the percentile concept, or the associated idea that people who report the same pain level can evidence substantially different responses to pain. However, attempts to lecture the patient concerning this concept may backfire. Even if the patient eventually gets the concept, the lecturing clinician runs the risk of alienating the patient (Patient: "My clinician talks down to me"). A response more consistent with the MI approach would be to reflect the patient's concern and to plan to discuss the possibility of differential adaptation to pain problems at a later time.

PATIENT: Anyone with as much pain as I have would have their life affected!

CLINICIAN: I have to agree with you. Pain problems have a big impact on people, and I think you are working hard to manage this as best you can right now.

AFFIRMING THE PATIENT

The MI clinician seeks to affirm the patient at every opportunity. Affirmations, in the form of direct compliments and praise, provide a more positive environment for change by increasing rapport, enhancing patient self-esteem, encouraging patient responsibility, and reinforcing patient self-motivational statements (Miller et al., 1992). Affirming statements may be contrasted with reflective statements: The former are sincere expressions of the *clinician's* positive responses to the patient, whereas the latter consist of efforts to reflect the *patient's* concerns.

HANDLING RESISTANCE

Most psychological models of pain, or any model that includes recognition of a psychological component in pain problems, place important emphasis on what the patient does and how he or she thinks about the pain problem (e.g., Turk, Meichenbaum, & Genest, 1983). Therefore, for a large number of people seeking help, something about what they are doing or thinking about the pain problem may be contributing to their difficulties. However, there are probably legitimate reasons (at least in the patients' minds) for using maladaptive coping strategies or thinking maladaptive thoughts concerning the pain. One of these reasons may be simply lack of information or lack of skills. If this were the whole story, however, simple skill training should be enough to assist all people with pain problems. Other reasons for maladaptive responding exist, and one of these is patients' "resistance" to trying new, adaptive approaches.

Miller and colleagues (1992) define resistance as a set of specific client behaviors, such as interrupting, arguing, sidetracking, or defensive responding, that appear to be associated with poor treatment outcome. A key MI concept in managing patients' resistant behaviors is to monitor interactions for such behaviors and then to *change strategies* when such behaviors emerge. Clinician responses that tend to evoke resistance, and that therefore should be avoided, include arguing, criticizing, warning a patient of negative consequences, active persuasion, analyzing or questioning possible reasons for resistance, confronting, or using sarcasm (Miller & Jackson, 1995; Miller et al., 1992). Any persuasion to be done is best done by the patient, not the clinician.

Four strategies for dealing with resistance are simple reflection, double-sided reflection, shifting focus, and rolling with resistance (Miller & Rollnick, 1991).

PATIENT: I never exercised before I had a pain problem. I don't see how I can do it now!

CLINICIAN: Before you had a pain problem, you did not see any reason to exercise. Now, with the pain, it seems like a real challenge to you. [By reflecting the patients concerns, the clinician avoids telling the patient "You can do it" and thereby avoids a series of "Yes, but" responses in which the patient systematically lists all his or her reasons for being unable to exercise. Acknowledging the perceived difficulty of exercising regularly can serve at least two purposes. First, it reflects what the patient is saying, and thus has the positive effects of accurate empathy. In addition, by re-

framing exercise as a "challenge" instead of the implied impossibility, the clinician may increase hope that such behavior is possible, and also help set up the patient for affirmation later ("You have successfully overcome this challenge").]

PATIENT: If I exercise, it will just make my pain problem worse.

CLINICIAN: Maybe it seems crazy to you that I think exercise might be worth another try, given some of the problems you've had with exercise in the past. [Although appropriate (i.e., gradually increasing and quota-based) reactivation is central to many chronic pain treatment programs, many patients express significant worry and concern about exercise. These concerns are realistic, given their previous attempts to exercise. Reflection allows such a patient to hear that the clinician understands and acknowledges this concern.]

PATIENT: It is hard for me to imagine going without my pain medications.

CLINICIAN: You are worried about being able to manage your pain without medications, yet you also seem to be considering it. What are your worries, and also why are you even considering this at this time? [That the patient states a difficulty thinking about going without medications suggests at least some effort to consider being medication-free. A double-sided reflection usually incorporates both sides of an argument. Double-sided reflective statements have at least two beneficial effects. First, they acknowledge that nearly any behavior change has both benefits and costs; to the extent that the patient may have previously been unwilling to consider behavior change, a balanced view represents movement in an adaptive direction. Second, encouraging the patient to consider both sides often elicits self-motivational statements, which can later be reflected back.]

PATIENT: I will never, ever give up my pain medications.

CLINICIAN: It seems to me that it is hard for you to imagine life without pain medications. A lot of people feel like this at first. But now is *not* the time to make any final decisions about how you want to handle this problem for the rest of your life. Today, let's just review what you are now doing to manage your pain. I hope that by doing this, I can begin to understand, from your perspective, which of these seem to be working. As we progress, I hope to learn if there are any coping strategies you are not currently using that you would be interested in learning more about. [It is important to avoid arguing strongly for a particular coping strategy. In order to avoid this, the clinician may choose to shift focus completely away from the issue when a patient expresses strong resistant statements, and to focus instead on an issue that is more likely to result in self-motivational statements.]

PATIENT: I will never, ever give up my pain medications.

CLINICIAN: You may be right. After we are through. you may decide to continue to seek prescriptions for pain medications. That choice will be yours to make. [A second way to manage confrontational statements is simply to acknowledge the possibility of their truth. By not arguing in response, a clinician avoids pushing a patient into expressing all the reasons for not changing. However, even when rolling with the resistance (essentially, agreeing with some component of what the patient is saying), the clinician has an opportunity to emphasize patient choice, as well as the *possibility,* that the patient may chose to engage in the adaptive behavior sometime in the future.]

REFRAMING

Reframing involves providing the patient with feedback that (1) puts the patient's maladaptive behavior in a generally positive light and (2) still allows for the possibility of behavior change. The rationale behind reframing is that if the patient does not have to defend his or her current pattern of responses, he or she will have more energy for changing those responses.

PATIENT: I will never, ever give up my pain medication.

CLINICIAN: You sound to me like a person who can really commit yourself to an action, once you decide that it is good for you.

SUMMARIZING

Toward the end of every session, it is important to set aside a time to summarize the basic content of the session for the patient. A summary serves the primary purpose of allowing patients to hear their own self-motivational statements again. Miller and colleagues (1992) point out that elements of resistant statements should also be included, so that a patient perceives that all his or her statements have been heard. Nevertheless, it is important to emphasize, as much as possible, the self-motivational statements that were elicited during the session.

SUMMARY OF PHASE 1 STRATEGIES

The eight Phase 1 strategies are eliciting self-motivational statements, listening with empathy, asking open-ended questions, presenting personal feedback, affirming the patient, handling resistance, reframing, and summarizing. These strategies are used by the MET clinician in the first session to enhance the patient's motivation to change—that is, to increase the probability that the patient will engage in an adaptive behavior change in the future. Because the clinician alternately leads and follows the patient in this process, the pace that the patient takes in moving toward the preparation and action stages is determined in large part by the patient. Rapid progression (e.g., within minutes), as indicated by a lack of resistant statements and frequent self-motivational statements, suggests that the patient may be ready to prepare to take action; in this case, the clinician should rapidly shift to Phase 2 strategies. Slower progress suggests that the patient is still in the contemplation stage and indicates that more time may be needed for Phase 1 intervention. Slow progress (e.g., a dearth of self-motivational statements) suggests precontemplation, again indicating the need for additional Phase 1 strategies.

Because the patient's responses to Phase 1 strategies provide information about readiness to change, these strategies are an excellent way to assess the patient's stage of change. In this way, MI can be considered both an assessment *and* an intervention approach. As the patient progresses through contemplation and begins to move to preparation, the clinician should switch strategies from those that enhance motivation (Phase 1) to those that strengthen a commitment to change (Phase 2).

Phase 2: Strategies That Strengthen Commitment for Behavior Change

The timing of the switch from Phase 1 to Phase 2 strategies is important. If the clinician switches strategies too early, while the patient is still in the precontemplation stage, then the patient will evidence resistance and progression to the preparation and action stages will be hindered. On the other hand, if the patient is already in the preparation stage, Phase 1 strategies that encourage contemplation may backfire by annoying the patient. Consider, for example, a smoker who has decided that he or she must quit smoking and who visits a health care provider in search of assistance. If the health care provider spends much of the time available for the visit reviewing with the patient all the reasons for quitting smoking, time is wasted that might have been used for reviewing strategies and developing a plan for quitting. On the other hand, consider a precontemplative smoker who visits a health care provider for a diagnosis and possible treatment of an ear infection. If the clinician attempts to assist the patient in developing a plan for quitting smoking, the patient is likely to evidence significant resistance ("I came here for an antibiotic, not a lecture!"). Fitting the motivational strategy to the patient, according to the stage of change the patient is in is an important component of MI.

Once the clinician has determined that the time is right to use Phase 2 strategies, he or she should (1) help the patient to develop a plan for change, (2) communicate free choice, (3) discuss the consequences of changing versus not changing, (4) provide information and advice as requested, (5) roll with resistance, (6) complete a change plan worksheet, (7) recapitulate, and (8) ask for a commitment. Each of these strategies, as they may be used with an individual who experiences pain and who is considering making some life change(s) to become better able to manage the pain, is discussed in the following sections.

DEVELOPING A PLAN FOR CHANGE

A primary goal of Phase 2 strategies is the development of a behavior change plan to which the patient can commit him- or herself.

"Given all of the things we've been talking about, what do you see as your options for making your life better? What do you think will work for you?"

"What are you now thinking about exercise [your medication use, the possibility that relaxation will be helpful, etc.]?"

The difference between these questions and Phase 1 questions should be obvious. Instead of eliciting self-motivational statements (Phase 1 strategy), the clinician is attempting to elicit specific ideas for behavior change. There is a shift from why the patient should consider change to *how* the patient will make changes. At this point, the clinician may consider offering direct suggestions. However, when advising a patient, it is best to (1) ask permission first, (2) couch advice in terms of freedom of choice, and (3) offer several ideas from which the patient can choose. The clinician should avoid attempts to convince the patient of the relative effectiveness of one approach over another. The clinician's primary role is to assist the patient in developing a plan that the patient can become committed to trying.

COMMUNICATING FREE CHOICE

To maximize self-motivation, and to facilitate the attribution of control to the patient, the clinician should provide frequent reminders of the patient's free choice in all aspects of his or her change plan.

"You are free to do whatever you think is best for you. Clearly, what you do will have consequences. I'm wondering whether you are interested in trying a quota-based exercise approach. What are your thoughts about the long-term consequences of trying this approach at this point?"

REVIEWING CONSEQUENCES OF CHANGE VERSUS NO CHANGE

Another effective way to strengthen commitment to change is to review with the patient the consequences of making the change versus not making the change. Most likely, the patient will realize that not making any changes means life as before. Such a life is unsatisfactory for many of the patients that clinicians see.

One way to do this is to ask the patient to review both the pros and cons of changing. Patients may choose to list in two columns on a piece of paper the benefits and costs (or pros and cons) of different options. Such lists—as long as the contents are generated by patients and not "fed" to them by clinicians, and as long as the benefits of behavior change outweigh the costs—should help strengthen patients' motivation to change or maintain a behavior change plan.

PROVIDING INFORMATION AND ADVICE

As patients with pain problems reach the preparation stage, or attempt to manage difficulties with a change plan that is in progress, they may ask for specific information and advice concerning how to proceed. Examples of informational questions asked by patients are as follows:

"Will I be pain-free after completing your program?"
"Will I have to continue to exercise after I am done with your program?"

Questions asking for advice may include the following:

"What do you think I should do?"
"I'm worse now than before I started. What should I do now?"

One way to respond is to provide information based on personal experience or research and then ask a follow-up question concerning what the patient wishes to do. Whenever possible, the clinician should offer a number of possible suggestions (a "menu") from which the patient can choose. This helps emphasize that it is the patient's responsibility to decide.

"I have seen people make different decisions; some have chosen to continue with their plan of increasing activity, while others have chosen to quit at this point. In my experience, those people who have done the best in the long run have been those who have kept at their plan. But I also think that you need to decide what will be best for you. What do you think your options are at this point, and what do you think the short- and long-term consequences of each of these are?"

If the patient continues to ask for advice, it is fine to provide it. Some resistance on the clinician's part to giving advice may help to ensure that the patient is interested in hearing what is being suggested and not seeking to hear information about which he or she can argue.

"I want you to understand that I support your right to decide for yourself what to do, and I'm a little worried that you might feel some pressure to follow any advice that I give. I would only want to make specific suggestions if I can also communicate that I believe you should do what *you* think is best for you."

If the patient expresses the desire to know what the clinician thinks may be best, especially after the clinician communicates some resistance to providing advice, then short and clear advice statements are best. Here are some examples:

"I think you should practice relaxation strategies 30 minutes a day for 3 months, and then decide whether to continue."
"I think you should reward yourself for exercising by spending some time, say 30 minutes, doing something just for you, like relaxing or sitting in a warm bath."

In general, it is always a good idea to follow up any information and advice with questions that gauge the patient's response. Such questions help to emphasize that it is the patient's responsibility to make a final decision as to what he or she is going to do next:

"Do you have any questions about what I said?"
"Does what I said fit with your own experience?"

ROLLING WITH RESISTANCE

It is as important to roll with resistance during Phase 2 as it is in Phase 1. Some ambivalence about change, despite the patient's statements indicating determination to try change, can be expected at every stage. Of course, a high level of resistance may indicate movement away from preparation and back into contemplation. In any case, resistant statements should still be responded to with reflection and reframing. At any stage, direct confrontation or challenging statements from the clinician should be avoided because of the resistant responses such communications elicit in patients.

USING A CHANGE PLAN WORKSHEET

Throughout Phase 2 (which may last only one session), the clinician may choose to keep notes of the information provided by the patient during this phase on a change plan worksheet (see Figure 4.2). This sheet can provide a structure for organizing the most important aspects of the patient's goals and reasons for making changes. Figure 4.2 presents the six issues addressed on the worksheet and discussed next.

"The Changes I Want to Make Are...." Clear goals are important to effective be-

havior change plans. The goals should be ones identified by the patient as important. However, among individuals suffering from chronic, nonmalignant pain, it is wise to avoid listing "decreased pain" as a primary goal. Although many patients identify pain relief as a primary goal at the beginning of treatment, few adaptive behaviors have been shown to have a profound influence on pain intensity in the short run. Moreover, two responses to pain that are thought to be maladaptive (pain-contingent use of opioid medications and pain-contingent rest) often have the short-term effect of decreasing pain experience. Thus, a primary goal of "decreased pain," placed in a prominent position on the change plan worksheet, may actually work *against* long-term positive adaptation. Patients who in-

CHANGE PLAN WORKSHEET

The changes I want to make are:

The most important reasons for making these changes are:

The steps I plan to take in changing are:

The ways that other people can help me are:
     Person   Possible ways to help

I know that my plan is working if:

Some things that could interfere with my plan are:

_____
Signature

FIGURE 4.2. Change plan worksheet. Adapted from Miller, Zweben, DiClemente, and Rychtarik (1992).

sist on keeping pain reduction on the worksheet may be willing to consider "minimization of pain in the long run" as one of several goals.

"The Most Important Reasons for Making These Changes Are . . ." Here is where the clinician can list the patient's review of the pros and cons of behavior change versus no behavior change. The clinician should be sure to emphasize those reasons for behavior change that the patient deems most important, especially those related to the patient's core values.

"The Steps I Plan to Take in Changing Are . . ." Under this heading, the clinician should list the ideas the patient has stated for making specific changes. Ideas initiated by the clinician may be included if the patient has endorsed these ideas as his or her own. The more specific these plans can be, the more helpful this section of the worksheet will be to the patient.

"The Ways Other People Can Help Me Are . . ." Pain clinicians have long recognized the importance of other people's responses to the patient in influencing patient functioning (e.g., Flor, Turk, & Rudy, 1989; Romano et al., 1992). Discussing with the patient, and with someone close to the patient (e.g., a spouse) if such a person is available, specific steps that the other person can take to assist the patient in making adaptive changes should increase the chances that such changes will actually occur.

"I Will Know That My Plan Is Working If . . ." Because making adaptive changes to pain problems can be challenging, it is important to identify signposts that indicate that the patient is going in the right direction. Such signposts can act as potential reinforcers for the efforts made, even if the final goal has not yet been reached.

"Some Things That Could Interfere with My Plan Are . . ." To the extent that patients can identify specific problems they may encounter, and come up with plans for addressing these problems, specific hurdles may be avoided altogether or at least more easily dealt with.

RECAPITULATING

The recapitulating strategy for Phase 2 provides benefits similar to those of the summarizing strategy for Phase 1. Patients get to hear once again their reasons for making change and their plan for change. The change plan worksheet, used by the clinician to keep track of the issues raised by the patient during Phase 2, may be used as a guide. Changes offered by the patient concerning recapitulation should be incorporated into the change plan worksheet. The patient should get a copy of the worksheet, and one should be included in his or her record.

ASKING FOR A COMMITMENT

The final strategy to employ with patients in Phase 2 is to ask them to commit themselves to the plan they have outlined. Miller and colleagues (1992) list several issues that may be worth exploring when obtaining a commitment. First, it is important to clarify what exactly a patient intends to do. This is a good time to review the change plan worksheet, beginning with the responses to the "The steps I plan to take in changing are . . ." stem. Are the steps, as listed, actually what the patient intends to do? The other components of the change plan worksheet should also be reviewed at this time, including perceptions of the benefits of change and the costs of inaction and concerns about what might interfere with making the change and how to deal with these obstacles. Following this review, the clinician should simply ask the patient for a commitment to follow through with his or her plan: "Are you ready to commit yourself to doing this?" If so, the clinician can ask the patient to sign the change plan worksheet, give the patient a copy, and retain a copy for the patient's records.

If the patient does not feel ready to commit to a plan of action at this time, the clinician should ask the patient what he or she would like to do now. Any pressure to "go ahead and try" some aspects of the plan (from the clinician) should be avoided. The patient may wish to think about the plan until the next visit or session. No patient should feel *pushed* into making a decision to change before he or she feels ready to do so, as this is likely to result in more rather than less resistance to change in the long run.

Phase 2 strategies should be used with patients who are in the preparation or action stages. The primary purposes of Phase 2 strategies are to develop a behavior change plan and obtain a commitment to this plan. The strategies themselves are as follows: helping the patient to develop a plan, communicating free choice, discussing the consequences of changing versus not changing, providing information and advice as requested, rolling with resistance, completing a change plan worksheet, recapitulating, and asking for a commitment. At the end of Phase 2, the patient should have a plan to make one or more specific behavior changes and should have expressed commitment to follow through on the plan. The next phase, Phase 3, involves following up with the patient on his or her efforts.

Phase 3: Follow-Through Strategies

On the premise that the most difficult obstacle to making adaptive behavior changes is lack of motivation to change, and not a lack of information or skills, Phases 1 and 2 of MET may be considered the most difficult and challenging for the clinician. Once motivation to change has been developed (Phase 1), and this motivation has been shaped into a clear plan of action and commitment to change (Phase 2), adaptive changes should occur. Phase 3, follow-up and follow-through, consists of only three basic strategies: reviewing progress, renewing motivation (if needed), and renewing commitment (if needed).

REVIEWING PROGRESS

The first thing to do in a follow-up session is to review the changes that have occurred since the last session. The clinician should review the specific commitment and plans made at the last session and explore the progress that has been made toward the plan. Any and all approximations of progress should be praised and reinforced as much as possible. Although the occasional patient appears annoyed with praise (making it necessary for the clinician to pro-

vide alternative creative reinforcers), most people appreciate acknowledgment of and praise for their efforts. It is appropriate to express such praise in as dramatic a way and for as long as the patient and session will permit.

RENEWING MOTIVATION

An assessment of motivation to change may include a review of the behavioral indicants of motivation (as reflected in what the patient has done since the last session), as well as the patient's responses to questions concerning reasons for making or maintaining changes. Any indications of a decrease in motivation to change can be met with Phase 1 strategies to renew motivation, if needed.

RENEWING COMMITMENT

Finally, Phase 2 strategies may be used to refine the change plan worksheet (if needed) and obtain a commitment to follow through on the new plan.

What if Motivational Interviewing Does Not Work?

What should the clinician do if all efforts to increase a patient's motivation to change and to solidify that motivation into a specific commitment fail? All clinicians have worked with patients in the precontemplative stage who continue to employ maladaptive coping strategies for pain management *and* appear to refuse to consider that what they are doing to manage the problem has a negative impact on their functioning. Such patients may not be interested in the MI approach and become so annoyed with the MI strategies and questions that they refuse to make or keep appointments. Although ambivalence to change exists in all patients, some simply may not have the patience to work with a clinician to develop motivation and commitment to try a new approach. With such patients, I still seek to plant a seed of adaptive responding, even if only during a single interaction.

"In the little time we have had to get to know each other, I hope you understand that I respect your right to make all decisions about how you will handle this problem. I hear you saying that you are convinced that another surgery has the best chances of making you feel better, and surgery is not something that we offer. If at some time in the future you become interested in considering other approaches to managing the pain, I want you to know that we are here to help you do that."

General Summary and Conclusions

The purpose of this chapter has been to introduce pain clinicians to the philosophy and strategies of MI. Although MI was initially developed to assist problem drinkers, this approach has been adapted to the treatment of other health-related problem behaviors (Miller & Rollnick, 1991). The MI approach appears to translate well to the treatment of pain problems, given the multiple motivational challenges that people who experience pain face in trying to develop and maintain adaptive responses to their problems. I have proposed that motivational problems may explain the lack of effectiveness of pain treatment programs for some individuals. Motivational problems may also explain relapse among some of the individuals for whom pain treatment was initially effective. For these individuals, the use of MI strategies may enhance the effectiveness of treatment among some and perhaps prevent relapse among others.

Moreover, the MI approach is consistent with current multidisciplinary pain treatment practice (Loeser & Turk, 2001). Multidisciplinary treatment emphasizes the encouragement of pain coping responses over which the individual has control, such as exercise, appropriate pacing of activities, non-pain-contingent activity, and avoidance of responses that are outside the direct control of the individual (e.g., pain-contingent opioid or sedative/hypnotic medication use, invasive procedures, and multiple medical tests).

MI, by emphasizing empathic listening, frequent patient affirmations, gentle persuasion, and avoidance of argument, significantly reduces patient resistance to clinician–patient interactions. Patients whom others might have described as "bitter, angry, resentful, and resistant" are much easier to deal with when MI strategies are used. As a clinician working in this field, I have found that efforts to incorporate MI strate-

gies into my interactions with patients have made my job much more pleasant.

It is possible that making the clinician's job more pleasant is the only impact that the use of MI strategies will have. However, I believe that this approach holds significant promise for increasing treatment effectiveness and patients' satisfaction with treatment, as well as for decreasing relapse. Models of empirical tests of MI strategies, comparing them to more traditional approaches, already exist in the literature (see Miller et al., 1993). Moreover, there has been a recent increase in the number of empirical tests of the transtheoretical model of change as it applies to persons with chronic pain problems, with the findings providing support for the utility of this model in persons with pain (e.g., Dijkstra, Vlaeyen, Rijnen, & Nielson, 2001; Jensen, Nielson, Romano, Hill, & Turner, 2000; Keefe et al., 2000; Keller, Herda, Ridder, & Basler, 2001). Pain clinicians and researchers have a long tradition of applying useful models and treatment strategies to ease the suffering of their patients. Perhaps MI will become one of these.

References

Bandura. A. (1977). Self-efficacy: Toward a unifying theory of behavioral change. *Psychological Review, 84*, 191–215.

Becker, N., Sjogren, P., Bech, P., Olsen, A. K., & Eriksen, J. (2000). Treatment outcome of chronic non-malignant pain patients managed in a Danish multidisciplinary pain centre compared to general practice: A randomized controlled trial. *Pain, 84*, 203–211.

Beitman, B. D., Beck, N. C., Deuser, W. E., Carter, C. S., Davidson, J. R., & Maddock, R. J. (1994). Patient stage of change predicts outcome in a panic disorder medication trial. *Anxiety, 1*, 64–69.

Bem, D. J. (1967). Self-perception: An alternative interpretation of cognitive dissonance phenomena. *Psychological Review, 74*, 183–200.

Bergner, M., Bobbitt, R. A., Carter, W. B., & Gilson, B. S. (1981). The Sickness Impact Profile: Development and final revision of a health status measure. *Medical Care, 19*, 787–805.

Bien, T. H., Miller, W. R., & Boroughs, J. M. (1993). Motivational interviewing with alcohol outpatients. *Behavioural and Cognitive Psychotherapy, 21*, 347–350.

Biller, N., Arnstein, P., Caudill, M. A., Federman, C. W., & Guberman, C. (2000). Predicting completion of a cognitive-behavioral pain management program by initial measures of a chronic patient's readiness for change. *Clinical Journal of Pain,* *16*, 352–359.

Brown, J. M., & Miller, W. R. (1993). Impact of motivational interviewing on participation and outcome in residential alcoholism treatment. *Psychology of Addictive Behaviors, 7,* 211–218.

DiClemente, C. C., & Prochaska, J. O. (1982). Self-change and therapy change of smoking behavior: A comparison of processes of change in cessation and maintenance. *Addictive Behaviors, 7,* 133–144.

Dijkstra, A., Vlaeyen, J. W. S., Rijnen, H., & Nielson, W. (2001). Readiness to adopt the self-management approach to cope with chronic pain in fibromyalgia patients. *Pain, 90,* 37–45.

Festinger, L. (1957). *A theory of cognitive dissonance.* Stanford, CA: Stanford University Press.

Flor, H., Turk, D. C., & Rudy, T. E. (1989). Relationship of pain impact and significant other reinforcement of pain behaviors: The mediating role of gender, marital status, and marital satisfaction. *Pain, 38,* 45–50.

Fordyce, W. E. (1976). *Behavioral methods for chronic pain and illness.* St. Louis, MO: Mosby.

Jensen, M. P., Nielson, W. R., Romano, J. M., Hill, M. L., & Turner, J. A. (2000). Further evaluation of the pain stages of change questionnaire: Is the transtheoretical model of change useful for patients with chronic pain? *Pain, 86,* 255–264.

Jensen, M. P., Turner, J. A., & Romano, J. M. (1991). Self-efficacy and outcome expectancies: Relationship to chronic pain coping strategies and adjustment. *Pain, 44,* 263–269.

Jensen, M. P., Turner, J. A., & Romano, J. M. (l994). Correlates of improvement in multidisciplinary treatment of chronic pain. *Journal of Consulting and Clinical Psychology, 62,* 172–179.

Jensen, M. P., Turner, J. A., & Romano, J. M. (2001). Changes in beliefs, catastrophizing and coping are associated with improvement in multidisciplinary pain treatment. *Journal of Consulting and Clinical Psychology, 69,* 655–662.

Karoly, P. (1980). Person variables in therapeutic change and development. In P. Karoly & J. J. Steffen (Eds.), *Improving the long-term effects of psychotherapy* (pp. 195–261). New York: Gardner Press.

Keefe, F. J., & Caldwell, D. S. (1997). Cognitive behavioral control of arthritis pain. *Medical Clinics of North America, 81,* 277–290.

Keefe, F. J., Lefebvre, J. C., Kerns, R. D., Rosenberg, R., Beaupre, P., Prochaska, J., Prochaska, J. O., & Caldwell, D. S. (2000). Understanding the adoption of arthritis self-management: Stages of change profiles among arthritis patients. *Pain, 87,* 303–323.

Keller, S., Herda, C., Ridder, K., & Basler, H. (2001). Readiness to adopt adequate postural habits: An application of the Transtheoretical Model in the context of back pain prevention. *Patient Education and Counseling, 42,* 175–184.

Kerns, R. D., & Rosenberg, R. (2000). Predicting responses to self-management treatments for chronic pain: Application of the pain stages of change model. *Pain, 84,* 49–55.

Kerns, R. D., Rosenberg, R., Jamison, R. N., Caudill, M. A., & Haythornthwaite, J. (1997). Readiness to adopt a self-management approach to chronic pain: The Pain Stages of Change Questionnaire (PSOCQ). *Pain, 72,* 227–234.

Loeser, J. D., & Turk, D.C. (2001). Multidisciplinary pain management. In J.D. Loeser, S. H. Butler, C. R. Chapman, & D.C. Turk (Eds.), *Bonica's management of pain* (3rd ed., pp. 2069–2079). Philadelphia: Lippincott Williams & Wilkins.

Lorig, K., Chastain, R. L., Ung, E., Shoor, S., & Holman, H. R. (1989). Development and evaluation of a scale to measure perceived self-efficacy in people with arthritis. *Arthritis and Rheumatism, 32,* 37–44.

McCarberg, B. H., & Barkin, R. L. (2001). Long-acting opioids for chronic pain: Pharmacologic opportunities to enhance compliance, quality of life, and analgesia. *American Journal of Therapeutics, 8,* 181–186.

Miller, W. R. (1983). Motivational interviewing with problem drinkers. *Behavior Psychotherapy, 1,* 147–172.

Miller, W. R. (1996). Motivational interviewing: Research, practice, and puzzles. *Addictive Behaviors, 21,* 835–842.

Miller, W. R., Benefield, R. G., & Tongigan, J. S. (1993). Enhancing motivation for change in problem drinking: A controlled comparison of two therapist styles. *Journal of Consulting and Clinical Psychology, 61,* 455–461.

Miller, W. R., & Jackson, K. A. (1995). *Practical psychology for pastors: Toward more effective counseling.* Englewood Cliffs, NJ: Prentice-Hall.

Miller, W. R., & Rollnick, S. (1991). *Motivational interviewing: Preparing people to change addictive behavior.* New York: Guilford Press.

Miller, W. R., Zweben, A., DiClemente, C. C., & Rychtarik, R. G. (1992). *Motivational enhancement therapy manual: A clinical research guide for therapists treating individuals with alcohol abuse and dependence* (DHHS Publication No. ADM 92–1894). Washington, DC: U.S. Government Printing Office.

Moore, J. E., Von Korff, M., Cherkin, D., Saunders, K., & Lorig, K. (2000). A randomized trial of a cognitive-behavioral program for enhancing back pain self care in a primary care setting. *Pain, 88,* 145–153.

Portenoy, R. K. (1996). Opioid therapy for chronic nonmalignant pain. *Pain Research and Management, 1,* 17–28.

Prochaska. J. O., & DiClemente, C. C. (1982). Transtheoretical therapy: Toward a more integrative model of change. *Psychotherapy: Theory, Research and Practice, 19,* 276–288.

Prochaska, J. O., & DiClemente, C. C. (1992). Stages of change in the modification of problem behaviors. In M. Hersen, R. N. Eisler, & P. M. Miller (Eds.), *Progress in behavior modification* (pp. 184–214). Sycamore, IL: Sycamore Press.

Prochaska, J O., DiClemente, C. C., & Norcross, J.

C. (1992). In search of how people change: Applications to addictive behaviors. *American Psychologist, 47,* 1102–1114.

Rollnick, S., & Miller, W. R. (1995). What is motivational interviewing? *Behavioural and Cognitive Psychotherapy, 23,* 325–334.

Rogers, C. R. (1957). The necessary and sufficient conditions for therapeutic personality change. *Journal of Consulting Psychology, 21,* 95–103.

Rogers, C. R. (1959). A theory of therapy: Personality and interpersonal relationships as developed in the client-centered framework. In S. Koch (Ed.), *Psychology: The study of a science. Vol. 3. Formulations of the person and the social context* (pp. 184–256). New York: McGraw-Hill

Romano, J. M., Turner, J. A., Friedman, L. S., Bulcroft, R. A., Jensen, M. P., Hops, H., & Wright, S. F. (1992). Sequential analysis of chronic pain behaviors and spouse responses. *Journal of Consulting and Clinical Psychology, 60,* 777–782.

Schofferman, J. (1993). Long-term use of opioid analgesics for the treatment of chronic pain of nonmalignant origin. *Journal of Pain and Symptom Management, 8,* 279–288.

Treasure, J. L., Katzman, M., Schmidt, U., Troop, N., Todd, G., & de Silva, P. (1999). Engagement and outcome in at the treatment of bulimia nervosa: First phase of a sequential design comparing motivation enhancement therapy and cognitive behavioural therapy. *Behaviour Research and Therapy, 37,* 405–418.

Turk, D. C. (1990). Customizing treatment for chronic pain patient: Who, what, and why? *Clinical Journal of Pain, 6, 255–270.*

Turk, D. C., Meichenbaum, D., & Genest, M. (1983). *Pain and behavioral medicine: A cognitive-behavioral perspective.* New York: Guilford Press.

Turk, D. C., & Rudy, T. E. (1991). Neglected topics in the treatment of chronic pain patients: Relapse, noncompliance, and adherence enhancement. *Pain, 44,* 5–28.

Vlaeyen, J. W. S., Teeken-Gruben, N. J. G., Groossens, M. E. J. B., Rutten-van Molken, M. P. M. H., Eek H., van Pelt, R. A. G. B., & Huets, P. H. T. G. (1996). Cognitive-educational treatment of fibromyalgia: A randomized clinical trial. Part I. Clinical effects. *Journal of Rheumatology, 23,* 1237–1245.

Wells-Parker, E., Kenne, D. R., Spratke, K. L., & Williams, M. T. (2000). Self-efficacy and motivation for controlling drinking and drinking/driving: An investigation of changes across a driving under the influence (DUI) intervention program and of recidivism prediction. *Addictive Behavior, 25,* 229–238.

5

Integrating Relational Psychodynamic and Action-Oriented Psychotherapies: Treating Pain and Suffering

Stephen C. Basler
Roy C. Grzesiak
Robert H. Dworkin

In this chapter, we present an integrative psychotherapy model based on recent developments in relational psychodynamic psychotherapy. The approach we describe is integrative, providing a theoretical and clinical framework in which active interventions aimed at behavioral change complement, rather than inhibit, clinical attention to the relational and dynamic issues emphasized in psychodynamic psychotherapy. As such, it addresses both the chronic pain patient's need for improved coping with diverse stressors and the relational patterns that contribute to maladaptive coping and shape the idiosyncratic meanings and suffering that are superimposed on the pain sensation. We believe that this approach, which incorporates a biopsychosocial view of development, has the potential to expand the breadth and depth of our understanding of chronic pain patients and is a treatment that addresses both pain and suffering.

In the first edition of this volume, psychodynamic psychotherapy was presented as a treatment option primarily for a limited subset of chronic pain patients who had failed to respond adequately to cognitive-behavioral interventions because of unresolved developmental conflicts and trauma (Grzesiak,

Ury, & Dworkin, 1996). The integrative psychodynamic model we present here is intended to be applicable to all patients with chronic pain and seeks to augment, rather than replace, existing psychological treatments. Accordingly, this chapter was written with two audiences in mind. The first consists of cognitive-behavioral practitioners who would like additional tools with which to optimize their use of the therapy relationship and address treatment resistance, past and present interpersonal variables, and the idiosyncratic meaning of pain for the patient. Our second audience includes psychodynamic therapists who recognize that the multiple challenges faced by patients with chronic pain and their families require active treatment interventions but who are concerned about how to incorporate these approaches within a psychoanalytic treatment model.

We have two objectives in this chapter. First we discuss both the relational dynamics that impair coping with chronic pain and the negative consequences of chronic pain on interpersonal relationships and, consequently, overall adjustment and life satisfaction. Our underlying assumption is that pain—like all life events—occurs in a relational context. Current and past relationships, including relationships with treatment providers, play an ongoing and interactive role in the development, course, and treatment of chronic pain. With some patients the interactive role of past and present relational variables looms large; with others it is a less significant part of the interactive mix of tissue damage, psychosocial vulnerability, and socioeconomic status, to list just a few of the factors that contribute to the experience of chronic pain. Unfortunately, relational variables have been underused as a resource that can be harnessed to maximize treatment response and the alleviation of suffering.

Our second objective is to present a model that emphasizes the role of past and present relational dynamics and incorporates them into a treatment approach that addresses the unique needs of each patient with chronic pain. Although originating in psychodynamic psychotherapy, this model parallels the increasing efforts among cognitive, behavioral, and family systems therapists to develop approaches to integrating treatments that were once thought to have irreconcilable differences in their understanding of human development and the mechanisms of therapeutic change.

Many of these integrative efforts emphasize relational variables, including the qualities of individuals' interpersonal relationships across the lifespan as well as the relationships they establish with their therapists. Relational approaches have made significant changes in conceptualizing the psychotherapy relationship, especially with respect to such qualities as authenticity, mutual influence, and the co-creation of meaning. The relational model can incorporate existing cognitive-behavioral therapy techniques (see Turk, Chapter 7, this volume). Psychotherapy with a psychodynamic orientation can therefore now be used to treat a wider group of chronic pain patients and not just be considered the "treatment of last resort" for the most treatment-resistant patients.

The story of each patient with chronic pain poignantly captures the seemingly contradictory human experience of being fundamentally alone even as our lives are influenced by our past and present relationships. Chronic pain is a solitary experience that cannot be felt, seen, or even independently confirmed. On the other hand, chronic pain can have a profound impact on relationships at work, at home, and with friends. Isolation and conflict are common, as is drastic change in social roles and the patient's ability to participate in mutually rewarding relationships. Likewise, although the idiosyncratic meaning of the pain experience and, therefore, the quality of a person's suffering, is difficult to articulate to another, it is largely shaped by the sum total of the individual's past and present relational experiences.

In the first section, we provide a brief overview of the classical psychoanalytic theory of development and treatment. Our focus is on its application to chronic pain and the limitations of this model in addressing adequately the needs of these patients. We then describe the emergence of a relational approach within psychodynamic theory and the manner in which the increased therapist participation that follows from this model enables use of the action-oriented techniques that are a staple of cognitive and behavioral therapies. An examination of the role of relational variables in the lives of patients with chronic pain follows. These include the early relationship patterns that create a vulnerability to dysfunctional coping and that promote progression to chronicity as well as the relational consequences of pain for interpersonal relationships and social roles. This section concludes with a relational focus on healthy and adaptive responses to pain and disability. In the final section of the chapter we discuss clinical applications. These include assessment of coping and relevant relational variables, goal setting and treatment planning, establishing the therapy relationship and treatment frame within a relational model, and incorporation of action-oriented techniques that specifically target the development of more adaptive behaviors.

Classical Psychoanalytic Approaches to Chronic Pain

Because the limitations of medicine in explaining chronic pain were apparent at an early point, it was only natural that psychoanalysis—which provided a model for explaining all of human behavior—would address the vexing problem of unexplained pain and physical suffering. Freud proposed that the underlying motivational force was the gratification of biologically based, instinctual drives. Chronic pain that could not be accounted for by tissue damage was viewed as the result of a drive that the individual is not able to gratify in a socially acceptable manner. When such repressed urges threaten to emerge into consciousness, severe anxiety results and the resolution, however maladaptive it may appear to the outside observer, is a psychic compromise that can include the development of physical or emotional symptoms. However, even Freud believed that at its source, the origin of chronic pain was an actual physical insult that the unconscious seized upon because it served to crystallize a dynamic conflict and could be used to partially gratify drives and conflicts through the subjective experience of pain and its accompanying disability and emotional responses.

The overriding goal of psychoanalytic treatment has been for patients first to become aware of and later to renounce unconscious impulses and conflicts and then to obtain partial gratification through sublimation in adult roles and relationships. With pain, the analyst made interpretations based on the patient's free associations, which provided insight into the reason that the symptom of pain developed and the function that it served in terms of both primary and secondary gain. Change in behavior, although assumed to be an eventual outcome of treatment, was not a primary goal and was often considered "acting out," an escape from the rigors of analysis by gratifying wishes and soothing anxiety. Interpretations were considered to be objective because the rigid treatment model prohibited the analyst's involvement in the therapeutic relationship and considered him or her a detached, neutral observer whose insight was not distorted by personal investment and who did not contaminate the unfolding of transference distortions by being a "real" person in the patient's life.

Critics dismissed psychoanalytic psychotherapy for chronic pain as being inefficient, ineffective, not grounded in research, or, at best, appropriate for only a small group of nonresponders. Proponents of dynamic psychotherapy have countered that cognitive-behavioral therapy has failed to live up to earlier hopes in treating these patients—as have many medical treatments—and often addresses only a limited portion of the chronic pain experience. Specifically, by not considering idiosyncratic developmental experiences, the cognitive-behavioral therapist cannot fully understand the patient's adaptation or maladaptation to physical injury, his or her treatment resistance, and the myriad transference and countertransference phenomena that occur in every type of treatment relationship. Cognitive-behavioral therapists may therefore fail to fully understand the personal meanings of pain and disability that contribute greatly to the suffering superimposed on the pain sensation.

Until recently, this is where the debate ended. Adherents of each school defended their own approach and criticized or dismissed the rest. Of course, the reality has been that many therapists have been creatively modifying the psychoanalytic treatment frame for years and that psychodynamic therapy as conducted by practicing clinicians has evolved well beyond the classical Freudian psychoanalysis presented in textbooks.

A Relational Psychodynamic Approach to Personality Development and Psychotherapy

Although there have been dramatic changes during the past two decades, psychodynamic theory—and especially its clinical application—has never been as monolithic as some critics charge. From the start, there were challenges from within psychoanalysis regarding even the most fundamental assumptions, such as Freud's assertion that discharge of instinctual drives is the underlying motivational force for behavior, with actual relationships playing a subordinate role and only important to the extent that they provide the external vehicle for expression and gratification of internal impulses. For example, by the 1920s Melanie Klein was referring to internalization of early relationships and relationship patterns. Although object relations were conceptualized as *repositories* of instinct-based drives, this perspective paved the way for the examination of the role of actual relationships in development. Sullivan made a dramatic break with classical analysis in the 1930s when he suggested that it is not the individual psyche but the interpersonal field that is the essential unit of study, and therefore treatment. This view was followed by the rise of the object relations school, the basic tenet of which was that "libido is not pleasure seeking but object seeking" (Fairbairn, 1952). Bowlby's (1969) attachment theory, although positing an instinctual source, provided much needed empirical support for the argument that a primary and irreducible motivation of humans (and primates) is attachment to others.

More recently, Stephen Mitchell has been instrumental in weaving these varied strands together and was the leading spokesperson for a psychodynamic relational theory of development and treatment. Mitchell (1988) argued that in relational models, "We are portrayed not as a conglomeration of physically based urges, but as being shaped by and inevitably embedded within a matrix of relationships with other people, struggling both to maintain our ties to others and to differentiate ourselves from them" (p. 3).

The implications with respect to our understanding of human development and the therapeutic relationship of this major break—not shift—from psychoanalysis can hardly be overstated, and this model has led to a school of psychodynamic psychotherapy that is congenial to therapist participation, not adamantly opposed to it.

A Relational Model of Development

Mitchell (1988) coined the term "relational matrix" to describe complex, internalized modes of relating to others. These include affectively laden images and representations of the individual (self), others (object), and patterns of self-in-interaction with others (the interpersonal transaction) that are the end product of significant early relationships interacting with an individual's other environmental experiences and genetic predispositions (e.g., temperament, intelligence, and physical constitution); in essence, a biopsychosocial model of development. Operating largely at an unconscious level, a relational matrix shapes our affect, cognitions, and behavior, especially in the interpersonal realm, and therefore constitutes the person's personality. In contrast to cognitive-behavioral or systems models, the intrapsychic is not eliminated but, rather, subordinated to the interpersonal and interactional world.

Classical psychoanalytic theory posits that we start as an individual entity, only adding others to suit our biological, internally derived needs. In contrast, relational theorists assert that we are relational from the beginning, noting that some of the early important bodily sensations such as holding, soothing, and feeding are interpersonal (Aron, 1998). Indeed, linguists and those studying cognition have demonstrated that we think primarily within the structure of language, a fundamentally relational process. Even self and identity, which had been viewed by psychoanalysts as reflecting the person's autonomy, are reconceptualized as developing in a relational context and as shaped and maintained throughout life by our relationships (Kohut, 1971). We are not a self alone; we are a self *in relation* to others (J. B. Miller, 1976).

In classical analytic theory, personality originates in the interaction between biological impulses and the external world during approximately the first 5 years of life. In contrast, the relational psychodynamic view increases emphasis on the present environment—especially the actual qualities of current relationships—in ongoing healthy or pathological adaptation. The relational matrix provides a template, largely unconscious, that the person uses to choose, shape, view, and perhaps distort current relationships. These current interactional patterns are then reinternalized and serve to validate the individual's assumptions about themselves, others, and their interactions with others.

In the relational model, there is a complex interaction between the internalized expectations of others—whether spouse, friend, employer, physician, or therapist—and their actual qualities, rather than the absolute distortion of the other person assumed in the classical analytic understanding of transference. The past is only replicated because the environment is selected and molded *and allows itself to be molded* in response to the expectations and demands that constitute our internalized relational matrix. Consider, for example, a patient who believes that others will not have empathy or understanding for his experience—that is, for the suffering pain has caused. Such an individual is likely to present in a detached and hostile manner. Consequently, others really will be unable to understand the patient's experience, will not wish to understand it, and will also be less inclined to respond with empathy, all of which will confirm the validity of the patient's beliefs about himself in relation with others.

Why would such a patient not welcome assistance? Behaving, interacting, and perceiving in accord with one's internalized relational matrix provides a sense of predictability, stability, and safety and is an efficient way to process the voluminous interpersonal data encountered daily by all people. In addition, such patterns of viewing others and interacting with them were established because at an earlier, developmentally significant time they were the most successful adaptation available. As adults, we organize and shape our world in a manner that is predictable. Homeostasis is sought, even at the cost of higher levels of functioning. With the aforementioned patient, significant others in the past may have reacted to the expression of needs, emotions, or suffering with indifference or even wrath. In a relationally oriented treatment, it would be seen as inevitable that the initial reaction of the therapist will be shaped by the patient to approximate the responses by significant others in his past and present relational world. The therapeutic relationship enables examination of the contributions of both the therapist and the patient to their interaction. Patients are likely to feel validated when their concerns and beliefs are not dismissed as projections but are explored to develop a shared understanding of how people co-create and shape their interactions with others.

An emphasis on the actual qualities of peoples' relational worlds has major implications with respect to considering their responses to persistent pain and impaired physical functioning. To maintain normal functioning, people have an ongoing need for the relationships they have established.

Therefore, sustained disruption in patients' relational homeostasis, such as often occurs with pain and disability, can have a substantial impact on their sense of self, coping abilities, and overall well-being.

Relational Psychodynamic Treatment

In relational psychotherapy, an individual's psychic development is viewed as emerging from and intrinsically interwoven in a interpersonal milieu. Maladaptive behavior and deficits in coping are treated within the context of a relational model that replaces the "one-person" intrapsychic model of psychoanalysis with a "two-person" interactional therapy relationship that seeks to increase the flexibility and range of the patient's relational roles. The relational therapist facilitates an authentic therapy relationship involving mutual and reciprocal influence, which becomes the primary instrument by which therapeutic goals are realized, whether they are changes in dysfunctional coping, personality and behavior, relationships, or symptomatology.

Features of the patient's relational matrix inevitably evoke certain behaviors, thoughts, and emotions in the therapist (and vice versa), and these "enactments" are welcomed and explored together. Removing the limiting and unrealistic constraints of the classically prescribed blank screen and embracing an interactional view of psychotherapy is more validating to the patient, builds trust, and gives the therapist a broader range of interventions to facilitate new experiences for the patient. In a relationship of openness and safety, patients have the opportunity to experiment with new relational experiences, harnessing experiential learning to potentiate insight and change. This opportunity includes new ways for patients to view and interact with others, and new ways for them to see themselves and themselves in interaction. Frank (1990, 1999) and Wachtel (1997) have built on the relational model, incorporating action-oriented interventions specifically aimed at concrete behavioral change outside of treatment. When the impact of these interventions on the therapeutic relationship is explored, they do not inhibit but rather enhance the relationally modified psychodynamic goals of insight and new relational experiences, making this a truly integrative treatment model.

Because the relational matrix provides the bridge for integrating psychodynamic and cognitive-behavioral approaches, we next review a selection of relational themes to which clinicians should attend in considering the development, maintenance, and successful treatment of chronic pain.

The Interplay of Relational Themes in the Development, Maintenance, and Treatment of Chronic Pain

Psychosocial antecedents, concomitants, and consequences of chronic pain have received increasing attention (e.g., Dworkin & Banks, 1999; Gatchel & Turk, 1999). In this section, we argue that many of what are considered "psychosocial" variables are relational or relationally mediated. We believe that antecedent interpersonal relationships, through their influence on subsequent relational patterns and assumptions about self and others, can create a vulnerability to developing a chronic pain syndrome by several different pathways. In addition, early relationship dynamics help shape patients' idiosyncratic meanings of their pain and, therefore, the quality of suffering superimposed on the pain sensation. Finally, notwithstanding relationally mediated vulnerability, the losses and changes in relationships and relational roles that are concomitants and consequences of chronic pain can be devastating and constitute a large part of the impaired quality of life and misery that many patients experience.

The major contribution of the relational psychodynamic model in understanding chronic pain patients is in capturing the interplay between past and present as it occurs in the individual's experience of the present. Vulnerabilities based on relational experiences of the past, combined with the effects of the real stressors of injury and pain on the individual's present life and relationships, reciprocally influence each other in a vicious circle of increasingly maladaptive coping, further deterioration of emotional and physical health, depletion of healthy sources of social support, and increased reliance on the ever diminishing secondary gain of the sick role.

Consider a patient who was raised by emotionally detached and critical parents. Seeking familiarity, as an adult such an individual might be more likely to select a spouse who replicates these traits and who reacts to pain and injury with withdrawal, indifference, and criticism. Not working, the patient is isolated from others who could provide support. The adversarial and often suspicious approach taken by insurance companies and others may augment this pattern, as does the invisible nature of pain, which hinders validation and understanding by others. While struggling with multiple stressors, and expecting criticism or at best indifference, it is difficult for the patient to seek help. The patient becomes guarded with treatment providers who, in turn, become more suspicious and less emotionally invested in his or her care and well-being, repeating the early parental dynamics and confirming the patient's assumptions about himself in relation to others.

For the sake of clarity, we have divided this section into past and present relational themes, acknowledging that this artificial categorization risks diluting one of the key arguments of this chapter, the continual interplay between the past and present in the relational matrix.

Relational Antecedents of Chronic Pain

It is easy to forget that patients presenting at pain management centers or who are referred for psychological treatment are an unrepresentative sample. The world is full of people with persistent pain and chronic illness—"silent sufferers" (Brena & Koch, 1975) as well as "adaptive copers" (Turk & Rudy, 1988)—who continue to work and love and play and generally function well, despite their physical limitations. In our biopsychosocial model of pain, a biological vulnerability (the diathesis of diathesis–stress models) is a necessary but not sufficient condition for the development of chronic pain, which only occurs when various psychosocial processes are also present. These psychosocial factors are diverse and include stressful life events, ongoing social support, and personal dispositions, which include personality and psychopathology (Dohrenwend & Dohrenwend, 1981). Relational antecedents—early experiences with significant others and the internalized relational patterns that develop as a result—influence all these psychosocial factors: our perception and experience of stressful life events, our ability to develop and use social supports, and our normal and maladaptive personality traits.

Complex interactions and inherent limitations of research design make it difficult to clarify the role psychosocial factors play in the etiology of chronic pain. Studies of patients cannot reliably differentiate the antecedents of chronic pain from its concomitants and consequences, for example, whether depression is a cause or a consequence of chronic pain or whether current suffering selectively influences the recall of traumatic childhood events. Only prospective research designs can identify causal antecedents of chronic pain, and because such studies are difficult to undertake, there is a relative paucity of compelling data addressing the psychosocial antecedents of chronic pain.

Nevertheless, the results of the few studies that have been reported are consistent with clinical observations and lead us to believe that early relationships with parents and others play a role in explaining why pain does or does not progress to chronicity. Engel (1951, 1959), for example, developed the concept of the pain-prone patient, noting that people with chronic pain seemed to share several early life experiences. These experiences included physically or verbally abusive parents; harsh or punitive parents who overcompensated with rare displays of affection, cold or emotionally distant parents who were only warm and solicitous when the child was ill, a parent who suffered from chronic illness or pain, and various other parent–child interactions involving guilt, aggression, or pain (Grzesiak, 1994).

The results of a study that examined the relationship between an operationally defined set of risk factors involving childhood psychological trauma and the outcome of spinal surgery (Schofferman, Anderson, Hines, Smith, & White, 1992) are consistent with Engel's (1959) observations. The following were considered risk factors: (1) physical abuse by a primary caregiver, (2)

sexual abuse by a primary caregiver, (3) alcohol or drug abuse in one or both caregivers, (4) abandonment (loss of a primary caregiver), and (5) emotional neglect/abuse by primary caregivers. The authors investigated 100 consecutive patients who had undergone spinal surgery and found that of those who recalled none of these traumas, 95% had successful postsurgical outcomes. On the other hand, only 15% of patients who recalled three or more of these risk factors had a successful outcome. In a similar study, Schofferman, Anderson, Hines, Smith, and Keane (1993) found an association between these childhood trauma risk factors and chronic low back pain.

In Schofferman and colleagues' (1992, 1993) research, the psychosocial risk factors that contributed to poor outcome and the development of a chronic pain syndrome either directly involved significant past relationships or occurred within a relational context. They involved some form of interpersonal experience, such as a loss, trauma, or neglect, and likely included the development of internalized ties to past significant others and a modeling of their characteristics in the present.

Personality disorders appear to provide additional risk factors for developing a chronic pain syndrome and for being refractory to treatment (Gatchel & Weisberg, 2000). A relational model views personality as comprising the internalization of prior relational experiences (in combination with temperament, intelligence, and other variables) and their manifestation in present behavior, relationships, affects, and cognitions. Accordingly, personality disorders are the extreme maladaptive end of a continuum of relational functioning and often interfere with the individual's ability to develop and maintain supportive relationships.

Relational antecedents may create a vulnerability to developing chronic pain and a propensity to experience suffering when it occurs. But how does this happen? We discuss several processes that we believe illustrate how prior relationships, through their effect on the development of psychic structure and future relational patterns, contribute to a vulnerability to developing chronicity in response to injury and pain.

RELATIONAL PATTERNS THAT INTERFERE WITH
SOCIAL SUPPORT

Some people function well during times of stability but fail to recover from an acute illness or injury because it is difficult for them to accept and benefit from the support of others, or because their relational roles are brittle and rigid in response to crisis. Maladaptive coping and emotional distress in response to injury or acute pain can lead to a chronic pain syndrome. Unfortunately, these patients have often been overlooked—especially by psychoanalysts—in favor of those whose symptoms appear to symbolically express some intrapsychic conflict or repressed wish. Our clinical experience leads us to believe that this relational pattern is found in a significant proportion of patients with chronic pain—although such people are probably less likely than other patients to appear for psychological treatment because of the nature of their relational dynamics. Their appearance and compliance in treatment might therefore occur as a result of varying levels of duress from outside sources, whether family, employers, agencies, or other treatment providers, or after their functioning has become so impaired that they can no longer refuse assistance. Openly identifying any outside pressures that are contributing to their participation in treatment helps establish a treatment frame of open disclosure and increases the likelihood that patients will assume responsibility for their participation in treatment.

The therapist must move slowly and cautiously in deepening the therapeutic relationship, responding to cues from the patient that are often nonverbal (e.g., missed sessions). With all patients, but especially this group, "more is better" does not always apply regarding expressions of empathy and support by the treatment provider. These may be threatening and elicit anxiety for these patients and lead to increased suspicion and even premature termination of treatment. Interventions that are concrete and emphasize the patient's autonomy are recommended, especially early in treatment. However, depending on whether a patient has compensating resources, it may be necessary to directly address his or her mal-adaptive interpersonal pattern to prevent early withdrawal from treatment. As is discussed later, this often best happens through careful and sensitive exploration of the relationship between the clinician and the patient. The following are four overlapping relational dynamics that interfere with deriving benefit from social support.

Distrust of Vulnerability and Intimacy. The patient's salient relational dynamic involves issues of distrust, that is, feeling unsafe or having a sense of being threatened when in a position of vulnerability or intimacy. This feeling prohibits the individual from using the support of others to recover or regain functioning and prevent chronicity.

Although sexual and physical abuse have often played a role, an extreme traumatic event is not necessary for this relational dynamic to develop. Relational events and variables more often shape the enduring psychic structure and personality much like the flow of water shapes a stone—bit by bit through a constant pattern of subtle pressures and influences. A clinician must probe carefully to tease out these less readily apparent but more common relational patterns, which might include emotional neglect, abandonment, betrayal, and abuses of power or a critical and denigrating approach by an early significant other. Such dynamics may be further revealed by carefully evaluating the patient's reactions to supportive comments and interventions early in the treatment.

These patients are often described as treatment resistant, help rejecting, guarded, and even hostile. Competing internalized relational needs may further complicate the picture. Although intimacy and vulnerability may evoke diffuse anxiety and a desire to withdraw, there may also be longing for nurturance and support. The result may be an approach-avoidant style of interaction in which patients have begun numerous treatment relationships that are ended abruptly or trail off for unclear reasons. The clinician may draw the erroneous conclusion that prior treatments—whether medications, psychotherapy, or procedures—were not administered in an effective manner.

A middle-age female had been through multiple and largely unsuccessful treatments for back pain including surgery, nerve blocks, medication, and physical therapy and was referred for psychotherapy as part of her multidisciplinary pain management program. She limped into the initial session with the aid of a cane, sporting a leather jacket, crew cut, and tattoos, sat on the edge of her chair, and glared in silence, ready for battle. Already squirming, the therapist began to explain what behavioral medicine treatment could offer, buying time and perhaps hiding with a detailed and quite possibly patronizing explanation of various techniques and skills. He was abruptly interrupted by the patient, who challenged, "I have been through this for years, this is my life, how the hell do you think you can get rid of my pain with your bag of tricks!"

Although recoiling physically, the therapist was surprised to realize that he did not feel the threat that one might expect with her remarks, attitude, and body language. Instead, he felt energized in the way therapists often do when deeply engaged with their patients in an authentic interaction. He felt permission—even a challenge and responsibility—to respond in a similarly direct manner. This was not to deny the reality that her confrontational approach also served a defensive role, circumventing efforts by the therapist to learn more about her. However, by the end of the session, she could respond to this feedback, not with hostility but with an acknowledging smile.

The patient opened the second session stating, "You didn't kick me out or play dead last session when I tried to scare you away. You passed. Ask away." Over the course of the session, the patient revealed that as a child she had been criticized and demeaned by both parents in a cruel fashion that capitalized on any weakness or sign of vulnerability. She grew up to be street smart and fiercely independent. However, in her significant relationships she felt completely subjugated to the needs and control of others, leading ultimately and repetitively to her leaving the relationship. Her interactions with friends were characterized by her talking tough but giving beyond her means, and with her being uncomfortable in receiving any support but then feeling used and resentful. In another self-fulfilling vicious cycle, she often engaged others through trading humorous insults, which invariably left her wounded and kept others from revealing themselves to her.

Over the years, the patient increasingly turned to alcohol, drugs, and suicidal behavior in attempting to ward off depression without being vulnerable by relying on others. After reaching her greatest level of dysfunction, the patient found a more adaptive means to obtain a positive identity through excessive work. Although this may have contributed to her injury, being unable to work was a huge threat to her stability. She was forced to turn to medical providers, social service agencies, friends, and family for tangible and emotional support. This was so difficult and anxiety provoking that she continually sabotaged her efforts to use the support of others in the service of her recovery.

Unfortunately, there may be valid reasons that explain why chronic pain patients are being wary or angry that have little to do with their relational dynamics. Previous providers may have been overly optimistic about expected treatment benefits and may have even responded to treatment failure by blaming the patient, which is also a common reaction of family and friends who are, of course, unable to experience the patient's pain. Then there is the often adversarial nature of insurance and workers' compensation systems, which can leave the patient feeling ignored and perceived as malingering. In distinction to psychoanalytic approaches that emphasize projective distortions and cognitive approaches that stress logical errors, the relational psychodynamic model considers it likely that there is an element of accuracy in a patient's perceptions of interpersonal situations and relationships, even if he or she also played a role in shaping these interactions.

Exaggerated Need for Autonomy. The predominant relational variable for these patients is not distrust but an exaggerated and inflexible investment in viewing the self as competent and autonomous. The dominant early relational dynamic was not abuse but was more likely the absence of critically needed emotional nurturance and guidance and possibly a message that one must be competent and function without assistance. Although autonomous functioning might not appear to be a relational dynamic, relational theories of development and functioning argue that our identity is not only initially formed in relationships but maintained and shaped throughout life in a relational context. This is true even when a person's particular identity and behavior suggest a dominant theme of rugged individuality and autonomous functioning.

A considerable number of chronic pain patients have experienced neglect or abandonment as a child, often as a result of parental substance abuse or mental illness, and place great value on being self-sufficient. Functioning autonomously may also maintain an internalized symbolic tie to a parent who modeled excessive independence from others, and there may be a driven increase in activity following an injury as the individual attempts to shore up a deteriorating sense of self-worth. Blumer and Heilbronn (1989) have described a trait they term "ergomania"—a conflicted work ethic that they believe is an important premorbid characteristic of many chronic pain patients and which may play a role in its development. They suggest that ergomanic pain patients have a history of excessive work performance, relentless activity, self-sacrifice, and the precocious assumption of adult responsibilities, as well as a marked difficulty trusting caretakers, including health care providers.

Need to Be Care Provider. Although overlapping with the previous dynamic, these people emphasize being the provider in relational roles and transactions. Early experiences often included having to take care of others in a manner that was inappropriate for their level of development. This caretaking could range from a relatively normative situation, such as an older child having responsibility for younger siblings, to more pathological variations in which the parent relied excessively on a child for emotional or physical support. These patients may have a family history of substance abuse or mental illness, especially when they filled the family role of competent caregiver.

Such people often experience painful guilt when they are in the role of receiving and may fear that they will be abandoned by others because they have become a burden and no longer have anything of value to offer. Description of pain and suffering may

be followed by self-deprecating remarks about their seeking sympathy and whining. Exquisitely sensitive to the needs of others, they can adroitly maneuver treatment such that the clinician has a belated realization that the patient has shifted focus away from himself and onto the clinician. Conflict and distress stem not just from the patient's inability to relinquish the caregiver role but from the inability of significant others in the patient's relational world to shift from their customary role of receiver of support to that of provider. Successful adaptation requires the patient with pain and his or her significant others to shift roles in response to the loss of physical capabilities.

Deficits in Using Social Support. These people often grew up in families in which the members were detached from each other and functioned as independent individuals living separate lives under the same roof. Approaching others for support when faced with a crisis was never modeled and did not become a part of their interpersonal repertoire. Ironically, turning to others for support may represent a loss of an internalized tie to a detached parent, because it is a new way of seeing oneself in a relationship. These people may have never developed or may have lost over time the ability to identify their own needs as well as to communicate them to others. In treatment they often respond well to communication training, role play, and modeling.

INTERNALIZED RELATIONAL PATTERNS
EXPRESSED IN THE "SICK ROLE"

For some patients, a chronic pain syndrome and its associated relational roles—many of which are aspects of what has been termed the "sick role"—are not the end result of a breakdown in functioning or coping. Instead, they represent an attempt by patients to establish familiar ways of viewing themselves and interacting with others that are attained in the roles and interpersonal transactions associated with having chronic pain. With some, this seeming contradiction may reflect a conflict between two mutually exclusive relational roles—that is, genuinely wanting to get better and function autonomously versus a largely unconscious investment in the chronic pain relational configuration, especially being sick and nurtured. This conflict may have arisen from competing and mutually exclusive relational roles in the individual's relationships with each one of his or her parents. The expression of these contradictory roles in the present maintains an internalized tie to both parents, at a high cost in functioning.

Pain and disability may prevent the symbolic or actual surpassing of a parent who may have been threatened and responded with rejection when the patient as a child demonstrated the emergence of competence and autonomy. Being disabled may also maintain an internalized or real tie to parents who cannot allow the patient to function autonomously because they themselves cannot relinquish the role of provider. This relational pattern may be manifest in the selection of a spouse who needs to nurture the patient as a parent would a helpless child. For such patients, to see themselves as someone who can get better and be successful, although it may be consciously desired, would require the loss of the connection to the parent or spouse via the sick role, as well as the anxiety that would accompany a departure from familiar relational territory. For some patients being sick and impaired was the only way they were able to gain attention or nurturing from parents who were inattentive (Basler & King, 1997). Having had parents who were not attuned to their needs, as adults they have a chronic sense of deprivation, coupled with a largely unconscious belief that they will not receive support unless they are visibly sick and distressed.

Although these patients appear compliant with treatment and perceive themselves in this way, they often seem to unwittingly sabotage their treatment in subtle ways. Responses of significant others and clinicians may fluctuate between extremes of overinvolvement that are out of proportion to the patient's impairment and a marked lack of empathy and minimization of the patient's genuine distress and disability. Acceptance of pain is often not a salient therapeutic issue with these patients, although their roles and relational needs may be partly gratified by diligent attempts to pursue additional treatment. It is difficult to have these patients recognize that they might have to become more autonomous, whether or not

their pain improves, and that they must take ultimate responsibility for their pain and its treatment, a key element of psychological approaches to pain management (Turk, Meichenbaum, & Genest, 1983).

These patients are not malingering, although they are often incorrectly accused of symptom exaggeration because of their seeming comfort in the chronic sick role. Although they may be aware that their treatment is hampered because they find the sick role gratifying, and may even acknowledge this in the context of a trusting relationship, these people can also genuinely want a more productive life. Depending on their degree of psychological insight, they will be more or less aware of this conflict and the fear that largely stems from their relational conviction that they cannot function autonomously and require the care of others. Unfortunately, this diminished sense of personal responsibility only worsens the longer they are disabled.

Furthermore, because significant others are often invested in the patient's dependency, they can resist efforts by the patient and treatment team to increase autonomous functioning and loosen the patient's allegiance to the sick role. It is therefore important to interview spouses and others who these patients may have selected or shaped to respond positively to their needs for care and support. Although they may be less likely than other chronic pain patients to develop depression or anxiety, if the continued stability of their relational world is threatened (e.g., financial reasons, discharge from care, and caregiver burnout), they may quickly develop depression or anxiety, which can solicit renewed care by others.

Some treatment approaches emphasize aggressive efforts to eradicate any reinforcement of pain behavior. One patient recalled that the staff of a pain center emphasized this approach by wearing buttons proclaiming "Pain Is Boring!" Such methods are undoubtedly helpful for some patients, but punitive responses to patients whose relational roles satisfy a profound need to be nurtured does not lessen their distress and will not change their behavior. In addition, there is the risk that such people will superficially comply with treatment because of their need to maintain relationships with their care providers. In this case, little real change will occur and it can be expected that relapse would be likely after completing treatment.

RELATIONAL THEMES INVOLVING THE MEANING
OF PAIN AND SUFFERING

The first two antecedent relational themes discussed involve the influence of premorbid relational patterns on engagement and progression in treatment. In contrast, this theme concerns the influence of prior relational experiences on shaping the unique meaning of pain for each patient. Clinicians should attend carefully to this issue because it can have a major influence on the subjective suffering superimposed on the pain sensation and, therefore, on psychological distress and life satisfaction.

The meaning that patients give their pain may not appear to be relationally mediated on the surface but may on closer examination reflect important, albeit subtle, relational themes. Consider pain during childbirth and cancer, two examples commonly used to contrast the importance of meaning in understanding experiences of pain and suffering. The relational significance of childbirth is readily apparent, and, in many instances, it enables tolerance of great physical pain. Childbirth is therefore one example of how the meaning of pain may reduce rather than augment suffering.

The relational themes of cancer pain may be less obvious. The pain of cancer raises the specter of progressive impairment in functioning with loss of certain relational roles and increased dependence on others. And cancer pain, of course, is often associated with fears of death, a unique relational theme involving permanent separation and aloneness. The relational meanings of pain in these two examples, as with all pain, can be complex. With regard to childbirth, is the baby wanted? Is the marriage in trouble? Has the couple struggled for years to conceive a child? With cancer, has the family reacted with denial or distancing? Has the patient addressed unresolved conflicts with loved ones? Is the patient anticipating being reunited with loved ones who have died?

When the meaning superimposed on the pain sensation increases subjective suffering, it can be expected that the risk for depression, anxiety, and other psychiatric symptoms increases considerably. In turn, the cognitive distortions associated with depression can further accentuate negative meanings, potentially creating a vicious circle. It is also possible, of course, that depression came first, determining the negative meanings associated with the pain, such as guilt and punishment, and that the patient will not attach the same meaning to his or her pain once depressive symptoms have resolved.

Relational Varieties of Suffering. Suffering can be accentuated because pain represents a loss. Although losses of present relationships and roles are most obvious, they may trigger the reexperiencing of previous losses that have not been adequately grieved. Consider a patient who presented with distress over head pain that was considered out of proportion to the physical findings. The picture became clearer as well as more complicated when she revealed, while providing her developmental history, that her mother had died of a brain tumor.

Pain and suffering can be seen as punishment, either punishment deserved or punishment unjustly administered; it may become apparent in treatment by the presence of guilt-laden themes or material offered by patients that is unusual or seems tangential to their pain experience.

A patient presented with migraine headaches that had been present for several years. Although there was no reason to question the severity of his headaches, the degree of disability seemed excessive. Furthermore, his suffering had an unusual depth and his emotional distress had an incongruent quality in the view of the therapist. When the patient first described kneeling naked on the floor of his shower with the water running and howling in anguish, the therapist had an image of one who has just learned of some unspeakable and unbearable tragedy. Later in treatment, the patient disclosed that many years ago his best friend had died of head injuries from an accident for which he held himself partially responsible. Unfortunately, it was difficult to fully explore the importance of this material to the patient's suffering and distress because of his belief that to do so would be tantamount to saying that his headaches were due to "psychological problems."

A second example demonstrates that the belief that suffering is punishment, although distressing, can also provide comfort by suggesting that atonement is possible. This particular patient saw his pain as validation that a higher power is concerned about his life.

"Years ago, a whole slew of hurdles simultaneously parted, clearing the way for me to pursue training in the ministry, which I felt strongly to be my calling. At the last minute, I balked. That was when my back pain and other medical problems began. I don't see my God as an exclusively punitive God, but he certainly lets things happen, perhaps to let me know he is now, and will continue to be, involved in my life. That is the only way I can make any sense or gain any understanding or acceptance of this pain."

Similar to the sick role, maintaining an internal tie to a significant other may also be served by suffering, which may involve the symbolic expression of anger or of punishing a significant other, such as the patient who bitterly remarked, "My father said I wouldn't amount to anything and would wallow in my misery. Well, here it is, Dad, does it make you happy?!"

Relational Consequences of Chronic Pain

In this section we discuss the substantial adverse relational impacts that injury, disability, and pain can have on patients and their families, independent of their premorbid relational patterns or coping style. These psychosocial consequences include changes and losses in relational roles, which can disrupt a complex homeostasis of familiar relational patterns involving the patient and significant others and further compromise their emotional adjustment. Indeed, the results of research suggests that psychosocial factors generally play a larger role in characterizing the chronic pain experience than biological processes (Gatchel & Turk, 1999; Turk & Rudy, 1988).

In initiating treatment, we attempt to normalize both the patient's and family's feelings of being overwhelmed, emphasizing that "pain is stressful and it is a family affair." It is a testament to the resilience of our patients and their families that, although they may stumble at first, most rally, make adjustments, and generally adapt fairly well. The stages of an individual or systems adaptation to a crisis often proceed from an initial, temporary loss of normal coping abilities to eventual adjustment, but many characteristics of the chronic pain experience complicate the reestablishment of homeostasis and adequate functioning. The stressors of chronic pain are multiple, substantial, sustained, interactive, and unpredictable. Unpredictability makes adaptation especially difficult, because the situation is constantly shifting. These psychosocial consequences of chronic pain reverberate throughout so many spheres of individual and family life that the cumulative effect can even produce maladaptive responses in an individual in a supportive environment whose coping is not otherwise hindered by any of the dysfunctional relational patterns described previously. Turk (2000) reflects this pattern when he notes, "It is not surprising that a large number of chronic pain patients are depressed. It is interesting to ponder: how is it that all such patients are not depressed?"

The following narrative was delivered in frustration during a session early in treatment.

"I haven't worked in a year. People at my job used to call and invite me to office functions. That has pretty much stopped. My supervisor and I used to talk so openly. Now, it is tense and I'm not sure how much to tell her and wonder sometimes if she even believes me. I still get to church occasionally but I can't volunteer or do anything extra. My friends try to keep in touch, but I hesitate to commit to anything ahead of time because I never know how I am going to feel. I don't have much good to say, people don't always want to hear you complain. I get sick of hearing myself. Anyway, I am so out of the loop, what do I have to talk about? Some of them have taken it personally, and I have blown up at a few who offered the kind of advice that makes me think they either don't have a clue what I am going through or think I am not trying very hard. To think I used to be the go-getter, the one who arranged the social calendar! After I get the kids off to school, I am at home by myself most of the day. It gives me too much time to think. What do you do? Exercise, really pushing it. That used to be such an outlet. That's out.

"My husband works all day and has to do most of the cooking, shopping, and work around the house. He's been great, but it takes a toll on him. We are both on edge as it is and I don't want to burden him with my complaining at the end of the day. Thanks to the pain and our moodiness, his being worn out, and me gaining weight and not feeling very sexy or alive, our physical relationship has all but shut down. My parents are getting older and I used to help them out. Now they are giving us money, watching our kids, and driving me to doctor appointments. Even though we dance around the topic, the question on everyone's mind is 'How is mom feeling today?' I do have a whole new set of friends, if that's what you want to call them. Doctors, specialists, physical therapists, my lawyer, insurance people, folks at social services, the workers compensation board, and bill collectors!"

This is hardly an atypical or extreme example. Indeed, this patient is still coping fairly well, although one can see what could be the beginning of a vicious circle involving a narrowing of her range of engagement with the world and the salience of the pain in her interpersonal interactions. There are at least four broad and overlapping categories of relational consequences of chronic pain that such patients experience—isolation, relational conflict, losses of relational roles, and new roles and relationships.

ISOLATION

As with the foregoing patient, chronic pain usually has an impact on almost all significant relational roles at the point of referral for psychological treatment. Patients are not working, hesitate to commit to social engagements or community responsibilities, and may have had friends, colleagues, and even family members gradually withdrawing from them. At home, they may spend a great deal of time in bed, have altered sleep patterns, and no longer regularly participate in family events. It is also likely that they have less interaction with their spouse, who may have had to increase work outside the home as well as assume additional household responsibilities, leaving him or her emotionally depleted. Furthermore, many patients on disability hesitate to go out even briefly to run errands, exercise, or socialize, fearing that their degree of disability will be contested or that others will conclude that they are malingering.

The overall trajectory is toward reduced energy to devote to a decreased amount of time spent interacting with a shrinking sphere of relationships. Clinicians who inquire about patients' relationships routinely hear them also describe an emotional distance in the presence of others and a belief that important persons in their life are not capable of understanding the multiple reverberations of chronic pain on their lives. In a relational model, an important lifelong component of our attachment needs is the sense that our subjective experience—especially our suffering—is understood by significant others, beginning with, ideally, responsive parents but also continuing throughout the lifespan. Patients may react to the sense of not being understood or believed by further withdrawal. Unfortunately, social isolation increases the risk of depression and depression increases social withdrawal, a destructive circle that can feed on itself.

Emotional isolation is worsened by feeling detached from society at large and from daily involvement in adult roles, activities, and responsibilities. These contribute not only to a sense of being an active and important participant in a rich tapestry of relational roles but also to a sense of belonging to something larger, something that encompasses family, community, and society.

RELATIONAL CONFLICT

The stress that accompanies chronic pain, including the new responsibilities placed on significant others and the unpredictability and overall disruption in familiar routines, all provide abundant opportunities for conflict in the patient's significant relationships. Quite understandably, others may have difficulty with what they often describe as "changes in personality," referring to the patient's passivity, defensiveness, and irritability. There may be an implication—to which patients are acutely sensitive—that they are not "doing enough" or have "given up." Although these beliefs may be partially true, they may also be a result of the difficulty that others have in appreciating some of the negative effects of chronic pain (e.g., difficulty concentrating and fatigue). There is also the human reaction of anger and blame in response to feelings of helplessness in being unable to alleviate the suffering of a loved one. In addition, the patient's negative affect is often directed toward those who have had to sacrifice the most because they are a safe target and the patient resents being dependent. Consequently, it is often valuable in treatment to provide an opportunity for patients to acknowledge appreciation to significant others for the additional load they have had to assume.

Relational conflict may be exacerbated by problematic aspects of the premorbid relational patterns. For example, some patients cannot accept their limitations or have difficulty communicating them and commit to responsibilities that they cannot realistically complete. They may engage in activities that are not within their physical capabilities, putting others in the unwelcome role of policing their activity. Conversely, the patient may create resentment by handing over more of their responsibilities than is really necessary. Another scenario involves the spouse who has been dependent and who, in fact, was selected by the patient as a partner because this relational role complemented the patient's need to be nurturing. Suddenly, the tables are turned and the spouse must now enter the work force and care for the patient, with conflict resulting from the difficulty both patient and spouse have with their now reversed relational roles.

In addition, the patient's interactions with various bureaucracies may have an adversarial and even litigious dimension. Although the anger the patient and family express toward others may partially be a response to feeling helpless or scared, there is often some reality given the environments within which they must interact. Teasing apart responses to feeling helpless from understandable anger and then helping patients to identify the sources of their emotions and assume greater responsibility for their recovery is an ongoing clinical challenge.

How patients and their significant others respond to relational conflict depends on a variety of factors, including the flexibility of their relational roles and the extent of their compensating resources, as well as skills in communication and conflict resolution. Unfortunately, many characteristics of the chronic pain experience complicate open communication. In a typical scenario, family members experience considerable stress but do not seek validation of this stress from the patient for fear of further burdening him or her. This feeling can lead to resentment, worsened by difficulty in understanding the limitations imposed by pain. The patient in turn wants to acknowledge the help provided by others but feels defensive, which can be accentuated by awareness of the other's unspoken resentment. Often, such situations deteriorate into angry outbursts or, much worse, icy silence and emotional distancing.

Openly disagreeing with and challenging the significant other is preferable to withdrawal and avoidance of sensitive topics. In working with families and couples, we try to promote communication, build morale, and put everyone on the same team by normalizing the conflict and asserting that the stressors of their situation require them to be better than the average family at communication and negotiation.

LOSSES OF RELATIONAL ROLES

Ideally, adults manifest various roles and relationships not only in keeping with their internalized relational patterns but also in ways that complement the relational patterns of significant others. This manifestation of roles contributes to a feeling of predictability and continuity over time. Unfortunately, the chronic pain experience involves substantial losses and disruptions in these interactions.

In a later section, we discuss the importance of obtaining an overview during the initial assessment of the patient's relational roles and how they have been affected by pain and disability. However, it is often difficult to capture the essential qualities of all of a person's relational roles—one can be a parent, spouse, child, friend, patient, and employee. Such categories provide frameworks for understanding patients that are generic, but there are innumerable variations of the roles. Descriptions of the actual behaviors associated with relational roles may not reveal the idiosyncratic meanings, satisfaction, and identity obtained by the individual in performing these roles.

Mutuality is an important component of many adult relationships. It can be considered the degree to which a relationship involves exchanges of emotional and tangible support and a depth of emotional expression, intimacy, and attunement, all of which serve to create a vital reciprocity in which both parties are meaningfully engaged. Mutuality is not exclusively determined by verbal content and can be present with adults who sit together in silence and in relationships in which both individuals share intimate details of their lives. Many patients feel that they are a burden with little of value to offer. Unless the role of being a chronic pain patient fits a premorbid relational pattern, the decreased capacity for mutuality in relationships will cause distress and demoralization in patients and the significant others in their lives. How can patients give to others when what consumes their thinking is their pain and its impact? Is mutuality possible when one is preoccupied with suffering and unable to be spontaneously available and attentive to others? Reductions in the mutuality inherent in many relational roles can also contribute to alterations in a patient's identity, which is formed and maintained in interaction with others and can gradually change from a self-perception of competence to one of helplessness.

NEW ROLES AND RELATIONSHIPS

Many pain patients' day-to-day activities become centered on their pain; "in addition to depression, patients develop associated chronic invalid behaviors . . . . [They curtail their] social activity...become increasingly homebound, and their chief interaction with others, in the home as well as out of it, is via the sick role" (Sternbach, 1989, p. 244). They have frequent appointments with health care providers, as well as meetings with attorneys and various agencies, as they attempt to negotiate the maze of workers' compensation and other assistance programs. These new relational roles can become increasingly dominated by the theme of an impaired patient being provided with medical care and assistance. This domination often becomes pervasive, and the cumulative influence can reinforce passivity and self-preoccupation. Healthy behaviors may also be explicitly or implicitly discouraged, as when patients fear that others will think they are malingering if they are active. Indeed, it could be argued that pain behaviors—for example, grimacing and limping—may reflect the person's need to communicate to significant others his or her legitimacy and the presence of a real but otherwise invisible impairment.

The Relational Matrix of the Adaptive Coper

Of course, some patients do respond adaptively and are able to maintain productive lives and healthy relationships. Although severity of the initial injury, persisting tissue or nerve damage, and pain severity may contribute to distinguishing adaptive copers from those who have maladaptive responses, it is unlikely that such biomedical variables fully explain the differences. An examination of the chronic pain patient who is coping well provides a transition to discussing treatment because the objectives of treatment can be identified by describing the characteristics of those who have successfully adapted to pain. As we have seen, dysfunctional aspects of a chronic pain relational matrix include extreme or exaggerated roles, roles that are brittle or unresponsive to changed needs or capacities, and a narrow repertoire of relational roles.

In contrast, a healthy and adaptive relational matrix is characterized by flexibility and responsiveness to change, reciprocity, and a diverse range of available roles. Relational needs can be adequately expressed and satisfied in a range of relationships and are therefore less vulnerable to disruption in homeostasis when stress occurs. Such people can take risks and try new relational roles. In addition, by retaining roles and responsibilities of which they are still capable, the individual's self-esteem is supported and significant others are less likely to feel taken advantage of. When these patients present for psychological treatment, it is likely that they have taken the initiative, seeking to fine-tune some aspect of the way they cope with pain or address an emerging problem before it significantly impairs functioning. They take responsibility for the success of their treatment and can readily make use of interventions, implementing and adjusting them to fit their needs.

One of our patients was recently married and his career was in full swing when an automobile accident resulted in a spinal cord injury and paralysis from the waist down. This formerly independent man recounted that during an initial period of grieving and withdrawal, he had the surprising realization that the most effective way to remain strong and function at a high level was to seek out and accept the concrete and emotional support of others. In addition, he decided there were certain roles and responsibilities he had to let go, such as extensive physical work around the house and other roles in his culture more typically performed by men. This was not just to preserve his limited physical stamina and his long-term health but also to spare those around him the anxiety of needing to police his activity.

Fortunately, his wife and extended family were able to communicate their needs and concerns openly and to make necessary adaptations, and they were not overly invested in either the patient maintaining his previous responsibilities or in taking over all his functions for him. There was reciprocal give and take as well, with the patient assuming responsibility for bills, paperwork, and cooking so that his wife could do more of the physical chores. Regarding work, the patient reluctantly gave up having his office at the work site and convinced his employer to make modifications to his routine so that he had more flexibility in response to pain flare-ups, pacing his work schedule by working at home.

We do not wish to suggest that these changes and adaptations came easily or smoothly. The patient described a trial-and-error process with periods of grieving before he could accept losses of certain roles and activities and move forward. In fact, he sought out psychological treatment, not just for specific pain management skills (which he had researched prior to his initial session) but because he found himself slipping into some previous routines, such as working long hours at a stretch to finish a pro-

ject, habits he realized he could no longer afford.

Treatment of Chronic Pain Patients Using an Integrative Relational Psychodynamic Model

Regarding treatment using the integrative psychodynamic relational model, first, we elaborate on the therapeutic rationale, specifically the essential features of an interactional psychotherapy relationship as well as the processes by which change in psychic structure, adaptive behavior, and other therapeutic objectives are achieved in this model. Second, we focus on how this treatment is actually conducted with chronic pain patients and on tailoring the model to meet the unique needs of these individuals.

Achieving Therapeutic Objectives Using a Two-Person Treatment Model

"All relational approaches agree on the importance of the treatment relationship as a new and positive one. That is, interpersonal patterns formed in infancy and early childhood are perpetuated and can be transformed as they are reenacted in the therapeutic relationship. A central therapeutic element of each involves the therapist's efforts to reach the patient meaningfully, empathically, or reparatively as [one] who strives to identify and understand, rather than to repeat with him or her the patient's pathological relational patterns" (Frank, 1990, pp. 739–740)

Classical psychoanalytic theory conceptualizes the individual's symptomatology and behavior in response to an event—such as physical injury—as a compromise that provides an opportunity to resolve or gratify an internal conflict or drive. The treatment frame of psychoanalysis is anchored in the analyst's neutrality and anonymity, so that he or she can objectively observe expressions of this intrapsychic material. The patient projects their transference distortions onto this "blank slate" and the analyst's interpretations facilitate the development of the patient's insight.

In contrast, relational models view the person's internalized relational matrix as formed from an ongoing search for human connection and attachment. All aspects of functioning throughout life are inextricably interwoven in a relational milieu. Therefore, it follows that physical injury and pain, or any life event or stressor, occur and are influenced within the context of a relational world. The quality of engagement of the individual with significant others—including the therapist—greatly influences the adaptive and maladaptive aspects of their response to the stressor.

Relationally oriented therapists contend that the therapist is a real person who communicates something to the patient with every action, emotion, or expression made or not made. In this view, we cannot *not* communicate. For example, a blank stare without comment after a patient has emotionally recounted his struggle with chronic pain does not communicate therapist neutrality but is a communication that the patient will appropriately attempt to interpret. Whether intended or not, it can hardly be considered a distortion if the patient concludes that indifference or disbelief was behind the therapist's response. The psychotherapy relationship, even with its asymmetries of self-disclosure and therapeutic focus, is a real relationship. The therapist must therefore be open to the possibility, indeed, the inevitability, that the patient's experience reflects, at least in part, something real in their relationship.

In this approach, the relational components of psychotherapy provide the foundation for and mechanisms of therapeutic change. The following are several aspects of the therapeutic relationship that are used in relational approaches to achieve therapeutic objectives.

INTERACTION, MUTUALITY, AND INTERSUBJECTIVITY

The psychotherapy relationship in relational models is viewed as a two-person interaction in which there is mutual influence, in marked contrast to the one-person model of psychoanalysis which emphasizes the mental events experienced by a person considered in isolation from the person's social world. Further, every interaction can be seen as an expression of intersubjectivity, the

condition in which the mental state or experience of both patient and therapist are due partly to the influence of the other, leading to the mutual co-creation of meaning as the therapeutic endeavor proceeds (Frank, 1999; Stolorow & Atwood, 1992).

ACTIVE PARTICIPATION

Compared to analytic models, there is an increase in the range and modes of participation by the relational therapist to facilitate new and more adaptive relational experiences for the patient. As Frank (1992) argues, "The task of the therapist is to engage *actively* with the patient in a relationship in which pathogenic patterns are re-experienced, thereby providing an opportunity to transform them" (p. 60).

REAL RELATIONSHIP

In relational psychodynamic therapy, there is also an increased emphasis on the real relationship, in which the therapist strives, first of all, to be warm, concerned, authentic, and responsive; such a relationship facilitates a safe atmosphere in which the patient is most likely to self-disclose, engage with the therapist, and take risks. This therapeutic stance is different from the abstinence and nonresponsiveness that are characteristic of psychoanalytic approaches.

What guidelines are used by the relational therapist to establish and maintain this type of psychotherapy relationship? Certainly, an increased level of active participation by the therapist is not a prescription for unexamined interventions and self-disclosure or the spontaneous expression of any emotion, without prior careful and informed consideration of their impact on the patient. Making interventions in therapy solely because they are unique or daring suggests a disconnection from the patient by a therapist who is no longer engaged in a truly reciprocal interaction. In fact, much more vigilance is required because relational therapists do not rely on a rigidly defined technique that emphasizes therapist anonymity. The therapist must simultaneously attend to the multiple levels of meaning and behavior in the overall treatment and in the specific ongoing interaction.

Neutrality and abstinence are replaced with constant attention to the subtleties of the relationship. This attention involves the therapist considering the patient's interactions in and out of the session in view of a developing understanding of the patient's relational matrix, as well as attending to the thoughts and feelings that are elicited in the treatment relationship with the patient.

In determining the therapeutic value of self-disclosure or emotional expression, the therapist must consider the specific purposes that will be served for the treatment. Foremost among them is promoting an authentic psychotherapy relationship in which the patient feels safe and validated and which facilitates the widest range of relational experiences. Clearly, self-disclosure or any other intervention in therapy is not for the gratification of the therapist and must follow the guiding principle of "do no harm."

The Role of Therapist Variables in the Psychotherapy Relationship

How do therapists gain awareness of their own unique relational patterns that influence their participation in therapy relationships? Insight is most useful when it is gained experientially, accompanied by affect and behavior. Therefore, we are limited by the boundaries of our lived relational experiences that, fortunately, can be expanded through psychotherapy and clinical supervision and, especially, by continually taking risks and experimenting with new relational experiences in our own lives. That being said, as therapists we must acknowledge that regardless of our training and experience, we are subject to the same resistances and anxieties as our patients are when encountering new experiences and ways of viewing ourselves and others.

There are some relational variables that are commonly shared by psychotherapists, such as an interest in human behavior and a strong belief in the possibility of personal change and growth. For many, early relational experiences trained them to be highly attuned and responsive to the needs and emotions of others (A. Miller, 1981). The identity derived from helping others is the driving force behind much clinical work and there may be important personal reasons why one is drawn to work with chronic pain patients.

These honorable ideals form the basis for commitment to and genuine engagement with patients. However, the daily experience of clinical work with chronic pain patients can be overwhelming as therapists learn the intimate details of lives that are often tragically disrupted. Some patients have previously led productive lives and may have backgrounds that are not dissimilar to that of the therapist. What are some possible therapist reactions to the suffering of pain patients? Therapists may begin to feel as helpless and frustrated as their patients or that they have failed as clinicians. They may blame bureaucracies, insensitive employers, families, and others in response to their own and not their patients' needs. Conversely, therapists may assuage their feelings of helplessness by subtle blaming of the patient and by doubting his or her sincerity or commitment to recovery. Finally, therapists may become numb to their patients' experiences of suffering. This re-creates for the patient the responses of significant others who have had similar reactions. Perhaps an even more damaging aspect to this numbing is that it removes the therapist from a full engagement with the patient in the here and now, the very cornerstone of relationally focused psychotherapy.

Openly acknowledging these reactions to ourselves and our colleagues helps to prevent their derailing a therapeutic relationship. As clinicians we must focus attention on our own reactions in psychotherapy and thereby increase our empathic understanding of our patients' relational worlds by learning how others experience and react to them. This focus also increases our understanding of the reactions of patients' significant others, who spend far more time with and are more personally invested in the patients but who do not have the benefits of professional training to help them understand their feelings. Finally, therapists working with pain patients must also strive to be aware of patient characteristics that are linked to their own personal experiences. For example, a clinician may be too helpful (or too detached) with an older patient if his own parents are aging and becoming more dependent. Here again, the important factor is that being aware is more useful—and more possible—than striving to eliminate ourselves and our responses from the therapy relationship.

A Relational Perspective on Interpretation and Insight

"The patient's unconscious conflicts and fantasies come alive in the interactive play between the analysand's experience and the analyst's experience. One does not have to choose. Attention paid to interaction in the analytic relationship does not diminish or distract from the exploration of the patient's unconscious: it potentiates and vitalizes it" (Mitchell, 1997, p. 19).

Because the patient's experience can only be viewed through the lens of the therapist's own relational matrix, two-person models dispense with the analytic goal of making an objective, correct interpretation of the patient's experience. How then does the relational therapist help the patient gain greater self-awareness? To change, patients undoubtedly need increased awareness of the ways that patterns of behavior, cognitions, and affect are maladaptive or otherwise limit the responsiveness and flexibility of their interactions with others. The therapeutic value of insight is not discarded under a relational model; instead, insight is redefined from objective truth to one of many possible explanations obtained within a relational context. Mitchell (1997) argues that "interpretations are never merely informational events; they are always relational events; they transform relationships. . . . Conversely, actions and interaction always contain implicit interpretative statements and concepts . . ." (p. 16).

To further experientially derived insight, the relationally oriented therapist fosters a therapeutic relationship of safety and engagement. Inevitably, the behavior and affect of the therapist will be shaped in response to pressures emanating from the patient and in a manner that approximates relational patterns with significant early figures in the patient's life. Unlike analytic models in which this would be an undesirable countertransferential response, such enactments can be viewed as part of being human, and welcomed as opportunities for insight potentiated by emotionally immediate relational experience (Frank, 1999).

By facilitating a therapeutic environment of curiosity and openness, exploration of the enactment is encouraged. The therapist's contribution to the interaction is acknowledged, as is the fact that like all interpersonal responses, it is shaped and perceived by the patient's relational matrix. This approach represents a new definition of transference and countertransference responses in which they are bidirectional and involve mutual influence. There is no presumption of an objective perspective on what transpires in the relationship. Rather, therapist and patient together co-create a variety of inherently subjective meanings in the course of their interactions. Ideally, this process leads to greater insight on the part of patients regarding how they view themselves in interaction with others and how this view contributes to their behaviors, coping, and symptoms.

INSIGHT, CHANGE, AND NEW RELATIONAL EXPERIENCES

We have focused on therapeutic enactments in which the patient gains insight regarding his or her relational matrix as it is manifested in the therapeutic relationship. Insight, however, is a necessary but not a sufficient condition for the patient to alter dysfunctional relational patterns, even when the insight is experientially obtained. Change in psychic structure requires *new* relational experiences; interactions which break free—however briefly—from the limitations of familiar relational patterns and perceptions of the self in interaction.

One way this change occurs is by therapists not allowing themselves to be unduly shaped by the patient's internalized relational matrix in their interaction with the patient. Due to the therapist's inherent subjectivity, the therapist must be highly attuned to multiple, simultaneous aspects of a therapeutic interaction, as well as be as aware as possible of his or her own reactions. Wachtel (1987) referred to this effort on the part of the therapist when he noted that "the virtue of the analytic interaction lies in how it both replicates *and* deviates from other significant interactions in the patient's life. Such a combination of replication and deviation need not be approached in an artificial or manipulative way. It happens inevitably, whether one intends it to or not; the force field of the patient's emotional pull on the one hand, and the effects of training and self-reflection on the other, see to that" (p. 17).

New relational experiences can also be initiated by the patient. Typically, these new relational experiences occur first in the therapeutic relationship and, subsequently, in relationships and roles in the patient's world outside therapy. When we discuss incorporating action-oriented techniques in a relational model later, it will be seen that new relational experiences for the patient are often an intended by-product of interventions specifically aimed at more adaptive behaviors.

This most important stage of psychotherapy is also the most difficult and requires courage and persistence on the part of the patient. Even as people consciously make genuine efforts to better adapt to their environments, at the more automatic, unconscious level there is considerable pressure to maintain the familiar relational matrix—whether or not these relational patterns are adaptive—to preserve both a sense of predictability and relational ties to past significant others. Furthermore, well-intentioned significant others provide continual, subtle pressures to maintain the familiar in their relationships with the patient.

Skill, timing, and self-awareness on the part of the therapist are required to overcome the patient's resistance and make possible new relational experiences. Fortunately, co-creating and exploring together the variety of meanings of the enactments that inevitably occur in therapy energize both therapist and patient (as do all authentic interactions). The patient's hope for reduced symptoms and better adaptation, combined with a secure therapeutic relationship, facilitates initial forays into unknown and often frightening new relational territory. When a new relational experience does occur, it has affective, cognitive, and behavioral components that have two important consequences. First, the experience is internalized and, ideally, modifies the patient's relational matrix. Second, by providing something new that contrasts with the familiar, the relational experience can increase the patient's insight—the new relational experience provides a new perspective on customary relational patterns, and hence, allows them to be viewed more clearly.

Incorporating Action-Oriented Interventions in a Relational Treatment Model

Most relational psychodynamic clinicians have restricted their increased participatory role to interpersonal interactions in the therapy session. Furthermore, like classical analysis, most do not focus on behavior change but rather emphasize change in psychic structure or internalized relational configurations—with the implicit belief that adaptive behavior will eventually follow. A premorbid dysfunctional relational matrix no doubt contributes to chronicity in many pain patients and must be addressed in any comprehensive treatment. However, a treatment model that does not also emphasize more adaptive behavior is untenable for most patients with chronic pain who are in great need of improved methods of coping with pain and the suffering it has caused.

Fortunately, Wachtel (1997) and Frank (1999) have presented relational models of psychotherapy that include the use of action-oriented techniques aimed specifically at more adaptive behavior. Experiential aspects of the psychotherapy relationship, insight, and behavior change are all used concurrently in their integrative treatment models without one compromising or undermining the other. Frank (1999) argues that if there is full consideration and exploration of the consequences of an action-oriented intervention for the psychotherapy relationship, then the intervention will facilitate, not hinder, the attainment of insight. Ideally, insight and new relational experiences occur in tandem and each serves to potentiate the other in a "virtuous circle."

Interventions leading to more adaptive behavior in the patient's life may include establishing a more flexible repertoire for interacting with others and fulfilling daily obligations. Frank (1999) notes that relationally oriented therapists have in common with behavior therapists the belief that change does not happen merely through insight or by altering maladaptive thinking but by lived, affect-laden experiences, whether these are new behaviors or new relational experiences. An integrative relational psychotherapy implements interventions aimed at behavioral change that reflect the dual objectives of increasing adaptive behavior and in so doing changing psychic structure (i.e., the relational matrix).

Cognitive and behavioral clinicians might use the same techniques but would focus on the new behaviors and not necessarily on the potential that new relational roles and expectations have for increasing patients' understanding of their relational matrix. If the scope of inquiry is limited to the behavior, therapists miss a valuable opportunity to deepen and enrich the therapeutic benefit of new relational experiences. Indeed, some cognitive therapists have recognized that attending to the patient's responses to the psychotherapy relationship provides an opportunity to examine important behaviors and cognitions occurring within the treatment itself (Safran & Segal, 1990).

Implementing an Integrative Relational Model in the Treatment of Chronic Pain

The clinical application of this model is based on understanding the relational antecedents that can create a vulnerability to developing a chronic pain syndrome, as well as the psychosocial impact of chronic pain on the patient's life, especially with respect to relationships and relational roles. More detailed discussion of this and similar relational treatment models can be found especially in Frank (1990, 1992, 1993, 1999) and Mitchell (1988, 1997, 2000) and in Wachtel's (1997) cyclical psychodynamic approach and Basch's (1980, 1988, 1995) developmental spiral.

FACTORS THAT INFLUENCE PATIENT PARTICIPATION IN PSYCHOLOGICAL TREATMENT

The therapist must be aware of factors that influence the initial approach of the pain patient to psychological treatment in general and, more specifically, to participation in the psychotherapy relationship. Foremost among these are the patient's relational patterns that, as discussed in the next section, are assessed by conducting a relational inventory. Patients' initial presentations are also, of course, influenced by the history of their chronic pain experience prior to refer-

ral for psychological treatment. This history includes the course of the injury, pain, and disability; the associated psychosocial stressors; and the treatment history. Beyond a factual chronology, however, it is important to determine how they and their significant others characterize their response to the various treatments they have had and their interactions with medical providers, employers, insurance agencies, and others. How a patient portrays (and shapes) these relationships will provide important information on his or her relational patterns and roles, although the therapist also considers the potential contribution of other persons and aspects of the patient's situation. Therefore, an initial angry or suspicious presentation on the part of the patient is not automatically attributed to projection or cognitive distortion but may be an understandable reaction to previous experiences or the present treatment situation.

It is almost always preferable for the psychotherapy referral to be made early in the patient's overall treatment so that it can be implemented in conjunction with other treatment modalities. An exception may be made for those patients who are exclusively focused on finding a "cure" for their pain and who view any approaches emphasizing coping and adjustment as "giving up." Unless this belief is addressed at the beginning of treatment, participation in the psychotherapy relationship will be impeded by the patient's resistance, with missed sessions, noncompliance with assignments, and an overall stance of noninvolvement with the therapy. Some patients evaluated shortly after an injury may also have an open and hopeful attitude toward psychological treatment, viewing it as one of many simultaneous therapeutic modalities and as an example of the comprehensive care they are receiving.

Nevertheless, there is often a sequential rather than concurrent use of treatment modalities, and psychological treatment usually follows the failure of other modalities to bring adequate relief. In these not infrequent situations, patients may understandably present as resistant and discouraged, having concluded that they have been referred for a treatment of last resort. Referral for psychological services late in the treatment of chronic pain also makes it more likely that patients (and their support system) are depleted, demoralized, and depressed. They may be unable to sufficiently engage in the therapeutic relationship until accumulated psychosocial stressors are addressed and they obtain some measure of relief from psychiatric symptoms.

What patients have been told about their referral and any knowledge they have about psychological treatments for pain influence their expectations, fears, and initial interactions with the therapist. Patients draw their own conclusions when little has been explained and they have limited or inaccurate knowledge of psychological treatment. They may conclude that their medical providers believe that the pain is "all in their head," that they are exaggerating their pain, or that their medical providers have given up and do not wish to work with them. Consequently, they may approach treatment with hostility and suspicion, which, in the self-fulfilling process that is a cornerstone of relational models, can shape the therapist's evaluation of the patient and also his or her interactions with the patient. Conversely, patients may have been given inaccurate or misleading information, leading to expectations such as "you are going to teach me strategies to make the pain go away." This is problematic not only because it exaggerates the therapist's ability to reduce pain and communicates that this will be the primary goal of treatment but also because it implies that the therapist will be doing something to the patient, which is inconsistent with having the patient assume an active role in treatment. In such cases, the patient may come to the relationship with an eager but passive receptivity to treatment.

The patient's motivation for complying with a recommendation for psychological treatment is another important influence on interactions with the therapist and participation in the therapy relationship. Does the patient fear that refusing psychological treatment will lead to a termination of medical benefits or disability payments? Does the patient believe that cooperation with treatment means he or she accepts that the pain is all in the head? Is the patient agreeing to see a psychologist in order to placate a spouse or other family member? Does a family member

have an agenda, for example, a hope that the therapist agrees the patient is avoiding his or her household responsibilities?

INITIAL CONTACT: ESTABLISHING THE TREATMENT FRAME AND COLLECTING THE RELATIONAL INVENTORY

Because the psychotherapy relationship itself is the major therapeutic intervention in a relational model, treatment commences with the first interaction. The psychotherapy relationship that the relationally oriented therapist seeks to develop is likely to be quite different from those with other health care providers, in which the patient is often expected to be passive, if not deferential. Therefore, the therapist must quickly strive to model an interactive and participatory treatment relationship. To reassure patients, we often start by emphasizing that we believe their pain has a physical basis. We go on to say that psychologists are involved in the treatment of chronic pain both because there are effective treatment techniques, such as relaxation training and hypnosis, that psychologists have been trained to administer and because many patients find themselves in a vicious circle of pain and stress, which it can be helpful to discuss with someone who is familiar with chronic pain.

We often join with the patient's resistance by downplaying the role of psychological factors as causes of chronic pain, but we also normalize psychosocial stress and psychological symptoms as common consequences of chronic pain. Describing these before they are reported by patients may help them begin to feel that the therapist understands their experience. We also make a point of identifying areas of strength, communicating that we see health as well as distress and that it will be important to draw on this competence as treatment progresses. To this end, we often reframe the situation, inquiring, "How is it that you and your family have held up so well in the face of this prolonged stress? What has worked for you, and what is special about your family?"

Beginning to establish rapport and the proper treatment frame is only one of many competing tasks to be accomplished during the initial assessment. In contrast to many other psychotherapy relationships, treatment of the patient with pain is not self-contained but is usually one part of an array of treatment modalities with a complex history that must be collected by the therapist. In addition, because patients often have an inadequate understanding of why they were referred, providing education and addressing their concerns about why they were referred to a psychologist are essential.

While attending to these tasks, it is also essential for the therapist to be formulating and refining a relational inventory for the patient. Practically speaking, this task entails collecting a history of significant relationships and relational roles—paying particular attention to repeating themes, which shed light on the largely unconscious assumptions and expectations that shape how patients perceive their relational world. Learning as much as possible about patients' premorbid relational patterns, as well as the relational and other psychosocial changes that resulted from their injury and pain, enables the clinician to view current functioning in its relational context and to better understand previous responses to treatment. In what ways are the reactions of the patient and significant others to pain and disability a manifestation of prior relational patterns? Have the individual and support system been able to reestablish some degree of homeostasis, however fragile? Healthy, flexible, and responsive relational patterns are especially important to assess, as, of course, are those that are rigid, brittle, or dysfunctional. Some of the relational changes may be apparent simply in the context of the interview situation, such as the once independent woman who must now be driven to appointments by her spouse or adult child.

The degree of structured inquiry depends largely on therapist style. Typically, we ask patients to tell us about themselves, beginning with their childhood. Medical history and treatment are collected at the point in the patient's narrative at which health became problematic. Although many patients race through their premorbid history, asserting that it has little to do with their chronic pain, they are—almost without exception— eager to describe how their world has changed since the onset of their pain. Of course, they have varying abilities to identify and articulate the less tangible, qualitative aspects of the impacts on their relationships and relational roles. Because recall of past relationships is influenced by a person's current psychological state, it is almost always helpful to have significant others provide an additional perspective on the patient and his or her relationships and interactions before and after the onset of pain.

Important relational information may also be obtained by direct observation of the patients' interactions with others, including, for example, their contacts with clinic staff and their behavior in the waiting room. Likewise, referring providers may provide important information on how the patient interacts with and is perceived by others, especially if the therapist has worked with the provider and has a sense of how he or she typically relates to patients.

Most important from a relational perspective, therapists must attend to their own reactions to the patient, including their emotions, thoughts, and behaviors. Is a reaction out of character to the material being presented? Is there an uncharacteristic feeling of being put off by the patient's report of great suffering? Or, conversely, does the therapist feel great sadness in response to a seemingly straightforward presentation? Is the therapist more solicitous than typical, for example, offering the patient a glass of water when it has not been requested? Paying careful attention to all the reactions elicited by the patient provides important information, and relational clinicians go beyond traditional approaches to countertransference by considering how the experiences of both the patient and the therapist are simultaneously being shaped by and shaping each other in the relationship. In other words, beyond attending to the patient's influence on the clinician, they also consider how the patient's behavior, cognitions, and affect are shaped by the clinician's relational matrix. For example, does the clinician selectively reinforce the patient's more passive responses or those which are more assertive?

NEGOTIATING THE GOALS OF TREATMENT

At the completion of the assessment, the therapist has a preliminary model of the patient's enduring patterns of relationships, as well as of the changes in these relationships that have occurred as a result of pain and disability. Along with the other information obtained, this model provides ideas and direction regarding a tentative hierarchy of treatment needs to be discussed with the patient. The therapist may also be able to make some initial predictions regarding how the patient is likely to respond to the engagement required for an effective psychotherapy relationship, and also to the various specific interventions that are used with chronic pain patients.

Treatment planning and goal setting serve as the transition from the assessment phase to treatment and are an important but often neglected process. Although a discussion of treatment goals often follows from the assessment, this is not always the case, especially when the patient is unclear about psychological treatment. We seek to create a context for the discussion of treatment goals that is both hopeful and realistic, emphasizing that psychological treatment is not undertaken just because everything else has failed; rather, it provides additional strategies for patients to minimize the disruptions that have been caused by chronic pain, along with the various other treatment methods that might be appropriate given their needs. We add that our overall goal is to give the patient as many tools as possible to regain control of his or her life—a goal that accentuates the patient's active role in the treatment we are embarking on together. This in itself is an important albeit difficult objective in treatment of patients with chronic pain, who have often been subtly encouraged by health care providers, family, and others to respond to the chronic pain experience by relying on others to get things done. Continued therapeutic progress is facilitated to the extent that initial therapeutic efforts emphasize the importance of the patient's initiative. Importantly, from a relational perspective, any discussion of therapeutic goals that is open and interactive both strengthens the therapeutic relationship and is in itself as therapeutically important as the specific treatment goals ultimately agreed upon.

Most people suffering from chronic pain do not attend pain management clinics for psychotherapy—they come for pain relief. How then does the therapist respect the patient's goals and also present a treatment model that emphasizes the patient's rela-

tionships and, especially, the psychotherapy relationship? Of course, clinicians are continually educating and reframing the scope of the pain problem and the corresponding treatment goals. Patients come seeking pain relief and clinicians respond with inquires about coping, losses, and acceptance; patients come to treatment to be given something or have something done to them, and their role in treatment is redirected to make them active participants with ultimate responsibility for the benefits they obtain.

To assist in balancing patient and therapist objectives, we modify a therapeutic approach initially developed by Klerman, Weissman, Rounsaville, and Chevron (1984) to treat depression that has now been applied to a variety of other psychiatric disorders. Interpersonal psychotherapy emphasizes that regardless of etiological factors, depression occurs in an interpersonal context and that improving relational skills and the quality of relationships can aid in recovery and prevent recurrences. Substituting chronic pain for depression, we emphasize to patients that pain undoubtedly has a physical cause but that it has probably had a negative impact on the patients' relationships and their ability to fulfill various roles and responsibilities, which will only worsen the distress caused by their chronic pain. We might also offer a tentative observation that some of the patient's characteristic relational patterns might be decreasing their ability to cope with chronic pain in the most effective way possible. Depending on the patient's receptivity, we might further speculate that these patterns could play a role in the therapy relationship, which we would welcome as an opportunity to take a firsthand look at how the patient's interactions and coping with pain might be improved. We conclude by noting that an important part of psychotherapy will be to examine the patient's ability to make optimal use of social relationships in coping with his or her pain and disability.

Some problems necessitate immediate attention, such as certain psychiatric disorders. A substantial percentage of chronic pain patients suffer from major depression, posttraumatic stress disorder, and panic disorder (Dworkin & Caligor, 1988, Dworkin & Gitlin, 1991), but these disorders must be explored carefully. Questions about psychiatric symptoms may be interpreted by patients as indicating that the therapist thinks that their pain is caused by psychological problems. Although the presence of a psychiatric disorder often becomes obvious during the initial assessment without a specific series of questions that might put the patient on the defensive, in other cases a more structured assessment of psychiatric symptoms and history will be necessary. Many chronic pain patients argue that their psychological distress would disappear if only their pain syndrome was treated effectively. Successful treatment of chronic pain may alleviate a psychiatric disorder in some instances (Maruta, Vatterott, & McHardy, 1989), but when a pain syndrome and a psychiatric disorder occur together, it is usually necessary to treat these disorders concurrently.

Some situations require immediate attention, for example, extreme family conflict, substance abuse, destructive conflict with another treatment provider, and acute stressful events that could derail treatment. A concurrent social work referral can help remove stressors that interfere with the patient's engagement in treatment. If not available, an alternative strategy is to draw on whatever resources the patient has—for example, family, friends, other providers—not just to resolve the crisis but to help the patients see that they have an active support network. Because this requires that the therapist be directive and problem solving at the very time when he or she is attempting to establish a relational treatment frame that emphasizes the patient's competence, care should be taken to emphasize that this type of active involvement in the patient's life is temporary. When the therapist ultimately relinquishes this crisis resolution role and becomes less active, it is important to discuss how the patient has experienced it; depending on patients' prior experiences with treatment providers and others, this relinquishment may be interpreted as rejecting, as a response to something they have (or have not) done, or as an indication that the therapist is also "giving up" on them.

COMBINING A RELATIONAL FOCUS WITH BEHAVIOR CHANGE

Fortunately, a choice does not need to be made between the therapeutic objectives of greater awareness of the patient's relational matrix and more adaptive interpersonal behavior. As discussed earlier, the integrative relational model incorporates action-oriented interventions that target more adaptive functioning, and a relational focus does not preclude addressing a wide range of treatment needs and objectives in psychotherapy with chronic pain patients (Frank, 1999; Wachtel, 1997).

With some patients, the initial life history sessions evolve directly into a psychodynamic, relationally focused psychotherapy in which there may be little need for the integration of cognitive-behavioral interventions and techniques (e.g., relaxation training). However, because these techniques have almost always been discussed in the initial description of the treatment, it is important to explore whether this is a result of patient resistance or a relational enactment. Nevertheless, we generally follow the patient's lead not only because the patient is more likely to be engaged in a direction he or she has chosen but also because relief of the suffering that accompanies pain can sometimes be achieved by treating any suffering that the patient has brought to psychotherapy that is not related to pain.

More typically, after reviewing the patient's life history and treatment history in a variable number of sessions in which a major goal is establishing rapport, we then begin training in self-regulatory techniques (i.e., relaxation, hypnosis, and biofeedback) (Arena & Blanchard, Chapter 8, and Syrjala & Abrams, Chapter 9, this volume). While this occurs, we continue to discuss the negative impacts of the patient's pain on his or her relationships with family and friends, on his or her ability to work and participate in other activities, and on his or her mood.

With a relational psychodynamic model of treatment, self-regulatory and other action-oriented interventions are sometimes introduced later in treatment than would be true in cognitive-behavioral therapy. This is because of the attention that is paid to the meaning of using action-oriented interventions and to their impact on the therapy relationship, as well as the need to explore how the interventions can be used as a vehicle for new relational experiences. This delay is offset by an increase in the overall benefit that derives from applying these interventions in a relational context and by the greater compliance with their use that accompanies careful discussion of the patient's response to the intervention.

At first glance, the self-regulatory strategies that are often used in the treatment of patients with chronic pain would not appear to offer opportunities for new relational experiences. However, consider the patient who by regularly practicing relaxation exercises becomes able to remain calm in response to a sudden increase in pain. This patient has a new experience of self-mastery, as opposed to previous feelings of being a helpless victim who relies on others during exacerbations of pain. On a more concrete level, by using relaxation exercises this patient may also become able to resume formerly gratifying social activities, a tangible change in behavior that could have a far-reaching impact on his interpersonal relationships and support.

Just as treatment begins during the initial assessment, psychotherapy involves a continual process of reassessment and subsequent reordering of treatment goals by the therapist and the patient, some of it explicit and some implicit. Interventions double as trial balloons that provide further information for this ongoing reassessment, and adjustments are then made based on the patient's response and other signs of engagement with the treatment. Indeed, an approach that simultaneously targets adaptive behavior and change in psychic structure does not lend itself well to a standardized treatment protocol. For example, incorporating a specific action-oriented technique for one patient might be contraindicated for another based on the relational meaning of the intervention.

Treating Chronic Pain Patients in a
Psychotherapy Relationship:
An Open System

More so than with most psychotherapy, the treatment of chronic pain patients does not occur in a vacuum. The therapist is likely to interact with other medical providers, employers, attorneys, insurance companies, and, of course, anxious family members. Physicians inquire about patient suitability for invasive procedures or risk of substance abuse, employers want to know about suit-ability for work, and agencies request disability determinations. Treatment of chronic pain is best conducted in a multidisciplinary context; to draw a firm boundary preventing contact with these people can be unrealistic and not in the best interests of the patient.

Such contact presents a fundamental challenge to the inviolate confidentiality of the therapeutic relationship and to the patients feelings of safety and trust. Can patients be open and trusting with therapists when they are also terrified of returning to work and want the therapist to form a particular judgment on this or some other question related to compensation or level of functioning? The patient's willingness to be honest and reveal what he or she is thinking and experiencing in the treatment relationship may be influenced by a desire to make a certain impression.

Although maintaining the confidentiality of the therapeutic relationship is paramount, ongoing therapeutic issues are raised by the many requests that therapists receive for information about the patient. Open communication that ideally includes patients feeling enough trust to communicate their true feelings, and penetrating discussion of all requests for information about the patient from others can be grist for the relational mill.

Furthermore, pain is a family affair. The psychosocial stressors that affect chronic pain patients and their families provide many instances in which it becomes desirable to involve family members in treatment. The therapist's interaction with family members may determine whether they become a valuable resource and ally in achieving the goals of treatment or a force that undermines the patient's progress in treatment. Significant others, especially the spouse, have a closely interlocking array of relational roles with the patient, and the upheaval of chronic pain can be devastating to them as well as the patient. Indeed, the spouses of chronically ill patients may have as much psychiatric symptomatology caused by the impact of the patient's illness as the patients themselves. Of course, these effects on a spouse then become an important part of the overall negative impact of chronic pain on the patient's relational world.

Even a limited degree of knowledge of the spouse's relational patterns and roles can help the therapist anticipate potential sources of resistance when trying to facilitate more adaptive behavior by the patient. Depending on the relational matrix of significant others, they can resist the patient's beginning to engage in more adaptive behaviors and relational roles in a way that is difficult for the therapist to overcome. For example, they may be overly invested in being a caregiver for a helpless patient. Conversely, they may need to be the recipient of the patient's care and cannot adjust to a situation in which they must provide care as a result of the patient's impaired function.

Case Example

A middle-age woman was evaluated at a pain treatment center for back pain. Since first injuring her back 5 years earlier, she had almost continuous pain, largely nonresponsive to surgery or medications. She had been seen at the clinic on several previous occasions for a variety of pain complaints with inconsistent follow-up care. Her referring surgeon felt that her most recent exacerbation of pain was out of proportion to physical findings and suggested that nonsurgical interventions could be useful.

During her initial psychological evaluation, she was pleasant but generally passive, at times becoming vague and evasive in a shy, almost coy manner. Despite the severity of her pain, there had been no previous behavioral medicine treatment, physical therapy, rehabilitation, or nerve blocks, interventions often used in treating pain patients. Psychological treatment was recommended, although her noncommittal response led the psychologist to be surprised when she called several months later for treatment.

In the interim, she had left her job in the human services field. She offered little input regarding treatment goals and the therapist shifted focus to compiling an inventory of relational patterns and roles. The patient's parents were preoccupied with running several businesses and, impaired by mental illness, her mother often left the patient's care to babysitters. As a child, the patient believed she was her father's favorite, although he was critical and, when disappointed, predicted she would never amount to anything.

The patient also reported vague recollections of inappropriate and sexually tinged experiences as a young child, perhaps involving touching by a babysitter, another male, or, alluded to but never stated directly, possibly her father. Although having no access to details or dates, she remembered a distinct shift when she began to strongly dislike being touched in an affectionate manner. Subsequently, as a young adult she was promiscuous, but only when intoxicated, which led to her getting into dangerous situations, one of which led to a date rape. Several attempts to hurt herself as a young adult followed relationship losses, which were hidden from her parents and did not lead to treatment.

Variations of the relational themes of unmet needs for nurturance, rejection, and abandonment established in early interactions with parents were replicated in subsequent relationships. Promiscuity and superficial relationships gradually gave way to isolation and self-sufficiency, and she protected herself from intimacy and combated loneliness with all-consuming involvement in work and alcohol use. She began working in the human services field, invigorated by making a difference in other's lives and she felt included as an integral team member in a close-knit and committed organization. Unfortunately, when recurring pain and injuries led to more frequent work absences, she felt passed over and abandoned by the staff and interpreted it as another personal failure.

After several sessions, the therapist formulated a working understanding of her past and present interpersonal relationships and their representation in her relational matrix. Throughout life, she experienced unfulfilled longings for support from others but believed herself to be inadequate and undeserving of sustained love and attention. Intense ambivalence regarding intimacy stemmed from a conviction that devastating rejection was sure to follow. Fantasizing about complete acceptance, she invariably sabotaged relationships in a manner that replicated her past experiences. Her approach–avoidant relational style and sudden withdrawals to preempt abandonment confirmed the correctness of her beliefs about herself and others. In addition, her excessive giving but her rejection of offers of help caused her to experience relationships as depleting.

Several aspects of these patterns had a negative impact on the treatment of her chronic pain. She reacted to her intense longing to be cared for by others with an excessive investment in being self-reliant. This self-reliance led to great difficulty accepting treatment and support from medical providers, family, coworkers, and friends following her initial injury. In a self-fulfilling manner, this pattern contributed to the development of a chronic pain syndrome that was accompanied by great emotional distress. The persistence of her pain and distress were interpreted by the patient as another episode in a long series of failures. At an unconscious level, her suffering may have served to maintain internalized ties to the significant others who had predicted she was inadequate and likely to fail.

Treatment Goals

In a relational approach, specific treatment goals are subsumed within two broad objectives: (1) greater awareness of dysfunctional relational dynamics and an increased flexibility in relational roles and (2) behavioral change aimed at symptom relief and more adaptive coping. Improved coping for this patient would include becoming more assertive in seeking and accepting the support of others in dealing with her numerous psychosocial stressors, including the lack of health insurance, inadequate utilization of health care, dangerously depleted finances, and increasing self-destructive behavior, including substance abuse. Skill acquisition and self-regulatory training specifically targeting pain management would also be important objectives.

Engaging in these adaptive behaviors and action-oriented interventions would entail the patient's participation in an expanded array of new relational interactions. Positive reactions of others to her new social participation would lend further momentum to the process of modifying existing internalized relational patterns. Healthier relationships would potentiate increased self-awareness, which would, in turn, further the development of more flexible behavior, a positive

feedback loop that would ultimately lead to a more functional relational matrix and less suffering.

Despite dysfunction, areas of strength that could be used in the treatment of this patient include intelligence, sense of humor, psychological mindedness, a survivor mentality, spirituality, and a strong work ethic. Furthermore, while self-absorbed due to her suffering, she repeatedly expressed a desire for her life to make a difference, which was supported by her work history and passion for helping others.

Therapeutic Resistance and Engagement

The dynamics in the psychotherapy relationship paralleled her relationships early in life. For example, the patient initially responded with characteristic passivity to the therapist's attempts to establish a collaborative psychotherapy relationship. This response was accentuated by the cumulative impact of ongoing psychosocial stress, which had overwhelmed her coping skills, contributing to depressive and anxious symptoms, social withdrawal, and substance abuse. Interventions early in treatment aimed specifically at providing relief from these symptoms so that she could better participate in treatment regrettably required that the therapist temporarily become more directive.

As we discussed earlier, behavior is characterized by a conscious effort to meet certain goals while simultaneously shaping the world to replicate familiar patterns, even if it interferes with developing a more satisfying way of living. For example, although she no doubt earnestly desired symptom relief, the patient repeatedly and without consulting providers discontinued medications before their full therapeutic efficacy could be evaluated. Therefore, an ongoing effort in psychotherapy was helping her work collaboratively with staff, identifying and reporting side effects and treatment response to various medications. In a similar fashion, although the patient was intensely anxious and preoccupied about her diminishing financial resources, it was later discovered she had not applied for any benefits. In treatment sessions, she lamented being victimized by the injustices of the workers' compensation system, which prevented her from obtaining adequate health care and necessary hip surgery. However, an inquiry by the billing office revealed that she had not even applied for benefits after her most recent injury and had previously hindered attempts to obtain coverage by missing hearings, letting deadlines for appeal expire, and not responding to inquiries.

Throughout the treatment, the patient expressed frustration with what was being emphasized, regardless of whether it happened to be an action-oriented intervention or a discussion of relational themes and the therapy relationship. However, when the therapist succumbed to her pull to change course, hoping that her level of engagement would increase, she would not become any more collaborative. Without compromising ideals of remaining genuine in the therapy relationship, the therapist—although frustrated—resisted judgmental responses, which would only serve to replicate in the session a familiar relational pattern. Instead, he strove to respond in a way that was different from what the patient had come to expect from others. By communicating understanding of her struggles, he hoped to modulate her own self-deprecation regarding the difficulty of changing her familiar behavior patterns. An atmosphere of acceptance would provide opportunities for improved intimacy in the therapeutic relationship, increasing her openness to exploring her characteristic and any newly developing relational patterns in what for her had been foreign territory—being in a vulnerable relationship with another person.

The therapist tried hard to not respond to the patient's repeated provocations with pessimism about her prospects, as had others in her past. Inevitably, he was unwittingly shaped to contribute to enactments in which familiar relational patterns were replicated in the therapeutic relationship. For example, at times he responded to the patient's intense need for nurturance by vacillating between extremes of overinvolvement and withdrawal. The initial effect on the patient was to confirm her belief that she would eventually be abandoned if she became close to another. The therapeutic goal, however, was not to avoid enactments but to engage in an examination of the contribution of both parties and consider alternatives to the familiar relational pattern.

The patient pulled for similar responses with others outside treatment (e.g., with her uninvolved attorney), and although she avoided support from family and friends, their subsequent detachment nevertheless confirmed her convictions. She was largely oblivious to her contributions to this dynamic until well into treatment.

Throughout therapy, the patient had brief periods of frenzied activity and wildly optimistic aspirations, such as her dream that she would emerge from several years of unemployment and single-handedly create a comprehensive social service agency. These dreams only temporarily interrupted her relentless prediction of failure; a continual therapeutic challenge was to modulate her tendency to respond to the slightest setback (e.g., inadequate relief from medications) with an almost triumphant assertion that it was further proof she would never improve. Prolonged periods of immobilizing anxiety, withdrawal, and treatment noncompliance followed such self-interpretations of setbacks.

The patient repeatedly predicted that the therapist would eventually agree she was beyond hope, and seemingly trying to provoke this reaction, she would remain silent in sessions for weeks at a time, wearing sunglasses to avoid eye contact. She would occasionally behave as if the rejection had already happened, leaving angry messages asserting that she did not need the clinician's help. The therapist tried hard not to respond to these continual provocations and reaffirmed his commitment to her treatment, and the patient eventually became able to acknowledge that she really did not want to end therapy but needed to test his commitment to her.

Turning Point

One year into treatment, a serious crisis occurred that ultimately became an important therapeutic turning point. At the time, the therapist was in the process of leaving the pain clinic, and although he made arrangements to see the patient at another clinic and in the interim provided sessions without charge through his private practice, she perceived the change as if it was a personal rejection. She increasingly neglected self-care, avoided contact with others, and self-medicated with alcohol. She was withdrawn in sessions and increased the seriousness and frequency of veiled suicidal threats, delivered with a tone of hostility toward the therapist.

After a consultation, the therapist came to the realization that his treatment of the patient had, in fact, been affected by his preoccupation with the change in his job, and that he had given the patient inconsistent signals. For example, he made a concerted effort to initiate a referral for case management services. However, despite familiarity with this process, he did not monitor its status and there was a considerable delay. In addition, he also wondered if he had been responding to the cumulative effect of her passivity with increasing resignation. He recalled having been more likely to fall back on repeated assurances of his understanding of her situation or on empty speeches attempting to put a positive light on her progress; these were not based on the actual clinical situation and did not reflect an authenticity in his relationship with the patient, which fueled her fears of the therapist's eventual abandonment.

Shortly thereafter, the therapist responded decisively to her further deterioration, sending a crisis team to her apartment, which resulted in her psychiatric hospitalization. Although he initially wondered if this necessary action had irreparably damaged their relationship, her initial distress quickly gave way to relief. A positive therapeutic effect continued even when he set conditions on their continued work together. These were aimed at ensuring her safety but, equally important, refocused the therapy, which had gradually shifted from addressing the importance of change to responding to a series of crises. The therapist also insisted on a plan to eliminate abuse of alcohol and pain medication.

Initially surprised by her positive reaction, he realized that his recent interventions had been experienced by the patient as a powerful demonstration of genuine concern for her by another individual. These interventions also communicated a belief in her potential and an affirmation of her intrinsic value as a human being. The therapist's success in this instance in not complying with her relational patterns provided a new relational experience, creating a small foothold from which the patient could edge slowly toward taking greater responsibility for continuing the process, first within the therapy relationship and gradually in relationships outside treatment. Tentatively at first, she began to risk the anxiety of leaving familiar patterns and roles. By persisting with these interactions and rejecting familiar, deeply-rooted impulses, she discovered that she was not as likely to be rejected as she had feared.

More relevant to her chronic pain, new relational experiences meant that she could begin to accept the support of others. Previously, her relationships had been structured in accordance with a developmentally immature and rigid dichotomy in which the choices were limited to the extremes of complete dependence on another or absolute self-sufficiency. An evolving belief that it is possible to accept support and still be ultimately responsible for oneself eventually led to a more mature view of the importance of mutuality in adult relationships. Embracing a relational pattern based on the reciprocally giving and receiving support, although healthy and sustainable, nevertheless came with a cost. Accompanying these desired changes in her relational patterns, the patient experienced a sense of loss because her changed relational matrix required that she alter her internalized relational ties to her parents as well as the fantasy of someday receiving the support they could not or would not provide.

Nevertheless, the positive feedback among new behaviors, affirming reactions from others, and increased self-awareness gained momentum. For the first time since initiating treatment, the therapist's efforts to secure the help of agencies and other providers was met with the patient's active and sustained cooperation. Facilitated by an exceptionally persistent and empathic case manager, the patient obtained an array of social services, and the lessening of various psychosocial stressors stabilized the patient and better enabled her to focus and participate in her treatment. Importantly, increased comfort accepting the support of others seemed to stimulate greater effectiveness in her ability to soothe and take care of herself. She began using progressive muscle relaxation techniques that she had previously resisted and, no longer needing to self-medicate, stopped drinking entirely.

About this time, the therapist became more aware of ways that other providers had shifted into treatment patterns with this patient that were not unlike those he had experienced. He was surprised to fully realize for the first time how uninvolved her primary physician had been in her care over the past 2 years. Independently of and almost simultaneously with this realization, the patient arrived for a session announcing she had decided to transfer her care to a family practice physician, who then immediately requested the therapist's records and input into her treatment.

The patient responded with renewed initiative, finding a surgeon and making arrangements for long-awaited surgery. She decided to move closer to a friend so that she could obtain help during her postsurgical recovery. Fearing that she would lose her now valued network of supportive friends, church, and therapist, she was able to discuss these concerns with the benefit of increased awareness of her relational patterns. A plan was developed to address these concerns by soliciting the advice and feedback of the therapist and others. Regular contact and support were maintained through e-mail, phone calls, and her return twice a month, in which she stayed for several days with friends and attended extended psychotherapy sessions.

Conclusions

In this chapter, we have attempted to demonstrate the importance of certain relational themes in the perpetuation and exacerbation of persistent pain. We have distinguished the sensation of pain from the development of a chronic pain syndrome, which often involves unremitting suffering having its origins in untoward early developmental experiences. Although there is increasing interest among psychoanalytically oriented psychotherapists in the contributions that cognitive-behavioral therapy can make to psychodynamic psychotherapy (e.g., Frank, 1999; Wachtel, 1997), unfortunately, cognitive-behavioral therapists have not demonstrated commensurate interest in the contribution that psychodynamic perspectives can make to their approach to treatment. Certainly, these therapists attend to the idiosyncratic beliefs, maladaptive schemas, dysfunctional thoughts, and dysphoric moods of their patients. However, we believe that attention to relational psychodynamic issues—including developmental conflicts, resistance, and, especially, the transference and countertransference aspects of the therapeutic relationship—could substantially increase the effectiveness of all therapy with chronic pain patients.

Psychodynamic approaches to psychotherapy that are relational in orientation can be especially helpful to clinicians working with pain patients, because they allow for the application of cognitive-behavioral techniques without interfering with or minimizing the importance of exploring the meaning of a patient's pain and suffering. Indeed, we believe that relational issues play an important role in all interventions—not just in psychodynamic psychotherapy—and that an increased understanding of these issues can assist therapists in working with resistant, noncompliant, and unresponsive patients. As we view it, the essence of a relational psychodynamic approach is attention to three sets of relationships—developmental relationships, especially with parents; ongoing relationships, especially with family and friends; and the relationship that is established between the patient and the therapist. An increased awareness of these aspects of patients' lives deepens the therapist's capacity to understand a patient's interpersonal needs and conflicts and in so doing creates a context that can facilitate the amelioration of pain and suffering.

We conceptualize the chronic pain experience as the result of a complex combination of factors, reflecting processes of both the body and the mind. In reviewing our cases, we have become aware that in the successful treatment of patients with pain and suffering the individual comes to accept his or her pain (McCracken, 1998). By this we mean that pain and illness are accepted as an important but not self-defining part of the person's life, and as an unfortunate and only partially controllable aspect of the human condition. We cannot specify how a relational psychodynamic psychotherapy contributes to this process whereby the mind no longer disavows the body's pain and illness. However, we do know that when this process occurs, the chronic pain patient becomes a person with persistent pain—one who is no longer disabled but able to remove pain from the center of awareness and to replace suffering with meaning.

References

Aron, L. (1998). The clinical body and the reflexive mind. In L. Aron & F. S. Anderson (Eds.), *Relational perspectives on the body* (pp. 3–37). Hillsdale, NJ: Analytic Press.

Basch, M. F. (1980). *Doing psychotherapy.* New York: Basic Books.

Basch, M. F. (1988). *Understanding psychotherapy: The science behind the art.* New York: Basic Books.

Basch, M. F. (1995). *Doing brief psychotherapy.* New York: Basic Books.

Basler, S. C., & King, D. A. (1997). "He's sick, but I'm the one who hurts": Our work with a medically ill older couple. In S. McDaniel, J. Hepworth, & W. Doherty (Eds.), *The shared experience of illness* (pp. 334–343). New York: Basic Books.

Blumer, D., & Heilbronn, M. (1989). Dysthymic pain disorder: The treatment of chronic pain as a variant of depression. In C. D. Tollison (Ed.), *Handbook of chronic pain management* (pp. 197–209). Baltimore: Williams & Wilkins.

Bowlby, J. (1969). *Attachment and loss: Volume one.* New York: Basic Books.

Brena, S. F., & Koch, D. L., (1975). "Pain estimate" model for quantification and classification of chronic pain states. *Anesthesiology Reviews, 2,* 8–13.

Dohrenwend, B. S., & Dohrenwend, B. P. (1981). Life stress and illness: Formulation of the issues. In B. S. Dohrenwend & B. P. Dohrenwend (Eds.), *Stressful life events and their contexts* (pp. 1–27). New York: Prodist.

Dworkin, R. H., & Banks, S. M. (1999). A vulnerability–diathesis–stress model of chronic pain: Herpes zoster and the development of postherpetic neuralgia. In R. J. Gatchel & D. C. Turk (Eds.), *Psychosocial factors in pain: Critical perspectives* (pp. 247–269). New York: Guilford Press.

Dworkin, R. H., & Caligor, E. (1988). Psychiatric diagnosis and chronic pain: DSM-III-R and beyond. *Journal of Pain and Symptom Management, 3,* 87–98.

Dworkin, R. H., & Gitlin, M. J. (1991). Clinical aspects of depression in chronic pain patient. *Clinical Journal of Pain, 7,* 79–94.

Dworkin, R. H., & Grzesiak, R. C. (1993). Chronic pain: On the integration of psyche and soma. In G. Stricker & J. R. Gold (Eds.), *Comprehensive handbook of psychotherapy integration* (pp. 365–384). New York: Plenum Press.

Engel, G. L. (1951). Primary atypical facial neuralgia: An hysterical conversion symptom. *Psychosomatic Medicine, 13,* 375–396.

Engel, G. L. (1959). "Psychogenic" pain and the pain-prone patient. *American Journal of Medicine, 26,* 899–918.

Fairbairn, W. R. D. (1952) *An object-relations theory of the personality.* New York: Basic Books.

Frank, K. A. (1990). Action techniques in psychoanalysis. *Contemporary Psychoanalysis, 26,* 732–756.

Frank, K. A. (1992). Combining action techniques with psychoanalytic therapy. *International Review of Psychoanalysis, 19,* 57–79.

Frank, K. A. (1993). Action, insight, and working through: Outlines of an integrative approach. *Psychoanalytic Dialogues, 3,* 535–577.

Frank, K. A. (1999). *Psychoanalytic participation: Action, interaction and integration.* Hillsdale, NJ: Analytic Press.

Gatchel, R. J., & Turk, D. C. (Eds.). (1999). *Psychosocial factors in pain: Critical perspectives.* New York: Guilford Press.

Gatchel, R. J., & Weisberg, J. N. (Eds.). (2000). *Personality characteristics of patients with pain.* Washington, DC: American Psychological Association.

Grzesiak, R. C. (1994). The matrix of vulnerability. In R. C. Gzesiak & D. S. Ciccone (Eds.), *Psychological vulnerability to chronic pain* (pp. 1–27). New York: Springer.

Grzesiak, R. C., Ury, G. M., & Dworkin, R. H. (1996). Psychodynamic psychotherapy with chronic pain patients. In R. J. Gatchel & D. C. Turk (Eds.), *Psychological approaches to pain management: A practitioner's handbook* (pp. 148–178). New York: Guilford Press.

Klerman, G. L., Weissman, M. M., Rounsaville, B. J., & Chevron, E. S. (1984). *Interpersonal psychotherapy of depression.* New York: Basic Books.

Kohut, H. (1971). *The analysis of the self.* New York: International Universities Press.

Kohut, H. (1984). *How does analysis cure?* Chicago: University of Chicago Press.

Maruta, T., Vatterott, M. K., & McHardy, M. J. (1989). Pain management as an antidepressant: Long-term resolution of pain-associated depression. *Pain, 36,* 335–337.

McCracken, L. M., (1998). Learning to live with the pain: Acceptance of pain predicts adjustment in persons with chronic pain. *Pain, 74,* 21–27.

Miller, A. (1981). *The drama of the gifted child.* New York: Basic Books.

Miller, J. B. (1976). *Toward a new psychology of women.* Boston: Beacon Books.

Mitchell, S. A. (1988). *Relational concepts in psychoanalysis.* Cambridge, MA: Harvard University Press.

Mitchell, S. A. (1997). *Influence and autonomy in psychoanalysis.* Hillsdale, NJ: Analytic Press.

Mitchell, S. A. (2000). *Relationality from attachment to intersubjectivity.* Hillsdale, NJ: Analytic Press.

Safran, J. D., & Segal, Z. V. (1990). *Interpersonal process in cognitive therapy.* New York: Basic Books.

Schofferman, J., Anderson, D., Hines, R., Smith, G., & Keane, G. (1993). Childhood psychological trauma and chronic refractory low-back pain. *Clinical Journal of Pain, 9,* 260–265.

Schofferman, J., Anderson, D., Hines, R., Smith, G., & White, A. (1992). Childhood psychological trauma correlates with unsuccessful lumbar spine surgery. *Spine, 17*(Suppl.), S138–S144.

Sternbach, R. A. (1989). Acute versus chronic pain. In P. D. Wall & R. Melzack (Eds.), *Textbook of pain* (2nd ed., pp. 173–177). Edinburgh: Churchill Livingstone.

Stolorow, R., & Atwood, G. (1992). *Contexts of being: The intersubjective foundations of psychological life.* Hillsdale, NJ: Analytic Press.

Turk, D. C. (2000, July–August). *Is pain mind or brain?* Paper presented at Medicine Meets Millennium, World Congress on Medicine and Health, Hannover, Germany.

Turk, D. C., Meichenbaum, D., & Genest, M. (1983). *Pain and behavioral medicine: A cognitive-behavioral perspective.* New York: Guilford Press.

Turk, D. C., & Rudy, T. E. (1988). Toward an empirically derived taxonomy of chronic pain patients: Integration of psychological assessment data. *Journal of Consulting and Clinical Psychology, 56,* 233–238.

Wachtel, P. L. (1987). *Action and insight.* New York: Guilford Press.

Wachtel, P. L. (1997). *Psychoanalysis, behavioral therapy, and the relational world.* Washington, DC: American Psychological Association.

6

Operant Conditioning with Chronic Pain: Back to Basics

Steven H. Sanders

Operant conditioning is an empirically based behavioral model of learning for all forms of voluntary animal and human responses, as well as more automatic or generalized emotional responses (e.g., crying, withdrawal, facial grimacing, and fight-or-flight responses). The learning model of operant conditioning asserts that all overt behaviors are significantly influenced by their consequences and the surrounding context in which they occur (for reviews, see Goldfred & Davidson, 1994; Iverson, 1994; Lattal, 1992).

Fordyce (1976) and his colleagues were the first to systematically extend and apply the operant conditioning model to chronic pain. Their pioneering work generated an explosion of research and clinical trials that clearly established that operant conditioning concepts and procedures could be used with chronic pain patients to produce significant functional and behavioral improvement (see Compas, Haaga, Keefe, Leitenberg, & Williams, 1998; Morley, Echelston, & Williams, 1999; van Tulder et al., 2000).

In this chapter, I review and describe the operant conditioning method with chronic pain. I present a detailed review of the application of operant conditioning with chronic

pain patients as it is currently being implemented in interdisciplinary clinical programs. Likewise, although the focus of the chapter is on operant conditioning and learning, such a learning model should not be viewed as the only form of learning and conditioning effects on chronic pain patients. As has been demonstrated and discussed for a number of years (Sanders, 1985; Staats, Hekmat, & Staats, 1996), learning and conditioning effects on patients with clinical pain are multilevel and interactional, which involves operant, respondent (Hollis, 1997; Montgomery & Kirsch, 1997), and observational (Bandura, 1986; Schanberg, Keefe, Lefebvre, Krebich, & Gil, 1998) learning effects from antecedent and consequence stimulus conditions, often occurring in a social context.

Operant Fundamentals

Pain and Well Behavior

Overt "pain behaviors" and more adaptive overt "well behaviors" exhibited by chronic pain patients have been the focus of most research and clinical practice. Although it is important to note that overt pain behaviors are only part of the pain presentation (Turk & Matyas, 1992), there is general consensus that these overt behaviors are an important part of the clinical presentation. The other responses also occurring in someone experiencing clinical pain include neurophysiological and cognitive–subjective responses (see Sanders, 1985, for an expanded discussion). Regardless of these other more internal responses, the overt expression of pain through behavior constitutes the most salient and clinically relevant aspect of a patient's presentation. The most common overt pain behaviors can be categorized as follows:

1. Verbal pain responses, such as expressions of hurting, moaning, sighing, and expressions of pain through subjective intensity ratings.
2. Nonverbal motor pain behaviors, such as limping, using a cane or brace, grimacing, guarding, and rubbing.
3. General activity level, sitting, and lying down.
4. Consumption of medications and use of other therapeutic devices to control pain.

The common defining quality of all pain behaviors is their capability to be reproduced by relevant tissue damage or irritation (Sanders, 1985).

Overt "well behaviors" are typically just the opposite or reverse of pain responses. They can be categorized in the same four areas as the pain responses and include such things as verbal expressions of reduced pain level, reduction in the use of medications and other aids for pain control, increase in standing and walking behavior, increase in work behavior, smiling, and social–recreational overt behaviors. Many of the well behaviors are incompatible with pain behaviors, with both overt pain and well behaviors the fundamental target for clinical intervention.

Reinforcement–Punishment–Extinction

Reinforcement

Within the operant conditioning model, the fundamental paradigm is that of "reinforcement" (for in-depth discussions, see, for example, Fordyce, 1976, 2000a, 2000b). The reinforcement paradigm involves contingently following an overt behavior with the *application* (positive reinforcement) or *removal* (negative reinforcement) of a consequence, which results in the maintenance and increase in the occurrence of that overt behavior. Positive reinforcement consequences typically are things the person enjoys or derives pleasure from (e.g., food, social contact, and music). Negative reinforcement consequences are unpleasant experiences or aversive situations such as, pain, social stress, worrying, calls from creditors, and fear. This negative reinforcement paradigm is also known as escape–avoidance conditioning (Grant, 1964), with generalized emotional responses, such as crying, physical withdrawal, facial grimacing, and so forth, often involved. Such generalized emotional responses are not only influenced by their consequences but also initiated and maintained by respondent–classical conditioning effects. Behaviors in this negative reinforcement, escape–avoidance conditioning paradigm typically occur to permit the person to escape or avoid the unpleasant experience. Such behavior is extremely resistant to change and may persist indefinitely, particularly if it is an avoidant response to an expected unpleasant consequence. From a host of animal studies (see Sidman, 1962), as well as a growing volume of more recent research with pain patients (Vlaeyen & Linton, 2000; see Vlaeyan, de Jong, Sieben, & Crombez, Chapter 10, this volume), the negative reinforcement–escape–avoidance conditioning paradigm plays a major role in the development and maintenance of overt pain behaviors. To change such overt pain behavior requires the specific application of operant conditioning techniques as well as some respondent and classical conditioning methods (Vlaeyen & Linton, 2000).

Punishment

In the punishment paradigm, overt behavior is contingently followed by an aversive-unpleasant experience. If the aversive-unpleasant experience or consequence is strong enough and applied consistently, the overt behavior that precedes it will be reduced in frequency or might cease altogether under certain circumstances. There are a host of possible punishers; however, the most common includes social ridicule, interpersonal discord, stress, loss of social attention or recognition, loss of material possessions or resources, and the experience of pain (nociception) itself. Likewise, the punishment paradigm is present when an overt behavior results in the removal of an enjoyable or pleasurable experience, contingent upon emission of the overt behavior.

Extinction

The systematic removal of the contingent relationship between an overt behavior and its positive or negative consequences is called extinction. If a contingent positive or negative reinforcer is removed, the overt behavior usually shows a reduction. On the other hand, if contingent punishment is removed, the overt behavior may show an increase.

The major exception to this extinction effect is seen with learned escape–avoidance behavior, where even with removal of the contingency, the escape–avoidance behavior tends to persist indefinitely. To change such avoidant behavior, it is often necessary to prevent or limit the behavior from occurring so the individual can experience and thus learn that the absence of this avoidant response does not result in the occurrence of the anticipated aversive-negative consequence (see Sidman, 1962; Vlaeyan et al., Chapter 10, this volume).

Discriminative Stimulus Control

Various stimuli in one's environment can acquire discriminative or cue-like properties. Given repeated pairings with the target behavior and a contingent consequence, these stimuli acquire the ability to alert or signal the person that emission of a given overt behavior is likely to result in a certain consequence. Many overt pain behaviors are controlled by discriminative stimuli (see Keogh, Ellery, Hunt, & Hannent, 2001; Paulson & Altmaier, 1995; White & Sanders, 1986). The influence of these discriminative stimuli can be quite strong in directing the emission of a variety of overt behaviors. This is particularly true with regard to escape–avoidant

overt behaviors where there may not be any actual consequence to the avoidant behavior. In this situation, the discriminative stimuli serve as the main controlling factors.

Conditions for Effective Usage

Certain conditions are typically needed for operant conditioning methods to be effective. First, it is important to identify specific overt behaviors and effective positive or negative consequences for these behaviors. Consequences need to be applied consistently and contingently upon the occurrence of the target overt behaviors. Although immediate application of a consequence is preferable, it is not critical as long as the patient is aware that the administration is contingent upon emission of the target behavior.

The concept of "shaping" the occurrence of a given overt behavior is quite important. Specifically, shaping refers to systematically reinforcing successive approximations of a given overt behavior until the complete response is seen (Reynolds, 1968). Shaping is most applicable in trying to increase overt well behaviors, which often will not spontaneously occur without the application of shaping and reinforcement principles.

Another general condition for effective usage is the combination of operant techniques with other learning-based and behavioral procedures for maximum effectiveness. Although operant methods can produce specific changes alone, they work best if combined with other procedures, such as relaxation training, modeling, and desensitization procedures for escape–avoidance and fear responses (see Goldfred & Davidson, 1994; Spiegler & Guevremont, 1998; Warren, 2001).

Functional Behavioral Analysis

Within the operant conditioning model, the first fundamental step is the systematic analysis of overt behaviors and their controlling antecedent (discriminative) and consequent (reinforcing or punishing) stimulus conditions. This information is commonly obtained through direct observation of the patient, behavioral assessment questionnaires, and self-monitoring by the patient (see Goldfred & Davidson, 1994;

Schwartz, Jensen, & Romano, 2001; Sharp & Nicholas, 2000).

Application of Operant Conditioning to Chronic Pain Patients

Why

It is important to understand why operant conditioning techniques with chronic pain patients are necessary, particularly as clinical pain is, for the most part, an internal, subjective experience. Other than an obvious answer that operant conditioning methods have clearly demonstrated the ability to produce significant improvement in patients (Morley et al., 1999), other studies underscore some more broad-based reasons.

Connally and Sanders (1991) have shown that although chronic pain patients exhibiting high rates of overt pain behaviors can benefit from interdisciplinary pain rehabilitation, less improvement is noted. In addition, high levels of overt pain behavior have been found to be significant risk factors for establishing a failure to return to work and chronic disability in low back injuries (Sanders, 2000).

Thus, the presence of overt pain behaviors and the need to reduce them have important clinical and functional value. Given the poor relationship between overt activity level and subjective pain intensity (Linton, 1985), those clinical interventions that focus on just reducing subjective pain intensity and nociception do little to ensure a reduction in pain behavior or reciprocal increase in general activity level and other well behaviors. Likewise, research has demonstrated significant differences in overt pain behavior and function among low back pain patients with similar physical findings from different cultures and countries (Sanders et al., 1992). Such findings further suggest rather potent and important social, cultural, and environmental factors influencing overt pain and well behaviors that appear independent of the level of nociception and actual injury.

When

The following conditions typically need to be satisfied for operant conditioning to be applied effectively: (1) overt pain behaviors are present; (2) salient positive and negative reinforcers or punishers can be identified; (3) there is sufficient environmental control to contingently apply antecedent and consequent stimulus conditions; (4) the patient is not experiencing any major non-drug-related cognitive-learning impairment; and (5) the patient is willing to participate actively.

Table 6.1 outlines those basic conditions suggesting that an overt pain behavior is at least partially influenced by operant conditioning (see Fordyce, 1976, 2000a; Sanders, 1985). One can assume that operant conditioning effects are present and probably significant if at least three of the basic indications in Table 6.1 are present. Even if none of the indicators are present, operant conditioning may still be useful in any treatment protocol designed to increase more adaptive well behaviors, such as walking without a cane, exercising, laughing, or working. Also, the presence of basic indicators in Table 6.1 does not exclude the concurrent presence of ongoing nociception from tissue damage or irritation.

Where

For those patients showing poor cooperation or the presence of potent controlling conditions in the natural environment, an inpatient setting is the most effective venue. For most other patients, it is quite possible

---

TABLE 6.1. Basic Indications for Operant Conditioning Effects in Chronic Pain Patients

1. Overt pain behavior is chronic (3 months or longer).
2. Overt pain behavior occurs as a function of the environment, time of day, or person(s) present (e.g., in the clinic, at night, and with spouse present).
3. Overt pain behavior is acknowledged by others (family, friends, etc.).
4. Overt pain behavior is sometimes followed by positive or negative reinforcers.
5. Overt pain behavior is in excess of known physical findings.
6. Patient exhibits significant concern about increased pain with increased physical activity or return to work.

to apply operant conditioning successfully in an outpatient arena with the cooperation of the patient and family. A thorough functional behavioral analysis typically provides an answer to this question. This is even true for changing the overt pain behavior of medication usage. Such patients require frequent monitoring to be successful as outpatients; however, it is still quite feasible. An exception to this feasibility is the patient showing excessive use of other medications, such as sedative-hypnotics or alcohol.

How

Table 6.2 summarizes basic recommendations for applying operant conditioning to chronic pain patients (see Fordyce, 1976,

2000a; Keefe, 1994). As the table denotes, the first step is an assessment of a patient using a functional behavioral analysis approach. Likewise, any pathophysiology needs to be identified to incorporate in goal setting for realistic change. If possible, the patient should be asked to either sample or monitor some of his or her own overt behavior, such as standing or walking time, exercise repetitions, use of medication, and subjective pain intensity. There are a number of well-tested and clinically useful monitoring formats available (e.g., Collins, Moore, & McQuay, 1997; Jensen, 1997; Sanders et al., 1996). Also, it is advisable to have more direct observation of relevant pain and well behaviors. There are several sophisticated and highly structured observa-

---

TABLE 6.2. Summary of Recommendations for Applying Operant Conditioning to Chronic Pain Patients

Assessment

1. Perform a functional behavioral analysis on patient to identify relevant overt pain and well behaviors, controlling antecedent and consequent stimuli, and level of patient and family cooperation.
2. Identify the extent of physical pathology present and incorporate it in setting realistic goals for behavioral change.
3. Continue to monitor amount of behavioral change during treatment to allow meaningful decisions about effects.

Treatment

1. Use extinction to reduce overt pain behaviors (with response prevention if these are escape–avoidance behaviors), plus positive and negative reinforcement to increase well behaviors.
2. For reducing medication-taking behavior, use time-contingent delivery while reducing the amount of medication per dose or day.
3. For increasing general activity level, uptime, and physical exercise, use initial baseline levels and gradually increase these at preset amounts (determined with patient cooperation), with abundant reinforcement.
4. Use the concept of shaping or gradual change for well behaviors whenever possible.
5. Once behavioral increases are occurring consistently, slowly reduce the application of positive and/or negative reinforcement to a less frequent, varying schedule of about 50 percent occurrence for a given behavior.
6. Apply operant methods to *each* relevant overt pain and well behavior across as many different environmental conditions and people as possible to maximize generalization and discriminative stimulus efforts.
7. Eliminate or reduce as many external controlling stimulus conditions maintaining overt pain behaviors outside the treatment environment as possible.
8. Enlist the cooperation of the patient and family whenever possible to directly apply operant conditioning methods to change behavior.
9. Give operant methods time to work *and* be sure to follow patients for at least three to six months after active treatment to facilitate maintenance of change.
10. Use operant conditioning methods in concert with other psychological and physical treatments (e.g., relaxation, physical therapy, antidepressant and anti-inflammatory medications) within an interdisciplinary treatment approach.

tional and automatic recording systems (Bussmann, van DeLaar, Neeleman, & Stam, 1998; Lewis, Lewis, & Cumming, 1995). These are not typically used that often in clinical practice because of their complexity and cost. Most direct behavioral observational systems employ a rather straightforward checklist filled out at various times by members of the clinical staff and the patient's family. Two of the more widely used observational rating scales include the UAB Pain Behavior Scale (Richards, Nepomuceno, Riles, & Suer, 1982) and the Pain Behavior Checklist (Turk, Wack, & Kerns, 1985). Whenever possible, direct observation methods should be administered at least at the beginning, middle, and end of active treatment.

The treatment recommendations in Table 7.2 are generic and applicable across a variety of chronic painful conditions. Changing the use of pain medications is addressed in Recommendation 2, with this behavior at least a partial escape–avoidance response for increased pain. To change the use of pain medication, a form of response prevention is often needed to eliminate the contingency between taking the medication and escape–avoidance of nociception and physical withdrawal symptoms. This response prevention involves applying medicine on a time-contingent basis versus pain and withdrawal symptom basis (see Burkson & Gotestam, 1987). Although some patients may be able to reduce medication usage without changing administration to a time-contingent schedule (Rouse, Williams, Richardson, Pither, & Nicholas, 1994), time-contingent medication schedules and reductions are advisable most of the time.

Recommendation 8 underscores the need to involve both the family and the patient in behavioral change. Contemporary operant conditioning recognizes the possibility for self-application of techniques (Spiegler & Guevremont, 1998; Warren, 2001). Thus, the idea of patients reinforcing themselves when engaging in more appropriate behavior is not only quite feasible but desirable. The last treatment recommendation in Table 7.2 highlights the critical need to incorporate operant conditioning methods within an interdisciplinary rehabilitation approach (Sanders, Harden, Benson, & Vi-

cente, 1999). Such an interface allows maximum effect.

Case Example

The following case describes a patient treated in an interdisciplinary pain rehabilitation program following empirically based practice guidelines (Sanders et al., 1999), using operant conditioning techniques, along with other psychological intervention and medical and physical therapy treatments.

Identification and Chief Complaint

The patient was a 41-year-old single male with 2 years of college. He presented with a 2-year history of low back pain with radiation into the right lower extremity. The pain onset occurred subsequent to a lifting injury at work. The patient described his pain as a bilateral aching, grabbing sensation in the lumbar region with secondary shooting pains and some dysesthesia in the right lower extremity. His medical diagnostic workup indicated disc protrusion at the lumbar 4–5 vertebrae without any frank herniations. The patient also showed multiple myofacial trigger points in the lumbar region and some secondary dermatoma sensory loss in the right lower extremity, consistent with mild nerve fiber irritation at the lumbar 4–5 disc space. Orthopedic evaluation indicated the patient was not a surgical candidate. He had undergone three lumbar epidural steroid injections with only time limited pain relief. At the time of the referral, the patient was not working and was on workers' compensation.

The patient also showed some depressive symptoms, including feelings of sadness, indecision, poor appetite, and sleep disturbance. He also exhibited mild to moderate anhedonia and met the criteria for a major depression diagnosis.

Functional Behavioral Analysis

The patient's overt pain behaviors included noticeable gait distortion, guarding, grimacing, verbal complaints of pain, complaints of inability to function at home and at work, expressions of fear that increased activity would injure him and significantly increase pain, work avoidance, use of pain medications, and prolonged lying down and sitting at home. Time spent walking or standing (uptime) was estimated to be less than 2 hours per day by both the patient and his wife. Controlling antecedent discriminative stimuli included movement, home environment, presence of health care professional, any discussion of returning to work or increased activity, and secondary nociception from his nerve fiber irritation and myofacial trigger points. Consequent stimuli included reduction and avoidance of the following: nociception, fear and anxiety regarding increased pain and additional injury, possible side effects from drug withdrawal, and physical demands and stress in his work environment. The patient was also receiving some positive reinforcement regarding economic gains with most of his original salary and benefits continuing under the worker's compensation system.

The patient and his wife expressed interest in trying to make changes in his current behavioral pattern, while his employer expressed a willingness to work with him regarding returning to work in some modified capacity. The patient was asked to begin daily monitoring of his medication intake and subjective pain intensity levels rated every 6 hours. His general activity level was assessed using a weekly activity checklist completed by program staff.

Operant Conditioning Treatment

The patient was seen on an outpatient basis 3 days a week for 6 weeks, approximately 4 hours per treatment day. His wife was also seen on a weekly basis to provide information and education regarding appropriate responses to his behavior at home and education regarding long-term home management. The patient's pain behaviors were put on extinction regarding any social reinforcement in the treatment center or at home. Staff members and the patient's wife were advised not to offer any assistance or social attention with the occurrence of various pain behaviors. In contrast, overt well behaviors (i.e., general activity increases, verbal expressions of feeling better, increase in exercise tolerance, reduction in quantity of pain medications consumed, and verbal expressions of desire to return to work) were consistently followed by social attention and praise. The patient's pain medication protocol was changed with the application of time-contingent delivery and gradual reduction in doses over the 6-week treatment period (see Kasser, Geller, Howell, & Wartenberg, 2001, for details on medication reduction and detoxification protocols).

The escape–avoidance pain behaviors of lying down and sitting, minimal guarded walking with distorted gait, and verbal expressions of fear regarding increased pain and injury with increased activity and returning to work were targeted for specific interventions. The patient was started on a low-level walking program on an indoor track, using a normal gait. Initially he was physically assisted to help with a normal gait; this help gradually was eliminated. Likewise, the patient's walking activity was gradually increased, with successful increases reinforced by verbal praise and passive physical therapy interventions, such as ultrasound and massage. In addition to walking, the patient engaged in other strength-building and flexibility-building exercises with gradual increases at preset levels and reinforcement as with the walking behavior over time. He was started on a gradually increasing activity assignment schedule for standing and walking and general activity outside the home. These actions were reinforced by verbal praise from the staff and his wife and other pleasurable events, including his favorite meal, watching a certain enjoyable television program, and a back massage from his wife. Other functional activities and well behaviors were slowly added to the protocol and included such things as walking up and down stairs and driving.

To reduce any avoidant response regarding returning to work and conditioned fear associated with it, the patient engaged in some simulated work behavior introduced gradually and also revisited his work site to discuss with his employer, in concert with physical therapy center, any job modifications necessary for him to accomplish return to work. These modifications were incorporated in his work-specific behavior at the center for practice and repetition, followed by a great deal of social reinforcement. Approximately midway through the patient's treatment, the reinforcement schedule was changed to intermittent application. Approximately 50% of the occurrences of overt well behaviors were reinforced.

Other Concurrent Treatments

Alone with the operant conditioning methods, the patient also received other psychological, and physical treatments as part of his interdisciplinary pain rehabilitation. These treatments included relaxation techniques (see the Syrjala and Abrams, Chapter 9, this volume) and participation in educational groups (see Keefe, Beaupre, Gil, Rumble, & Aspnes, Chapter 11, this volume), which included social modeling effects, home-based physical exercise instruction, with a gradual increase in demands both in the center and at home, and use of nonsteroidal anti-inflammatory and antidepressant medications to help with his mood and sleep. Possible vocational options were identified and outlined, including both his existing work and other work options.

Treatment Outcome

At 6-month follow-up, the patient showed significant improvement in his overall function. Estimated daily uptime was reported at 6 hours per day, with a 40% increase in overall muscle strength and stamina. He had stopped using all opioid-based medications and reported a 60% increase in his general activity level. Subjective pain intensity was rated at 20% below his pretreatment level, and the patient's mood was rated as within normal limits. The patient's sleep showed significant improvement with approximately 7 hours of uninterrupted sleep per night. Overt pain behaviors showed a 75% reduction. He had resumed full-time modified work.

Operant Conditioning in the 21st Century

As this chapter illustrates, operant conditioning methods are a fundamental part of successful pain rehabilitation programs for chronic pain patients, particularly in today's health care market. Interventions that only reduce subjective pain intensity without demonstrating an improvement in general function do not really meet the needs of chronic pain patients. Improvement in physical function and reduction in health care usage, which operant conditioning can certainly influence, must be part of outcome objectives for as many chronic pain patients as applicable.

In spite of the clear efficacy of operant conditioning and other behavioral–psychological intervention, there has been a dangerous focus on more pharmacological and procedural methods with chronic pain patients over the last 5 years (Sanders, 2001). Indeed, the survival of operant conditioning and other behavioral interventions is at stake, with the real potential for their extinction. It is imperative that psychologists and other health care professionals do all that is possible to prevent this from happening, particularly, given the overwhelming evidence for behavioral–psychological treatment efficacy with chronic pain patients.

In addition to working within the health care arena to sustain and revitalize the application of operant conditioning and other methods, there is a need for continued research on the effects and limits of operant conditioning with chronic pain patients. Use of behavioral methods in the natural home environment, thus reducing the need for an intense in-center treatment, is an area of potential advancement (see, e.g., Cott, Ansel, Goldberg, Fabich, & Parkinson, 1990; Rowen & Andrasik, 1996). Likewise, the early application of psychological methods in more of a secondary preventive fashion is an area that has a great deal of promise (Marhold, Linton, & Melin, 2001).

The more broad-based sociocultural/environmental factors (e.g., political and economic policies, medical community practices, and cultural and religious practices) that influence overt pain and well behaviors clearly need a great deal more research and attention (Blyth, March, Brnabic, Jorm, Williamson, & Cousins, 2001; Sanders et al., 1992). It may well be that these more broad-based sociocultural factors that influence overt pain and well behaviors are quite powerful and controlling. This can be viewed as a learning-conditioning model at the cultural level. More research in this area could be quite useful regarding patient selection and the probability for improvement within a certain environmental context.

The preceding areas represent just a sample of those within the operant conditioning conceptual model that need more research leading toward improved application. Assuming efforts are successful in preventing the elimination of learning-based techniques with chronic pain patients, there is a potentially rich future for operant conditioning. Given successful political and research efforts, expanded application of operant conditioning and other psychological methods has the real potential to make a significant reduction in debilitating pain behaviors and an increase in productive well behaviors for millions of chronic pain patients throughout the world.

References

Bandura, A. (1986). *Social foundations of thought and action: A social cognitive theory.* Englewood Cliffs, NJ: Prentice-Hall.

Blyth, F. M., March, L. M., Brnabic, A. J. M., Jorm, L. R., Williamson, M., & Cousins, M. J. (2001). Chronic pain in Australia: A prevalent study. *Pain, 89,* 127–134.

Burkson, D., & Götestam, K. G. (1987). Effects of on-demand or fixed-interval schedules in the treatment of chronic pain with analgesic compounds: An experimental comparison. *Journal of Consulting and Clinical Psychology, 55,* 213–218.

Bussmann, J. B. J., van DeLaar, Y. M., Neeleman, M. P., & Stam, H. J. (1998). Ambulatory accelerometry to quantify motor behavior in patients after failed back surgery: A validation study. *Pain, 74,* 153–161.

Collins, S. L., Moore, R. A., & McQuay, H. J. (1997). A visual analog pain intensity scale: What is moderate pain in millimeters? *Pain, 72,* 95–97.

Compas, B. E., Haaga, D. A., Keefe, F. J., Leitenberg, H., & Williams, D. A. (1998). Sampling of empirically supported psychological treatments for health psychology: Smoking, chronic pain, cancer, and bulimia nervosa. *Journal of Consulting and Clinical Psychology, 66,* 89–112.

Connally, G. H., & Sanders, S. H. (1991). Predicting low back pain patient's response to lumbar sympathetic nerve blocks in interdisciplinary pain rehabilitation: The role of pretreatment overt pain behavior and cognitive coping strategies. *Pain, 44,* 139–146.

Cott, R., Anshel, H., Goldberg, W. M., Fabich M., & Parkinson, W. (1990). Non-institutional treatment of chronic pain by home management: An outcome study with comparison groups. *Pain, 40,* 183–194.

Fordyce, W. E. (1976). *Behavioral methods for chronic pain and illness.* St. Louis, MO: Mosby.

Fordyce, W. E. (2000a). Operant and contingency management. In J. Loeser, S. Butler, C. R. Chapman, & D. C. Turk (Eds.), *Bonica's management of pain* (3rd ed., pp. 1745–1750). New York: Lippincott.

Fordyce, W. E. (2000b). Learned pain: Pain as behavior. In J. Loeser, S. Butler, C. R. Chapman, & D. C. Turk (Eds.), *Bonica's management of pain* (3rd ed., pp. 478–482). New York: Lippincott.

Goldfried, M. R., & Davidson, G. C. (1994). *Clinical behavior therapy.* New York: Wiley.

Grant, D. A. (1964). Classical and operant conditioning. In A. W. Melton (Ed.), *Categories of human learning* (pp. 1–31). New York: Academic Press.

Hollis, K. L. (1997). Contemporary research on pavlovian conditioning: A "new" functional analysis. *American Psychologist, 52,* 956–965.

Iverson, G. L. (1994). Will the real behaviorism please stand up? *The Behavioral Therapist, 17,* 191–194.

Jensen, M. P. (1997). Validity of self-report and observation measures. In T. S. Jensen, J. A. Turner, & Z. Wiesenfeld-Hallin (Eds.), *Proceedings of the 8th World Congress on Pain* (Vol. 8, pp. 637–661). Seattle, WA: IASP Press.

Kasser, C., Geller, A., Howell, E., & Wartenberg, A. (2001). *Detoxification: Principles and protocols* [Online]. Available: www.asam.org.

Keefe, F. J. (1994). Behavior therapy. In P. D. Wall & R. Melzak (Eds.), *Textbook of pain* (3rd ed., pp. 392–406). Edinburgh: Churchill Livingstone.

Keogh, E., Ellery, D., Hunt, C., & Hannent, I. (2001). Selective attentional bias of pain-related stimuli among pain fearful individuals. *Pain, 91,* 91–100.

Lattal, K. A. (Ed.). (1992). Reflections on B. F. Skinner and psychology [Special issue]. *American Psychologist, 47,* 1269–1533.

Lewis, B., Lewis, D., & Cumming, G. (1995). Frequent measurement of chronic pain: An electronic diary and empirical findings. *Pain, 60,* 341–347.

Linton, S. J. (1985). The relationship between activity and chronic back pain. *Pain, 21,* 289–294.

Marhold, C., Linton, S. J., & Melin, L. (2001). A cognitive-behavioral return-to-work program: Effects on pain patients with a history of long-term versus short-term sick leave. *Pain, 91,* 155–163.

Montgomery, G. H., & Kirsch, I. (1997). Classical conditioning and the placebo effect. *Pain, 72,* 107–113.

Morley, S., Echelston, C., & Williams, A. (1999). A systematic review and meta-analysis of randomized control trials of cognitive behavioral therapy for chronic pain in adults, excluding headaches. *Pain, 80,* 1–13.

Paulson, J. S., & Altmaier, E. M. (1995). The effects of perceived versus inactive social support on the discriminative cue function of spouses for pain behaviors. *Pain, 60,* 103–110.

Reynolds, G. S. (1968). *A primer of operant conditioning.* Glenview, IL: Scott Foresman.

Richards, J. S., Nepomuceno, C., Riles, M., & Suer,

Z. (1982). Assessing pain behavior: The UAB Pain Behavior Scale. *Pain, 14,* 393–398.

Rouse, J. A., Williams, A. C., Richardson, P. H., Pither, C. E., & Nicholas, M. K. (1994). Opiate reduction in chronic pain patients: A comparison of patient-controlled reduction and staff-controlled cocktail methods. *Pain, 56,* 279–288.

Rowen, A. B., & Andrasik, F. (1996). Efficacy and cost-effectiveness of minimal therapist contact treatments of chronic headaches: A review. *Behavior Therapy, 27,* 207–234.

Sanders, S. H. (1985). The role of learning in chronic pain states. In S. F. Brena & S. Chapman (Eds.), *Clinics and anesthesiology: Pain control* (pp. 57–73). Philadephia: Saunders.

Sanders, S. H. (2000). Risk factors in the development and management of low back pain in adults. In K. S. Rucker, A. J. Cole, & S. M. Weinstein (Eds.), *Low back pain: A symptom based approach to diagnosis and treatment* (pp. 299–311). Boston: Butterworth & Heinemann.

Sanders, S. H. (2001). Chronic pain rehabilitation: Should and can it be saved? *American Pain Society Bulletin, 11,* 5–17.

Sanders, S. H., Brena, S. F., Spier, C. J., Beltrutti, O., McConnel H., & Quintero, O. (1992). Chronic low back pain patients around the world: Cross-cultural similarities and differences. *Clinical Journal of Pain, 8,* 317–323.

Sanders, S. H., Harden, R. N., Benson, S. E., & Vicente, P. J. (1999). Clinical practice guidelines for chronic non-malignant pain syndrome patients, II: An evidence-based approach. *Journal of Back and Musculoskeletal Rehabilitation, 13,* 47–58.

Sanders, S. H., Rucker, K. S., Anderson, K. O., Harden, R. N., Jackson, K. W., Vicente, P. J., & Gallagher, R. M. (1996). Guidelines for program evaluation in chronic non-malignant pain management. *Journal of Back and Musculoskeletal Rehabilitation, 7,* 19–25.

Schanberg, L. E., Keefe, F. J., Lefebvre, J. C., Kredich, D. W., & Gil, K. M. (1998). Social context of pain in children with juvenile primary fibromyalgia syndrome: Parental pain history and family environment. *Clinical Journal of Pain, 14,* 107–115.

Schwartz, L., Jensen, M. P., & Romano, J. M. (2001). Development and primary validation of an instrument to assess spouse responses to pain and well behavior in chronic pain patients: The spouse response inventory. *Health Psychology, 13,* 313–320.

Sharp, T. J., & Nicholas, M. K. (2000). Assessing the significance others of chronic pain patients: The psychometric properties of significant other questionnaires. *Pain, 88,* 135–144.

Sidman, M. (1962). Operant techniques. In A. J. Bachrach (Ed.), *Experimental foundations of clinical psychology* (pp. 170–210). New York: Basic Books.

Spiegler, M. D., & Guevremont, D. C. (1998). *Contemporary behavior therapy.* Pacific Grove, CA: Brooks/Cole.

Staats, P. S., Hekmat, H., & Staats, A. W. (1996). The psychological behaviorism therapy of pain: A basis for unity. *Pain Forum, 5,* 194–207.

Turk, D. C., & Matyas, T. A. (1992). Pain related behaviors: Communication of pain. *American Pain Society Journal, 1,* 109–111.

Turk, D. C., Wack, J. T., & Kerns, R. D. (1985). An empirical examination of the "pain behavior" construct. *Journal of Behavioral Medicine, 8,* 119–130.

van Tulder, M. W., Ostelo, R., Vlaeyen, J. W., Linton, S. J., Morley, S. J., & Assendelft, W. J. (2000). Behavioral treatment of chronic low back pain: A systematic review within the framework of the Cochrane back review group. *Spine, 25,* 2688–2699.

Vlaeyen, J. W., & Linton, S. J. (2000). Fear-avoidance and its consequences in chronic musculoskeletal pain: A state-of-the-art. *Pain, 85,* 317–332.

Warren, M. P. (2001). *Behavioral management guide: Essential treatment strategies for adult psychotherapy.* Northvale, NJ: Jason Aronson.

White, B., & Sanders, S. H. (1986). The influence on patients' pain intensity ratings of antecedent reinforcement of pain talk or well talk. *Journal of Behavior Therapy and Experimental Psychiatry, 17,* 155–159.

7

A Cognitive-Behavioral Perspective on Treatment of Chronic Pain Patients

Dennis C. Turk

Despite advances in the understanding of anatomy and physiological processes and innovative and technically sophisticated pharmacological, medical, and surgical treatments, pain continues to be a perplexing puzzle for health care providers and a source of significant distress for pain sufferers and their families. No treatments are currently available that consistently and permanently relieve pain in all people.

Patients with chronic and recurrent acute pain (e.g., migraine) often feel rejected by the elements of society who exist to serve them. They lose faith and become frustrated and irritated with the health care system that may initially create expectations for cure but turns its back on the pain sufferer when the treatments prove to be inadequate. At the same time that returning to work and earning a full income seem less possible, bills for unsuccessful health care mount. In time, chronic pain sufferers may begin to feel that they are being blamed by their physicians, employers, and even family members when their pain condition does not respond to treatment. Third-party insurance payers may even suggest that the individual is fabricating his or her pain to receive financial gain (e.g., disability compensation).

Thus, the emotional distress that is commonly observed in chronic pain patients may be attributed to a variety of factors, including fear, inadequate or maladaptive support systems and other coping resources, treatment-induced (iatrogenic) complications, excessive use of potent medications, inability to work, financial difficulties, prolonged litigation, disruption of usual activities, and sleep disturbance. Moreover, the experience of *medical limbo*—the presence of a painful condition that eludes diagnosis and implies either psychiatric causation or malingering on the one hand or an undiagnosed progressive debilitating disease on the other—is itself a source of significant stress and can aggravate a premorbid psychiatric condition or initiate psychological distress.

The person who has a chronic pain condition resides in a complex and costly world that is populated not only by a large number of sufferers but also by their family members, health care providers, employers, and third-party payers (insurance companies, government). Family members feel increasingly hopeless and distressed as medical costs, disability, and emotional suffering increase while income and available treatment options diminish. Health care providers grow increasingly frustrated as available medical treatment options are exhausted while the pain condition worsens. Employers, who are already resentful of growing workers' compensation costs, pay higher costs while productivity suffers because the employee frequently calls in sick. Third-party insurance payers watch as health care costs soar with repeated diagnostic testing for the same chronic pain condition. In time, those involved may question the legitimacy of the person's pain reports, particularly when no medical diagnosis substantiates the complaint. Some may suggest that the patient is complaining in an attempt to gain attention, avoid undesirable activities, or seek disability compensation. Others may suggest that the pain is not real but attributable solely to psychological factors (i.e., psychogenic).

People with persistent pain become enmeshed in the medical community as they migrate from doctor to doctor, laboratory test to laboratory test, and imaging procedure to imaging procedure in a continuing search to have their pain diagnosed and successfully treated. For many people, pain becomes the central focus of their lives. As they withdraw from society, they lose their jobs, alienate family and friends, and become more and more isolated. The quest for relief often remains elusive.

In contrast to acute pain, persistent pain confronts people not only with the stress created by the presence of pain but with a cascade of ongoing problems that compromise all aspects of their lives. Given this scenario, it should hardly be surprising that patients experience feelings of demoralization, helplessness, hopelessness, anxiety, frustration, anger, and depression. Living with persistent pain conditions requires considerable emotional resilience and tends to deplete people's emotional reserves, and taxes not only the sufferer but also the capacity of family, friends, coworkers, and employers to provide support.

A number of studies have demonstrated that even the most powerful medications, sophisticated surgical interventions, and innovative neuroaugmentation procedures (e.g., spinal cord stimulators and implanted drug delivery systems) do not totally eliminate pain and disability for all patients with chronic pain conditions (cf. Turk & Okifuji,

1998). This is not completely surprising given the long duration of pain and the impact that disabling symptoms have on all domains of life. Treating only the physical components of pain by trying to eliminate the cause or by blocking pain pathways fails to address the important psychological factors that become enmeshed with the chronicity of symptoms. In the absence of cure, the most appropriate treatment will be one that addresses cognitive, affective, and behavioral factors associated with chronic pain and not solely physical ones (see, e.g., Gatchel, Chapter 21, this volume).

In this chapter I describe a cognitive-behavioral (C-B) approach to pain management. This approach is not a replacement for more traditional health care but can be used to supplement interventions such as surgery and as part of a comprehensive approach to rehabilitation. It is important to keep in mind that at least for the foreseeable future, chronic pain is a chronic disease that will not be cured. Thus, pain sufferers need to learn methods and skills that can help them function better and improve the quality of their lives despite their pain. They also require continuity and ongoing support even when treatment has terminated. It is best to think of chronic pain as a disease similar to diabetes or asthma. In the absence of cure, the pain sufferer has to manage and his or her disease has to be managed over long periods.

Cognitive-Behavioral Model

The C-B model has become the most commonly accepted conceptualization of pain (cf. Chapters 18–26, this volume; Morley, Eccleston, & Williams, 1999; Turk & Okifuji, 1999) as it appears to have heuristic value for explaining the experience of and response to chronic and acute recurrent pain. The applicability of the C-B conceptualization has not been carefully examined in acute pain states, yet there is no reason to believe that the underlying features of the model would not apply to acute pain.

The C-B model incorporates pain sufferers' fear avoidance (see Vlaeyen, de Jong, Sieben, & Crombez, Chapter 10, this volume) and contingencies of reinforcement (see Sanders, Chapter 6, this volume) but suggests that cognitive factors, in particular expectations rather than conditioning factors, are of central importance. Thus, the model is a hyphenated one—C-B. It does not ignore the important role of contextual factors and principles of learning theory but rather incorporates them within an integrated perspective on pain sufferers and pain management. The C-B model proposes that so-called conditioned reactions are largely self-activated on the basis of learned expectations rather than automatically evoked. The critical factor for the C-B model, therefore, is not that events occur together in time or are operantly reinforced but that people learn to predict them based on experiences and information processing. They filter information though their preexisting knowledge and organized representations of knowledge (e.g., cognitive schema; cf. Turk & Salovey, 1985) and react accordingly. Their responses, consequently, are based not on objective reality but on their idiosyncratic interpretations of reality. Because interaction with the environment is not a static process, attention is given to the ongoing reciprocal relationships among physical, cognitive, affective, social, and behavioral factors.

According to the C-B model, then, it is the pain sufferer's perspective, based on his or her idiosyncratic beliefs, appraisals, and unique schemas, that filter and interact reciprocally with emotional factors, social influences, and behavioral responses, as well as sensory phenomena. Moreover, patients' behaviors elicit responses from significant others (including health care professionals) that can reinforce both adaptive and maladaptive modes of thinking, feeling, and behaving.

Assumptions of Cognitive-Behavioral Treatment

There are five central assumptions that characterize the C-B perspective on treatment (Turk & Okifuji, 1999). The first assumption is that all *people are active processors of information rather than passive reactors to environmental contingencies.* People attempt to make sense of stimuli from the external environment by filtering information through organized schema derived from their prior learning histories and by general heuristics that guide the processing of information. People's responses (overt as well as covert) are based

on appraisals and subsequent expectations and are not totally dependent on the actual consequences of their behaviors (i.e., positive and negative reinforcements and punishments). Thus, from this perspective, *anticipated* consequences are as important in guiding behavior as *actual* consequences.

A second assumption of the C-B perspective is that one's *thoughts (e.g., appraisals, attributions, expectancies) can elicit or modulate affect and physiological arousal, both of which may serve as impetuses for behavior. Conversely, affect, physiology, and behavior can instigate or influence one's thinking processes.* Thus, the causal priority depends on where in the cycle one chooses to begin. Causal priority may be less of a concern than the view of an interactive process that extends over time.

Unlike orthodox behavioral models (operant and respondent conditioning) that emphasize the influence of the environment on behavior, the C-B perspective focuses on the reciprocal effects of the person on the environment as well as the influence of environment on behavior. The third assumption of the C-B perspective, therefore, is that *behavior is reciprocally determined by both the environment and the individual.* People not only passively respond to their environment but elicit environmental responses by their behavior. In a real sense, people create their environments. The person who becomes aware of a physical event (symptoms) and decides the symptom requires attention from a health care provider initiates a set of circumstances different from the person with the same symptom who chooses to self-manage.

A fourth assumption is that *if people have learned maladaptive ways of thinking, feeling, and responding, then successful interventions designed to alter behavior should focus on maladaptive thoughts, feelings, physiology, and behaviors and not one to the exclusion of the others.* There is no expectancy that changing thoughts, feelings, or behaviors will necessarily result in the other two following suit.

The final assumption of the C-B perspective is that *in the same way as people are instrumental in developing and maintaining maladaptive thoughts, feelings, and behaviors, they can, are, and should be considered active agents of change of their maladaptive modes of responding.* People with chronic pain, no matter how severe, despite their common beliefs to the contrary, are not helpless pawns of fate. They can and should become instrumental in learning and carrying out more effective modes of responding to their environment and their plight.

From the C-B perspective, people with pain are viewed as having negative expectations about their own ability to control certain motor skills without pain. Moreover, pain patients tend to believe they have limited ability to exert any control over their pain. Such negative, maladaptive appraisals about the situation and personal efficacy may reinforce the experience of demoralization, inactivity, and overreaction to nociceptive stimulation. These cognitive appraisals and expectations are postulated as having an effect on behavior leading to reduced efforts and activity that may contribute to increased psychological distress (helplessness) and subsequently physical limitations (Jensen & Karoly, 1992). If we accept that pain is a complex, subjective phenomenon that is uniquely experienced by each person, then knowledge about idiosyncratic beliefs, appraisals, and coping repertoires become critical for optimal treatment planning and for accurately evaluating treatment outcome (Turk, Meichenbaum, & Genest, 1983).

Biomedical factors that may have initiated the original report of pain play less and less of a role in disability over time, although secondary problems associated alterations within the nervous system with deconditioning may exacerbate and maintain the problem. Inactivity leads to increased focus on and preoccupation with the body and pain and these cognitive-attentional changes increase the likelihood of misinterpreting symptoms, overemphasis on symptoms, and the perception of oneself as being disabled. Reduction of activity, fear of reinjury, pain, loss of compensation, and an environment that, perhaps, unwittingly supports the *pain-patient role* can each impede alleviation of pain, successful rehabilitation, reduction of disability, and improvement in adjustment. As has been noted, cognitive factors may not only affect the patient's behavior and indirectly his or her pain but may actually have a direct effect of physiological factors believed to be associated with the experience of pain (e.g., Flor, Turk, & Birbaumer, 1985).

People respond to medical conditions in part based on their subjective representations of illness and symptoms (cognitive schemas). When confronted with new stimuli, the person engages in a *meaning analysis* that is guided by the schemas that best match the attributes of the stimulus. It is on the basis of the person's idiosyncratic schema that incoming stimuli are interpreted, labeled, and acted on.

People build fairly elaborate representations of their physical state, and these representations provide the basis for action plans and coping. Beliefs about the meaning of pain and one's ability to function despite discomfort are important aspects of the cognitive schemas about pain. These representations are used to construct causal, covariational, and consequential information from their symptoms. For example, a cognitive schema that one has a serious, debilitating condition, that disability is a necessary aspect of pain, that activity is dangerous, and that pain is an acceptable excuse for neglecting responsibilities will likely result in maladaptive responses. Similarly, if patients believe they have a serious condition that is quite fragile and a high risk for reinjury, they may fear engaging in physical activities. Through a process of stimulus generalization, patients may avoid more and more activities and may become more physically deconditioned and more disabled.

People's beliefs, appraisals, and expectations about pain, their ability to cope, social supports, their disorder, the medicolegal system, the health care system, and their employers are all important as they may facilitate or disrupt the patient's sense of control. These factors also influence patients' investment in treatment, acceptance of responsibility, perceptions of disability, support from significant others, expectancies for treatment, acceptance of treatment rationale, and adherence to treatment recommendations

Cognitive interpretations also will affect how patients present symptoms to significant others, including health care providers and employers. Overt communication of pain, suffering, and distress enlists responses that may reinforce pain behaviors and impressions about the seriousness, severity, and uncontrollability of the pain. That is, reports of pain may lead physicians to prescribe more potent medications, order additional diagnostic tests, and, in some cases, perform invasive procedures. Family members may express sympathy, excuse the patient from usual responsibilities, and encourage passivity, thereby fostering further physical deconditioning. It should be obvious that the C-B perspective integrates the operant conditioning emphasis on external reinforcement and respondent view of learned avoidance within the framework of information processing.

People with persistent pain often have negative expectations about their own ability and responsibility to exert any control over their pain and they avoid activities that they believe will exacerbate their pain or contribute to additional injury (Vlaeyen, Kole-Snijders, Boeren, & Van Eek, 1995; see Vlaeyen et al., Chapter 10, this volume). Moreover, they often view themselves as helpless. Such negative, maladaptive appraisals about their condition, situation, and personal efficacy in controlling their pain and problems associated with pain reinforce their overreaction to nociceptive stimulation, inactivity, and experience of demoralization. These cognitive appraisals are posed as having an effect on behavior, leading to reduced effort, reduce perseverance in the face of difficulty, and activities and increased psychological distress.

The specific thoughts and feelings that patients experience prior to exacerbations of pain, during an exacerbation or intense episode of pain, as well as following a pain episode, can greatly influence the experience of pain and subsequent pain episodes (see, e.g., Jensen, Turner, Romano, & Lawler, 1994; Turk & Okifuji, in press). Moreover, the methods patients use to control their emotional arousal and symptoms are important predictors of both cognitive and behavioral responses.

The C-B perspective on pain management focuses on providing patients with a repertoire of techniques to help them gain a sense of control over the effects of pain on their lives as well as actually modifying the affective, behavioral, cognitive, and sensory facets of the experience. Behavioral experiences help to show patients that they are capable of more than they assumed, enhancing their sense of personal competence. Cognitive techniques (described later) help to place affective, behavioral, cognitive, and sensory responses under the patient's control. The assumption is that long-term maintenance of behavioral changes will occur only if the patient has learned to attribute success to his or her own efforts. There are suggestions that these treatments can result in changes of beliefs about pain, coping style, and reported pain severity, as well as direct behavioral changes. Furthermore, treatment that results in increases in perceived control over pain and decreased catastrophizing also is associated with decreases in pain severity ratings and functional disability (Sullivan, et al., 2001; Turner & Aaron, 2001). The most important factor in poor coping may be presence of catastrophizing rather than differences in the nature of specific adaptive coping strategies (Jensen, Romano, Turner, Good, & Wald, 1999; Jensen et al., 1994).

Cognitive-Behavioral Treatment

When patients with chronic pain come to a mental health professional, they have received multiple evaluations and a range of treatments provided by a host of health care providers. A common feature across all patients, regardless of medical diagnosis, is that the array of interventions did not adequately ameliorate their suffering. Thus, it is not surprising that when these patients are seen by a mental health professional, they feel demoralized and frustrated and believe that their situations are hopeless, yet they continue to seek *the* cure for their suffering. This is the background against which any therapeutic regimens that will be offered must be viewed.

Self-management and rehabilitation require a great deal of patient self-management and the onus of treatment success is transferred from the therapist to the patient. Patient motivation and willingness to become an active participant are critical to successful outcomes. Upon referral, it cannot be assumed that all patients are, indeed, motivated. Thus, the therapist must assess patient motivation and when necessary help foster motivation (see Jensen, Chapter 4, this volume).

Cognitive-behavioral therapy (C-BT) is designed to help patients identify, evaluate, and correct maladaptive conceptualizations and dysfunctional beliefs about themselves and their predicament. In addition, patients are taught to recognize the connections linking cognition, affect, and behavior along with their joint consequences. Patients are encouraged to become aware of and to monitor the impact that negative symptom-engendering or exacerbating thoughts and feelings may play in the maintenance and increase of maladaptive behaviors. The C-B therapist is concerned not only with the role that patients' thoughts play in contributing to disability, and to their effects on symptoms, but also with the nature and adequacy of the patient's behavioral repertoire. The strategic plan of a C-B intervention then is to facilitate patients' reconceptualizations of their plight. Patients initially believe that their illness is exclusively a medical problem. They view their symptoms as overwhelming and over which they have no personal control. The C-B approach is designed to be optimistic, emphasizing both the effectiveness of the intervention and patients' abilities to alleviate much of their suffering even if they cannot exert total control over their disease and physical limitations.

At the outset of treatment and continuing throughout, attempts should be made to discuss symptoms (physical limitations) and impact on the sufferers' lives as well as how others' lives may be affected by the problem created by the presence of symptoms (limitations). That is, the therapist conveys to the patient that he or she will work *with* the patient to achieve the best possible outcome given the constraints imposed by any physical limitations, but the therapist will not do anything *to* the patient. It is preferable to have this discussion with significant others present so that their misinformation and their concerns and fears can be identified and addressed as well.

Throughout the rehabilitation process, symptoms are reconceptualized so that patients come to view their situation as amenable to change by combined psychologically based and physically based approaches. Thus, there is an attempt to change the patient's beliefs about his or her condition. The treatment program is designed to teach patients a range of cognitive and behavioral skills and to assist them in dealing with maladaptive thoughts and feelings as well as noxious sensations that may precede, accompany, and follow the experience of symptoms or symptom exacerbation and thereby escalate emotional suffering.

Many behavioral (reinforcement, exposure) as well as cognitive techniques (e.g., cognitive restructuring, problem-solving training, and coping skills training, described below) are used. Other techniques based on these models (e.g., biofeedback, extinction of inappropriate illness behaviors, and reinforcement of activity) provide opportunities for patients to question, reappraise, and acquire self-control over maladaptive thoughts, feelings, and behaviors (e.g., avoidance), and physiological responses as well as adaptive skills.

The C-B approach is a collaborative endeavor that attempts to foster an increased sense of self-efficacy and self-motivation (Bandura, 1997). It is important to emphasize that the patient must be willing to work with the therapist and other members of the rehabilitation team. In this way, C-BT is quite different from what patients have come to view as appropriate treatment for their symptoms or impairment (medical problems). The therapist must be prepared to discuss the discrepancy between the patients' conceptualization of their problems, beliefs, and expectancies for treatment and the specific rationale for C-BT. Even if not acknowledged, there is no doubt that patients harbor some misconceptions and reservations about what appears to be a radical departure from conventional physically based treatments, and if these are not addressed by the therapist, the treatment is destined to fail as the patient will be unmotivated to become actively engaged. Even the most ideal treatment plan has little likelihood of success if the patient does not continue to engage in the prescribed behaviors once discharged.

The C-B perspective can be a basis for some physical as well as psychological interventions. When physical therapists or nurses work with disabled individuals they can use the same principles enumerated (Turk, Okifuji, & Sherman, 2000). The emphasis is on helping the patient to reconceptualize their situation and their own role in improving their physical functioning as well as in positive adaptation and accommodations to limitations imposed by their physical impairments. Table 7.1 summarizes the major features of C-BT for chronic pain patients.

TABLE 7.1. Characteristics of Cognitive-Behavioral Approach to Pain Management

- Problem-oriented
- Educational (teach self-management, problem solving, coping, and communication skills)
- Collaborative (patient and health care provider work together)
- Makes use of in clinic and home practice to consolidate skills and identify problem areas
- Encourage expression of feelings and then control of feelings that impair rehabilitation
- Addresses the relationship among thoughts, feelings, behavior, and physiology
- Anticipate setbacks and lapse and teaches patients how to deal with these

Aims and Objectives of Cognitive-Behavioral Interventions

Given the overview of the C-B perspective discussed earlier, we can now consider what the implications of this perspective are for developing interventions for use with people with diverse chronic pain diagnoses. Table 7.2 summarizes the goals of treatment. The objectives and each component of the treatment should be directed toward accomplishing these objectives.

We can now consider some of the specific components of the intervention. Treatment consists of four interrelated components: (1) reconceptualization, (2) skills acquisition, (3) skills consolidation, and (4) generalization and maintenance. Ongoing assessment proceeds throughout the treatment process.

Cognitive Reconceptualization

People are constantly thinking, evaluating, and appraising information and their situation. The thoughts that people have can greatly influence their mood, their behavior, and some of their physiological processes. Conversely, a person's mood, behaviors, and physiological activity can influence his or her thoughts. Thus, it is important for pain sufferers to become aware of the thoughts and feelings associated with their pain episodes. Cognitive restructuring is a method that encourages people to identify and change stress-inducing thoughts and feelings that are associated with the pain they experience.

It is hard for many people with persistent pain to accept that their thoughts and emotions can actually affect their bodies. To convince themselves of this fact, it is useful to have them self-monitor the thoughts and feelings that precede, accompany, and follow a pain episode or pain flare-up. When patients monitor their thoughts, they frequently identify a number of thoughts and beliefs that might lead to increased muscle tension and increased emotional distress. For example, patients may find that they have some of the following thoughts:

"I feel as though I can't take it any more."
"I can't do anything when my pain is bad."
"I don't see how this pain is ever going to get better."
"I shouldn't have to live this way."

These types of thoughts are maladaptive. They can increase pain through increased muscle tension and preventing efforts to cope with the situation. Using a diary (see Figure 7.1), pain sufferers can record when

TABLE 7.2. Goals of a Cognitive-Behavioral Approach

- Reconceptualization of patients' views of their problems from overwhelming to manageable (*combat demoralization*)
- Convince patients that skills necessary for responding to problems more adaptively will be included in treatment (*enhance outcome efficacy*)
- Reconceptualization of patients' views of themselves from being passive, reactive, and helpless to active, resourceful, and competent (*foster self-efficacy*)
- Ensure that patients learn how to monitor their thoughts, feelings, behaviors, and physiology and learn interrelationships among these (*break up automatic, maladaptive patterns*)
- Teach patients how to use and when to use adaptive overt and covert behaviors required for adaptive response to problems associated with chronic pain (*skills training and use*)
- Encourage patients to attribute success to their own efforts (*self-attribution*)
- Anticipate problems and discuss these as well as ways to deal with them (*facilitate maintenance and generalization*)

DATE/TIME	SYMPTOMS (How bad, 0–10?) SITUATION (What were you doing or thinking?)	HOW DID YOU FEEL? (How bad, 0–10?)	WHAT WERE YOU THINKING?	WHAT DID YOU DO? WITH WHAT RESULT?

FIGURE 7.1. Record of Symptoms, Feelings, Thoughts, and Actions.

their pain was particularly severe, what the situation was at the time of the pain, including what they thought about and felt prior to the exacerbation of pain or pain episode, during the episode, and after the episode as well as what they tried to do to help alter their pain. Examination of these diaries can help the therapist and patient identify maladaptive patterns of thoughts, feelings, behaviors, and symptom flare-ups.

Once specific associations of thoughts, emotions and pain are identified, the patient can consider alternative thoughts and strategies that might be used in similar circumstances. He or she can try these alternative thoughts and record the effects. For example, when a patient is reminded of the growing financial pressures by his wife, he may have a tendency to blame himself and think he has become a failure because of his inability to provide financially for the family. Thinking that he is a failure contributes to his feelings of helplessness and hopelessness, increases autonomic arousal, and eventually may exacerbate his pain. Many different thoughts and techniques can replace these distorted, self-defeating ones. This patient needs to consider the possibility that his wife is not blaming him; rather, she is trying to get them both to develop a plan to manage their finances. By viewing the situation less negatively, he can limit the impact that stress has on his pain.

The crucial element in successful treatment is bringing about a shift in the patient's repertoire from well-established, habitual, and automatic but ineffective responses toward systematic problem solving and planning, control of affect, behavioral persistence, or disengagement when appropriate. Table 7.3 outlines several essential functions in the reconceptualization process.

Reconceptualization involves continually reorienting the patient from his or her belief that symptoms or physical impairments are overwhelming, unmanageable, all-encompassing sensory experiences resulting solely from tissue pathology to a belief that symptoms and impairments as experiences can be differentiated, systematically modified, and controlled by the patients themselves. Again, it is the patient's beliefs about his or her condition and not the objective functional limitations that is of primary concern. Reconceptualization of maladaptive views is the framework of C-BT and provides validity and incentive for the development of proficiency with various coping skills employed in symptom control.

Cognitive restructuring focuses on identification of anxiety-engendering and other

TABLE 7.3. Functions of the Reconceptualization Process

- It provides a more benign view of the problem than the patient's original view.

- It translates patients' physical and psychological symptoms into difficulties that can be pinpointed as specific, addressable problems rather than problems that are vague, undifferentiated, overwhelming, and uncontrollable.

- It recasts problems in forms that are amenable to solutions and thus the reconceptualization should foster hope, positive anticipation, and expectancy for success.

- It prepares patients for interventions contained within the treatment regimen that are directly linked to the conceptualization proposed.

- It creates a positive expectancy that the treatment being offered is appropriate for the patient's problems. People are constantly thinking, evaluating, and appraising information about their situation. Thoughts can greatly influence mood, behavior, and physiological processes, and conversely, mood, behavior, and physiological activity influence thought processes. Thus, it is important for chronic pain sufferers to become aware of the thoughts, feelings, and behaviors that are associated with their pain and recognize that thoughts can affect psychological functioning and pain responses.

maladaptive appraisals and expectations and subsequent consideration of more appropriate alternate modes of interpretation. It is designed to make patients aware of the role thoughts and emotions play in potentiating and maintaining stress and physical symptoms. The therapist elicits the patient's thoughts, feelings, and interpretations of events; gathers evidence for or against such interpretations; identifies habitual self-statements, images, and appraisals that occur; tests the validity of these interpretations; identifies automatic thoughts that set up an escalating stream of negative, catastrophizing ideation; and helps examine how such habitual thoughts intensify stress and interfere with performance of adaptive coping responses. Table 7.4 provides a set of steps involved in cognitive restructuring.

TABLE 7.4. Steps in Cognitive Restructuring

1. Verbal set: rationale and overview of the procedure

2. Identification of patients' maladaptive thoughts during problematic situations such as during exacerbations of pain, when emotionally aroused, when feeling stressed.

3. Introduction and practice of coping thoughts

4. Shifting from self-defeating to coping thoughts

5. Introduction and practice of positive or reinforcing thoughts

6. Home practice and follow-up

Using these steps, the therapist encourages patients to test the adaptiveness of specific thoughts, beliefs, expectations, and predictions. Patients' actual performance may be used as a way to assist in cognitive restructuring. That is, self-monitoring of successful accomplishment of home practice tasks can be used to combat patients' maladaptive beliefs about the helplessness of their situation or their own functional limitations.

The therapist can make use of *imaginal recall* to assist in the process of cognitive restructuring. For example, patients may be asked to relive in their mind's eye one or more recent experiences of stress as if they were running a movie in slow motion in their mind, eliciting thoughts and feelings around specific events and responses. A number of questions might be used to guide the patient, for example,

"Is their anything common about these situations?"
"What thoughts and feelings preceded, accompanied, and followed the situation?"
"How did you cope with the situation?"
"How did it resolve?"

The therapist helps the patient to discriminate between functional symptoms (e.g., hyperventilation-induced chest pain) and disease-based symptoms (e.g., angina on effort) and to respond appropriately to each (see Mayou, Chapter 24, this volume).

Through self-monitoring, the therapist

helps patients identify when they are becoming stressed, assists them to become aware of low-intensity cues, examines the contribution of their thoughts, and deautomatizes the connection between events and arousal or distress. The therapist may ask patients to monitor symptoms but not to over react by assuming that all unusual or noxious sensations are attributable to worsening of disease.

As noted, treatment is viewed as a collaborative process by which the therapist carefully elicits the troublesome thoughts and concerns of patients, acknowledges the bothersome nature, and then constructs an atmosphere in which the patient can critically challenge the validity of his or her own beliefs. Rather then suggesting alternate thoughts, the therapist attempts to elicit competing thoughts from the patient and then reinforces the adaptive nature of these alternatives. Patients have well-learned and frequently rehearsed thoughts about their condition. Only after repetitions and practice in cuing competent interpretations and evaluations will patients come to change their conceptualizations.

Significant others are important as they may unwittingly undermine patients' changing their conceptualizations. The therapist should attempt to ascertain how significant others respond to the patient and when their manner of response is inappropriate to help the patient alter these conceptualizations. This clarification may be accomplished by encouraging the patient to discuss the response of significant others openly. It may be desirable to have the patient practice with the therapist how he or she will conduct this discussion.

Throughout treatment, it is important to permit and even to urge patients to express their concerns, fears, and frustrations, as well as their anger directed toward the health care system, insurance companies, employers, social system, family, fate, and perhaps themselves (Okifuji, Turk, & Curran, 1999). Failure to address these issues will inhibit motivation and success. During the reconceptualization process, symptoms are explained briefly with a simplified explanation of the role of stress on physical functioning. Often, physicians have been inattentive or dismissive of the patient's concerns, and an expression of genuine interest will help engagement. Caution should be exercised in suggesting that psychological factors or psychiatric illness play a causal role in symptoms. For many patients, such suggestions imply that they are imagining or exaggerating symptoms, are at fault for being ill, or are going insane. Common ground can be established by discussing the role of *stress* in medical conditions. Consider the following discussion with a patient who has chronic musculoskeletal pain:

"When people get upset, there is an unconscious tendency to tense their muscles. Muscle tension can create symptoms such as those that you experience. You have noted that you have been under a lot of pressure on your job lately. It is quite possible that the heavy demands of your job at this time are promoting the symptoms that you have been experiencing. There are a number of ways that you can affect your symptoms. We can consider some alternatives and see whether the symptoms are alleviated or improved. Does this make sense to you?"

The last question is crucial; the patient is not likely to be motivated to participate in a treatment that is not consistent with his or her conceptualization of the cause of the symptoms. To reduce defensiveness, it may be useful to state to the patient:

"When we have explained the relationship between stress, muscle tension, autonomic arousal, and symptoms to some people, they have been skeptical. What we have told them is that when we become upset, there is a tendency for our muscles to increase the level of tension, to become tight, and for stress hormones to increase making us feel more aroused and anxious. Have you ever noticed this happening to you?"

If the patient says "no," the therapist might note that muscle tension often happens without our being aware of it. He or she might even use biofeedback to demonstrate the effect of stress on muscle tension. Offering examples from everyday life can also be helpful—*how does one feel and what one does experience after a near miss in an automobile accident?* The therapist would then proceed to note that tense muscles and stress hormones can affect one's emotional states as well as exacerbate symptoms.

For some patients, stress may have a less direct effect on their physical symptoms but will be related to emotional distress. In either case, the therapist can note that there is a great deal that can be done by pain sufferers to control their levels of arousal and emotional distress once it is identified as a problem. Control is presented in a way the patient can understand using personally relevant examples.

Patients are encouraged to review stressful episodes and to examine the course their symptoms followed at that time. For example, a recent conflict with a spouse might be examined to determine whether the patient's getting upset had any effect both on the physical and psychological symptoms experienced. Imaginal presentation or recall of previous symptomatic exacerbations can be especially useful at this juncture. Patients can be asked not only to recall the situation but also their thoughts and feelings. With the help of the therapist, they can then discover the impact of thoughts and feelings on the experience of symptoms. In this manner, the therapist engages patients in a dialogue. The patient's maladaptive thoughts and feelings should be used by the therapist to illustrate how such thinking may influence inappropriate behavior and contribute to a worsening of the problem.

The therapist works collaboratively with the patient to link maladaptive, self-defeating thoughts with the patient's pain experience. Examples include thoughts such as the following:

"I feel so frustrated and angry with my doctor [employer, claims adjustor, family, self]."
"I can't do anything when my pain is bad."
"I shouldn't have to live this way."

These maladaptive thoughts typically fall within a common set of cognitive errors that affect pain perceptions and disability. A cognitive error may be defined as a negatively distorted belief about oneself, one's situation, or the future (Lefebvre, 1981). Table 7.5 lists a set of some of the most common cognitive errors made by pain patients.

Cognitive errors, frequently observed in chronic pain sufferers, can be related to emotional difficulties associated with living with pain. Variability in pain report and disability in chronic pain sufferers may be accounted for by maladaptive thoughts; in contrast, physical factors appear to contribute little to variability in pain and dis-

---

TABLE 7.5. Some Common Thinking Errors

- *Overgeneralization*: Extrapolation from the occurrence of a specific event or situation to a large range of possible situations. For example, "The failure of this coping strategy means none of them can work for me."

- *Catastrophizing*: Focusing exclusively on the worst possibility regardless of its likelihood of occurrence. For example, "This pain in my back means my condition is degenerating and my whole body is falling apart."

- *All-or-none thinking*: Considering only the extreme "best" or "worst" interpretation of a situation without regard to the full range of alternatives. For example, "If I am not feeling perfectly well, I cannot enjoy anything."

- *Jumping to conclusions*: Accepting an arbitrary interpretation without a rational evaluation of its likelihood. For example, "The doctor is avoiding me because he thinks I am a hopeless case."

- *Selective attention*: Selectively attending to negative aspects of a situation while ignoring any positive things. For example, "Physical exercises only serve to make me feel worse than I already do."

- *Negative predictions*: Assuming the worst. For example, "I know this coping technique will not work" or "If I lose my hair as a result of chemotherapy my husband will no longer find me attractive."

- *Mind reading*: Instead of finding out what people are thinking, make assumptions. For example, "My family does not talk to me abut my pain because they don't care about me."

TABLE 7.6. Challenging Maladaptive Negative Thinking

Challenge	Specific questions
What is the evidence?	What is the evidence to support these thoughts, assumptions, or conclusions?
What are alternative views?	How might someone else view this situation? If this were happening to someone else, how would I view it?
Is the thinking distorted?	Are you only attending to the dark side of things? Are you assuming that you can do absolutely nothing to change things?
What action can you take?	Where does thinking like this get you? What can you do to change the situation or how you feel?

ability. Once cognitive errors that contribute to pain perception, emotional distress, and disability are identified they become the target of intervention. Patients are usually asked to generate alternative, adaptive ways of thinking and responding to minimize stress and dysfunction (e.g., "I'll just take one day at a time," "I'll try to relax and calm myself down," and "Getting angry doesn't accomplish anything, I'll try to explain how I feel."). Patients may be asked to practice these alternatives at home and to review them during therapy sessions. The therapist will also praise patients for their efforts and suggest that they should positively reinforce themselves for the effort and not necessarily for the result, as changing habitual ways of thinking can take time. Table 7.6 includes a set of questions that can be used to target and challenge different cognitive errors.

Home Assignments and Practice

Home assignments are especially useful both for assessing and treating of chronic pain patients. Table 7.7 includes a listing of the purposes of home assignments.

An important feature of the C-B approach is the active involvement of patients and significant others outside the therapy sessions and the clinic. Home assignments and practice should be mutually agreed on. They provide important feedback to both patients and therapists. Successful completion of these assignments can be reinforced and maladaptive patterns that inhibit rehabilitation can be identified and addressed di-

TABLE 7.7. Purposes of Patient Home Activities

- To assess various areas of the patient's life and how these influence and are affected by the pain problem
- To assess the typical responses of significant others and the patient to pain, pain behaviors, and functional limitations
- To make the patient and significant other more aware of the factors that exacerbate and alleviate suffering
- To help the patient and significant others identify maladaptive responses to pain and pain behaviors
- To consolidate the use of coping skills, communication skills, and physical exercises
- To increase activity levels
- To illustrate to the patient and significant others that progress can be made in living with pain with reduced suffering
- To serve as reinforcers and as enhancers of self-efficacy as the patient achieves his or her goals
- To identify impediments to self-management
- To assist the clinical team, including the patient and significant others, in evaluating progress and in modifying goals

rectly. Table 7.8 summarizes a set of factors to consider when developing and implementing home practice assignments.

During treatment, each assignment is targeted toward observable and manageable tasks, starting with those that are most readily achievable and progressing to more difficult ones. The purpose of graded tasks is to enhance patients' sense of competence and to reinforce their continued efforts. Mastery experiences gained through performance accomplishments have the greatest impact on establishing and strengthening expectations. They provide the most information about actual capabilities and thereby challenge maladaptive beliefs about the lack of self-control and self-efficacy.

Self-Management Strategies

A wide variety of techniques appear to assist patients who are living with their pain while reducing suffering and disability. These strategies or skills can be broadly categorized as self-management and are used to help patients control and manage pain, factors that trigger pain, and distress associated with the pain. Some of these strategies are self-regulatory skills (e.g., relaxation training, biofeedback, and attention diversion) that allow the pain sufferer to self-regulate or control physiological responses that may be involved in pain production. Other self-management strategies are stress-management skills (e.g., problem solving) that allow the pain sufferer to effectively manage stress-inducing thoughts, behaviors, and emotions that trigger pain and maladaptive responses. With self-management strategies, instead of being a passive recipient of a medical intervention (e.g., medication and anesthetic nerve block), the individual plays an active role in learning and applying skills to manage the episodic or persistent pain problem.

There are many potential benefits from the use of self-management strategies. As patients learn to self-regulate physiological responses and manage stressful situations, they can develop an increased sense of personal control over the pain and the factors that influence pain and combat demoralization.

Skills Acquisition

In all cases, it is essential for patients to understand the rationale for the specific skills

---

TABLE 7.8. Factors to Consider When Setting Up Home Practice

- *Customize* the task to the patient's needs and style. Whenever possible, set the task collaboratively with the patient. This should increase commitment to adhere with instructions.
- Design the practice tasks so they are *appropriate* for the patient's level of education, gender, physical, and psychological abilities
- Try to create a *"no-lose" situation.* When possible make sure patient will succeed. Set standards slightly below what you believe they can reasonably do. Increase task demands as patient succeeds. For example, if walking more than 200 yards is the current limit, begin with a task of walking 150 yards for 2 days increasing to 200 yards for 2 days, 225 yards for 2 days, and so on until an appropriate limit is reached.
- *Explain* the rationale for each home practice task.
- Make instructions for home practice tasks as *concrete and specific* as possible. For example, practice relaxation exercises for 10 minutes once at 8:00 in the morning and once at 8:00 in the evening.
- Ask patient to *write down* each home practice task, to read the list back to you, and to explain the rationale.
- Ask the patient to *anticipate* what factors (including thoughts and feelings) that might interfere with their ability to successfully complete the home practice.
- Ask the patient what he or she *can do* if impediments to successful completion of home practice arise.
- Ask patients to *record* when they practice and what occurred. Ask them to bring recording sheets to next session
- *Review* home practice at next session. Modify requirements as needed.

being taught and the tasks they are being asked to perform. Unless patients understand the rationale for treatment components and have opportunities to raise issues and sources of confusions about them, they are less likely to persevere in the face of obstacles, benefit from therapy, or maintain therapeutic gains.

In rehabilitation, this is true for both physical and psychological interventions. For example, physical therapists should explain the rationale for specific physical exercises being taught, explain concepts of pacing so that patients will not *over do* exercises to reserve strength and protect from exacerbations of symptoms, discuss the differences between hurt or fatigue and harm, and discuss the possibility of *flare-ups* and relapse along with how these might be addressed. In this manner, physical therapists can adopt a cognitive-behavioral perspective rather than the more conventional physical–mechanistic approach that they have been taught. Mental health professionals can serve an important role as consultants to other health care providers, assisting them to take a broad perspective, one that focuses on the person and not exclusively on the symptom or physical diagnosis.

Cognitive and behavioral treatment makes use of a whole range of techniques and procedures designed to bring about alterations in patients' perceptions of their situation, their mood, their behavior, and their abilities to modify these psychological processes. Techniques such as progressive relaxation training, problem-solving training, distraction skills training, and communication skills training, to name only a few, have all been incorporated within the general C-B framework.

A number of specific skills have been reported to be useful in helping patients cope with their symptoms. At this point, research does not provide much guidance in how to select from among them. Perhaps more important than the specific tactics selected from those that have proven useful are the strategic goals of enhancing self-control and intrinsic motivation. The manner in which the various skills are described, taught, and practiced may be more important than the skills per se.

Again, it is essential for therapists to keep in mind the patients' perspective and how they perceive each skill and assignment. The therapist's skills and the relationship that is established between therapist and patient grease the gears of treatment; without a satisfactory therapeutic alliance, treatment will grind to a halt. Treatment should not be viewed as a rigid process with fixed techniques. There is a need to individualize the treatment program for specific patients; however, the C-B rationale described previously remains constant.

PROBLEM SOLVING

A technique that is closely aligned with and incorporated into cognitive restructuring (described earlier) is problem solving. Problem solving consists of six steps, each of which is related to specific questions or actions (Tables 7.9 and 7.10) and a problem-solving orientation has been shown to be particularly useful in treating chronic pain patients (Shaw, Feuerstein, Haufler, Berkowitz, & Lopez, 2001). An important first step is to identify the situations that are associated with pain. Self-monitoring can help identify the links between thoughts, feelings, and pain and thereby identify the problem (see Figure 7.1). By using problem-

---

TABLE 7.9. Steps of Problem Solving

- Define the source of distress or stress reactions as problems to be solved
- Set realistic goals as concretely as possible by stating the problem in behavioral terms
- Generate a wide range of possible alternate courses of action to reach each goal
- Imagine and consider how others might respond if asked to deal with a similar problem
- Evaluate the pros and cons of each proposed solution and rank order the solutions from least to most practical
- Rehearse strategies and behaviors by imagery, role reversal, or behavioral rehearsal
- Try out the most feasible solution
- Expect some failures, but reward self for having tried
- Reconsider the original problem in light of the attempted solution
- Recycle as needed

TABLE 7.10. Problem-Solving Questions
and Actions

Steps	Questions/actions
Problem identification	"What is the concern?"
Goal selection	"What do I want?"
Generation of alternatives	"What can I do?"
Decision making	"What is my decision?"
Implementation	"Do it!"
Evaluation	"Did it work? If not, recycle."

solving strategies, patients can target situations that trigger muscle tension associated with their pain.

Once a problem has been identified, the patient can begin to enumerate a set of solutions. Patients evaluate the likely outcomes of implementing each possible solution. Patients may then try their strategies and evaluate the outcome. If they are not satisfied with the first strategy, they can review the other options that they generated and decide to try another one. There is no one perfect solution, but some are more effective than others at a particular point in time. After using successful problem-solving approaches, patients can increase their confidence in their ability to handle stressful situations. Generalization should be encouraged as new problems will likely arise. Initial success will also provide patients with disconfirmation of their lack of control, increase motivation, and provide information that can alter their cognitive schema of hopelessness and helplessness to control and adapt to chronic pain.

RELAXATION

Perhaps the most common and practical techniques to manage pain are controlled breathing and muscle relaxation. It is helpful to begin relaxation exercises early in treatment because they are readily learned by almost all patients and appear to the patient to be physically oriented and thus credible.

The teaching and practice of relaxation is designed not only to help patients learn a response that is incompatible with muscle ten-

sion but also to help patients develop a behavioral coping skill that can be used in any situation in which adaptive coping is required. The practice of relaxation strengthens patients' beliefs that they can exert some control during periods of stress and symptoms and that they are not helpless or impotent.

The therapist should discuss with patients how to identify bodily signs of physical tenseness, the stress–tension cycle, how occupying one's attention can short-circuit stress, how relaxation can reduce anxiety because it enables patients to exert control, how relaxation and tension are incompatible states, and finally, how unwinding after stressful experiences can be therapeutic.

Relaxation can be used for its direct effects on specific muscles, for reduction of generalized arousal, for its cognitive effects (as a distraction or attention diversion strategy), and for its value in increasing the patient's sense of control and self-efficacy. Patients should be reminded that relaxation can be used in any situation in which adaptive coping is required. There is a wide range of different relaxation techniques (e.g., biofeedback, imagery, and controlled breathing; see Arena & Blanchard, Chapter 8, and Syrjala & Abrams, Chapter 9, this volume) geared toward assisting patients to learn how to deal with stress and, in particular, how to reduce site-specific muscular hyperarousal. Moreover, relaxation also includes active efforts such as aerobic exercise, walking, and engaging in a range of pleasurable activities that are consistent with the patient's interests and physical limitations.

Throughout the practice of relaxation, the therapist continues to take the collaborator's role. This is important for developing the conceptualization of relaxation as a self-management skill, thereby facilitating self-control of stress, affective distress, and at times physical symptoms. Because failure during the initial stages of treatment can seriously undermine the patients' confidence and motivation, the therapist should assume a role that fosters the patients' perception of success. This support can be accomplished by frequently acknowledging patients' efforts and progress. All possible indications and reports of success by the patient should be reinforced.

Following each session, patients should be provided specific home practice assignments to perform, self-monitor, and record (see Table 7.11). At the beginning of each subsequent session, the therapist reviews the self-monitored practice charts with the patient to identify problems and to reinforce effort as well as success.

After patients have become proficient in relaxation, it is useful to have them imagine themselves in various stress or conflict situations and to visualize themselves employing the relaxation skills in those situations. The therapist may describe coping versus mastery examples derived from other patients. That is, the therapist may describe how patients reported trying to relax, having problems, and then overcoming them. In this way, patients become aware that problems might arise; however, they can confront these problems as well as see that they are not the only ones who have difficulties. Patients are informed that relaxation is a skill and like any skill requires practice.

In subsequent sessions, the therapist teaches patients that one can relax not only by tensing and releasing muscle groups as in progressive relaxation, or by means of some passive activities such as controlled breathing, but also by means of absorbing activities such as physical activity (e.g., walking and swimming), hobbies (e.g., knitting and gardening), and so forth.

Because many pain problems have musculoskeletal or neuromuscular components, learning to reduce and control muscle tension can be effective for several reasons. When pain is due to muscle spasm, muscle relaxation procedures may directly reduce pain by decreasing or preventing this process. Engaging in muscle relaxation may also reduce the anxiety and distress that accompany persistent pain or trigger pain episodes. Relaxation can improve sleep, which may have secondary benefits; it is much easier to cope when rested than fatigued. Finally, muscle relaxation may also distract the patient from noxious sensations.

All too often, therapists and patients fail to understand the fact that relaxation is a state of mind as well as a state of the body. Mental relaxation may be as important as physical relaxation.

There are many types of relaxation and no one "best" approach has been demonstrated to be more effective than any other. The patient can learn different approaches in order to find one that is most useful. If one approach does not seem to be effective, others can be tried (for more details on relaxation, see Syrjala & Abrams, Chapter 9, this volume).

COGNITIVE COPING SKILLS TRAINING

Coping is assumed to occur by spontaneously employed purposeful and intentional acts, and it can be assessed in terms of covert and overt behaviors. Cognitive coping strategies include various means of distracting oneself from pain, reassuring oneself about one's own capabilities or about the likelihood that the pain will diminish, seeking information, and problem solving. Coping strategies are thought to alter both the perceived intensity of pain and the ability to tolerate pain while continuing daily activities.

There does not appear to be any one best coping skill to manage pain and disability. Rather than teaching patients a specific set of coping strategies, it may be more helpful for the patient to learn about several that can then be used in combination.

ATTENTION DIVERSION

Attention is a major precursor of perception and therefore of concern in examining and changing behavior. Patients in pain are often preoccupied with their bodily symptoms. Every new sensation is seen as an indication of deterioration or a new problem resulting from increased exercise and activity. There has been some debate as to whether diverting attention is actually positive or negative let alone doable when in severe pain (e.g., Leventhal & Everhardt, 1979; see also Vlaeyen et al., Chapter 10, this volume). However, many people in pain find that because of their isolation, they have nothing to focus on but their pain and their misery. Preoccupation with one's own body can lead to increased awareness and overestimation of sensory information. For example, many athletes often do not experience pain during the intense activity of the game but after the game, when they become aware and attend to their injuries—they experience pain. Taking one's mind off of pain by attending to something else may lead to reduced perceptions of pain and reduce levels of stress arousal, at least in some circumstances.

People who have persistent pain often try to distract themselves by reading books, watching television, engaging in hobbies, or listening to music. Using thoughts and imagination can also help people distract themselves from their bodies and pain. This is not a new idea, as there are numerous personal accounts of people describing the use of distraction to control pain.

A great deal of research based on attentional focus has been conducted on the relative efficacy of various cognitive distraction techniques. Fernandez and Turk (1989) concluded that no one coping strategy was consistently more effective than any other; however, the imaginal strategies as a set seem to be more effective than those strategies that did not include any imagery.

Prior to a description of specific cognitive coping strategies, patients should be told how attention can influence perception. The therapist can suggest that people can fully focus their attention on only one thing at a time and that we can control, to some extent, what is attended to, although at times it may require a good deal of effort.

The therapist might ask patients to close their eyes and to focus attention on some part of their body. The therapist then notes some ambient sound such as the ventilation system and suggests that while attending to their body, they were not aware of the sound of the air conditioning. The therapist calls attention to the sound of ventilation but then reminds them that they have stopped focusing on their body. The therapist also might call their attention to some part of their body that they were not attending to such as the gentle pressure of their watch on their wrist. The point is that there is environmental (internal and external) input that remains out of conscious attention until the patient focuses directly on it. The objective is to communicate to patients that people commonly employ various methods to get some degree of control over the focus of their attention.

As noted, no one category or type of cognitive coping technique has proven to be universally effective. Thus, providing patients with education and practice in the use of many different ones may be the best approach. A variety of cognitive coping images and attention diverting tasks may be reviewed in an attempt to find several that are most appealing to individual patients.

Imagery is one useful strategy for helping patients to relax and distract themselves from pain (see Syrjala & Abrams, Chapter 10, this volume). It is important to customize any images to the patient by, for example, asking patients to identify specific situations that they find pleasant and engaging. A detailed pleasant image can be created with the patient. One feature that seems especially important is to involve all senses—vision, sound, touch, smell, and taste. There is no one best image to use. Rather, it is important for each person to develop his or her own set of images, ones that they can vividly imagine and that they find pleasant. Some people may have difficulty with generating a particularly vivid visual image and may find it helpful to listen to a taped description or purchase a poster on which they can focus their attention as a way of assisting their imagination.

Clearly, no one would suggest that a pain sufferer should be inactive and fantasize about pleasant situations the majority of the time. Rather, imagery can be used as a technique when one is tired or alone, such as after waking in the middle of the night and having difficulty falling back to sleep. Using images to distract oneself is a skill and like all skills they improve with practice. The more success in making use of a skill, the greater the feeling of self-control, which can serve to decrease muscle tension, reduce production of stress hormones, and lower pain severity.

Imagery and other cognitive coping strategies are usually combined with other techniques such as cognitive restructuring, relaxation, and problem solving and would not be suggested as the sole treatment approach for dealing with persistent pain. Once again, the most important goal is to provide the patient with some sense of control and to change his or her maladaptive, thoughts, appraisals, and beliefs and thereby a fundamental change in their self-schemas and their schemas about the controllability of pain. Enhancement of functioning despite initial fear can provide a powerful disconfirmation of helplessness and hopelessness and alteration in patients' self-schemas. Actual behavior is likely to be more potent mode for change of subsequent behavior than exclusive reliance on verbal exhortations and persuasive efforts by the therapist.

Regardless of the coping skill used, the emphasis should be placed on self-control and resourcefulness as opposed to helplessness and passivity. Actively employing coping skills can alleviate the isolation that provides only an opportunity to focus on pain and misery.

ASSERTIVENESS AND COMMUNICATION SKILLS TRAINING

Assertiveness training is often an important intervention for enabling patients to reestablish their roles, particularly within the family, and thus to regain a sense of self-esteem and potency. Through role playing of existing tension-producing interpersonal transactions, the patient and therapist can identify and modify maladaptive thoughts, feelings, and communication deficiencies underlying nonassertiveness while practicing more adaptive alternatives. The patient may find assertiveness training useful in addressing reactions from family members and health care providers that may be opposing the patient's self-management objectives. Involvement of significant others in treatment should contribute to improved maintenance and generalization of outcomes (see Kerns, Otis, & Wise, Chapter 12, this volume).

EXERCISE AND ACTIVITY PACING

Physical exercise and activities are important not only for building muscle strength, flexibility, and endurance but also in bolstering a person's sense of control over physical functioning. Again, behavioral change challenges maladaptive beliefs of incapacity and helplessness. In addition, physical exercise may facilitate the release of endorphins and consequently reduce perception of pain.

Patients should begin physical exercises at a level that is reasonably comfortable and gradually increase the levels of activity. For example, at first it only may be possible for a back pain sufferer to walk one-half block before his back begins hurting. In this case he may start with one-quarter block and then over several days or weeks increase the distance.

When muscles have not been used for long periods they may hurt when exercised. Most of us learned that if something hurts we should stop doing it, but for those who are out of shape or suffer with chronic pain, pain onset or aggravation does not necessarily mean that harm is being done. It may be that pain is the result of using muscle that has been weakened from disuse. People with chronic pain need to learn that hurt and harm are not equivalent.

It is important for people with chronic pain to learn to pace their activities. It is equally important that they learn to rest only after attaining specified activity goals rather than when they experience pain. A goal for each day should be planned and recorded. It is helpful to keep charts of the activities so that progress can be monitored. A simple graph can be constructed with the days of the week along a horizontal line at the bottom of a sheet of paper and the amount of activity on a vertical line along the left-hand edge of the paper. Then each day a recording can be made of the amount of the specific activity (e.g., walking distance, number of sit-ups) that was achieved for that day. In time, the benefits of exercise will be evident not only in the recordings on paper but also in feeling physically and emotionally more healthy.

Skills Consolidation

During the skills-consolidation phase of C-BT, patients practice and rehearse the skills they have learned during the skills-acquisition phase and continue to apply them outside the clinic. Therapist can facilitate progress by engaging the patient in mental rehearsal, during which the patient imagines using the skills in different situations, role playing, and role reversal. An important feature of rehabilitation is patients' ability to make use of skills learned during treatment in their natural environment. Thus, home practice of each of skills covered during the skills-acquisition phase of treatment is critical. When patients practice skills at home it is useful to have them record their experiences including any difficulties that might arise. Once problems are identified, they should become targets for discussion.

ROLE PLAYING AND ROLE REVERSAL

Role playing is useful not only in the rehearsal of new skills but also in the identification of potential problem areas that may require special attention. Most typically, patients are asked to identify and participate in a role-play situation indicative of a particular problematic area for them.

In a variation on role playing, role reversal, the patient is asked to role play a situation in which the therapist and the patient reverse roles. Patients are instructed that it is their job to assume the role of the therapist, and the therapist will assume the role of another person with a similar physical diagnosis to the patient who has not received the specific skills training. This exercise is employed as it is known from research on attitude change that when people have to improvise, as in a role-playing or role-reversal situation, they generate exactly the kinds of arguments, illustrations, and motivating appeals that they regard as most salient and convincing. In this way, they tailor the content of their roles to fit their unique motives, predispositions, and preferences. In such situations, they not only emphasize those aspects of the training that are most convincing but also focus on less conflicting thoughts, doubts, and unfavorable consequences. In short, these exercises contribute to self-persuasion as well as permit the therapist to determine areas of confusion and potential difficulties.

Preparation for Generalization and Maintenance

The generalization and maintenance phase serves at least two purposes: (1) it encourages the patient to anticipate and plan for the posttreatment period and (2) it focuses on the necessary conditions for long-term success. Specifically, relapse prevention gives the patient the understanding that minor setbacks are to be expected but that they do not signal total failure. Rather, these setbacks should be viewed as cues to use the coping skills at which they are already proficient. It is important for the patient not to think of his or her responsibility as ending at termination of treatment but as entering a different phase of maintenance. Emphasis is placed on the importance of adherence to recommendations on an ongoing basis.

To maximize the likelihood of maintenance and generalization of treatment gains, C-B therapists focus on the cognitive activity of patients as they are confronted with problems throughout treatment (e.g., failure to achieve specified goals, plateaus in progress on physical exercises, and recurrent stresses). These events are employed as opportunities to assist patients to learn how to handle such setbacks and lapses because they are probably inevitable and will occur once treatment is terminated.

In the final phase of treatment, discussion focuses on possible ways of predicting and avoiding or dealing with symptoms and symptom-related problems following treatment termination. It is helpful to assist patients to anticipate future problems, stress, and symptom-exacerbating events and to plan coping and response techniques before these problems occur—*relapse prevention*. In this way, patients learn that lapses are probably inevitable and rehabilitation is not a cure. Discussion of relapse must unfold delicately. On the one hand, the therapist does not wish to convey an expectancy of treatment failure, but, on the other hand, the therapist wishes to anticipate and assist the patient to learn how to deal with potential recurrences or problematic situations that may occur.

Briefly, relapse prevention involves helping the patient learn to identify and cope successfully with factors that may otherwise lead to relapse. Patients are asked to identify high-risk situations (nonsupportive spouse, conflict with child) and the types of coping and behavioral responses that may be necessary for successful coping. Table 7.11 contains a list of some things that can be done in an attempt to prevent or reduce relapse.

It is important to note that all possible problematic circumstances cannot be anticipated. Rather, the goal during this phase, as for the entire treatment strategy, is to enable patients to develop a problem-solving perspective in which they believe that they have the skills and competencies within their

TABLE 7.11. Steps to Prevent Relapse

- Discuss the importance of adherence to home practice throughout treatment, not just at termination.
- Address patient's understanding of recommendations, why necessary, be specific.
- Be proactive, help patient to anticipate problems (e.g., identify high-risk situations that may undermine efforts).
- Teach how to deal with problems, setbacks, flare-ups, side effects, and lapses in effort.
- Encourage self-reinforcement and use of charts to self-monitor behavior and progress.
- Provide explanation of need and importance of recommendations and home practice with significant others (e.g., family members).
- Enlist assistance of significant others.

repertoires to respond in an appropriate way to problems as they arise. In this manner, attempts are made to help the patient to learn to anticipate future difficulties, develop plans for adaptive responding, and adjust his or her behavior accordingly. Successful responses should further enhance patients' sense of self-efficacy and help to form a *virtuous circle* in contrast to the *vicious circle* created and fostered by inactivity, passivity, physical deconditioning, helplessness, and hopelessness that characterize people with chronic illnesses.

During the final sessions, all aspects of the treatment should be reviewed. Patients should be engaged in discussions of what they have learned and how they have changed from the onset of treatment and recognition of how the patient's own efforts contributed to the positive changes. The therapist is also encouraged to use patient self-monitoring charts to foster self-reinforcement of accomplishments. The goal is to help patients realize that they have skills and abilities within their repertoires to cope with their circumstances without the need to contact their therapists and without becoming dependent on others. The therapist emphasizes that change has been achieved and can be maintained only if patients continue to accept responsibility for their lives. Patients should no longer view themselves as *patients* but as *competent people* who manage their physical symptoms and discomfort.

Concluding Comments

People have prior learning histories that precede the development of their current pain. Based on these experiences, they have developed cognitive schema that consist of all information acquired over their lifetimes. These cognitive schemas serve as the filters through which all subsequent experiences are perceived and to which they are responded. Thus, it is essential that people with chronic pain be viewed as integrated wholes, not body parts that are damaged and requiring repair. Failure to attend to cognitive and affective influences, either by a narrow focus on physiology and anatomy, as is the case in the traditional medical model, or exclusively on environmental influences, as is emphasized in operant models, will prove to be inadequate. People are more than physical parameters or pawns of reinforcement contingences. Rather they observe, anticipate, and interpret internal and external stimuli. Moreover, people exist in a social environment and contextual factors also play an important role in the pain experience. Because chronic pain is by virtue of its sole defining characteristic *chronic*, and because there is no cure, it is essential that treatment focus on people's adaptation to the symptoms and accompanying problems and not just the symptoms.

This chapter described a C-B perspective and a treatment approach based on this perspective. *The perspective is more important than the techniques used.* The goals are independent of treatment modalities. The emphasis is on helping patients assume increased control over their own pain and their own lives, become empowered, and become less dependent on the health care system. The C-B perspective and approach should not be viewed as an alternative to traditional medical treatments or operant conditioning. Rather, the C-B perspective itself is important in how we think about people with any chronic diseases, regardless of our preferred interventions. Cognitive and behavioral methods can be used in conjunction with other treatment approaches as part of a comprehensive rehabilitation program.

Those who use physical modalities must be aware of the messages they convey to patients about their pain and their responsibility. They must consider how this information will be filtered and processed and influence rehabilitation. If the message conveyed by the health care provider is that the patient's pain is solely a physical problem that needs to be fixed by the health care professional, there will be little incentive for the patient to engage in a treatment that requires active participation. The implicit messages that patients receive as they travel the path to different health care providers is that there is some derangement in their physical apparatus and that they should continue on what will likely be a fruitless and frustrating quest to find someone who can eliminate their pain. The promise of new drugs and methods is seductive but each new failure ultimately contributes to the demoralization of the pain sufferer.

Acknowledgments

Preparation of this chapter was supported in part by grants from the National Institute of Arthritis and Musculoskeletal and Skin Diseases (AR/AI44724, AR47298) and the National Institute of Child Health and Human Development/National Center for Medical Rehabilitation Research (HD33989). I acknowledge the careful reading and helpful comments of Dr. Elena S. Monarch on an early version of this chapter.

References

Bandura, A. (1997). *Self-efficacy: The exercise of control*. New York: Freeman.

Fernandez, E., & Turk, D.C. (1989). The utility of cognitive coping strategies for altering pain perception: A meta-analysis. *Pain, 38*, 123–135.

Flor, H., Turk, D. C., & Birbaumer, N. (1985). Assessment of stress-related psychophysiological responses in chronic back pain patients. *Journal of Consulting and Clinical Psychology, 54*, 354–364.

Jensen, M. P., & Karoly, P. (1992). Pain-specific beliefs, perceived symptom severity, and adjustment to chronic pain. *Clinical Journal of Pain, 8*, 123–130.

Jensen, M. P., Romano, J. M., Turner, J. A., Good, A. B., & Wald, L. H. (1999). Patient beliefs predict patient functioning: Further support for a cognitive-behavioral model of chronic pain. *Pain, 81*, 95–104.

Jensen, M. P., Turner, J. A., Romano, R. M., & Lawler, B. K. (1994). Relationship of pain-specif-

ic beliefs to chronic pain adjustment. *Pain, 57*, 301–309.

Lefebvre, M. F. (1981). Cognitive distortion and cognitive errors in depressed psychiatric low back pain patients. *Journal of Consulting and Clinical Psychology, 49*, 517–523.

Leventhal, H., & Everhart, D. (1979). Emotion, pain and physical Illness. In C.E. Izard (Ed.), *Emotion and psychopathology* (pp. 263–299). New York: Plenum Press.

Morley, S., Eccleston, C., & Williams, A. (1999). Systematic review and meta-analysis of randomized controlled trials of cognitive-behaviour therapy and behavior therapy for chronic pain in adults, excluding headache. *Pain, 80*, 1–13.

Okifuji, A., Turk, D. C., & Curran, S. L. (1999). Anger in chronic pain: Instigators of anger, targets and intensity. *Journal of Psychosomatic Research, 61*, 771–780.

Shaw, W. S., Feuerstein, M., Haufler, A. J., Berkowitz, S. M., & Lopez, M. S. (2001). Working with low back pain: Problem-solving orientation and function. *Pain, 93*, 129–137.

Sullivan, M. J. L., Thorn, B., Haythornthwaite, J. A., Keefe, F., Martin, M., Bradley, L. A., & Lefebvre, J. C. (2001). Theoretical perspectives on the relation between catastrophizing and pain. *Clinical Journal of Pain, 17*, 52–64.

Turk, D. C., Meichenbaum, D., & Genest, M. (1983). *Pain and behavioral medicine: A cognitive-behavioral perpsective*. New York: Guilford Press.

Turk, D. C., & Okifuji, A. (1998). Treatment of chronic pain patients: Clinical outcome, cost-effectiveness, and cost-benefits. *Critical Reviews in Physical Medicine and Rehabilitation Medicine, 10*, 181–208.

Turk, D. C., & Okifuji, A. (1999). A cognitive-behavioral approach to pain mangement. In P. D. Wall & R. Melzack (Eds.), *Textbook of pain* (4th ed., pp. 1431–1444). London: Churchill Livingstone.

Turk, D. C., & Okifuji, A. (in press). Psychological factors in chronic pain: Evolution and revolution. *Journal of Consulting and Clinical Psychology*.

Turk, D. C., Okifuji, A., & Sherman, J. J. (2000). Psycholoigcal factors in chronic pain: Implications for physical therapists. In J. W. Towney & J. T. Taylor (Eds.), *Low back pain* (3rd ed., pp. 353–383). Baltimore: Williams & Wilkins.

Turk, D. C., & Salovey, P. (1985). Cognitive structures, cognitive processes, and cognitive-behavioral modification: I. Client issues. *Cognitive Therapy and Research, 9*, 1–17.

Turner, J. A., & Aaron, L. A. (2001). Pain-related catastrophizing: What is it? [Commentary]. *Clinical Journal of Pain, 17*, 65–71.

Vlaeyen, J. W. S., Kole-Snijders, A., Boeren, R., & van Eek, H. (1995). Fear of movement/(re)injury in chronic low back pain and its relation to behavioral performance. *Pain, 62*, 363–372.

8

Biofeedback Training for Chronic Pain Disorders: A Primer

John G. Arena
Edward B. Blanchard

Psychological interventions in traditionally medical realms have increased at an exponential rate in the past three decades. One of the principal reasons that such interventions have become widely accepted by the medical community is their effectiveness in dealing with traditionally refractory medical problems such as chronic pain. Chronic pain is the most frequent cause of visits to primary care health settings (Sobel, 1993), and it is probably the most frustrating challenge for traditional medically oriented health care providers to deal with. Cousins (1995) reports that estimates are that the health care costs of chronic pain exceed the costs of cancer, coronary artery disease, and AIDS combined. The two psychological techniques generally believed to have proven the most effective with people suffering from chronic pain syndromes are biofeedback and various forms of relaxation therapy (see Syrjala & Abrams, Chapter 9, this volume); such treatments have usually been classified under the rubric "psychophysiological interventions" (see, e.g, Arena & Blanchard, 2001; Blanchard & Arena, 1999; Gatchel & Blanchard, 1993).

In this chapter, we present a "how-to" guide for clinicians interested in using one type of psychophysiological technique with chronic pain patients: biofeedback training. We deal with the three major types of chronic pain in which psychophysiological interventions have been used most often—namely, chronic tension headache, chronic vascular headache, and low back pain. For each, we first describe the chronic pain disorder and then describe in detail how to conduct biofeedback therapy for patients suffering from that syndrome. We purposely assume that the clinician has little knowledge about biofeedback. In addition, we emphasize five special groups of headache sufferers: the elderly headache patient; the pediatric headache patient; the headache sufferer with high medication usage; the patient with chronic, daily headache; and the pregnant headache patient. Finally, in our concluding remarks, we describe how the procedures used with the pain disorders discussed here can be extrapolated to most other pain problems. It is our intention to make this chapter as clinically useful as possible; thus we include as many "clinical hints" as practicable, and, rather than reviewing the treatment literature in depth, in most instances we refer the reader to recent reviews.

What is Biofeedback?

"Biofeedback," as it is commonly employed, is a procedure in which the therapist monitors through a machine the patient's bodily responses (such as muscle tension, surface skin temperature, heart rate, blood flow, or electrodermal response) and then "feeds back" this information to the patient, generally through either an auditory modality (a tone that goes higher or lower depending on, say, muscle tension's going higher or lower) or a visual modality (now usually a computer screen, where, for example, surface skin temperature is graphed on a second-by-second basis during each minute). Through this physiological feedback, it is hoped that a patient will be able to learn how to control his or her bodily responses. A more formal definition of biofeedback is "any technique which increases the ability of a person to control voluntarily physiological activities by providing information about those activities" (Olton & Noonberg, 1980, p. 4). Probably the simplest example of the use of a biofeedback device is a child's looking at himself or herself in a mirror, trying to find the best way to smile or frown.

Tension-Type Headache

What Is Tension-Type Headache?

Tension headache is generally described as a bilateral "dull ache," "pressure," or "cap-like pain" that is usually located in the forehead, neck, and shoulder regions. The headache typically occurs from 2 to 7 days a week and can last from 1 hour to all day. A small proportion of tension-type headache sufferers have continuous headache.

Most investigators who work in the area of headache would define chronic tension-type headache as having lasted for at least 1 year; most would also want patients to characterize the headache as significantly interfering in their lives. Clinicians who deal with headache patients should use a standardized set of inclusion and exclusion criteria for diagnosis, such as those proposed by the Headache Classification Committee of the International Headache Society (1988).

Etiology of Tension-Type Headache

Although traditional views on the etiology of chronic tension-type headache attribute the disorder to sustained contraction of skeletal muscles in the forehead, neck, and shoulder regions, recent psychophysiological investigations that have empirically tested this theory have arrived at conflicting, and for the most part negative, results; the majority of studies have not demonstrated any difference between controls and tension headache sufferers in forehead or neck electromyographic (EMG) activity (see, e.g., Arena, Blanchard, Andrasik, Appelbaum, & Myers, 1985; Arena, Hannah, Bruno, Smith, & Meador, 1991; Arena & Schwartz, forthcoming).

A second major theory of the etiology of tension-type headache is that tension and migraine headache are variants of the same disorder and that the headache is attributed to a dysfunctional vasomotor system (see, e.g., Blanchard & Andrasik, 1987; Wolff, 1963). There has been a surprising paucity of research into this theory in recent years, however. The vascular theory of tension-type headache appears to have fallen out of favor because of two simultaneously occurring factors. First, Wolff, the father of headache research and main advocate of the blood flow abnormality theory in tension headache, stopped publishing in the early 1960s. Second, in 1962 the Ad Hoc Committee on the Classification of Headache published inclusion and exclusion criteria that attributed tension headache solely to muscle tension. Given the research findings that appear to call into question the theory of sustained muscle contraction, it would appear that the vascular theory of tension headache warrants further research.

Psychophysiological Interventions for Chronic Tension-Type Headache and a Proposed Mechanism of Treatment

Psychophysiological treatments for chronic tension-type headache have been found to be as effective as pharmacological interventions (Blanchard, 1992). The two primary kinds of psychophysiological interventions used for tension-type headache are some form of relaxation therapy, generally progressive muscle relaxation therapy, and

EMG biofeedback. A number of review articles (e.g., Arena & Blanchard, 2000; Blanchard, 1992; Blanchard & Arena, 1999)
have consistently demonstrated that approximately 50% of tension-type headache
sufferers are significantly improved both
statistically (significant pre–post group differences) and clinically (50% or greater reduction in headache activity) through either
of these techniques, and most studies find
that there is no difference in outcome when
the two treatments are directly compared.

The failure to demonstrate support for
the theory that sustained levels of muscle
tension cause tension-type headache is especially troubling for biofeedback clinicians.
The rationale for biofeedback treatment is
that because these headaches are caused by
elevated levels of muscle tension, when tension headache sufferers are taught to decrease their muscle tension levels, there
will be a corresponding decrease in their
headache activity. This lack of support for a
straightforward psychophysiological etiology means that clinicians and researchers
must look for mechanisms other than, or in
addition to, psychophysiological ones that
are responsible for improvements in their
tension headache sufferers.

In our opinion, the most sophisticated
and methodologically elegant study to date
that has examined alternative change mechanisms underlying improvements in tension-
type headache was conducted by Holroyd
and colleagues (1984). In that study, 43 college students who suffered from tension-
type headache were randomly assigned to
one of four possible biofeedback conditions
in a 2 × 2 factorial design. In the first factor,
although all subjects were led to believe that
they were decreasing their forehead EMG
levels, only half the subjects were given
feedback contingent upon decreased EMG
activity; the other half were given feedback
contingent upon increasing EMG activity.
The second factor consisted of a high success group (bogus video displays demonstrating high-success compared to the rest of
the subjects in the experiment) or a moderate-success group (bogus video displays indicating moderate success compared to the
rest of the group). Results indicated that it
made no difference whether subjects learned
to increase or decrease their muscle tension

levels; the high-success feedback group
showed substantially greater improvements
in headache activity (53%) than did the
moderate-success group (26%).

Rokicki and colleagues (1997) replicated
to some extent their 1984 work, using a
young adult population of 30 tension-type
headache subjects who were given a combination of relaxation therapy and EMG
biofeedback. Improvements in headache activity were correlated with increases in self-
efficacy induced by biofeedback training.

Blanchard, Kim, Hermann, and Steffek
(1993) gave progressive muscle relaxation
therapy to 14 tension-type headache sufferers. At the end of each session, they were
also given computerized bogus feedback regarding their performance: six were led to
believe that they were highly successful in
the relaxation task, whereas eight were informed that they were only moderately successful. Patients who perceived themselves
as highly successful at relaxation reported a
greater amount of improvement in their
headache activity, as measured by the daily
headache diary, than did those with perceptions of moderate success. These findings
extend the results of the Holroyd and colleagues (1984) study, because they were obtained on a treatment-seeking sample of
adults who were in their mid-30s and who
had suffered from headaches an average of
over 10 years.

Preliminary results from the Arena laboratory (Arena, Bruno, Rozantine, Garner &
Meador, 2002) also strongly support the
work of Holroyd and his colleagues: People
given high-success feedback were much like-
lier to be successful at EMG biofeedback
(mean reduction in headache activity
pre–post = 53.2%) than those given moderate-success feedback (who had a mean *increase* in headache activity of 2.3%). Similarly, as in the Holroyd and colleagues
(1984) study, whether tension headache
subjects were taught to increase or decrease
EMG levels during biofeedback training
made no difference in treatment outcome
(37.7% decrease in pre–post headache activity for those who were taught to increase
their EMG activity, versus 42.9% decrease
for those taught to decrease their muscle
tension levels). These results were obtained
on a treatment-seeking sample of adults

who were over age 30 and had headaches for at least 10 years.

The Holroyd and colleagues (1984) and Rokicki and colleagues (1997) studies demonstrated the importance of cognitive mediating factors such as perceived success and self-efficacy in biofeedback training, and the Blanchard and colleagues (1993) and Arena, Bruno, and colleagues (2002) findings essentially replicated the Holroyd and colleagues study's conclusions using a treatment-seeking, typical tension-type-headache-age population. These findings taken together as a whole are strongly supportive of a cognitive self-efficacy component being the primary change mechanism involved in successful psychophysiological treatment for tension headache. They suggest that clinicians who work with tension headache patients should attempt to put their patients' results in the best light possible. They should be as optimistic as they can be, deemphasizing the patients' difficulty in grasping the response and magnifying even small successes. From an ethical perspective, however, we would certainly not recommend that clinicians "fake" data to lead patients to believe they are being successful.

EMG Biofeedback Training for Chronic Tension-Type Headache

EMG BIOFEEDBACK "HOOKUP"

There is not sufficient space here to describe in detail the complexities of the EMG signal or basic biofeedback instrumentation and safety issues. Prior to conducting biofeedback on any patient, however, the clinician should familiarize him- or herself with such basics by reading a standard text such as Schwartz and Associates (1995) or Basmajian and DeLuca (1985). It is strongly urged that the novice biofeedback therapist, prior to attempting biofeedback therapy, receive training from a licensed health care provider familiar with biofeedback or become certified in biofeedback by the Biofeedback Certification Institute of America.

The immediate question that the clinician must deal with is this: On which muscle group should the sensors be placed (forehead, neck, shoulder, etc.)? Unfortunately, the research is rather vague on this point. One approach to answering this question

would be to conduct a psychophysiological assessment, measuring the major muscle groups purported to be implicated in tension headache, and then placing the sensors during biofeedback training in the region that exhibits the most elevated muscle tension. There are a number of problems with this strategy, however. First, to our knowledge, there have been no studies demonstrating the clinical utility of this type of psychophysiological assessment. Second, one immediately runs into technical questions such as these: Does the clinician conduct the psychophysiological assessment during baseline (resting) conditions or during stressful conditions? What exactly constitutes the baseline conditions (reclining or standing, eyes open or eyes closed, etc.)? Similarly, what stressful condition does one use—stressful imagery, electric shock, an exercise step-up test? What happens if neck muscles show elevated tension during stressful imagery but not during baseline or in response to electric shock? Third, what if the patient tells the clinician that the pain is located in the neck and shoulders but the psychophysiological assessment indicates that there are muscle activity elevations only in the forehead? (We do not have space in this chapter, unfortunately, to provide answers to these rhetorical questions. Interested readers may wish to refer to Arena & Schwartz, in press, for some guidelines.) Finally, nearly all of the biofeedback tension headache outcome research is conducted with the sensors placed on the forehead region (Arena, Bruno, Hannah & Meador, 1995). For exact sensor placements for muscle groups, clinicians should refer to standard texts such as Lippold (1967). For clinical purposes, however, we generally just swab the forehead with alcohol (during which time the eyes are closed); then, instructing the patient to stare straight forward, we place the two active sensors on the forehead, in line with the pupil of each eye. The reference (ground) sensor is placed in the center of the forehead, between the two active sensors. For upper trapezius (neck and shoulder) placement, we have the patient shrug his or her shoulder(s) and place the active leads over the belly of the muscle between the spine and the shoulder joint, approximately 1–2 inches apart; the reference sensor is placed between the two active ones. Figure 8.1 graphically depicts the upper trapezius muscle site placement.

Clinical Hints. Three things are important to note regarding electrode placement. First, we use only disposable EMG sensors to ensure against infection. Second, to decrease anxiety, we call electrodes by the more innocuous term "sensors." Third, also to decrease anxiety, we inform our patients that there is no danger of being harmed during EMG biofeedback training and that the sensors are not sending any electricity into the body; they are only picking up the muscles' electronic patterns.

RATIONALE AND STRATEGIES GIVEN
DURING INITIAL SESSION

As stated previously, we believe that with tension headache sufferers, the rationale, strategies, and therapist–patient interactions are paramount in achieving positive treatment outcome. We would advise strongly against attempting to describe a complex rationale such as self-efficacy to patients; rather, we describe the theory of sustained levels of muscle tension. We say something like this:

"It's traditionally been assumed that the type of headache you have—tension headache—is caused by very high levels of muscle tension in your forehead, neck, and shoulder areas. These muscles have been tense for a long time. Through biofeedback training, you will learn to decrease your muscle tension levels. When you do this, it's hoped that you will get a decrease in your headaches."

We inform patients that stress plays a role in their headaches by leading to elevated muscle tension, and that it is essential to deal with their stress as well as their muscle tension, as these are interrelated. (We routinely provide a number of cognitive-behavioral strategies regarding stress; see Turk, Chapter 7, this volume.)

We emphasize that these techniques are self-regulation skills that will allow the patients to prevent a headache from occurring. We stress to them that they need to incorporate these skills into their lifestyle—that they are making a lifestyle change rather than receiving a "treatment" from a therapist. In this way, something is not being done to them; they are learning how to employ these skills for themselves. Again, this increases the likelihood of enhancing self-efficacy.

We next give the patients a number of possible strategies from which to choose. We emphasize that learning the biofeedback response is purely an idiosyncratic process and that what works for others may not work for them. We customarily describe seven possible biofeedback strategies:

1. *Relaxing imagery.* The patient imagines a pleasant scene, such as walking through the woods on an autumn evening and listening to the leaves crunch with each

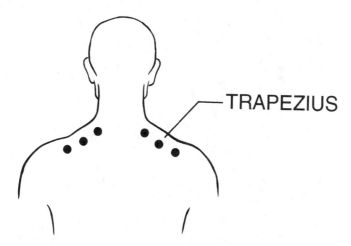

FIGURE 8.1. Electrode placement for bilateral upper trapezius EMG biofeedback training.

step, or lying on a beach listening to the waves as they roll in and roll back out again. We routinely tell patients to avoid any possible sexually stimulating imagery, because this is arousing rather than relaxing, and to switch to another image if they are having trouble decreasing their muscle tension with a particular image. We also tell them not to imagine themselves engaging in any vigorous physical activity, and to try to feel as if they are actually in the scene rather than just imagining a movie playing in front of them (here we also suggest that they try to involve every sensory modality, such as smell, sound, and touch). Finally, we tell them that, if at all possible, it is best to be by oneself in the image, as the presence of other people is often arousing.

2. *Relaxing (autogenic) phrases.* Relaxing phrases, repeated over and over again, can be an effective strategy. Although there are standardized phrase lists (e.g., Arena & Blanchard, 1996; Blanchard & Arena, 1999), we have found that relaxing phrases are most effective with biofeedback training when the patients think up their own phrases. We emphasize to patients that they have to repeat these phrases numerous times (50–100) rather than just once or twice. We also instruct them that sometimes these procedures do not work initially but may work over repeated sessions. (See the section on thermal biofeedback for vascular headache, below, for additional details on autogenic phrases.)

3. *Deep breathing procedures.* The patient, with eyes closed, concentrates on diaphragmatic breathing (breathing by expanding the lungs fully while keeping the shoulders and chest relaxed, allowing the abdomen to expand) and repeats a relaxing word such as "relax," "calm," or "peaceful" when exhaling. We tell patients to limit the pace of breathing to no more than 12 breaths a minute, and preferably to keep it to between 6 and 8 breaths per minute. We have found that for a substantial minority of patients words that have nothing to do with relaxation, such as "amber" or "stream," are often effective. Some people like to pair this strategy with relaxing imagery—for example, if they are imagining a beach scene, they pace their breathing with the rhythm of the waves (inhalation with wave coming in, exhalation with wave go-

ing out). It is important to inform patients—especially those whose breathing is faster than 30 breaths per minute—that they may feel quite strange when they get their breathing down into the relaxed range. We tell them that this will pass as time goes on, and that they will actually begin to enjoy the novel feelings of relaxation (e.g., heaviness and floating).

Clinical Hint. Research has demonstrated (MacHose & Peper, 1991) that is nearly impossible to breath diaphragmatically if one is wearing tight jeans or clothing (e.g., belts and jeans). We remind patients to wear loose-fitting pants or jeans.

4. *Awareness of sensations.* Some people are able to lower their muscle tension levels simply by concentrating on and becoming aware of the sensations of tightness and tension in their forehead, neck, and shoulders—in other words, by focusing on what it is like when those muscles relax, loosen up, and unwind. We tell them that as the muscles become relaxed, they may feel warmth, heaviness, and looseness in the muscles that they have not felt before.

5. *Mental games.* Some patients find that focusing on a color ("warm" earth colors, such as yellow, green, or blue, seem to work best) helps to relax them and decrease their muscle tension levels. Others actually play a game in their mind, such as tic-tac-toe, bowling, cards, or basketball.

6. *Concentrating on the auditory feedback.* Some individuals just ignore all the preceding strategies and simply concentrate on the feedback tone. They even report imagining the tone going down when they practice in their everyday environment without a portable biofeedback device.

7. *Nothingness.* Some patients report that if they can make their minds blank and think of nothing—actually stop thinking—they can relax and lower their muscle tension. This is indeed difficult for most people to do, and fewer than 2% of people can achieve it. However, if the patient can enter into a state of nothingness, it will probably lower his or her muscle tension levels.

During the first session, we usually tell a patient to pick only one strategy and stick with it throughout the entire session. We keep the initial session short—a 3- to 5-minute adaptation period ("Just sit quietly with your eyes closed") and a maximum of 12 minutes of biofeedback. (In later sessions, we increase the biofeedback portion to a maximum of 25 minutes.) We emphasize to patients that this is a difficult response to learn and that it will take some time before they can lower their muscle tension reliably; we tell the patients not to get discouraged if they cannot control their EMG levels immediately. Often, we tell patients that during the first few sessions they should expect to do exactly the opposite of what they are striving for—that in all likelihood they will increase, rather than decrease, their muscle tension. This gives us as therapists a rare opportunity for a "no-lose" situation, and potentially a great chance to enhance feelings of self-efficacy and success. If the patients increase their muscle tension, we say, "That was to be expected for a first session." If they stay the same or actually decrease their muscle tension, we praise them for succeeding during the first session: "It's very rare to do as well as you've done today; that's a great sign."

During the first session, we instruct each patient to let the response occur rather than make it occur—to be passive rather than try to force the forehead or neck muscles to relax. We tell patients that when people have difficulty with biofeedback, it's often because they are trying too hard to obtain the response ("I want you to try very hard not to try very hard"). We go through the various forms of feedback and let them choose which type of visual and auditory feedback they like. Finally, although we restrict our research protocols to 12 to 16 sessions, it is not unusual for our clinical patients to run up to 24 sessions. In some few instances, we have gone up to 36 sessions. These instances have generally involved advancing to another muscle group (if starting with the forehead, then going to neck and shoulder biofeedback training, or vice versa), and special generalization training.

COACHING AND THERAPIST ATTITUDE

The first and most important thing for a therapist to determine about coaching is whether a patient wants and can benefit from it, which is truly idiosyncratic. From our clinical experience, about 25% of patients do not want to be coached at all. These patients are usually easily identified, as they will most likely tell us, "I can do it better if you just leave me alone," or we can infer that attitude from nonverbal cues. A few patients (about 5%) want us to give them constant coaching. The vast majority of patients want and need some coaching but not all the time. For these people, we usually coach a lot during the first biofeedback session; then, during successive biofeedback sessions, we coach a bit at the beginning of each biofeedback phase and then once every 5 minutes or as necessary (e.g., the patient is doing the opposite of the desired response, or has suddenly had an "Ah ha" experience and has learned how to control the response).

Any therapist who has ever coached anything already knows two important things: the way to coach a biofeedback session and the fact that a coach's verbal repertoire is extremely limited (especially when the coach cannot use expletives!). A therapist should be prepared for three general situations:

1. The patient has decreased his or her muscle tension levels. Here are some possible responses: (a) "That's fantastic! Keep up the good work." (b) "I want you to remember what you are doing now, so you can tell me later at the end of the session." (c) "Real good! Try to allow the tone to go even lower."

2. The patient has not been able to decrease his or her muscle tension levels. Possible responses include the following: (a) "That's OK. It's as important to find out what makes your muscle tension go up as it is to find out what makes it go down." (b) "I want you to remember what you're doing now, so you can tell me later at the end of the session." (c) "That's OK. You can only go up so far before you have to start going down." (d) "You seem to be at an impasse; you might want to switch to a different strategy."

3. The patient seems frustrated or appears to be trying too hard. Possible responses are as follows: (a) "That's to be expected. Remember, I told you that this is a very difficult response to get. If it was easy, you wouldn't need me or the machines."

(b) "Let's take a break. Sometimes all you need is a few minutes to clear your mind, and then you come back like gangbusters." (c) "Remember, this is a skill like learning to drive. At first it's difficult, but with practice and time you become more skilled. Pretty soon, the response will become automatic, just as driving becomes automatic." (d) "You may want to think of yourself as a scientist, who in a somewhat detached manner tests theories and tosses them in or out, depending upon whether or not they work."

Interestingly, the limited research on coaching and therapist presence during a biofeedback session indicates that learning is retarded when there is a great deal of coaching (Borgeat, Hadd, Larouche, & Bedwani, 1980). As a rule, we would suggest that coaching be done on a limited basis, as it will help to generalize the response to the "real world," for in everyday situations patients do not have a therapist accompanying them. Limited coaching will also prevent patients from becoming dependent on the therapist.

Some people, especially the elderly who have vision or hearing problems, can benefit from tactile stimulation as coaching. Usually such stimulation takes the form of a slight pressure on the wrist or hand, or a slight pat on the back.

The importance of coaching, and especially of therapist attitude, cannot be overemphasized. As Holroyd and colleagues (1984) demonstrated, imparting to the patient the perception of success is perhaps the essential change mechanism underlying improvement in biofeedback training for tension headache. It is imperative for the therapist to convey enthusiastically to each patient that he or she is doing well in the biofeedback training. A number of researchers have emphasized the importance of other therapist factors, such as perceived warmth and competence, as being essential in biofeedback training (Taub & School, 1978). However, the empirical evidence does not support these assumptions (Blanchard et al., 1983), possibly because the therapists in that study were nearly all rated as warm and competent. We would certainly urge therapists to try to be perceived as positive, warm, and competent.

POSTSESSION FEEDBACK

At the end of each session, we always ask patients what strategy they found to be the most effective (if any were effective), as well as to rate (on either a 0–10 or a 0–5 scale) their degree of relaxation and their level of overall body tension now as compared to at the beginning of the session. At both the beginning and end of each session, it is important to explore any situationally stressful events that may have been occurring recently in a patient's life, especially any that have occurred just prior to the onset of the training session (e.g., argument with spouse, difficulty at work, upcoming test, or deadlines). If patients are unable during the training session to decrease their muscle tension levels, we frequently point out at the end of the session that these factors may have contributed to their inability to relax that day. It is always useful to have patients rate their headache level (on either a 0–10 or a 0–5 scale) prior to and following the biofeedback training. This rating can then be used to help give the patients some understanding of how they were performing (i.e., to relate headache activity level to ability to decrease muscle tension levels during biofeedback, as well as to contrast baseline levels from session to session with pain levels from session to session). Moreover, frequently patients are unable to control their muscle tension levels effectively but their headache activity decreases during the session. When this happens, it can be used to give the patients a perceived sense of self-control over their pain and to enhance self-efficacy.

HOMEWORK

Home practice has traditionally been considered an essential element of all psychophysiological interventions for chronic headache (Blanchard & Andrasik, 1985; Blanchard, Nicholson, Radnitz, et al., 1991). We usually begin home practice for biofeedback once patients have demonstrated that they can reliably produce the desired biofeedback response in the office setting. Home practice can be conducted in many ways. The simplest form of homework is to instruct the patients to practice the office strategy that seems to work the best at home and in other real-world locations, such as the job, the supermarket, and so forth (we usually instruct them to do so at least 10 times a day). We want them to practice it when they are brushing their teeth, waiting for a traffic light to change, taking a coffee break, or the like. We tell the patients that the biggest problem they will have in the beginning is simply to remember to practice the biofeedback during the day ("If you can remember to practice, you've got 95% of the problem licked"). We ask them to choose something they do 10–20 times a day and allow that to be the cue to remind them to practice. Some of our patients have practiced every time they look at themselves in a mirror, open and close a door, answer the telephone, or see a specific color. If this proves too troublesome, we ask them to buy colorful "stick-ons" (purple half-inch dots seem to work best) and place them in strategic areas as reminders to practice their biofeedback skills. In other instances, we ask patients to obtain a wristwatch that beeps every 30 minutes or carry a small kitchen timer with them and let the beep or alarm be a reminder to practice.

We sometimes ask patients with a great deal of noticeable muscle tension to use a small pocket mirror during home practice as a biofeedback aid ("Try to smooth out your forehead as much as you can"). Small portable biofeedback devices are available for less than $300, and we routinely lend these to our patients during the course of treatment. It is important to note, however, that there has been no research examining the utility of biofeedback home practice for chronic tension-type headache, and only one study (Blanchard, Nicholson, Taylor, et al., 1991) has compared home practice versus no home practice for relaxation therapy (this study found only a trend for relaxation therapy to be more effective with home practice than without). In spite of this paucity of data on the usefulness of homework in biofeedback training for tension headache, for the face validity alone, we would still urge clinicians to place great emphasis on home practice.

GENERALIZATION OF THE BIOFEEDBACK
RESPONSE TO THE "REAL WORLD"

Generalization involves preparing a patient to, or determining whether or not the pa-

tient can, carry the learning that may have occurred during the biofeedback session into the "real world." There are many ways to test or prepare for generalization. The most common by far is a "self-control" condition, which is interspersed between a baseline and a feedback condition. The self-control condition involves asking the patient to control the desired psychophysiological response (e.g., "Please try to lower your forehead muscle tension") without any feedback. If the patient can control the response, the clinician may infer that between-session learning (i.e., generalization) has occurred. We routinely add such a condition to our biofeedback training after the second or third session. Another method of testing for generalization is to present the same stressor to the patient before and after treatment. If there is less arousal during and after a stressor at the posttreatment presentation, the clinician may infer that generalization has occurred. (Except in special circumstances, such as a pre and post cold exposure test for Raynaud's disease patients, we do not use this method.) A third, and potentially the most useful, way of preparing the patient to generalize the biofeedback response is to attempt to make the office biofeedback training simulate real-world situations. For example, in Augusta, we initially have each patient sit in a reclining chair. Once the patient has mastered the rudiments of biofeedback, we routinely progress to a comfortable office chair (with arms), an uncomfortable office chair (without arms), and, finally, a standing position. Finally, giving patients homework assignments to practice the biofeedback response in the "real world" is, of course, an excellent way of preparing them for generalization.

*Problems That Arise during
Biofeedback Training*

INTRUSIVE THOUGHTS

One major problem that patients seem to have with biofeedback training is the occurrence of intrusive ("busy") thoughts. We alert patients prior to the initial session that they may initially have problems with such thoughts entering their minds. We tell them simply to expect that these thoughts will occur. Some thoughts will be productive, such as, "Oh, how relaxed I am feeling," "I'm feeling more relaxed this time than before," and "My headache has definitely lessened and my neck feels less tense." Other thoughts will be unproductive, such as worries about problems at work, tasks that need to be finished, meals that have to be cooked, and so on. We then tell patients that it is essential that they do *not* attempt to stop those unproductive thoughts, because trying to stop them will only exacerbate the problem. We inform the patients that as they get better at the biofeedback procedures, the problem will lessen. We also tell them when they are practicing at home not to get frustrated when the thoughts occur, to let them play themselves out, and always to return to the biofeedback response when the thoughts are over.

These suggestions usually work with most people. With those people who are having severe intrusive thoughts after numerous sessions, we suggest a mild form of thought stopping:

"Imagine that these thoughts are like a freight train, and at the first thought they become chained or linked together. In order to stop them, try to imagine a stoplight that flashes, and in your mind say, `STOP!' Immediately replace that unproductive thought with a more productive thought, such as 'I am learning to relax myself more quickly,' or 'I am feeling the relaxation spreading throughout my muscles.'"

PANIC ATTACKS AND RELAXATION-
INDUCED ANXIETY

Although it is not frequently discussed, there is a subset of patients who experience increased tension and anxiety during biofeedback. In a few people, this anxiety may take the form of a panic attack. (For an excellent theoretical discussion of relaxation-induced anxiety, please see Heide & Borkovec, 1983.) Our clinical experience and the limited research available suggest that individuals who suffer from generalized anxiety or panic disorders, or those who are very anxious during the preliminaries to the first session of biofeedback or who report increased tension as a result of the biofeedback, are at increased risk for relaxation-induced anxiety and panic attack. Because

relaxation-induced anxiety can lead to patients' dropping out of treatment, it should be carefully assessed. For these subjects at high risk, we have them focus more on the somatic aspects of the biofeedback training instead of focusing on cognitive factors (e.g., stress how the muscles feel rather than how quiet their minds are). We also emphasize that they are always in control during the biofeedback training; they will always be aware of what is going on around them, what they are doing, and what we are saying.

In spite of all preparations, panic attacks may occur occasionally. These usually take the form of patients' opening their eyes during the biofeedback procedure, crying, stating that they feel nervous, and/or attempting to leave the therapist's office. There are three things a therapist should do in this situation: stay calm; reassure the patient, "I understand what you are going through, and these feelings will soon pass"; and try not to act as a dynamic, insight-oriented therapist (even if the therapist is one).

The essential thing for the therapist to do during a panic attack is to assume a calm demeanor. Novice therapists especially seem to have trouble with this; they often pick up on the intense affect of these patients and contribute to it with their own fears and concerns. It is important to remember that (to the best of our knowledge) no one has ever died from a panic attack, although they are quite frightening. The worst that could happen from the therapist's perspective is that he or she will have to take the patient to the local emergency room (and we have never heard of any therapist actually having to do this). Therefore, the therapist should stay calm, speak in a slow and low voice with a relaxed tone, and act as if things are going to be fine. Even if the therapist is extremely concerned and anxious, it should not be conveyed to the patient.

Next, before the patient can say what he or she is experiencing, the therapist should state what the patient is feeling. This lets the patient know that the therapist is understanding and competent, and that whatever else the therapist says will be accurate as well. We say something like this:

"Right now you're feeling really nervous, like something terrible is going to happen to you.

You maybe even feel as if you are going to die. Your heart is pounding, your thoughts are racing, you are breathing very rapidly and shallowly, your mouth is dry, you're sweating a lot, you can't catch your breath, your hands and feet are very cold, and you just want to get out of here. Don't worry; nothing that you feel now is permanent. It will all be over in a few minutes."

We usually get the patient a glass of water and a tissue and then wait for him or her to calm down. We then say: "Remember how you did the diaphragmatic breathing? Let's do it right now. I want you to breathe at the same rate that I am and notice how quickly you are starting to feel more calm and relaxed. Notice that your heart is now slowing down and you feel more in control." If at all possible, the patient should be prevented from fleeing the office, because flight can lead to avoidance of relaxation and to a pairing of biofeedback with becoming anxious.

It is important for a therapist, especially an insight-oriented psychotherapist, not to try to act as "supertherapist" and give the patient insight into why he or she is having these feelings. Not that those questions and insights are not important, but during or immediately following a panic attack is not the time to gather such information or impart such interpretations. They are best left for subsequent sessions. At this time, the therapist's main goal should be to calm the patient and demonstrate how even though the patient was anxious and felt that he or she was going to die, it did not happen, and the patient was able to calm down. From our experiences, we have found that questions such as "Have you ever felt these feelings before at any time in your life?" "During your childhood, were you ever in situations where you felt a loss of control similar to these feelings today?" or "Did any images come to mind when you became very nervous that reminded you of things when you were growing up?" are resented by patients experiencing a panic attack.

Usually, when the foregoing suggestions are followed, the patient will calm down and feel well enough to leave the office or continue discussion (we strongly recommend *not* continuing the biofeedback therapy during that session). The next session, we spend some time discussing with the patient how he or she felt and whether he or she wishes to continue with the biofeedback. Most patients who do not drop out of therapy will continue with the regimen. A small subset of patients will not wish to continue the psychophysiological intervention, and for those people we offer cognitive-behavioral therapy for pain (see Turk, Chapter 7, this volume) or another psychophysiological intervention, usually relaxation therapy (see Syrjala & Abrams, Chapter 9, this volume; see also Arena & Blanchard, 1996).

Relaxation Therapy for Chronic Tension-Type Headache

It is important to remember that although nearly all the headache literature treats biofeedback and relaxation therapy as separate interventions, most clinicians combine the two procedures when treating headache. With tension-type headache, however, we generally choose first to give an entire regimen of one intervention. Should a patient prove refractory to that treatment, we offer him or her a course of the other psychophysiological procedure. We have previously asserted that relaxation therapy, because it generally entails fewer sessions and does not require machinery, should be administered before biofeedback training. We have employed this strategy in our research (Blanchard, Andrasik, Jurish, & Teders, 1982; Blanchard, Andrasik, Neff, Arena, et al., 1982; Blanchard, Andrasik, Neff, Teders, et al., 1982; Blanchard, Andrasik, Evans, Neff, et al., 1985). Unfortunately, there have been no direct comparisons of this strategy with that of using EMG biofeedback first, followed by relaxation therapy for those refractory to biofeedback. Therefore, no empirical data at the present time confirm the validity of our assertion.

There are excellent references available for relaxation therapy in general (e.g., Lichstein, 1988; Smith, 1990), as well as references available for its specific application with tension headache (Arena & Blanchard, 1996; Blanchard & Andrasik, 1985). (See Syrjala & Abrams, Chapter 9, this volume, for a detailed review and description of relaxation therapy for pain.)

Vascular Headache

There are two primary headache disorders that are vascular in origin—migraine headache and cluster headache. The latter is a smaller problem in terms of prevalence and in terms of research from a psychophysiological viewpoint. We discuss it briefly before devoting the bulk of this section to migraine headache and its treatment with thermal biofeedback. In addition to both migraine and cluster headaches being vascular in nature, they share to some extent a proximal pain mechanism (see next section): Both types of headaches tend to be episodic. Thus, the vast majority of sufferers go from being headache free to having a headache of some duration (with intensity building fairly rapidly—in minutes to an hour or two) to again being headache free.

Cluster Headache

SYMPTOMS

Cluster headache tends to be much rarer than migraine (perhaps up to 10% as prevalent; Kudrow, 1980) and tends to be found predominantly in males. It is generally diagnosed by its distinctive temporal pattern. Most patients with cluster headache have episodic cluster headache; 5–10% have chronic continuous cluster headache. (See Lewis & Solomon, 1999, for an excellent monograph on cluster headache.) In episodic cluster headache, the patient is headache free for months to years and then enters a so-called cluster bout. During the cluster bout, the one-sided headaches appear fairly regularly, once or twice a day to every other day. The headaches are described as intense, excruciating pain; they last from 15 to 30 minutes to 2 to 3 hours. Many patients are so debilitated by this type of headache that it can take hours for them to return to a normal level of functioning. The cluster bout lasts several weeks to several months and then disappears. For some patients, there is a seasonal regularity to the onset of the cluster bout. This has led some to suspect that cluster headache is part of an allergic reaction, but research has not borne out this view (Kudrow, 1980).

Clinical Hint. During a cluster bout patients seem especially sensitive to alcohol, such that a single drink can trigger a headache. A therapist can thus try to help a patient become abstinent during the cluster bout. This sensitivity does not seem present between cluster bouts.

BIOFEEDBACK TREATMENT

There is only a limited literature on the psychosocial treatment of cluster headache, with most reports presenting data on one to five cases (see Blanchard & Andrasik, 1987, for a summary). A report by Blanchard, Andrasik, Jurish, and Teders (1982) has probably the largest series ($n = 11$). Only 2 of the 11 (19%) were helped somewhat, based on follow-ups of 20 to 30 months. For these two patients, the headaches were sometimes less intense and of shorter duration after treatment than before treatment. Subsequent cluster bouts were perhaps of shorter duration.

The treatment regimen responsible for these meager results was fairly intensive, involving 10 sessions of relaxation training over 8 weeks, followed by 12 sessions of thermal biofeedback over 6 weeks. (The biofeedback treatment protocol much like that described in this chapter.)

Clinical Hint. Given the relatively poor results of Blanchard, Andrasik, Jurish, and Teders (1982), we no longer take cluster headache patients, and we would advise the reader to be cautious about offering the procedures described in this chapter to the individual who suffers from the cluster headache.

There have been isolated case reports of the apparently successful treatment of chronic cluster headache (cluster headache without the usual regular remission of the cluster bout; the headaches are there continuously) with psychosocial procedures. For example, King and Arena (1984) successfully treated a 69-year-old male with chronic cluster headache with a combination of thermal biofeedback, relaxation home practice, and marital therapy. At a 15-month follow-up, his medication consumption was markedly reduced and his headaches were improved.

Migraine Headache

SYMPTOMS

As mentioned previously, migraine headache is episodic: The typical attack lasts from 2 to

3 hours to 2 to 3 days and is usually accompanied by sensations of nausea (and sometimes vomiting) and sensitivity to light and sound. A typical migraine headache starts as a one-sided headache but usually progresses so that the whole head is involved. Headache frequency varies from one to two headaches a year to three to four headaches a month. In our experience, patients seeking treatment usually have one or two headaches a month or more.

Up to half of patients with migraine headache also meet the criteria for tension headache. These unfortunate individuals have been labeled as having "mixed migraine and tension headache" or "combined migraine and tension headache." We have typically lumped both pure migraine and mixed migraine and tension headaches together under the label of "vascular headache" and treated them in the same fashion.

Clinical Hint. A key question to ask in diagnosing mixed headaches is this: "Do you have more than one kind of headache?" If the answer is "yes," we advise taking a separate description of each type of headache. One occasionally finds that the difference is primarily in intensity but that the phenomenology and temporal factors are the same. In this case, a diagnosis of mixed headache is not appropriate.

Treatment for Vascular Headache

Several generalizations seem warranted about the treatment of vascular headache (see Blanchard, 1993, or Blanchard & Arena, 1999, for a more detailed summary). For mixed headache, both thermal biofeedback and relaxation training are generally needed. Mixed headache sufferers, as a group, respond relatively poorly to relaxation training alone. In one study, just 22% of subjects with mixed headaches receiving only relaxation therapy met our criterion for clinically significant improvement, which we have defined as at least a 50% reduction in headache activity as documented by a daily headache diary (Blanchard, Andrasik, Neff, Arena, et al., 1982). Moreover, mixed headache sufferers in another study did not do as well as pure migraine sufferers with thermal biofeedback alone (Blanchard, Nicholson, Radnitz, et al., 1991); they required additional treatment with relaxation.

Our "standard" treatment for vascular headache has been a combination of relaxation training and thermal biofeedback. Across three separate samples of 50 or more patients each, treated with this combination over a 10-year period in Albany, Blanchard and his colleagues found that 52% of each sample met the success criterion of 50% reduction in headache activity (Blanchard, Andrasik, Appelbaum, et al., 1985; Blanchard, Andrasik, Neff, et al., 1982; Blanchard, Appelbaum, Nicholson, et al., 1990). This replicability is impressive.

Thus either relaxation alone or biofeedback alone seems poor for mixed headache and fair for migraine. Thermal biofeedback alone is adequate for migraine and for mixed headache, but the combination of relaxation and thermal biofeedback seems to work best for vascular headache.

One other point needs to be made about psychosocial treatments of primary headache disorders. The addition of a cognitive therapy component, especially cognitive stress coping therapy modeled after the work of Holroyd and Andrasik (1982), does *not* seem to improve overall outcome with vascular headache (Blanchard, Appelbaum, Radnitz, Morrill, et al., 1990), but it does seem to make a difference when added to a relaxation regimen with tension-type headache (Blanchard, Appelbaum, Radnitz, Michultka, et al., 1990). Other chapters in this volume discuss cognitive therapies for chronic pain.

Thermal Biofeedback

Thermal biofeedback as a treatment for migraine headache was initially described 30 years ago by Sargent, Green, and Walters (1972). The essence of this treatment is to teach patients to warm their hands with the assistance of relatively immediate sensory feedback. It is reasonably well established that this treatment involving volitional peripheral vasodilation is beneficial to sufferers of migraine headache. For a comprehensive review, see Arena and Blanchard (2001) or Blanchard and Arena (1999).

PRACTICAL CONCERNS

Treatment Duration and Spacing. When we treat migraine headache (and also mixed headache), treatment length is usually 8 to

12 sessions, once or twice a week. Our rec-ommendation is for twice-a-week sessions, at least for the first 2 weeks. There is an ap-parent skill-like component in learning pe-ripheral vasodilation, so that relatively massed training sessions seem to help early on. (This point has not, to the best of our knowledge, been empirically tested.)

Duration of Sessions. The actual feedback portion of the session should be relatively brief, in the range of 15 to 20 minutes. Sus-tained hand warming is subjectively difficult for patients. Patients who are beginning to show control tend to trail off or lose the control after about 15 minutes.

We do know that for acquisition of the vasodilation response and subsequent headache relief, a sustained or continuous trial of 15 to 20 minutes is superior to 10 to 20 brief 1- to 2-minute trials with 30-second breaks (Andrasik, Pallmeyer, Blan-chard, & Attanasio, 1984).

Feedback Instruments. The actual biofeed-back instrument is a fancy thermometer. The brand does not seem to matter much. The thermal biofeedback instrument con-sists of a temperature-sensitive probe or sen-sor, a thermistor, and an electronic device that converts the temperature signal to a feedback display. It seems that a fairly high degree of sensitivity is needed; the device should register changes of 0.1°F or 0.1°C.

We routinely let patients sample both vi-sual and auditory (a tone changing in pitch) feedback signals. Over 80% of patients re-ceiving thermal biofeedback choose the vi-sual display. The feedback display can be the pen on a voltmeter, a digital output, or bars on a video screen. The actual form of the visual feedback display does not seem to matter (Evans, 1988).

Thermistor Placement. The thermistor placement is somewhat arbitrary. We have routinely used the ventral pad of the last dig-it on the index finger of the nondominant hand. No empirical research of which we are aware shows an advantage for one place-ment over another. The thermistor should be held in close contact with the skin by either a Velcro band or paper tape. Care should be taken when tape is used not to encircle the finger fully and create a tourniquet.

Room Temperature. The patient should be comfortably seated in a relaxed posture. However, a recliner with a headrest is not necessary, as it is for good relaxation train-ing. The room should be reasonably warm, at least 72°F and preferably 75–78°F. It is hard for a patient to warm his or her hands in a cool or cold room. In this latter circum-stance, the patient is fighting a strong reflex (heat conservation by peripheral vasocon-striction).

Timing of Phases within the Session. We recommend that routine sessions (those af-ter the first one or two) should begin with at least 10 minutes devoted to adaptation and in-session baseline. (In Albany, New York, in the winter, Blanchard and colleagues use a longer adaptation period if a patient is freshly arrived from outdoors.) Next, we recommend a 3- to 5-minute self-control phase in which the patient is asked to warm his or her hands without the assistance of the feedback display. Data from this portion of the session enable the therapist to moni-tor progress toward the eventual goal of treatment—true volitional control of hand temperature without the assistance of exter-nal feedback.

Home Practice. We strongly urge headache patients to practice the hand-warming pro-cedures at home on a regular basis between clinic training sessions. Our normal recom-mendation is for at least 20 minutes of prac-tice a day, preferably in a single session (but we also encourage two 10-minute sessions as an alternative). We routinely give patients a small alcohol-in-glass thermometer as a home practice device; it can be read accu-rately to within 2°F, and possibly 1°F. Alter-natively, we have used electronic home train-ers with digital output; however, they cost $50 to $125, as compared to 50¢ for the thermometer. We ask patients to record be-ginning and ending temperatures as well as length of home practice sessions, as a way of checking on compliance and progress.

Evidence in support of the value of regu-lar home practice is scant. Blanchard and colleagues (1983) reported that a low level of continued home practice (vs. no practice) was associated with better maintenance of headache reduction and with other sympto-matic improvement.

In an empirical test of the role of home practice, Blanchard, Nicholson, Radnitz, and colleagues (1991) gave 46 vascular headache sufferers 12 sessions (two a week) of thermal biofeedback alone (with *no* adjunctive relaxation training). For half the subjects, instruction for regular home practice were included (and followed fairly well); for the other half, no mention was made of home practice, and patients' inquiries were politely rebuffed. There was no difference between the groups in headache relief, either statistically or in terms of the proportion of the sample who improved significantly. The major difference was in the temperature control data: Those patients practicing regularly appeared to master the volitional vasodilation response by about the sixth or seventh session, whereas those without regular home practice appeared to need 9 or 10 sessions to reach the same level of proficiency. Thus home practice seems to improve the efficiency of thermal biofeedback training but not the overall efficacy if enough treatment is provided.

INITIAL SESSION INSTRUCTION AND RATIONALE

We believe that the initial instructions and rationale given to the patient are important. Summarized here is the information we try to convey to migraine patients at the first treatment session. We begin by telling patients we want them to learn to warm their hands with the assistance of the biofeedback training, and then by acknowledging that the connection between hand warming and migraine relief is not obvious. We go on to say that to warm one's hands, the tiny blood vessels in the periphery must open up or dilate. This vasodilation is under the control of the autonomic nervous system—the branch of the nervous system that controls involuntary functions, such as how fast the heart beats. In particular, the sympathetic nervous system, the part of the autonomic nervous system that controls the "fight-or-flight" response, controls peripheral vasoconstriction and vasodilation. When there is sympathetic nervous system activity, or "sympathetic outflow," the blood vessels constrict. (We should note that it is not clear whether this is truly the mechanism involved; the evidence is mixed. For example, McCoy et al., 1988, found contrary evidence.) Thus patients are told that in essence, we are attempting to reduce sympathetic nervous system activity (outflow) and monitoring it by measuring hand temperature.

We also stress that this treatment is designed to bring about a "tonic charge," or generalized reduction, in sympathetic activity. Thus regular daily practice is important. The treatment is not especially designed as a phasic or short-term coping strategy. The overall goal is to reduce the frequency and intensity of headache (a prophylactic or preventive strategy), not to abort headaches or reduce their discomfort once they have begun.

An immediate question many patients have is how they are supposed to do this. It is good to anticipate this question by acknowledging it and admitting that no strategy is universally successful. Instead, we explain to the patients that the biofeedback setup or "loop" allows them to explore various strategies to find one that will work for them. It is thus a trial-and-error (or trial-and-success) process. Strategies that some people have used successfully include mental images of warm sun at the beach, watching the meter directly and trying to control it, or attending to the feeling of blood pulsations in the fingertips.

Clinical Hints. We believe that it is useful for the therapist to try to warm his or her own hands with the assistance of biofeedback, to be able to speak more authoritatively on this point.

Two other points need to be mentioned. First, patients need to relax to make it work. This treatment is not just a way to teach relaxation but to teach that relaxation is necessary and facilitative, but not sufficient, to achieve the hand warming. Second, we emphasize that the patients should *not try too hard* to warm their hands because the active striving elicits a sympathetic nervous system response and defeats the whole experience. Instead, patients should try to use *passive volition,* allowing the response to occur rather than trying to force it to occur.

Finally, patients should be warned that some people find the task difficult and frustrating at first. Thus, they should try not to be discouraged if it takes several sessions to begin to succeed. This forewarning can help prevent early discouragement and premature termination.

AUTOGENIC PHRASES

The initial description of thermal biofeedback training for migraine headache by Sargent and colleagues (1972) included the use of limited autogenic training (Schultz & Luthe, 1969)—in particular, training in relaxation, heaviness, and warmth. "Autogenic training" is a meditational form of relaxation that focuses on specific self-instructions.

We have routinely introduced limited autogenic phrases during the first two thermal biofeedback training sessions by describing them to our patients as one possible strategy to generate hand warming. Patients are cautioned that the phrases may or may not help them, but they are offered as one strategy within the trial-and-success framework. Table 8.1 lists the actual relaxation phrases.

To conduct this part of the training, we recommend that therapists tell patients that they will be giving them a series of phrases in the first person (see Table 8.1). The patients are to repeat the phrase verbatim (hence the use of the first person) to themselves; as the patients give themselves these self-instructions, they should try to have the experience described and notice the peripheral sensations. We routinely give each patient a copy of the phrases to use at home as he or she chooses.

Clinical Hint. Pacing, or timing, of the presentation of the phrases is important. There needs to be enough time for a patient to repeat the phrase mentally and try to generate the response. The therapist can measure the time roughly by repeating the phrase silently to him- or herself.

PRESENCE OF THERAPIST

A decision needs to be made on whether or not the therapist is in the room with the patient (which assumes an office arrangement that allows such a choice). In the work in Albany, a therapist was routinely in the same room with the subject for the first two sessions (when the autogenic phrases were used) and then in a separate room, but in voice contact, during the remainder. The

TABLE 8.1. Autogenic Phrases

"I feel quite quiet . . ."
"I am beginning to feel quite relaxed . . ."
"My ankles, my knees, and my hips feel heavy, relaxed, and comfortable . . ."
"My chest, my stomach, and my whole body, feel relaxed and quiet . . ."
"My breathing is deep, slow, and relaxed . . ."
"My hands, my arms, and my shoulders feel heavy, relaxed, and comfortable . . ."
"I can feel my neck and shoulders unwind, loosen up, smooth out, and relax more and more . . ."
"My neck, my jaws, and my forehead feel relaxed . . ."
"They feel comfortable and smooth . . ."
"My eyes feel heavy and relaxed . . ."
"My whole body feels quite heavy, comfortable, and relaxed . . ."
"My arms and hands are heavy and warm . . ."
"I can feel myself settling deep into the chair . . ."
"I feel quite relaxed . . ."
"My whole body is relaxed and my hands are warm, relaxed and warm . . ."
"My hands are warm . . ."
"Warmth is flowing into my hands, they are warm, warm . . ."
"My mind is quiet . . ."
"My mind is calm, relaxed and quiet . . ."
"I feel an inward quietness . . ."
"My mind is quiet and my whole body is relaxed and comfortable . . ."

only empirical research (Borgeat, Hade, Larouche, & Bedwani, 1980) suggests that leaving the subject alone with the feedback display promotes learning (or that the therapist's presence is a hindrance or distracter).

TRAINING TO A TEMPERATURE CRITERION

It has long been advocated by clinicians involved in the development of thermal biofeedback (especially Fahrion, 1977) that patients be trained to a specific temperature criterion. The recommended temperature is 95°F; the empirical basis for this temperature is not clear. There is some limited empirical evidence (Libo & Arnold, 1983) that patients trained to the 95°F criterion did better during a long-term (1-year) follow-up than did those who did not reach this level. Another criterion suggested by Sargent and colleagues (1972) is that the patient be able to produce a 1.5°F rise in hand temperature within 2 minutes. Again, the empirical basis for this criterion is unclear.

In our own work, the strongest overall correlation between temperature training parameters and headache reduction is with the number of sessions on which any temperature rise above in-session baseline is noted (Blanchard et al., 1983). We have also observed a discontinuity in outcome for patients who achieve 96°F or higher at any point during training. Those who reach this level have a significantly higher likelihood of experiencing a clinically meaningful reduction in headache activity (at least 50%) than do those who reach lower maximum levels (Blanchard et al., 1983). This apparent threshold was replicated in a later study on a new cohort of vascular headache patients (Morrill & Blanchard, 1989).

MANIPULATION OF ATTRIBUTIONAL RESPONSES

Given the powerful results of Holroyd and colleagues (1984) in showing that manipulation of the attributions made by tension headache sufferers profoundly affected headache reduction in EMG biofeedback, it was logical to see whether similar results would be obtained with vascular headache patients receiving thermal biofeedback.

In a study on 28 vascular headache patients receiving 12 sessions of thermal biofeedback with no home practice, Blanchard, Kim, Hermann, and Steffek (1994) tried an attributional manipulation similar to Holroyd and colleagues'. It was not universally successful in leading patients to believe that they were either highly successful or modestly successful at the hand-warming task. For the patients for whom the manipulation succeeded, the expected effects on headache relief were found. Patients who believed they were highly successful experienced greater headache relief than did those who believed they were only moderately successful.

LIMITED-CONTACT, HOME-BASED TREATMENTS AND TELEMEDICINE THERAPY

The availability of relatively low-cost, high-precision thermal biofeedback training devices lends itself to the possibility of a limited-therapist-contact, largely home-based treatment regimen. Blanchard and col-

leagues have published three separate studies (Blanchard, Andrasik, Appelbaum, et al., 1985; Blanchard, Appelbaum, Nicholson, et al., 1990; Jurish et al., 1983) evaluating a treatment regimen of three sessions (over 2 months) combining thermal biofeedback and progressive relaxation training. In all three instances, positive results were found for this attenuated form of treatment. Tobin, Holroyd, Baker, Reynolds, and Holms (1988) reported similar results.

We believe that some limited therapist contact is necessary so that patients understand the rationale for the treatment and that problems (trying too hard, thermistor misplacement, etc.) can be caught and corrected early. We also believe that detailed manuals to guide the home training and telephone consultation to troubleshoot problems are crucial in this approach. Given the national push for improving the efficiency of treatments, this approach has much to recommend it. We should also note that this home-based approach was not as successful as office-based treatment of essential hypertension with thermal biofeedback (Blanchard et al., 1987).

Arena, Dennis, McClean, and Meador (2002) recently reported a small ($n = 4$) uncontrolled study investigating the feasibility of an internet and/or telemedicine delivery modality for relaxation therapy and thermal biofeedback for vascular headache. Each subject was over the age of 50 and had suffered from headaches for more than 20 years. Subjects came into the clinic for treatment but never saw the therapist in person. Instead, all treatment was conducted through the use of computer terminals and monitors. The only difference between this treatment and office-based treatment was physical presence of the therapist. Results indicated that one of the subjects had treatment success (greater than 50% headache improvement) and two others had between 25 and 50% improvement. Thus, it seems that further exploration of the potential of telemedicine and Internet delivery of psychophysiological interventions is warranted.

Special Headache Populations

Most of what we have described thus far in this chapter is based on research and clinical treatment with the general adult headache population. There are, however, several special headache populations to which relaxation and biofeedback have been applied. This section describes these populations, and changes in standard treatment procedures that should be made for them.

Pediatric Headache

Migraine headache affects approximately 2.5% of the child and adolescent population in the United States, with the prevalence and incidence progressively higher with older cohorts within this attenuated age range (Stang et al., 1992).

There is now a sizable body of research attesting to the efficacy of thermal biofeedback with pediatric migraine (see Blanchard, 1992, Table 2, for a concise narrative summary). A meta-analysis by Hermann, Kim, and Blanchard (1993) comparing drug and nondrug treatments revealed that thermal biofeedback and propranolol appeared to be the treatments of choice, with both yielding high levels of headache relief. The average percentage of improvement in studies of thermal biofeedback with pediatric migraine is about 70%—substantially better than one finds with adults.

In adapting thermal biofeedback to a pediatric population, certain ideas seem relevant:

1. *Length of training session.* The attention span of pediatric patients, especially preadolescents, is somewhat limited. For that reason we recommend a 30-minute total session length, with the baseline and self-control phases reduced to about 2 to 3 minutes and the feedback portion reduced to about 12 minutes. Home practice should probably be monitored by parents of younger children, who seem not to remember this task readily.

2. *Feedback display.* The feedback display needs to sustain the pediatric patient's attention. Many patients in this age range are familiar with video games and computerized graphics; thus their expectations may be high. We recommend, in the absence of empirical data, that the therapist stay in the room with the patient to act as a coach.

3. *Home-based treatment.* Hermann (1994) has shown that a limited-contact thermal biofeedback regimen (four sessions over 8 weeks) is effective with a pediatric population. Sixty-nine percent of her 32 subjects showed clinically significant reductions in headache activity as documented by headache diaries.

Headaches of the Elderly

Although headaches are often thought of as disorders that afflict the young or middle-aged, epidemiological data show that over 9% of adults over the age of 65 have moderate to severe headaches from benign (i.e., migraine or tension-type headaches) causes (Cook et al., 1989). A recent epidemiological study (Prencipe et al., 2001) suggests that the Cook and colleagues (1989) data may be an underestimate. In this study, involving a two-phase survey and neurological examination carried out on all residents greater than or equal to age 65 in three rural Italian villages, 1-year prevalence rates were 44.5% for tension and 11.0% for migraine headache. Prevalence of headache did decrease steadily with age—57% for those ages 65–74, 45% for those ages 75–84, and 26% for those greater than age 84.

In the mid-1980s, conventional clinical wisdom held that older headache patients did not respond well to biofeedback training. This view was reinforced by an uncontrolled series of cases from Albany (Blanchard, Andrasik, Evans, & Hillhouse, 1985) that presented the data from 11 headache patients over the age of 60 who had been treated with various combinations of biofeedback and relaxation therapies. Only 2 of 11 (19%) showed clinically meaningful reductions in headache activity.

Uncontrolled studies by Arena and colleagues (Arena, Hannah, Bruno, & Meador, 1991; Arena, Hightower, & Chang, 1988) on elderly tension headache patients successfully challenged this conventional wisdom by showing very high levels of success with relaxation training (70% success in Arena et al., 1988) and frontal EMG biofeedback training (50% success in Arena et al., 1991). The key to this success by Arena and colleagues was adapting the treatments to the information-processing capacities of an older population. Instructions were repeated as necessary and presented more slowly; more handouts, often in larger type, were made available to guide home practice; and other alterations to make the treatments more age-relevant were made.

The Albany group profited from Arena's advice and incorporated these changes into the treatment protocols. A new uncontrolled series of elderly headache patients in Albany (Kabela, Blanchard, Appelbaum, & Nicholson, 1989) showed that four of eight (50%) tension headache patients improved and six of eight (75%) vascular headache patients improved. Interestingly, 5 of 16 patients eliminated all or almost all (80%+) of their headache medications. Such elimination alone is a major benefit for the elderly, who are often taking several medications chronically.

Finally, in a controlled study, Nicholson and Blanchard (1993) showed a significant advantage for treatment combining relaxation and biofeedback over headache monitoring in a population of older (age range = 61 to 80) headache sufferers when the treatments were tailored to the population and its information-processing capacities. With such changes, older headache patients readily respond to biofeedback and relaxation.

Chronic, Daily High-Intensity Headache

Blanchard, Appelbaum, Radnitz, Jaccard, and Dentinger (1989) identified a relatively refractory headache type that they labeled "chronic, daily high-intensity headache." People with this type of headache account for about 6% of patients seen at university-based headache clinics. They describe their headache as present essentially all the time (at least 27 out of 28 days) at a moderately severe to severe level of pain and distress. Thus, although these patients usually meet the nominal criteria for tension-type headache, their severity ratings are like those of migraine patients and show little variability. In a retrospective case-control analysis, Blanchard and colleagues found that only 13% of patients with chronic, daily high-intensity headache responded favorably to combinations of biofeedback, relaxation, and cognitive therapy. Moreover, this group of patients shows a higher degree of distress in standard psychological tests than do gender-matched and diagnosis-matched controls who had more variability to their

headaches but who received similar treatments.

Recently, Barton and Blanchard (in press) treated 16 patients with chronic daily headache of moderate to severe intensity with a combination of progressive muscle relaxation therapy, thermal biofeedback, and cognitive stress-coping therapy. All were to receive 20 sessions but four stopped treatment after 12 visits (but had received all three treatment components). Only 2 of 12 completers (17%) showed significant headache relief (50% or greater reduction in headache activity). Thus far, we have not developed successful treatments for this subset of headache patients.

High-Medication-Consumption Headache

Kudrow (1982) first called attention to a phenomenon he labeled "analgesic rebound headache." In a pioneering but poorly controlled study, he found that those patients who continued on high levels of regular analgesic medication responded much more poorly to amitriptyline than did comparable patients who were able to discontinue most of the analgesic. Mathew, Kurman, and Perez (1990) also found this relative refractoriness of patients who take high levels of all medications to be associated with poor response to behavioral treatments and a high dropout rate.

Michultka, Blanchard, Appelbaum, Jaccard, and Dentinger (1989) have identified a group of headache patients as having what they have termed "high-medication-consumption headache." This group was identified on the basis of daily records of medication consumption. Using the medication-scaling procedures of Coyne, Sargent, Segerson, and Obourn (1976) (over-the-counter analgesics such as aspirin and acetaminophen are scaled as 1, Fiorinal as 2, etc.), Michultka and colleagues identified patients with average weekly scores of 40 or greater across 4 consecutive weeks (this translates into roughly six aspirin per day, three Fiorinal per day, etc.). About 12% of headache patients met this criterion. Using retrospective case-control analysis, the authors found that high-medication-consumption headache sufferers did significantly poorer than diagnosis-matched patients taking lower levels of medication who received comparable behavioral treatments; only about 29% of the high-medication patients responded favorably.

In an uncontrolled case series, Blanchard, Taylor, and Dentinger (1992) developed a special protocol for 10 high-medication-consumption patients. After baseline headache and medication recording, a consulting neurologist gave the patients individually tailored schedules for discontinuing their medication. As the patients tried to decrease the medication, they were simultaneously given relaxation training and a great deal of psychological support (phone consultations, at least two visits a week) to assist in the detoxification process. Patients had also been carefully warned about the possibility of rebound headache.

After patients had decreased their medication as far as possible, they received standard biofeedback, relaxation, and/or cognitive therapy. Of the 10 patients, 8 had substantial decreases in medication, and 6 had clinically significant decreases in headache activity that were maintained at follow-ups of up to 1 year. Two patients experienced complete failure, despite two (and in one case three) attempts to reduce medication. Moreover, in two cases patients dropped out of treatment after successfully eliminating their medication. They were apparently content to tolerate their continued headaches.

Clinical Hints. It thus seems clear that high-medication-consumption headache cases can be helped, primarily by focusing first on reducing or eliminating the medications and then on treating the patients' residual headache. The key to the medication reduction step is a high level of support for the patients as they go through this process, especially during the period of increased headache severity and duration that is very likely to occur.

Headache during Pregnancy

Estimates are that up to 80% of women report onset of headaches with pregnancy, mostly during the first trimester (Scharff, Marcus, & Turk, 1997). It would appear that psychophysiological treatments such as relaxation and biofeedback would be efficacious for treating headaches during preg-

nancy, as pregnant women are not able to use most pain medications. There is now growing evidence to suggest that this is indeed the case.

In a pioneering study, Hickling, Silverman, and Loos (1990) gave five pregnant patients with severe vascular headaches between 4 and 12 sessions of biofeedback, relaxation therapy, and psychotherapy. During headache, and at follow-up evaluation between 4 and 17 months after pregnancy, all patients showed a marked reduction or complete cessation of headaches.

Marcus, Scharff, and Turk (1995), in a methodologically elegant series of studies, first demonstrated that a combination of relaxation therapy, hand-warming biofeedback, and physical therapy given to 19 pregnant women was successful in decreasing headache activity by 72.9%, with 15 of the 19 women obtaining clinically significant results of 50% or greater reduction in headache activity. In a second study, they then compared the combined treatment (*n* = 11) to an attention control group (*n* = 14) that received headache education and hand cooling biofeedback. The combined group was successful in decreasing headache activity by 81.2%, with 8 of the 11 women (72.7%) obtaining clinically significant reductions of 50% or greater. For the attention control group, 32.7% overall decrease in headache activity was obtained, with only 4 of the 14 subjects (28.6%) achieving significant clinical relief. These results were maintained on 1-year follow-up (Scharff, Marcus, & Turk, 1996). Thus, we feel that the available evidence suggests that biofeedback in combination with other techniques such as relaxation therapy and psychotherapy should be the first-line intervention for headache during pregnancy.

Chronic Low Back Pain

There are a number of theories concerning the relationship between muscle tension and chronic low back pain (Dolce & Raczynski, 1985; Nouwen & Bush, 1984). These theories can be broken down into two major models. The first of these is the "biomechanical theory," according to which the paraspinal muscles of the lower back are unduly lower than normal, or there is a left–right asymmetry in the lower back (in this case, one side of the back musculature is abnormally lower or higher than the other). This asymmetry is presumed to be the result of some mechanical or physical pathology, such as lesions, trauma, abnormal gait, poor posture, or the like. The second major model is the "stress causality theory," or "psychosocial stressor theory," in which back pain is presumed to be the result of increased paraspinal muscle activity caused by ineffective stress coping skills. There is limited evidence to support either of these two theories (Arena & Blanchard, 2001; Arena, Sherman, Bruno, & Young, 1989; Dolce & Raczynski, 1985; Nouwen & Bush, 1984). With low back pain patients, biofeedback has been used as a general relaxation and stress reduction technique, as well as a specific strategy to correct muscle tension abnormalities.

Psychophysiological Intervention with Chronic Low Back Pain

There is one major difference in the psychophysiological treatment of chronic low back pain and chronic headache: Whereas with chronic headache, treatments such as biofeedback and relaxation training can be the primary or even sole therapy, with chronic low back pain we feel that psychophysiological intervention should never be used alone. There are data to support this assertion. In 1992, Sherman and Arena exhaustively reviewed the biofeedback treatment of chronic low back pain (this review was limited to biofeedback as the *sole* treatment). They found that most of the studies suffered from a number of critical methodological and conceptual limitations, including small sample sizes *(n* ≤ 10), unspecified diagnosis, lack of inclusion and exclusion criteria, lack of adequate control groups, the mingling of acute and chronic low back pain, inadequate description of the biofeedback procedures, lack of clinical significance (i.e., what percentage of subjects were significantly helped?), and no or limited follow-up. Sherman and Arena concluded that biofeedback in and of itself had not been adequately demonstrated to reduce back pain sufficiently to the point where no further treatment was necessary. Arena and Blanchard (2001) came to similar conclusions regarding the methodological and conceptual limitations of the more recent low back pain studies but found that there had been enough additional research to now tentatively conclude that biofeedback could be employed as a sole treatment for low back pain but appeared to work better when combined with other modalities.

Psychophysiological interventions are essential components of nonsurgical chronic low back pain treatment. However, instead of being used by themselves, we feel they should be included in an overall multidisciplinary treatment program that can encompass such services as physical therapy, pharmacological management, kinesthetic therapy, recreational therapy, behavioral and cognitive-behavioral treatments, social work, nursing, vocational counseling, orthopedic/neurosurgical/anesthesiological treatment, and so forth. Indeed, when biofeedback and relaxation procedures are combined with such interventions, treatment effects are maximized (Flor, Fydrich, & Turk, 1992; Loeser & Turk, 2000).

As with a headache patient, it is essential for the nonphysician therapist to have a chronic low back pain patient medically screened prior to the onset of treatment and to coordinate treatment with the physician who is managing the patient. Indeed, the latter may be even more important with low back pain than with headache patients. In general, headaches do not change over the course of treatment, whereas low back pain can change drastically (as a result of age, trauma, disease, etc.) and may require medical intervention.

It is important to familiarize oneself with basic anatomy and physiology prior to working with low back pain patients. Any therapist who works with the lower back needs to have a text handy that has anatomical drawings of the bones, nerves, and muscles of the back. We use *Grant's Atlas of Anatomy* (Agur, 1991), as well as Clemente's *Anatomy* (Clemente, 1987). It is not possible in the space allocated to review all but the essentials. The spinal column runs from the skull to the coccyx and is divided into a number of regions: cervical (neck region), thoracic (upper back), lumbar (lower back), and sacral (hip region). Most back surgeries are done in or near the fourth and fifth lumbar vertebrae (L4–L5).

From the two major theories concerning the relationship of muscle tension and low back pain (see above), one could hypothesize two psychophysiological strategies with EMG biofeedback. The first would be to conduct a psychophysiological assessment, in which paraspinal and other muscles presumed to be involved in low back pain (upper trapezius, biceps femoris, etc.) would be measured. The therapist would then attempt through EMG biofeedback to correct any abnormality found (e.g., if abnormally low or high muscle tension was present, the therapist would teach the patient to increase or decrease the muscle tension to normal levels; if a left–right asymmetry was noted, the therapist would teach the patient to increase or decrease the muscle tension in the abnormal side). The second strategy would be to conduct frontal EMG biofeedback training as a general technique for enhancing muscle tension awareness, stress reduction, and relaxation training. In the review of the literature described earlier, Sherman and Arena (1992) concluded, "There is no evidence that use of biofeedback from muscle groups (to correct demonstrated muscle tension pattern abnormalities) is more effective than use of biofeedback from the frontal or general upper trunk regions (as part of general muscle tension awareness and relaxation training)" (p. 189). The studies that have been published since that review have not changed these conclusions.

In Georgia, Arena and his colleagues use a combination of both strategies with low back pain patients, based on clinical experience as well as assessment research (Arena et al., 1989; Arena, Sherman, Bruno, & Young, 1990). In that research, surface EMG recordings of bilateral paraspinal muscle tension were made on 207 subjects from the five low back pain groups described previously, and 29 nonpain controls, during six positions: standing, bending from the waist, rising, sitting with back unsupported, sitting with back supported, and prone. Results of both individual and group analyses revealed controls to have significantly lower overall EMG levels than the groups with intervertebral disk disorders and unspecified musculoskeletal backache. Control subjects during the standing position had significantly lower EMG levels than did all low back pain groups, and sub-

jects with intervertebral disk disorders had significantly higher EMG levels than did all other groups during the supported sitting position. It is especially important to note that the diagnostic groups did not differ from one another in the prone position. It is in this position that low back pain subjects and normals are measured in the majority of surface EMG studies. Another study (Arena, Sherman, Bruno, & Young, 1991) found that the paraspinal muscle tension levels of low back pain subjects did not change as a function of low or high pain levels (the previously described assessment was conducted twice—once in a low-pain state and once in a high-pain state—on 21 patients with intervertebral disk disorders and 25 subjects with unspecified musculoskeletal backache). This later study demonstrated that EMG levels alone are not substantially connected with the maintenance of chronic low back pain.

On the basis of this research and their clinical experiences, Arena and his colleagues use the following psychophysiological protocol with chronic low back pain patients. They first give a regimen of frontal EMG biofeedback, followed by upper trapezius EMG biofeedback, using a strategy of general relaxation therapy and muscle tension awareness. With chronic low back pain, Arena and his colleagues always teach patients to generalize the biofeedback response (in an attempt to make the office biofeedback training simulate real-world situations) after initially training the patients on a recliner or couch. Once the patients have mastered the rudiments of biofeedback, they then routinely progress to a comfortable office chair (with arms), an uncomfortable office chair (without arms), and finally a standing position. This strategy is followed for both frontal and upper trapezius training. This generally takes 12–16 sessions.

If the patient achieves significant relief with frontal and upper trapezius EMG biofeedback, at this point he or she terminates therapy. When the patient does not receive sufficient relief, Arena and his colleagues follow one of two treatment courses. If their patients obtain some reduction in pain through frontal and upper trapezius biofeedback, they continue with the general relaxation strategy by beginning relaxation therapy (see Syrjala & Abrams, Chapter 9, this volume, and Arena & Blanchard, 1996, for additional information on this procedure).

With those people who fail to achieve any relief with frontal and upper trapezius EMG biofeedback, or with those individuals who do not get sufficient relief from relaxation therapy, Arena and his colleagues then conduct a psychophysiological assessment, following the logic of the biomechanical theory of low back pain. This assessment consists of bilateral paraspinal (L4–L5) and biceps femoris (back of thigh) muscle tension readings in at least two positions: sitting with back supported in a recliner or other comfortable chair and standing with arms by sides. They use biceps femoris for the leg measure, because in their clinical work they have found more abnormalities in this region than in other leg sites, such as quadriceps femoris (front of thigh) or gastrocnemius (back of calf). The back of the leg is enervated by the sciatic nerve, and is usually the area where most patients say that their pain is referred from the lower back. For exact sensor placement for the paraspinal and biceps femoris muscles, see Basmajian and DeLuca (1985) or Lippold (1967). Figure 8.2 graphically depicts the paraspinal muscle site placement, as well as the biceps femoris muscle site placement.

The Augusta group looks for three possible muscle tension abnormalities in both the paraspinal and biceps femoris muscle groups: (1) unusually low muscle tension levels (this usually occurs only with nerve damage and resultant muscle atrophy), (2) unusually high muscle tension levels (this is the abnormality most frequently found), or (3) a left–right asymmetry, in which one side of the back or thigh muscles has normal muscle tension levels while the other side has unusually low or high readings. (Unfortunately, normative values are based on the equipment used. Readers should refer to their equipment reference manuals or run some non-pain controls to obtain their own norms.) In the first instance, they teach patients through biofeedback to increase their muscle tension levels in the respective muscle group(s); in the second instance, they teach them through biofeedback to decrease their muscle tension levels in the respective muscle group(s). When no asymmetry is found, as in these two instances, they usually give feedback from a single side during the biofeedback sessions. If an asymmetry is found (the third instance), they use biofeedback to increase or decrease the abnormal side. The goal is to bring both sides into the normal range.

Clinical Hints. It is essential to look at the gait and posture of every low back pain pa-

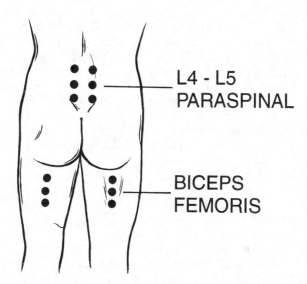

L4 - L5
PARASPINAL

BICEPS
FEMORIS

FIGURE 8.2. Electrode placement for bilateral paraspinal and biceps femoris EMG biofeedback training.

tient. Nearly all will have the neck forward, the gait slowed, and weight usually borne on the unaffected side. The therapist should have the patient walk, without making it obvious that the patient is being observed. Gait and posture abnormalities should be corrected through education, as well as through biofeedback. A full-length mirror used as a biofeedback device to correct exaggerated posture is helpful. In many instances of severe gait and posture abnormalities, a physical therapist referral is quite helpful.

Finally, with low back pain, it is imperative to deal with the cognitive-behavioral component as well as the psychophysiological one. Again, readers should refer to Turk, Chapter 7, this volume, for assistance in this area.

Conclusions

It has been our intent in writing this chapter to present the novice clinician with a reasonably detailed "how to" guide for conducting biofeedback with chronic headache and low back pain, as well as to provide the more advanced reader with an understanding of how two fairly experienced clinician–researchers approach some of the major pitfalls and questions that arise when biofeedback procedures are employed with chronic pain patients. We hope we have succeeded in our goal.

We also hope that the reader will modify the biofeedback procedures we use with chronic headache and low back pain for application to other pain disorders. This does not mean that the reader should charge blindly ahead and implement these procedures with every patient who presents with chronic pain; that would be neither ethical nor prudent. Rather, we anticipate that the procedures outlined in this chapter, *coupled with a careful reading of the available psychophysiological intervention literature* on the pain disorder in question, should enable the clinician to approach the pain problem with some level of expertise and comfort. It is important to scrutinize the existing literature carefully, both to avoid making obvious mistakes (e.g., treating a vascular disorder such as Raynaud's disease with EMG biofeedback rather than thermal) and to avoid repeating the failure of others (e.g., attempting to treat cluster headache with psychophysiological interventions or mixed headache with only relaxation therapy).

Although we have repeatedly stressed a common theme throughout this chapter, it bears repeating. Any psychophysiological treatment must be tailored to the needs of the individual patient. It is the clinician's job to be creative and flexible. For example, if a patient has trouble relaxing when caught in rush-hour traffic, the therapist can make an audiotape or videotape of the stressful event and have the patient practice the biofeedback exercises while the tape is playing. If a patient generally gets headaches after working on a computer, the therapist can connect the EMG sensors to the forehead and trapezius muscles, have the patient use a computer, and see whether the patient is inadvertently tensing those muscles or has poor posture while working at the task.

We hope we have demonstrated to clinicians that they should not put their basic clinical and common-sense skills "on the shelf" when they are using psychophysiological interventions. Too often, we have heard from both students and experienced clinicians that they "feel like technicians" when they perform procedures such as biofeedback and relaxation therapy. It is our experience that if such feelings occur, they are often an indication that a clinician has failed to grasp the complexities and nuances of a patient or a pain disorder. Although we have been searching now for quite some time, we have yet to see the "textbook" chronic pain patient. The fact that every patient is different from the others is what makes clinical work both engaging and rewarding.

Acknowledgments

This chapter was supported by a Department of Veterans Affairs Merit Review awarded to John G. Arena, and by National Institute of Mental Health Grant No. MH-41341 awarded to Edward B. Blanchard.

References

Ad Hoc Committee on the Classification of Headache. (1962). Classification of headache.

Journal of the American Medical Association, 179, 127–128.

Agur, A. M. R. (1991). *Grant's atlas of anatomy* (9th ed.). Baltimore: Williams & Wilkins.

American Academy of Orthopedic Surgery. (1996). *Common orthopedic procedures and codes: A reference guide* (2nd ed.). New York: Author.

Andrasik, F., Pallmeyer, T. P., Blanchard, E. B., & Attanasio, V. (1984). Continuous versus interrupted schedules of thermal biofeedback: An exploratory analysis with clinical subjects. *Biofeedback and Self-Regulation,* 9, 291–298.

Arena, J. G., & Blanchard, E. B. (1996). Biofeedback and relaxation therapy for chronic pain disorders. In R. J. Gatchel & D. C. Turk (Eds.), *Chronic pain: Psychological perspectives on treatment* (pp. 179–230). New York: Guilford Press.

Arena, J. G., & Blanchard, E. B. (2001). Biofeedback therapy for chronic pain disorders. In J. D. Loeser, S. D. Butler, C. R. Chapman, & D. C. Turk (Eds.), *Bonica's management of pain* (3rd ed., pp. 1755–1763). Baltimore: Williams & Wilkins.

Arena, J. G., Blanchard, E. B., Andrasik, F., Appelbaum, K., & Myers, P. E. (1985). Psychophysiological comparisons of three kinds of headache sufferers during and between headache states: Analysis of post-stress adaptation periods. *Journal of Psychosomatic Research,* 29, 427–441.

Arena, J. G., Bruno, G. M., Hannah, S. L., & Meador, K. J. (1995). A comparison of frontal electromyographic biofeedback training, trapezius electromyographic biofeedback training, and progressive muscle relaxation therapy in the treatment of tension headache. *Headache,* 35, 411–419.

Arena, J. G., Bruno, G. M., Rozantine, G., Garner, E. & Meador, K. J. (2002). *Effect of high versus moderate success and training to increase or decrease muscle tension on the treatment outcome of biofeedback training for tension headache.* Unpublished manuscript.

Arena, J. G., Dennis, N., McClean, R., & Meador, K. J. (2002). *A pilot study of the feasibility of a telemedicine delivery system for psychophysiological treatments for vascular headache.* Unpublished manuscript.

Arena, J. G., Hannah, S. L., Bruno, G. M., & Meador, K. J. (1991). Electromyographic biofeedback training for tension headache in the elderly: A prospective study. *Biofeedback and Self-Regulation,* 16, 379–390.

Arena, J. G., Hannah, S. L., Bruno, G. M., Smith, J. D., & Meador, K. J. (1991). Effect of movement and position on muscle activity in tension headache sufferers during and between headaches. *Journal of Psychosomatic Research,* 35, 187–195.

Arena, J. G., Hightower, N. E., & Chang, G. C. (1988). Relaxation therapy for tension headache in the elderly: A prospective study. *Psychology and Aging,* 3, 96–98.

Arena, J. G., & Schwartz, M. S. (forthcoming). Psychophysiological assessment and biofeedback baselines for the front-line clinician: A primer. In M. S. Schwartz (Ed.), *Biofeedback: A practitioner's guide* (3rd ed.). New York: Guilford Press.

Arena, J. G., Sherman, R. A., Bruno, G. M., & Young, T. R. (1989). Electromyographic recordings of five types of low back pain subjects and non-pain controls in different positions. *Pain,* 37, 57–65.

Arena, J. G., Sherman, R. A., Bruno, G. M., & Young, T. R. (1990). Temporal stability of paraspinal electromyographic recordings in low back and non-pain subjects. *International Journal of Psychophysiology,* 9, 31–37.

Arena, J. G., Sherman, R. A., Bruno, G. M., & Young, T. R. (1991). Electromyographic recordings of five types of low back pain subjects and non-pain controls in different positions: Effect of pain state. *Pain,* 45, 23–28.

Barton, K. A., & Blanchard, E. B. (in press). The failure of intensive self-regulatory treatment with chronic daily headache: A prospective study. *Applied Psychophysiology and Biofeedback.*

Basmajian, J. V., & DeLuca, C. J. (1985). *Muscles alive: Their functions revealed by electromyography.* Baltimore: Williams & Wilkins.

Blanchard, E. B. (1992). Psychological treatment of benign headache disorders. *Journal of Consulting and Clinical Psychology,* 60, 537–551.

Blanchard, E. B. (1993). Behavioral therapies in the treatment of headache. *Headache Quarterly,* 3, 53–56.

Blanchard, E. B., & Andrasik, F. (1985). *Management of chronic headache: A psychological approach.* Elmsford, NY: Pergamon Press.

Blanchard, E. B., & Andrasik, F. (1987). Biofeedback treatment of vascular headache. In J. P. Hatch, J. D. Rugh, & J. G. Fisher (Eds.), *Biofeedback: Studies in clinical efficacy* (pp. 1–79). New York: Plenum Press.

Blanchard, E. B., Andrasik, F., Appelbaum, K. A., Evans, D. D., Jurish, S. E., Teders, S. J., Rodichok, L. D., & Barron, K. D. (1985). The efficacy and cost-effectiveness of minimal-therapist contact, non-drug treatments of chronic migraine and tension headache. *Headache,* 25, 214–220.

Blanchard, E. B., Andrasik, F., Evans, D. D., & Hillhouse, J. (1985). Biofeedback and relaxation treatments for headache in the elderly: A caution and a challenge. *Biofeedback and Self-Regulation,* 10, 69–73.

Blanchard, E. B., Andrasik, F., Evans, D. D., Neff, D. F., Appelbaum, K. A., & Rodichok, L. D. (1985). Behavioral treatment of 250 chronic headache patients: A clinical replication series. *Behavior Therapy,* 16, 308–327.

Blanchard, E. B., Andrasik, F., Jurish, S. E., & Teders, S. J. (1982). The treatment of cluster headache with relaxation and thermal biofeedback. *Biofeedback and Self-Regulation,* 7, 185–191.

Blanchard, E. B., Andrasik, F., Neff, D. F., Arena, J. G., Ahles, T. A., Jurish, S. E., Pallmeyer, T. P., Saunders, N. L., Teders, S. J., Barron, K. D., & Rodichok, L. D. (1982). Biofeedback and relaxation training with three kinds of headache: Treatment effects and their prediction. *Journal of Consulting and Clinical Psychology, 50,* 562–575.

Blanchard, E. B., Andrasik, F., Neff, D. F., Saunders, N. L., Arena, J. G., Pallmeyer, T. P., Teders, S. J., Jurish, S. E., & Rodichok, L. D. (1983). Four process studies in the behavioral treatment of chronic headache. *Behaviour Research and Therapy, 21,* 209–220.

Blanchard, E. B., Andrasik, F., Neff, D. F., Teders, S. J., Pallmeyer, T. P., Arena, J. G., Jurish, S. E., Saunders, N. L., & Rodichok, L. D. (1982). Sequential comparisons of relaxation training and biofeedback in the treatment of three kinds of headache, or the machines may be necessary some of the time. *Behaviour Research and Therapy, 20,* 469–482.

Blanchard, E. B., Appelbaum, K. A., Nicholson, N. L., Radnitz, C. L., Morrill, B., Michultka, D., Kirsch, C., Hillhouse, J., & Dentinger, M. P. (1990). A controlled evaluation of the addition of cognitive therapy to a home-based biofeedback and relaxation treatment of vascular headache. *Headache, 30,* 371–376.

Blanchard, E. B., Appelbaum, K. A., Radnitz, C. L., Jaccard, J., & Dentinger, M. P. (1989). The refractory headache patient: I. Chronic, daily, high intensity headache. *Behaviour Research and Therapy, 27,* 403–410.

Blanchard, E. B., Appelbaum, K. A., Radnitz, C. L., Michultka, D. M., Morrill, B., Kirsch, C., Hillhouse, J., Evans, D. D., Guarnieri, P., Attanasio, V., Andrasik, F., Jaccard, J., & Dentinger, M. P. (1990). A placebo-controlled evaluation of abbreviated progressive muscle relaxation and relaxation combined with cognitive therapy in the treatment of tension headache. *Journal of Consulting and Clinical Psychology, 58,* 210–215.

Blanchard, E. B., Appelbaum, K. A., Radnitz, C. L., Morrill, B., Michultka, D., Kirsch, C., Guarnieri, P., Hillhouse, J., Evans, D. D., Jaccard, J., & Barron, K. D. (1990). A controlled evaluation of thermal biofeedback and thermal biofeedback combined with cognitive therapy in the treatment of vascular headache. *Journal of Consulting and Clinical Psychology, 58,* 216–224.

Blanchard, E. B., & Arena, J. G. (1999). Biofeedback, relaxation training and other psychological treatments for chronic benign headache. In M. L. Diamond & G. D. Solomon (Eds.), *Diamond's and Dalessio's the practicing physician's approach to headache* (6th ed., pp. 209–224). New York: Saunders.

Blanchard, E. B., Kim, M., Hermann, C., & Steffek, B. D. (1993). Preliminary results of the effects on headache relief of perception of success among tension headache patients receiving relaxation. *Headache Quarterly, 4,* 249–253.

Blanchard, E. B., Kim, M., Hermann, C., & Steffek, B. D. (1994). The role of perception of success in the thermal biofeedback treatment of vascular headache. *Headache Quarterly, 5,* 231–236.

Blanchard, E. B., McCoy, G. C., McCaffrey, R. J., Berger, M., Musso, A. J., Wittrock, D. A., Gerar-

di, M. A., Halpern, M., & Pangburn, L. (1987). Evaluation of a minimal-therapist-contact thermal biofeedback treatment program for essential hypertension. *Biofeedback and Self-Regulation, 12,* 93–103

Blanchard, E. B., McCoy, G. C., Musso, A., Gerardi, R. J., Cotch, P. A., Siracusa, K., & Andrasik, F. (1986). A controlled comparison of thermal biofeedback and relaxation training in the treatment of essential hypertension: I. Short-term and long-term outcome. *Behavior Therapy, 17,* 563–579.

Blanchard, E. B., Nicholson, N. L., Radnitz, C. L., Steffek, B. D., Appelbaum, K. A., & Dentinger, M. P. (1991). The role of home practice in thermal biofeedback. *Journal of Consulting and Clinical Psychology, 59,* 507–512.

Blanchard, E. B., Nicholson, N. L., Taylor, A. E., Steffek, B. D., Radnitz, C. L., & Appelbaum, K. A. (1991). The role of regular home practice in the relaxation treatment of tension headache. *Journal of Consulting and Clinical Psychology, 59,* 467–470.

Blanchard, E. B., Taylor, A. E., & Dentinger, M. P. (1992). Preliminary results from the self-regulatory treatment of high medication consumption headache. *Biofeedback and Self-Regulation, 17,* 179–202.

Borgeat, F., Hade, B., Larouche, L. N., & Bedwani, C. N. (1980). Effects of therapist active presence on EMG biofeedback training of headache patients. *Biofeedback and Self-Regulation, 5,* 275–282.

Clemente, C. D. (1987). *Anatomy: A regional atlas of the human body* (3rd ed.). Baltimore: Urban & Schwarzenberg.

Cook, N. R., Evans, D. A., Funkenstein, H., Scherr, P. A. Ostfeld, A. M., Taylor, J. O., & Hennekens, C. H. (1989). Correlates of headache in a population-based cohort of elderly. *Archives of Neurology, 46,* 1338–1344.

Cousins, M. J. (1995). Foreword. In W. E. Fordyce (Ed.), *Back pain in the workplace:Management of disability in nonspecific conditions. A report of the Task Force on Pain in the Workplace of the International Association for the Study of Pain.* Seattle, WA: International Association for the Study of Pain Press.

Coyne, L., Sargent, J., Segerson, J., & Obourn, R. (1976). Relative potency scale for analgesic drugs: Use of psychophysical procedures with clinical judgments. *Headache, 16,* 70–71

Dolce, J. J., & Raczynski, J. M. (1985). Neuromuscular activity and electromyography in painful backs: Psychological and biomechanical models in assessment and treatment. *Psychological Bulletin, 97,* 502–520.

Evans, D. D. (1988). *A comparison of two computerized thermal biofeedback displays in migraine headache patients and controls.* Unpublished dissertation, State University of New York, Albany.

Fahrion, S. L. (1977) Autogenic biofeedback treatment for migraine. *Mayo Clinic Proceedings, 52,* 776–784.

Flor, H., Fydrich, T., & Turk, D. C. (1992). Efficacy of multidisciplinary pain treatment centers: A meta-analytic review. *Pain, 49,* 221–230.

Gatchel, R. J., & Blanchard, E. B. (Eds.). (1993). *Psychophysiological disorders: Research and clinical applications.* Washington, DC: American Psychological Association Press.

Headache Classification Committee of the International Headache Society. (1988). Classification and diagnostic criteria for headache disorders, cranial neuralgias and facial pain. *Cephalalgia,* 8(Suppl. 7), 29–34.

Heide, F. J., & Borkovec, T. D. (1983). Relaxation-induced anxiety: Paradoxical anxiety enhancement due to relaxation training. *Journal of Consulting and Clinical Psychology, 51,* 171–182.

Hermann, C. U. (1994). *Pediatric migraine: A comprehensive assessment and treatment study.* Unpublished doctoral dissertation, University of Tubigen, Tubigen, Germany.

Hermann, C. U., Kim, M., & Blanchard, E. B. (1993, March 25–30). The efficacy of behavioral intervention in the treatment of pediatric migraine: A meta-analytic review. In *Proceedings of the 24th Annual Meeting of the Association for Applied Psychophysiology and Biofeedback* (pp. 149–154). Wheatridge, CO: Association for Applied Psychophysiology and Biofeedback.

Hickling, E. J., Silverman, D. J., & Loos, W. (1990). A non-pharmacological treatment of vascular headache during pregnancy. *Headache, 30,* 407–410.

Holroyd, K. A., & Andrasik, F. (1982). A cognitive-behavioral approach to recurrent tension and migraine headache. In P. C. Kendall (Ed.), *Advances in cognitive-behavioral research and therapy* (Vol. 1, pp. 275–320). New York: Academic Press.

Holroyd, K. A., Penzien, D. B., Hursey, K. G., Tobin, L. R., Holm, J. E., Marcille, P. J., Hall, J. R., & Chila, A. G. (1984). Change mechanisms in EMG biofeedback training: Cognitive changes underlying improvements in tension headache. *Journal of Consulting and Clinical Psychology, 52,* 1039–1053.

Jurish, S. E., Blanchard, E. B., Andrasik, F., Teders, S. J., Neff, D. F., & Arena, J. G. (1983). Home versus clinic-based treatment of vascular headache. *Journal of Consulting and Clinical Psychology, 51,* 743–751.

Kabela, E., Blanchard, E. B., Appelbaum, K. A., & Nicholson, N. (1989). Self-regulatory treatment of headache in the elderly. *Biofeedback and Self-Regulation, 14,* 219–228.

King, A. C., & Arena, J. G. (1984). Behavioral treatment of chronic cluster headache in geriatric patients. *Biofeedback and Self-Regulation, 9,* 201–208.

Kudrow, L. (1980). *Cluster headache: Mechanisms and management.* New York: Oxford University Press.

Kudrow, L. (1982). Paradoxical effects of frequent analgesic use. In M. Critchley, A. P. Friedman, S. Gorini, & F. Sicuteri (Eds.), *Advances in neurology: Vol. 33. Headache: Physiopathological and clinical concepts* (pp. 335–341). New York: Raven Press.

Lewis, T., & Solomon, G. D. (1999). Cluster headache. In M. L. Diamond & G. D. Solomon (Eds.), *Diamond's and Dalessio's The practicing physician's approach to headache* (6th ed., pp. 71–82). New York: Saunders.

Libo, L. M., & Arnold, G. E. (1983). Does training to criterion influence improvement? A follow-up study of EMG and thermal biofeedback. *Journal of Behavioral Medicine, 6,* 397–404.

Lichstein, K. L. (1988). *Clinical relaxation strategies.* New York: Wiley.

Lippold, D. C. J. (1967). Electromyography. In P. H. Venables & I. Martin (Eds.), *Manual of psychophysiological methods* (pp. 245–297). New York: Wiley.

Loeser, J. D. & Turk, D. C. (2000). Multidisciplinary pain management. In J. D. Loeser, S. D. Butler, C. R. Chapman, & D. C. Turk (Eds.), *Bonica's management of pain* (3rd ed., pp. 2069–2079). Baltimore: Williams & Wilkins.

MacHose, M., & Peper, E. (1991). The effects of clothing on inhalation volume. *Biofeedback and Self-Regulation, 16,* 261–265.

Marcus, D. A., Scharff, L., & Turk, D. C. (1995). Nonpharmacological management of headaches during pregnancy. *Psychosomatic Medicine, 57,* 527–535.

Mathew, N. T., Kurman, R., & Perez, F. (1990). Drug induced refractory headache: Clinical features and management. *Headache, 30,* 634–638.

McCoy, G. C., Blanchard, E. B., Wittrock, D. A., Morrison, S., Pangburn, L., Siracusa, K., & Pallmeyer, T. P. (1988). Biochemical changes associated with thermal biofeedback treatment of hypertension. *Biofeedback and Self-Regulation, 13,* 139–150.

Michultka, D. M., Blanchard, E. B., Appelbaum, K. A., Jaccard, J., & Dentinger, M. P. (1989). The refractory headache patient: II. High medication consumption (analgesic rebound) headache. *Behaviour Research and Therapy, 27,* 411–420.

Morrill, B., & Blanchard, E. B. (1989). Two studies of the potential mechanisms of action in the thermal biofeedback treatment of vascular headache. *Headache, 29,* 169–176.

Nicholson, N. L., & Blanchard, E. B. (1993). A controlled evaluation of behavioral treatment of chronic headache in the elderly. *Behavior Therapy, 25,* 395–408.

Nouwen, A., & Bush, C. (1984). The relationship between paraspinal EMG and chronic low back pain. *Pain, 20,* 109–123.

Olton, D. S., & Noonberg, A. R. (1980). *Biofeedback: Clinical applications in behavioral medicine.* Englewood Cliffs, NJ: Prentice-Hall.

Prencipe, M., Casini, A. R., Ferretti, C., Santini, M., Pezzella, F., Scaldaferri, N., & Culasso, F. (2001). Prevalence of headache in an elderly population: Attack frequency, disability, and use of medication. *Journal of Neurology, Neurosurgery, and Psychiatry, 70,* 377–381.

Rokicki, L. A., Holroyd, K. A., France, C. R.,

Lipchik, G. L., France, J. L., & Kvaal, S. A. (1997). Change mechanisms associated with combined relaxation/EMG biofeedback training for chronic tension headache. *Applied Psychophysiology and Biofeedback, 22,* 21–41.

Sargent, J. D., Green, E. E., & Walters, E. D. (1972). The use of autogenic feedback training in a pilot study of migraine and tension headaches. *Headache, 12,* 120–124.

Scharff, L., Marcus, D. A., & Turk, D. C. (1996). Maintenance of effects in the nonmedical treatment of headaches during pregnancy. *Headache, 36,* 285–290.

Scharff, L., Marcus, D. A., & Turk, D. C. (1997). Headache during pregnancy and in the postpartum: A prospective study. *Headache, 37,* 203–210.

Schultz, J. H., & Luthe, W. (1969). Autogenic methods. In W. Luthe (Ed.), *Autogenic therapy* (Vol. 1, pp. 1–245). New York: Grune & Stratton.

Schwartz, M. S., & Associates. (1995). *Biofeedback: A practitioner's guide* (2nd ed.). New York: Guilford Press.

Sherman, R. A., & Arena, J. G. (1992). Biofeedback in the assessment and treatment of low back pain. In J. Bazmajian & R. Nyberg (Eds.), *Spinal manipulative therapies* (pp. 177–197). Baltimore: Williams & Wilkins.

Smith, J. C. (1990). *Cognitive-behavioral relaxation training: A new system of strategies for treatment and assessment.* New York: Springer.

Sobel, D. S. (1993). Mind matters, money matters: The cost-effectiveness of clinical behavioral medicine. *Mental Medicine Update, 2,* 1–8.

Stang, P. E., Yanagihara, T., Swanson, J. W., Beard, C. M., O'Fallon, W. M., Guess, H. A., & Melton, L. J. (1992). Incidents of migraine headache: A population-based study in Olmstead County, Minnesota. *Neurology, 42,* 1657–1662.

Taub, E., & School, P. J. (1978). Some methodological considerations in thermal biofeedback training. *Behavior Research Methods and Instrumentation, 10,* 617–622.

Tobin, D. L., Holroyd, K. A., Baker, A., Reynolds, R. V. C., & Holms, J. E. (1988). Development and clinical trial of a minimal contact, cognitive-behavioral treatment for tension headache. *Cognitive Therapy and Research, 12,* 325–339.

Wolff, J. G. (1963). *Headache and other head pain.* New York: Oxford University Press.

9

Hypnosis and Imagery in the Treatment of Pain

Karen L. Syrjala
Janet R. Abrams

Hypnosis and imagery have been used for the past century to treat pain unrelieved by traditional medical treatments. Interest in these techniques has again risen over the last two decades, both as pain treatment becomes a widely practiced specialty and as the limits of traditional medical care are recognized. Inquiries into hypnosis as a pain treatment usually stem from either fears of the side effects of medical treatments or the lack of efficacy of medical treatments attempted. The fact that pharmacological and invasive methods do not alleviate all pain without undesired side effects makes hypnosis and other imagery strategies worth pursuing and worthy of scientific inquiry. Extensive randomized controlled clinical trials indicate that hypnosis and imagery are more effective than placebo or most other nonpharmacological strategies. In this chapter we describe the research and practical applications of mental imaging strategies to assist patients with unrelieved pain.

What Is It?

The distinctions between terms and mechanisms used to describe mental transformations in pain perception are gaining greater consistency. Hypnosis and imagery are generally agreed to be states of highly focused attention during which alteration of awareness, sensations, and the affective response to perceptions occur. Untested to our knowledge is the question whether hypnosis is an altered state of consciousness and distinct from imagery because of this. Hypnosis has been hypothesized to reduce pain by mechanisms including attention control and dissociation (Hilgard & Hilgard, 1983; Spiegel & Spiegel, 1978). More recently, both theories have received positive neurophysiological support. Spinal descending pathways and multiple cerebral regions, both in blood flow and electrical activity, have demonstrated change during hypnosis consistent with altered consciousness (Danziger et al., 1998; Kiernan, Dane, Phillips, & Price, 1995; Rainville et al., 1999). Greater change has been measured when analgesic suggestions are added to relaxation images. Finally, simple explanation remains elusive given the evidence that different individuals respond in opposing neurophysiological directions in response to effective hypnotic analgesia (Danziger et al., 1998).

Other strategies share more commonalities than differences with hypnosis. Upon reading, a clinician is hard pressed to prop-

TABLE 9.1. Strategies Associated with Imagery and Proven Effective for Pain Control in Randomized Controlled Trials

Progressive muscle relaxation
Passive (autogenic) relaxation
Meditation
Imagery or visualization
Hypnosis

erly designate which script is meditation, which imagery, and which hypnosis (see Table 9.1 for a list of associated strategies).

Imagery and visualization are synonymous in our use of the terms and generally indicate incorporation of visual images. Although imagery implies the use of "mental pictures," there has been no scientific demonstration that pictures are essential to effective pain control. In other words, a patient who says he does not actually picture an image, but rather hears sounds or has a particularly soothing thought or feels the music or warmth of a light moving through his body may receive as much benefit as the patient who can describe her visual images with great detail.

Hypnosis usually includes visual imagery but always implies a state of highly focused attention during which time one is susceptible to direct or indirect suggestions for reaching a goal (Hilgard & Hilgard, 1983). Suggestion may or may not be offered in imagery, relaxation, or meditation strategies. Certainly the intention to hypnotize is not required for hypnosis. Thus a suggestible person may be easily hypnotized using imagery or meditation, or even a highly focused conversation. Although trance is also considered an essential component, the ability to measure or define this has been elusive beyond intense focus, with a mind more receptive to suggestion.

What is the Role of Suggestion?

For the purposes of pain relief, suggestion is a central component of clinical efficacy. As such, suggestion may be much more important for a clinician to understand than the concept of trance. In essence, suggestion is, as it sounds, the conveying to a patient that something will be accomplished or experienced; this suggestion can be explicit or im-

plied; it can be direct or indirect. In other words, a clinician may simply act as though pain relief will, of course, be accomplished with treatment, and this can be a powerful suggestion. Alternatively, the clinician can suggest comfort and mastery over physical well-being, never mentioning pain as such. This suggestion is effective because it frames a positive goal to achieve rather than a negative goal of what to eliminate. Pain relief is an implicit suggestion as both patient and clinician know that this is the goal.

As a rule, we find positive suggestion—the indication of what *is* felt, whether comfort, cold, or activity—more broadly powerful than negative suggestion (e.g., "the pain will disappear"). Similarly, for many acute pain situations, where long-term coping with pain is not necessary, analgesic or sensory transformation suggestions are not even needed. Relief is obtained by actively moving the patients' mind to comfort and pleasure contradictory to negative symptoms. For chronic pain, focus away from pain is difficult to sustain when one must interrupt an intense, single focus to go about routine life activities. Thus chronic pain suggestions may focus on reducing pain or moving pain into background awareness rather than eliminating pain.

Although suggested analgesia may be more powerful in the hypnotic state than without hypnosis (McGlashan, Evans, & Orne, 1969), suggestion is an extremely powerful tool in any state. In essence, suggestion in its simplest form is the same as a placebo effect, which is increasingly recognized as a positive outcome of treatment to be maximized rather than eliminated (Turner, Deyo, Loeser, Von Korff, & Fordyce, 1994). Even such strategies as cognitive-behavioral reframing or distraction incorporate an element of suggestion in their method. Regardless of the choice of terminology or method selected, effects will be stronger if clinicians actively use suggestion to achieve comfort and to increase patients' sense of control over their own well-being.

Does Hypnotizability Matter?

Hypnotic susceptibility is defined as the degree of ability to experience images and to respond to suggestions following a hypnotic induction. Susceptibility can be measured by performance on standardized tests or, less formally, by methods described later. Responsivity to hypnosis on standard instruments is relatively stable and some believe that this is a trait, that there is little one can do to enable a low susceptibility person to have a hypnotic experience (Hilgard & Hilgard, 1965; Shor & Orne, 1962; Spiegel, 1985). Data do concur that high hypnotizable subjects reduce pain more than do low hypnotizable subjects in laboratory studies (e.g., Spanos, Kennedy, & Gwynn, 1984; Spanos, Radtke-Bodorik, Ferguson, & Jones, 1979), but even here, hypnotizability is not the best predictor of response (Price & Barber, 1987). For patients, with stronger motivating factors, response on standard measures is less useful as a predictor of benefit but still has an association with hypnotic analgesia (Barber, 1980; Frischholz, Spiegel, Spiegel, Balma, & Markell, 1981; Montgomery, DuHamel, & Redd, 2000).

Although there are conflicting and inconsistent clinical and laboratory reports on who is or is not a good candidate for hypnosis, assuming the patient wants to use hypnosis or imagery, almost anyone can benefit from individualized treatment. Among others, Diamond (1984) and Holroyd (1996) suggest that some capacity for hypnotic trance resides with most people. In this model, teaching and motivation can increase responsiveness to hypnosis (Spanos, Radtke-Bodorik, Ferguson, & Jones, 1979; Spanos, Robertson, Menary, & Brett, 1986). We agree that with some motivation from the patient and with individualizing the method to the response style of the patient, nearly all patients can benefit from these techniques. This requires the clinician usually to explore with a patient what the patient does and does not respond to (e.g., water, gardens, music, movement, warmth, and cold). Still the patient with more responsivity will likely respond more readily to any approach.

Who Benefits from What Method?

The goal of treatment is less to selectively apply these techniques than to blend the methods to be as effective as possible in the indi-

vidual situation. In practice, we avoid distinguishing terminology and adapt the method to the presentation of the patient. Some people feel uncomfortable being "hypnotized" because of their fear that the clinician or an evil force might take control of their minds (Hendler & Redd, 1986). They respond much better to the use of imagery and a focus on "self-imagery"—"you are controlling your own thoughts, you can stop whenever you like, you tell me what you would like to accomplish." For others the implied "magic" of hypnosis is a powerful expectation component. Our clinical trial data indicate that use of the phrase "relaxation with imagery" is equally effective as the phrase "hypnosis" when applied to identical procedures (Syrjala, Cummings, & Donaldson, 1992; Syrjala, Donaldson, Davis, Kippes, & Carr, 1995). For the practical purpose of reducing pain, we use an individualized approach with labels and language that fit the patient's request and personal style.

When Is Imagery or Hypnosis Helpful?

Numerous studies have indicated that imagery and hypnosis reduce many types of pain. Since World War II, clinicians have described hypnosis to help medically ill patients (Erickson, 1959; Sacerdote 1965, 1970) and have described effective analgesic and anesthetic strategies using hypnosis (Hilgard & Hilgard, 1983; Lang et al., 2000). When treating chronic pain, writers have suggested that hypnosis is effective in changing the pain experience by shifting attention to something other than bodily sensations (Crasilneck, 1979).

In meta-analysis of the efficacy of cognitive-behavioral methods for pain control, imagery/hypnosis demonstrated the strongest positive effects across studies with various types of pain (Fernandez & Turk, 1989). Other research has incorporated relaxation with imagery into interventions and found that the package is only as helpful as relaxation with imagery alone (Syrjala et al., 1995; Turner & Jensen, 1993). A recent meta-analysis reported that hypnosis for pain has a moderate to large effect size with 75% of lab and clinical participants receiving substantial analgesia (Montgomery et al., 2000). Thus imagery strategies repeatedly have demonstrated the greatest effect size of all cognitive-behavioral strategies tested for efficacy in pain control.

To date there are few controlled clinical trials using hypnosis or imagery for pain control with continuous pain rather than brief pain. Spiegel and colleagues randomly assigned breast cancer patients to either no treatment, support group, or support group with brief hypnosis. At 1 year, those in the hypnosis group reported the lowest pain levels although not significantly lower than those in the support-only group (Spiegel & Bloom, 1983). Syrjala, Cummings, and Donaldson (1992) and Syrjala and colleagues (1995; Syrjala, Davis, Abrams, & Keenan, 1992) have completed two clinical trials testing the efficacy of hypnosis/imagery and cognitive-behavioral skills for pain related to high-dose cancer treatment. Syrjala and colleagues found that patients could learn and apply hypnosis or imagery to pain management with two sessions of training followed by brief "booster" sessions. This strategy was as effective as a cognitive-behavioral package of skills that included imagery. With chronic benign pain, hypnosis, meditation, imagery, and relaxation have all demonstrated efficacy in providing relief; however, no studies indicate that one method is superior to others (Kabat-Zinn, Lipworth, & Burney, 1985; Turner & Jensen, 1993). Burn pain, migraine, and phantom limb pain have also responded to hypnosis (Olness, MacDonald, & Uden, 1987; Patterson, Everett, Burns, & Marvin, 1992; Sthalekar, 1993).

What Evaluations Improve Choice of Method and Outcome?

Before a clinician can responsibly develop a psychological treatment plan incorporating hypnosis or imagery, a patient needs to have a medical evaluation for diagnosis and determination of appropriate medical treatments. Although additional psychological assessment is valuable, the depth of this assessment depends in part on the duration of pain relief being sought. Brief imagery for a procedural pain may require only a brief assessment. Designing a strategy for management of chronic pain, whether benign or cancer-related, usually takes a more thorough assessment. The evaluation needs to be updated as needs change, depending, for instance, on treatment effects, course of the illness, cognitive shifts, and input from others such as family members. Further details on assessment of pain are available from other sources (e.g., Chapman & Syrjala, 2001; Turk & Melzack, 2001). Here we focus only on those aspects of evaluation directly related to planning hypnosis or imagery interventions.

Pain Assessment

A good description of the pain will help in developing hypnotic strategies and suggestions that can be tailored to the individual needs of the patient.

ETIOLOGY AND LOCATION

Knowledge of the natural course of a pain problem is needed along with awareness of specifically what anatomy is involved. These are particularly valuable if imagery includes shifts in the pain location or sensation.

TEMPORAL PATTERN

Is the pain brief, continuous, or intermittent? Treatment is likely to shift depending on whether the pain is fairly constant or is only present with movement, whether it is long in duration or sharp, sudden, unpredictable, or short-lived. Choice of imagery strategy will differ if the goal is to help a patient get through 20 minutes until medication takes effect, to get through an intense 5-minute pain that medication will not treat, or to reduce the life disruption caused by continuous pain. With a predictable, brief procedural pain, imagery can focus on actively distracting the patient from discomforts for the duration of the procedure. For a continuous or recurrent pain, mere distraction imagery will not be as effective in treating the pain (McCaul & Malott, 1984; Suls & Fletcher, 1985); a sensory transformation method is needed to integrate modified pain perception into one's ongoing life.

PAIN QUALITY

In the use of analgesic imagery, the patient's description of the qualities of the pain can assist in defining approach and content. Quality of the pain (stabbing, burning, aching) can be incorporated into the sensory transformation. For a brief burning or hot pain as in some postherpetic neuralgia attacks, we may use images of blowing freezing arctic air through the sensation. Both the control of breathing and the icy image that patients can do readily on their own helps when the clinician is not there and more extended focus may be difficult. For longer duration aching pains, analgesic suggestions may include strategies that acknowledge the pain and then take the patient through a process to transform and reduce the pain without attempting to eliminate it altogether. The patient imagines what the pain looks like and then modifies the image, sometimes in surprising ways.

For example, this is a simple image that patients with tension headache can learn quickly and then do on their own anywhere:

CLINICIAN: What words describe how the headache feels to you?

PATIENT: It feels like really intense pressure, like my head will explode.

CLINICIAN: Would you like a way to feel better that you can use when you start to get headaches? ["Sure."] How about if we try a short little experiment to see if your head can feel better? ["OK."] First take a couple deep breaths just to focused inside and get comfortable, you can close your eyes if you like, all that matters is that you are as comfortable as can be right now. (*Breathe deeply with the patient.*) Now let your mind go to how it feels when you have a headache. Notice the tightness like a balloon, see the balloon filled with pressure (*pause*). What color is the balloon that you see? [*Response*] And you can feel the pressure in your head like the air pressing and expanding tight against that balloon. The air has a color, what color is that pressurized air? Any color is fine just notice what color comes to mind. (*pause*) Now you can begin to let the air out of the balloon as you breathe out the tension. Listen to the sound as the air moves out, the pressure drops, seeing the [color] air as it moves away, as the air leaves the balloon in the same way the feelings in your head can blow out into the air, breathing out pressure, breathing in fresh blue air, or perhaps your fresh air is clear or another color, what color is your fresh clean air? (*pause*) OK, breathing in fresh soft [color] air, just enough to comfort-

ably replace as much air as you like as your head relaxes. Now as your head stays relaxed, watch as the [color] air you've gotten rid of mixes with the outer air, watch as it expands. Just letting it expand in its normal way until it's impossible to see where the [color] air is, as it just drifts away absorbed into the fresh air as you've drained all the pressure and replaced it with this easy fresh feeling you can carry through the day. And whenever you like, wherever you are, you'll find it easy to think of the balloon, the color of the air and feel the pressure leave you as it leaves the balloon, out with the [color] air, in with that refreshing, relaxing [color] air.

In a similar way, other pain perceptions can be changed through describing shifts in sensation, shape, colors, textures, or other qualities of a visualized pain.

PAIN SEVERITY

The severity or intensity of the pain is easily measured with a 0–10 scale from "no pain" to "pain as bad as can be." A baseline assessment and reassessment after the use of imagery can assist both the patient and clinician in evaluating the efficacy of treatment. In itself, this can act as a suggestion and motivator, reminding the patient that the time spent using the technique has a measurable effect even if pain does not disappear altogether. However, assessment immediately after treatment is not recommended if a goal is for extended pain relief. A clinician would not wish to return the patient's attention to pain after working hard to move attention away. Assessment at the next treatment session is likely to be more productive.

MEANING OF THE PAIN

What is the meaning of the pain to the patient? Does the person want the symptom diminished? Is the pain a sign of frustration, helplessness, or loss to the patient; is it needed to support a law suit or disability claim; is it a cause for anxiety and questions about whether a disease is progressing? In some of these situations, patients may receive special care or attention because of the pain. Possible ways the pain is a positive indicator or provides secondary gain may need to be evaluated. In understanding the meaning of the pain, it is helpful to ask patients what they believe is causing the pain, what will happen to the pain over time (will it get better, worse or stay the same forever), and what would happen to them if the pain went away (what would change in their lives, what activities would change). This has particular importance for chronic pain or when a patient seems to not be responding to any treatments and the clinician perceives a barrier.

TREATMENT AND EFFICACY

It is necessary to identify treatments attempted and their efficacy. What increases the patient's discomfort and distress, what reduces discomfort or distress? If treatments were stopped or refused, the reason may be important. In particular, ineffective past trials of hypnosis, relaxation, or imagery may greatly reduce the positive expectancy that is part of the effectiveness of hypnosis. A clinician's goal for a suffering patient should be optimal treatment. If such treatment can be accomplished with medication or a different procedure, education may be warranted to address fears, side effects, or lack of awareness of options. Patients and their family members at times turn to hypnosis and other complementary strategies as a way to avoid treatments they fear or resist, including both medical treatments and other behavioral approaches such as exercise. The evaluation should result not only in a plan for using imagery but also integration of all treatments, if possible.

Coping Style

The ways a person copes with pain or stress is useful to understand in selecting a methodology. As a general rule, "problem-focused" copers want to gather information, solve problems, and find something to do about the pain. "Avoiders" prefer not to think about problems, particularly the pain problem. "Catastrophizers" tend to have extreme thoughts in response to the pain such as "This is so terrible, I can't stand it, what if it just gets worse and worse, it's never going to stop." Of course, patients may not be only one of these but may use all these strategies to a different extent at different times. Clinical impression suggests

that problem-focused copers more readily use imagery strategies in which they can participate. Avoiders and catastrophizers are less likely to seek these methods, although they often respond well if the clinician uses hypnosis and is willing to take more control and to be more directive in the process. Avoiders particularly like to use pleasant place, escape types of images as they begin. We use this approach initially with these patients, and as confidence builds, we incorporate more sensory transformation and mastery images.

Even problem-focused copers, who in general are ready to participate in their pain relief, can require more care if they are concrete, inflexible, or very biologically minded. These are more often males who initially see imagery or hypnosis as too inexplicable and intangible. This type of person responds well to initial training with tense-release progressive muscle relaxation, where they experience something concrete happening, followed by brief imagery, combined with explanation of the biological mechanisms for effectiveness. The physical experience of contrast in perception from tense to relaxed is instructive to them, and then they have greater confidence in use of imagery without the formal relaxation.

Mental and Psychiatric Status

ALERTNESS, CONCENTRATION

Critical questions include: How alert is the patient? A sedated patient is more likely to fall asleep during the induction. Is the patient able to focus attention and is fatigue or agitation manageable? A patient with limited attention or concentration will need brief methods, will more likely need the clinician to be actively involved (vs. teaching self-hypnosis), and may benefit from more active imagery or storytelling that involves the patient providing some of the images. Patients with delirium are generally poorer candidates for these methods.

COGNITIVE CAPACITY AND STYLE

Clearly, language needs to be tailored to the comprehension of the patient. A highly elaborate confusion strategy as an induction may be ineffective in a patient with limited vocabulary or verbal skills whereas it may be ideal for a vigilant, highly verbal, cognitively oriented patient. Patients also have dispositions toward being visual, auditory, or tactile in their experiences. Using natural dispositions in the images or suggestions offered will certainly make things easier for everyone.

AFFECTIVE STATE

The emotional state of the patient is as important to assess prior to hypnosis as prior to any psychological method. The actively distressed patient may have difficulty focusing on imagery until distress is discussed and explored at least briefly. The depressed patient may seem to bring little motivation to the process. The sense of helplessness that accompanies depression can be assisted with the clinician initially taking more control then shifting imagery to reestablish mastery and a sense of control. However, clinical depression should be treated directly along with imagery for pain control. Similarly, the anxious or extremely tense patient is likely to have difficulty focusing attention. Shorter methods may be needed for the anxious person. We find tense-release progressive muscle relaxation again an effective beginning strategy for patients who will benefit from first taking control of the tension and then contrasting this to their relaxation. This is also helpful with patients who are not aware of the amount of tension they carry.

The phobic patient or those with panic need different considerations. If catastrophizing and anxiety reach a level of diagnosed panic, it is rarely possible to provide an induction. We move directly into breathing control, imagery, and suggestion and evaluate by response whether they benefit the patient. The content of imagery and suggestion is shaped to counter the content of thoughts and images during the panic. Pharmacological methods should be considered if panic recurs and imagery does not readily reduce symptoms. We see phobias develop particularly related to procedures that must be repeated again and again for which the patient had uncontrolled pain and an extreme feeling of loss of control. In these situations, we closely review the patient's recollections of the procedure, particularly the most difficult or painful parts. We then provide systematic desensitization using imagery to assist the patient in gaining control over the procedure and his or her thoughts and emotions during the procedure.

Motivation and Expectation

How invested is the patient in these methods working? How important is symptom reduction? What are the patient's expectations for pain reduction? Usually someone in acute pain is highly motivated. Those with chronic pain may have exhausted their positive expectations, thus their motivation to try new treatments that require their participation may be reduced. Before beginning an intervention, it is useful to ask about previous experience with hypnosis or imagery and current expectations of treatment. These aspects of expectancy do influence outcome and are worth maximizing when possible (Spiegel, 1997; Turner et al., 1994).

Control Need and Self-Efficacy

A sense of the patient's need or preference for control is useful in anticipating likely responses and in tailoring the intervention to these individual needs. Patients with strong needs for control respond best to being left in control. This control may be achieved both through indirect methods (discussed later) that allow them to determine their experience and also through use of a skills training model, teaching them to do imagery or self-hypnosis. Some of these patients are so vigilant during inductions that it is helpful to first explain the steps before beginning an induction.

At the other extreme is a patient who wants no control or active participation. Directive approaches may work better and save time with these people. Be alert to the patient who seems passive but in fact is quite in need of control.

Some fear of being controlled by hypnosis is normal. Fears can be reduced with addressing patient concerns directly. A clinician must explain that no one can force people to concentrate, to relax, or to do something counter to their beliefs. It is the patient who decides if he or she wants to enter a state of focused attention. We tell patients who are quite worried about being "controlled" that by merely opening their eyes, they can stop the experience at any time and we encourage them to experiment with this.

Family Involvement and Attitudes

If family is active in the patient's pain problem, their beliefs and attitudes may need to be considered. They can assist or hinder the process. Ideally, family members support the use of these methods but leave the responsibility for use with the patient. Some families may actively discourage an interested patient or may convey all their own fears about these approaches. Alternatively, families may be so invested in the use and success of the method that they badger the patient or leave the patient feeling like a failure if "success" is not achieved.

When family members are supportive and available, they may act as good "coaches" for patients, helping to use imagery when pain escalates and the clinician is not available. We have taught patients and their family members together and assisted the family in coaching. Scripts can be helpful to ease family member performance anxiety. Frequently, families are initially quite hesitant, believing there is something special in the voice or experience of the hypnotherapist. Gentle support and encouragement can often overcome this reluctance.

Religion and Culture

It is important to understand the role religion and culture have in the person's life. If religion is a central determinant of the patient's perspective, and especially if the person expresses any concern about imagery taking them from a focus on God, we readily bring God into the imagery to assist the patient.

Religion can be a powerful facilitator or inhibitor in hypnotic work. In our own and others' experience, some patients reject hypnosis because of religious beliefs or cultural perspectives (Schafer, 1976). Frequently this rejection includes all forms of imagery and relaxation because the religion or culture teaches that these methods allow evil forces to take control of the patient's mind (Vandeman, 1973). Numerous times we have had patients ask their clergy whether these methods are safe to use. With these people we are most likely to suggest that God or spiritual beliefs be incorporated into the imagery to help them. We never dispute a patient's beliefs nor do we try to convince people to try the method if they are uncomfortable for any reason.

Hypnotizability

In the clinical setting, susceptibility is rarely directly tested. Use of a standardized measure is actually not recommended because it can set the expectations of a low hypnotizable patient to be not responsive. If training is planned for a continuous pain problem, it may be useful to have some sense of the patient's susceptibility. Simple questions about absorption provide some clues. For instance, how readily does the patient become deeply absorbed in movies, is the patient able to picture or feel as if he or she is in a favorite places easily? The goal of assessment in this area is to establish the best approach for a patient rather than to set expectations or to determine who to treat.

Reassessment

As with any treatment, it is important to reassess the pain and the patient's experience. This reassessment can be done briefly, immediately after each session, with a general "how are you doing?" and a bit more extensively before the start of a new session until the patient and clinician are comfortable with the patient's response and with the efficacy of the method selected. It is helpful to assess any observations, discomforts, or preferences of the patient. Once patient and clinician are assured that the method is appropriate, it is usually best not to reassess regularly but to let the patient relate how he or she is doing in general, as assessment brings the patient's attention back to the pain that the imagery or hypnosis most likely drew the patient's mind away from. Returning to thoughts of the pain can decrease comfort and make patients understandably irritated.

What Is the Influence of Therapeutic Relationship and Clinician Style?

Any successful treatment requires a trusting environment. In addition, the clinician must present a calm and confident demeanor conveying the expectation that suggestions will be effective. When using this optimistic perspective, the practitioner communicates in a caring manner, "I'm not afraid of your pain, I'm here to relieve your pain, your pain will be relieved." The clinician becomes the guide in whom the patient can confide and express doubts or fears without transferring these doubts and fears to the clinician. This is not always easy. One of the most common reasons that clinicians trained in hypnosis do not use the technique is because of their own doubts and worries about whether the method will work. The burden seems heavily on the clinician to "make it work" similar to magic. One way to ease this burden is to adopt all the confidence expressed previously within the framework of recognizing that the decisions and efficacy ultimately will be up to the patient. Encouraging an experimental approach to the problem can be useful in easing a sense of burden. We might say to a patient, "I'm sure we will find something that helps you to be more comfortable, let's experiment with this and see how it works for you. You might be surprised at how well this works, but you tell me how well it works." Thus we suggest that the patient take an experimental attitude that it is likely to work but no one has failed if it does not. We leave room for the patient to decide and tell us while still making the positive suggestion of "how well it works."

How To Do It

Technique is similar across most imagery and hypnosis methods, although the time spent in each step may vary greatly depending on the needs of the patient and the situation. Hypnotherapists use many different specific processes successfully. The first full training session, for a continuous or repeated problem, takes 60–90 minutes including establishing a trusting relationship and assessment. For future sessions, 30 minutes is usually adequate for the analgesic imagery work itself.

Table 9.2 outlines the basic framework for hypnosis or imagery. We adapt this framework to the duration and intensity of pain as well as to the characteristics of a pa-

TABLE 9.2. Basics of Imagery or Hypnosis

Preliminary requirements:
Some attention capacity.
Limited disruptions within the setting.
Some interest, motivation by the patient.

Step 1: Capture the patient's attention.
Have the patient close or focus eyes.
Have the patient focus attention using:
Breathing
Simple, repeated image or words
Internal physical experience exploration

Step 2: Deepen the focus of attention, reduce awareness of external world (some or all of these can be used).
Induce relaxation by focusing on releasing tension in body locations.
Count to deepen relaxation with each number.
Move the patient into images of a safe, removed place.
Change sensory awareness.
Maintain intense interest through action in imagery or changes and surprises.

Step 3: Visualize.
Represent a situation or type of approach with words, images.
Involve all senses, watch as change:
Sight—colors, shapes, light
Smell
Sounds
Taste
Touch/feel—texture, softness, density, movement
Temperature

Step 4: Suggest.
Suggest images that accomplish goals:
Comfort, well-being
Change in sensations as pain decreases
Numbness, anesthesia
Make posthypnotic suggestions:
"You can accomplish these goals anytime you choose."
Use breathing or another image to anchor this suggestion (e.g., "Take three deep breaths and picture this image when you wish to return to this feeling of comfort").

Step 5: Return to alertness.
Count in reverse, deep breath, move arms, shoulders, legs to return the patient to being alert, refreshed, and to get blood flowing.

tient. When pain is chronic but mild to moderate, we select a method that teaches self-hypnosis, or we use a skills-training model as described later. If pain is severe, concentration is always more of a problem. We are then more likely to use brief inductions and relatively more direct suggestions. Alternatively, we may actively engage the patient in talking with us during the imagery to more fully maintain focus away from the pain. Storytelling of a favorite past experience into which we add movement and surprises can work well for someone with less responsivity or no time for preparative assessment and training, or even for someone afraid of losing control. If pain is unpredictable, intermittent, but brief, such as severe cramps or a post-herpetic neuralgia with intermittent shooting pain, brief imaging and controlled breathing may be adequate. We listen to the quality of the pain and facilitate selection of an image that the patient accepts and that modifies or counters the painful sensation. For procedural pain with significant anxiety, we prefer time to work with the patient prior to the procedure. We can then provide some desensitization, establish rapport, and develop trust that the patient will be safe with the clinician. Next we rehearse a pleasant but physically challenging activity that both counters the pain sensations and maintains active engaging of attention. However, we must add that some of the most successful hypnosis has been done with patients in acute distress, high motivation to complete a procedure, and no prior assessment or training.

Direct versus Indirect and Permissive Language

Direct approaches instruct the patient in what to do and how to feel (e.g., "close your eyes and take a deep breath, let it out slowly and notice how you feel more relaxed with each exhale"). Indirect methods offer the patient choices from which he or she selects experiences (e.g., "I wonder whether you will notice your right arm feeling heavy, or perhaps it is your left, perhaps both arms feel heavy, or is it a feeling of lightness, it really doesn't matter, however it is for you is fine, just notice how relaxed you can feel."). Indirect wording works

when patients might otherwise be saying to themselves, "No that's not what is happening." This approach does not rely on the clinician knowing exactly what the patient experiences.

Data indicate that indirect approaches, both in inductions and analgesic suggestions, are effective for more people than are direct suggestions (Alman & Carney, 1980; Barber, 1980; Fricton & Roth, 1985). On the other hand, with a highly responsive patient or someone who does not want any control, direct suggestions may provide greater effect and can be quicker to administer (Lynn, Neufeld, & Matyi, 1987). We tend to use indirect approaches when we have the time and a patient is not clearly highly responsive. When symptoms are severe or when the patient seems responsive and motivated, more direct, rapid measures, such as those described in the Brief Induction, can be effective (Appendix 9.1).

Introducing Hypnosis or Imagery

A clinician must convey the message that the pain is real. It is valuable to say this explicitly to patients, then briefly and simply explain the gate-control theory (Melzack & Wall, 1965). Next complete the evaluation as described earlier. If this is the method of choice for imagery context, explore the patient's most enjoyable place or favorite activity, where he or she feels safe, most focused, perhaps even energized. What it is about that place or activity that the patient finds most enjoyable? We have had many surprises in identifying favorite places or activities. It is always important to check out any assumptions. For instance, some people are afraid of water; some people have never been to a beach or mountain. Using their own place or activity always allows patients to bring much more of their own imagination to the experience to make it more authentic for them.

When ready to begin the induction, we explain:

"What we are about to do is very much like things that happen to all of us all the time when we daydream or focus intently on something. For example, driving from one place to another while you are lost in thought, you don't notice the familiar route, yet you arrive safely. If you needed to pay attention, you could bring your mind right back to driving, but in the meantime, your mind is far away. In the same way, some people can get so absorbed in a movie that everything around them fades away. It's as if, for a little while, the movie is all that is real. This is like deep relaxation or hypnosis. When you are intensely absorbed in an experience it is also easier to find relief from pain. Any experience that concentrates your attention away from the body can bring comfort."

Another effective example of how powerful the mind can be is to have the patient and clinician stand facing each other. As the therapist holds his arms at shoulder height and width the patient does the same. From half an arm's-length distance, patient and clinician grasp each other's forearm. The patient is told, "I am going to press on your arms until you bend them. Your job is to hold your arms straight without pressing toward me for as long as you can without stepping back." After this example the instruction is, "Now we are going to do the same thing, I will press on your arms without your moving. But this time I want you to imagine that your arms are pipes of steel, strong and totally unbending."

This simple demonstration can explain more about the power of the mind than many words. We then briefly review the steps the patient can anticipate, as described in Table 9.2.

Induction

The induction phase is a way to establish the focus away from bodily sensation or to transform sensations. The length of this phase depends on how long it takes the patient to enter into a focused or trance state. As has been emphasized throughout this chapter, the uniqueness and attitudes of the patient should be in large part the determining factor in making a decision about what kind of induction would be beneficial. Inductions can be as long as 30 minutes and used when the patient is new to the experience (see the script in Appendix 9.2 for an example of a longer induction). The simple act of asking whether the patient would like to feel more comfortable and of having the patient follow a direction from the clinician

(e.g., "Take a slow breath, in and out") may be adequate when a patient has severe pain. In this situation, the clinician is called on to be more directive and to demonstrate control for the patient whose pain is out of control. As patients become comfortable with the method and familiar with the trance state, they prefer shorter inductions. Brief inductions are also more effective when a patient does not have the attention span to maintain longer imagery or if the patient believes in the "magic" of hypnosis, seems relatively high in hypnotizability, and gives a lot of power to the clinician (see Appendix 9.1).

Early in the induction, many clinicians suggest that patients may find it easier to close their eyes, if this has not already happened. Closed eyes help patients stay absorbed in their mental experiences. Patients who do not wish to close their eyes may focus on an object or fixed place in the room. Most inductions then have the patient focus on deep, rhythmic breathing. Such breathing slows autonomic arousal, focuses the patient and clinician, and begins to reduce tension.

An important component of the induction is "pacing." The clinician needs to closely attend to the patient's responses. Initially, the clinician begins by making a suggestion (e.g., "Just become aware of your breathing . . . you might enjoy taking a deep breath and just noticing how it is to breath deeply and then let it out slowly."). We know that all people breathe, so the clinician is suggesting something the patient is already doing, known as pacing with the patient. Next, the clinician suggests that the patient take a deep breath or another action and observes whether or not the patient is following with him or her. The goal, particularly with indirect methods, is to stay with the patient and give suggestions with which the patient cannot disagree or that are close to what the patient is already doing so that the patient does not think, "Oh no, that's not what I feel." Any sharp discordance during the induction between what the clinician says and what the patient experiences will leave a patient less deeply focused. For this reason, indirect permissive methods that provide options but do not dictate experience are useful.

In our first session with patients who have no experience with any type of relaxing or imagery and who may exhibit some reluctance, we often teach progressive muscle relaxation as part of the induction (Bernstein & Borkovec, 1973). We explain to the patient that a natural response during pain or stress is to tense the muscles around the pain or stress. During the relaxation, warm images that are relaxing, such as sun, bath, or shower, may be added to the relaxation. In the next session we deepen the relaxation and focus, often with counting and an image that moves the patient toward his or her favorite place. The patient is then ready for imagery and analgesic suggestions.

For the imagery phase, we often use patients' favorite places. If we are relatively sure that a patient is comfortable with the procedure, we may leave the location open to the patient's choice at the time. If we wish to make sure patients are still with us, we suggest they lift a finger to signal when they are in this favorite place. Patients with moderate to severe continuous pain tell us that the escape to a comfortable, safe place, as time out from the pain, is as important as direct analgesic suggestions. We find that patients immensely enjoy this time out and this pleasure makes them more ready to use the method again. However, when we use only analgesic suggestions, the mental concentration required, without the pleasure, can leave some patients reluctant to use the methods when they feel pain but are also fatigued.

During this process we make suggestions to facilitate deepening the experience. Suggestions include the patients' being aware of all the details around them—these might be shapes, color and light, hearing sounds, feeling the air and sun against the face, smelling the air, and touching things nearby. We have patients walk in this place to feel their own body as healthy, whole, and knowing how to move and take care of itself even without conscious thought. To take the mind away from moderate to severe pain, we suggest physical activity within the imagery. We may bring someone else into the imagery by asking if patients can see someone else, someone coming toward them. We may expressly suggest a loved one or a wise inner guide. We suggest they listen to see if that person has something to say to them that can be helpful, something that can give them what they most need to hear right now.

This entire process can be done out loud as a conversation between the patient and clinician, with the clinician asking questions and the patient filling in the details. This keeps the clinician aware of and able to immediately respond to the patient's experience, while the patient is required to stay deeply involved in the imagery to be able to respond to the questions. We are most likely to use this oral method with patients who have difficulty creating their own images or concentrating on images, without tangential thoughts disrupting their focus. But this method can be effective for anyone.

Analgesic Suggestions

Once patients have enjoyed being in their special place, we bring in analgesic suggestions developed during the assessment of pain qualities. An effective option can be ice placed on the painful area. As it melts, the cold absorbs into the sensations until that area is numb or just tingles. Ice works well for several reasons. It is familiar to most people and ice can be brought into any imagery. In the mountains, snow can be used; at the beach or in a warm cozy house, an ice cold, refreshing drink can be used, with the ice taken out of the drink and placed where it would help the most. Many other analgesic options are available, as described in Table 9.3. Selecting several of these options and becoming comfortable with using them is more useful than knowing them all. No data indicate that any certain imagery is more valuable than another.

Posthypnotic Suggestion

Once comfort has been achieved, posthypnotic suggestions are built into the imagery. As we complete the imagery, we suggest that patients capture an image, thought, or feeling that, with a deep breath, can bring them back immediately to this feeling of comfort and ease. Thus whenever they need it, they can bring in the analgesic image and increase their comfort even more.

Finally, we count patients back to being alert and refreshed. Usually this counting is simple. As we count from 5 to 1, the patient becomes more alert and aware of the present with each number, then moves his or her hands, arms, and legs to increase blood flow and orientation.

TABLE 9.3. Hypnotic Suggestions for Pain Control

Most frequently used:

1. *Escape or distraction* by going to a favorite place:
   a. Include action for added intensity or involvement.
   b. Metaphors for dissociation may include flying above or away from the physical sensations, moving down a path or stairs and leaving behind more discomfort with each step.
   Advantages
      Most enjoyable.
      Takes the least effort from an energy-depleted patient.
   Disadvantage
      May provide shorter duration of pain relief.

2. *Blocking pain* through suggestions of anesthesia or analgesia:
   a. Often uses numbness via cold or anesthetic.
   b. Can use flipping switches in the brain or spinal cord to disconnect pain messages or switching channels.
   Advantages
      Includes a cognitive component the patient can use outside of hypnosis.
      Has potential to extend pain relief past the duration of hypnosis.
   Disadvantages
      Takes more active participation and concentration ability from the patient.
      May require more hypnotizability to be effective.

3. *Sensory tansformations*
   a. Go to the pain location and explore it; "open to the pain" rather than push it away; watch as the pain changes; usually it diminishes greatly.
   b. Take the pain description and introduce an image that can change as pain changes:
      Find the color of pain and change the color.
      Change the intensity of pain (e.g., reduce "8" to "3").
      Blow cold, arctic air through a hot, burning pain.
      Take a knotted, cramping pain and gather the knot into the fist and throw it away or unknot the pain, soften, and smooth it.
   Advantages
      Takes less energy and goes with the patient's focus of attention instead of fighting it.
      Can be done quickly without lengthy induction, especially for patients with acute onset, severe pain.
      Can be very effective.
   Disadvantages
      Does not seem to "get rid of the pain."
      Pain may initially seem worse, scaring the patient.

Less often used:

4. Move pain to a smaller or less vulnerable area (e.g., hand).

5. See yourself on a screen in front of you, next see another screen some distance away, see the pain projected on it, separate from you, able to see it with a new perspective, then describe it and how it changes; notice how it stays removed from yourself.

6. Substitute another feeling for the pain (e.g., itch or pressure).

7. Alter the meaning of the pain to make it less fearful or debilitating (e.g., itch, pressure, or burning are signs of treatment working, sensations are indications of healing).

8. Increase tolerance of pain or decrease perceived intensity of pain (e.g., use metaphor of dessert: "With each bite you are less aware of the taste, by the 68th taste it isn't bad, you just don't care about the flavor anymore, it's just there, but you don't notice").

9. Dissociate the body from the patient's awareness or move the mind out and away from the body.

10. Distort time so it seems to go by very quickly.

11. Suggest amnesia to forget pain and reduce fear of painful recurrences.

Skills-Training Model

When a patient has a relatively inflexible cognitive, vigilant style, or when pain is long term and patients need to develop methods for using imagery or hypnosis on their own, we use a skills-training model. Patients receive explanations about why the methods work and the steps of the procedure. They receive an individualized induction with the clinician. They are then given the printed material as seen in Appendix 9.3, provided with an audiotape of the session, and asked to practice at home with the suggestion that with practice the skills often become easier and more natural. A second session is provided within the next week. Problems are considered and addressed and a second induction is offered and audiotaped. The second session usually has less relaxation, with more imagery and suggestion. Again patients are encouraged to practice on their own both in quiet and, more briefly, during activities when discomfort may occur. From this point on, sessions are highly individual, tailoring the number of sessions and content of suggestions to the needs of the patient and the circumstances.

Mastery is an important component of any imagery. We always include reminders that these are patients' own experiences; they are the ones who have done it and now that they see how easily it can be done, they will be able to do it again.

In essence, most of our work is "self-hypnosis." We teach the patient so that he or she can use the intervention without the direct guidance of the clinician. This helps patients gain back some control when so often, in the medically ill patient, much control has been taken away. Patients are empowered by realizing their own internal resources, which they may not have known they had.

How to Adapt to Specific Needs and Problems

Throughout this chapter we have talked about the need to individualize intervention to adapt to specific needs and characteristics of the patient. Certain circumstances are common enough that some planning for how to manage them is possible (see Table 9.4 for details). We have discussed the im-

portance of assessing pain, coping style, control needs, fatigue, and distress, and adapting methods to these features of the patient. Age is another component that should be considered.

Children

The controlled clinical trial data on use of hypnosis or imagery with children confirms that these are successful strategies for assisting with pain control (Ellis & Spanos, 1994; Liossi & Hatira, 1999; Smith, Barabasz, & Barabasz, 1996). However, most of this efficacy has been demonstrated with acute, procedural pain rather than chronic pain (Katz, Kellerman, & Ellenberg, 1987; Kuttner, 1988). Nonetheless, these methods can be readily adapted to chronic pain problems and to self-hypnosis training (Kohen & Olness, 1993). Children often have an easier time responding to hypnosis than adults, most likely because of their ready access to imagination and fantasy (Barber & Calverley, 1963; Olness & Gardner, 1988). Children lack distinct boundaries between fantasy and reality and consequently can go into hypnosis without formal induction (Kohen & Olness, 1993). Strategies include telling of a favorite story or acting out through play, then incorporating hypnotic and posthypnotic suggestions for mastery, comfort, and analgesia, always using a language and image level appropriate for the child (Kuttner, 1988). Any child with the ability to attend to and enjoy books or stories is able to respond to imagery. If a child cannot think of a story the clinician can make one up, or can adapt a child's favorite TV show. Furthermore, children can help tell the story and can learn to use analgesic suggestions such as glove analgesia or pain switches, such as light switches, that they can flip. Children may initially disconcert the clinician because they tend to keep their eyes open and talk readily and yet can be fully involved in the process. Hilgard and LeBaron (1984) and Olness and Gardner (1988) discuss the use of hypnosis for pain control in children in detail.

Elderly

We know of no research on hypnosis or imagery specifically with the elderly. Clinical

TABLE 9.4. Adapting to Different Needs and Styles

Coping style

Avoidant	• "Don't want to think about it." • Start with escape images.
Biologically minded	• "Just give me drugs." • May help to start with progressive muscle relaxation to enhance awareness of physical change.
Support seeking	• May need talk first.
Intense control need	• Have most difficulty. • Need to give choice to them for what will work. • Use very permissive, indirect approaches.
Action focused	• Do well. • Extremely action-oriented, may respond well to progressive muscle relaxation as a first step so they "feel like they're doing something."

Age

Elderly	• May use fewer coping strategies. • May be less accustomed to using imagination. • May be more open to turning over control to medical providers, therefore may respond well to "hypnosis."
Children	• Use imagination easily. • Need action not passive images. • Need less formal inductions. • Storytelling may be ideal. • May not close eyes, but still be very responsive.

Fatigued or in severe pain

First:	• Use medications for better pain control. • Consider medication options for fatigue/depression.
Then:	• Use brief images; little induction is needed. • *As appropriate,* use touch on the hand, foot, or shoulder to help the patient focus; to anchor the patient away from the location of the pain; and to provide a competing sensation to the pain. • Begin simply; do only what is possible (e.g., breathing with an image of pain description changing; see Table 9.3, "Sensory transformations").

Highly distressed	• Have difficulty concentrating. • May become more anxious. • Need to talk out feelings first. • If feeling out of control, need signs that you are in control and believe the situation is manageable. • They can relax because you are in control and will make sure they are OK.

experience and coping literature suggest that these patients may be less flexible in coping and are more willing to see the doctor as powerful. They may not have actively used imagination in some time. In our experience, the elderly seem to respond well to more directive imagery that does not depend on them to create images. This strategy also uses the perceived power of the clinician to create change. However, this is a broad generalization that clearly does not apply to all elderly and needs to be evaluated individually.

Problems

Unanticipated responses can leave the clinician fearful of using hypnosis or imagery again. However, many problems can be solved if the practitioner is ready to adapt to them. Table 9.5 lists difficulties we have faced more than once, as well as some solutions that have worked well. Some of these issues were discussed earlier. Others are complex and need individual evaluation.

We have never seen an instance of a patient crying or becoming agitated that did not readily resolve with discussion. It is usually possible to check in with these patients during the imagery to see whether they can share their experience and whether they would like to stop or continue. Sometimes patients indicate that crying is simply a release and does not bother them; in this case we continue with the process and then review the event after completing imagery. Even if patients elect to stop imagery, they benefit from sorting out the thoughts or images related to the emotion. A decision can then be made about whether to do the imagery again. It is most important for the clinician to calmly let the patient know that this is normal and has happened to many people and the clinician is prepared to deal with it.

What if a patient falls asleep while in trance? Many people with chronic pain have sleep disturbances. Hypnosis can provide the relaxation needed so that they can have restful sleep. Patients in the hospital or using the methods at home can be instructed to simply continue with a deep restoring sleep. They awaken in the same way they awaken from a nap or a regular night's sleep. For patients who fall asleep in the office or who complain that they always fall asleep when trying to

TABLE 9.5. Problems and Solutions Encountered in Clinical Practice

Problem	Solutions
Lack of concentration	Use brief images. If preoccupied, talk about preoccupations. Perhaps try at a later time.
Unsupportive family	Talk to the family. Involve the family in helping the patient. Help the patient solve the problem.
Not practicing	Review what gets in the way. Problem solve. Try to remove guilt or "homework" associations so patient can claim the activity, not see it as externally imposed.
Skeptical patient	Encourage an experimenting attitude—"see what happens."
Religious patient	Discuss but be prepared to defer to patient beliefs. Assure that patient is always in control, can stop any time. Offer an option to observe first. Explore whether faith and help of God can be incorporated as a focus of imagery.
Crying, increased anxiety, or other negative effects	Ask if patient is OK and wants to stop or continue. Talk about it; start again if patient is comfortable. Open eyes if feel safer.
Falling asleep	For patients in severe pain with sleep deprivation, encourage to continue with a deep, restful sleep. Raise the tone of voice and incorporate suggestions for more active imagery. If patients complain of falling asleep during home practice, suggest practice sitting up and at a time of day when more alert.
Unresponsive patients	Explore whether the patient has control fears. Discuss what was experienced. Decide if worth trying again or if change in method is indicated. Reassure the patient that it often takes practice and gets easier with practice, or that you may need to try several approaches to find the one that works best for him or her.

practice at home, and therefore are not benefiting from the analgesic suggestions, several approaches are possible. In the office, it can help to raise the tone of one's voice and continue with imagery that is less focused on relaxation and requires more attention or mental action from the patient. For at-home practice, we usually instruct patients to sit up rather than lie down and to select a time of day when they are not too tired. As they are learning to use these methods, we want them to be able to focus without falling asleep.

Clinician Issues

Clinicians should use this psychological technique after they have some training and understand the basics of how and why it works and how to respond to some of the common issues discussed earlier. At the same time, continued practice is the only way to become skilled with these methods. Supervision or consultation should be used when learning clinical applications of these techniques.

Clinicians have expressed some of the following fears and concerns:

• What if the patient does not come out of a trance? This is extremely rare, but it is the clinician's responsibility to ensure that each patient is alert and fully out of hypnosis prior to allowing the patient to leave the office. For highly hypnotizable patients, it is helpful to directly state to the patient, "You are no longer hypnotized, you are completely alert and out of hypnosis."

• What if the patient has an extreme reaction? Rarely, traumatic material will surface without a lot of warning. This needs to be discussed and worked through, at least to the point of the patient feeling in control of his or her emotions, before the patient leaves. Working through intense emotional material is an important process that can be done through hypnosis, but it is beyond the scope of this chapter to elaborate on that process.

• What if I can't get the patient hypnotized (i.e., what if nothing happens?). These fears lessen as one sets realistic goals and does not promise the patient instant and total relief but, rather, an experiment to see what is useful to that specific person.

• How do I know if the patient was hypnotized? This is an easy fear to erase if one simply does not care or worry about the state and rather stays focused on the goal of pain relief.

Appendix 9.1. Brief Induction

Brief induction is for patients who are (1) responsive to hypnosis; (2) motivated with moderate to severe symptoms; (3) experienced and wish to have more rapid induction to the hypnotic state. Numerous methods are available which share similarities of focusing on the eyes, breathing, brief counting and letting the hand float or become heavy. The entire session can take a few minutes. This method can be taught to patients as an induction to self-hypnosis or can be used by the clinician prior to introducing suggestions for comfort and analgesia.

Induction: "We will count from 1 to 3. One: look up with your eyes as far as you can without moving your head. Up, up, that's right. Two: slowly close your eyelids, keep your eyes up, while you take a deep breath. Good. Three: as you let the breath out, let your eyes relax and let your body feel twice as relaxed. Fine. Now I will raise your hand. [Hold the hand about a foot off the lap.] Let your hand feel very heavy, as if bricks are attached to it. That's right, very heavy. [Wait until the arm and hand loosen and relax, give more suggestion if needed: "Very heavy, as if it's just too much trouble to hold it up, as if a huge weight is on it."] Now, as your arm drops to your lap you can feel twice as relaxed as before; deeply comfortable and relaxed. So relaxed you find it easy to accomplish what your mind wants to do today."

Next, add imagery or suggestions to accomplish goals.

Appendix 9.2. Comfort and Analgesia Script

When you are ready to begin, adjust your body so that you can feel as comfortable as possible, as you get ready to become even more relaxed and at ease. At any time you wish, make any adjustments or changes to help you feel even more comfortable. All that's important is for you to become as relaxed as you are ready to feel, letting go of any unnecessary tension as we go along, remembering that there is nowhere else you need to be right now, nothing you need to be doing, that this is your time to be here right now. To experience whatever you experience and perhaps to enjoy that experience in whatever way you feel it right now. You may find that at times your mind may wander. If it does that's fine, just gently bring back your attention to the sound of my voice, knowing that right now there's nothing to bother you and nothing to disturb you, that all you need to do is to listen to the sound of my voice and allow yourself to become as comfortable as you would like to feel right now.

Begin then to focus on your breathing. Really pay attention to what it feels like to breathe in and out, breathing in easily and deeply, holding the breath for a moment and then exhaling fully. And perhaps imagining that as you breathe in, you breathe in comfort and calmness and as you breathe out, you breathe out discomfort and tension. And you might imagine that with each breath your body becomes twice as relaxed, just breathing in and out, twice as relaxed. And at times you may hear some sounds from outside, and that's all right. You may notice that they don't really make any difference, they are just passing by, becoming part of your whole experience as you continue to focus inward, on your breathing and on the growing sense of comfort and calmness, just breathing in comfort and calmness, breathing out tension and discomfort, allowing yourself to be soothed by the steady rhythm of your breathing, in and out, with nothing to bother you and nothing to disturb you.

And as you enjoy this increasing sense of comfort, you may want to imagine a pleasant warmth beginning to spread through your body. Perhaps it's the warmth of a bath, or the sun or another warmth you enjoy. Soaking that warmth into your muscles as you soften all the parts of your body one after another. First the warmth over the top of your head, softening the muscles of your scalp, moving down through your forehead into all the small muscles of your eyes. Feeling all those small muscles as they soften and relax in the warmth. Allowing that feeling to absorb and relax the muscles of the cheeks and jaw and even the tongue. Feeling that flow of warmth moving down through your neck and into your shoulders smoothing the muscles and increasing your sense of comfort . . . the warmth continuing down into the right arm into the palm and through each finger. Then the left arm into the palm of the hand and fingers, feeling as the tension just flows away, as the warmth takes its place. And now the warmth spreading into your upper body, through your chest and abdomen

and down through your back, soothing and comforting all the muscles there.

That warmth flowing freely and easily down through the top of your legs, through your lower legs and into the feet and toes. Enjoying that warmth as it fills your whole body now, soothing and calming. Letting all the tension flow away, leaving only a feeling of comfort. Take a moment now to notice if there is any part of your body that you want to be more comfortable . . . and if there is, go to that area and focus your breathing on it, imagining breathing through that place, the breath moving through each cell, gently blowing away tightness and discomfort, just watching as the sensations change, finding all the nooks and crannies of concern or tension and watching as the peacefulness takes their place.

As you continue to enjoy this pleasant sense of ease, begin counting to yourself from 100 to 99, 98, 97, seeing each number move past you like on a movie screen, and with each number feeling twice as relaxed, 96, 95, continuing to see the numbers and count (pause) or perhaps the numbers hardly matter any more, finding yourself comfortable and as deeply relaxed as you'd like to feel right now, with an increased sense of peace and well-being that you feel when your body and mind are in tune and at ease, when you feel in charge of your own well-being.

And as you enjoy this feeling of deep comfort and well-being allow yourself to begin to create a special place of your choosing. A place where you feel safe and secure and content. It may be a place you've been before, it may be a place you'd like to go now, or a place only in your imagination. All that matters is that you find a place for you right now. And begin to notice that place. Notice if it is indoors or out. Observe what is all around you now. Take it in. Notice the colors, the different tones of the same color. Perhaps there are reds, or yellows, I'm certain somewhere there may be greens, and notice how many different greens are still green. The light and the dark shades, the light around you as it moves and changes.

Explore the shapes in your surroundings . . . perhaps you can reach out and touch things, notice what they feel like . . . are they soft or hard, rough or smooth, warm or cool. Enjoying each new thing you see or feel, enjoying being in this pleasant safe place experiencing it fully. And I wonder if you might be surprised by any of the smells in the air . . . perhaps the smells of life or energy or freshness, just taking a moment to smell the air and feel the air against your skin . . . notice if it is cool or warm or perhaps a bit of both . . . warmth from the sun or something else cool from the fresh air, it doesn't really matter what it is, whatever is there is just fine. And you can allow yourself to enjoy this fresh air as it refreshes your face and body. Taking in a deep cleansing breath, feeling the comforting coolness. And notice whether you can find something icy cold nearby. You may need to move around or look about you. It may be a refreshing drink with ice that you can take with you as you find a comfortable place to relax, or perhaps a glacial cold stream, even the cold of snow or a different cold however it is where you are.

But wherever it is, however it is for you, just explore that feeling of cold on your hand. As you touch it, keep it touching your hand, notice how the sensations change. First cold, then perhaps tingly or maybe numb, no feeling at all. You might even be curious to put that icy cold on a part of your body where you sometimes feel discomfort and notice how the feelings change, gradually the coldness seeps in . . . a tingling feeling perhaps . . . and then the feelings become less intense, perhaps even numb or no feeling at all, further away until it seems hard to remember. However it is for you, just less noticeable or less bothersome, just cool sensations around the edges perhaps, a soothing cool.

And you can hold this coolness there for as long as you like. And know that whenever you would like to come back to this comfort or numbness, you need only to close your eyes, take a deep breath, see this place in your mind, and bring back the feeling of fresh air in your face. Then you can bring this icy cool to any place on your body as you allow the sensations to change and you become more and more comfortable. And you might even be surprised at how easy this becomes for you, to just let the cold seep in and other feelings melt away.

And you can continue now to carry these feelings of comfort and ease with you as you move through the next hours or even the next days. Knowing that they are of your own creation; that these abilities to find greater comfort are within yourself. Realizing perhaps your own abilities to create or to change your experience. You might even notice that you are sometimes surprised with your own abilities, how much you can do with just a thought and focus and how easy it can be to be comfortable. And I wonder how long this comfort will last for you. Is it an hour, a day, a week perhaps? However long, becoming longer each time and easier each time to find this place and this feeling.

And then begin once again, to focus on your breathing, bringing with you these feelings of increased peacefulness and comfort. And in a moment I will begin to count from 5 to 1. And as I do, you can gradually come back to being aware of your surroundings, preparing to feel more alert and refreshed. Still relaxed, but energized and ready to continue with what you choose to do with this day. So when you open your eyes, you can feel refreshed and comfortable . . . fully alert. And now, 5, 4, beginning to be more aware of the sounds of the world around you, 3, taking in a deep refreshing breath, 2, moving your muscles to feel the blood flow, stretching your fingers, arms, legs, feeling aware of your body again, and 1, opening your eyes when you are fully ready...alert, refreshed, energized. Make sure that you are fully alert and awake now as you continue with the rest of your day.

Appendix 9.3. Instructions for Learning Relaxation with Imagery

These printed instructions may be given to patients along with audiotapes for home practice.

You can relax and take your mind to an enjoyable, comfortable place. This is an extremely powerful way of reducing pain, tension, anger, fear, and frustration. Emotions often accompany physical discomforts and make them worse.

Deep relaxation is a skill that needs *practice*. With practice now, you will be able to relax when and where you want to. You might even be surprised at how well you can use relaxation to increase feelings of well-being and comfort at any time.

A Three-Step Method of Relaxation

A three-step method of deep relaxation is described below. Patients tell us that the individual steps can each be helpful at different times, so you will want to practice each one. When you wish to really take a break and feel better, you can put all three steps together.

STEP 1—DEEP BREATHING

Deep breathing quickly sends a signal to your entire body to relax. Whenever you notice some tension in your body, or your emotions are in turmoil, you can use these steps:

1. Make your *position* (sitting, lying, or standing) as comfortable as you can.

2. Deeply *inhale* through your nose while counting slowly to 4.

3. As you inhale pull the oxygen into your abdomen, then through your entire chest and upward to your shoulders. Notice your chest moving up and your shoulders moving back as you breathe in deeply.

4. *Hold your breath* for a few moments.

5. *Exhale* through your mouth, making a relaxing whooshing sound like the wind as you blow out to a slow count of 4.

6. As you exhale let your breath go from the bottom of your abdomen up through your chest and all the way up to your shoulders. Notice your chest moving down and your shoulders moving forward as you breathe out all the air.

7. Imagine all the tension from your body being pulled into your lungs and being exhaled with your breath.

8. Continue deep breathing for several minutes.

9. Scan your body for any area which may remain tense. Focus on this area and imagine breathing directly in and out of this area.

10. When you have learned to relax yourself using deep breathing, practice it whenever and wherever you feel yourself getting tense.

STEP 2—MUSCLE RELAXATION

By relaxing your muscles one group at a time, you can relax your whole body. This is usually easier than trying to relax your whole body all at once. When you relax your muscles, start at the top of your head and move your attention to each muscle group. For example, you might relax in the following order:

Forehead, eyes, cheeks, and tongue
Neck
Shoulders
Right arm and hand
Left arm and hand
Chest
Abdomen
Right leg and foot
Left leg and foot

There are two common ways to relax these muscles:

1. Tense the muscle (not so much that it hurts, but enough to feel the tension). Let the tension go and feel the relaxation move in.

2. Bring your attention to the muscle and relax it while imagining tension draining away. Imagine the muscle as heavy and warm or use another image that substitutes relaxation for tension.

STEP 3—IMAGERY

Imagery is simply picturing something in your mind using shapes, colors, sounds, thoughts—anything that helps you to feel like you are there. In a relaxed state, your mind is most open to imagery. Imagery can also be a fun way to relax. You can use it just to take your mind away from its worries for a while and even to feel more in charge of what is happening to your body. Imagery can last just long enough to get a clear, positive picture in your mind, or it can last for 30 minutes of deep relaxation. There are lots of ways to do imagery. There is no right or wrong way.

A few tips from people who have used imagery successfully are:

1. Don't put any pressure on yourself to come up with images. Instead, just let your mind wander across memories of places you've enjoyed or places that seem like they would be enjoyable, safe, and relaxing.

2. Allow yourself to experiment with all your senses of sight, smell, taste, touch, and sound. Allow the imagery to be as real and involving as you can. See the shapes, colors, light. Feel the air. Touch objects and notice if they are smooth, hard, soft, fuzzy, warm. Notice if there are any tastes or scents. Is anything moving? Are other people there or do you prefer to be alone? Listen to the sounds. Change any parts you would like to be different.

3. Allow yourself to develop images to use at different times. You might see yourself going through something difficult, doing well and feeling calm. You might see yourself finished with something difficult, feeling strong, looking back on how well you did.

4. It's normal for your mind to wander. Sometimes it is just a sign that you are relaxing. Gently bring your mind back to the imagery. Do whatever works for you and don't be afraid to try a new idea if you find something isn't working.

5. When you are ready to stop, give yourself time to become alert, take a deep breath and stretch your muscles.

A Few Thoughts about Relaxing and Using Imagery

With practice you will be able to relax quickly even in difficult situations. Practice at least once a day with a tape or on your own. Find a comfortable, quiet place and go through your relaxation with imagery.

The steps for doing relaxation and imagery on your own are:

1. Deep breathe to start relaxing and to focus your attention.
2. Allow your muscles to relax from the top of your head to the bottom of your feet.
3. Take your mind to a favorite place using all your senses. Feel your body as comfortable, strong and healthy in that place.
4. Take a few deep breaths and stretch to bring your attention back to the present.

This is a special time for you, a time out from all of your usual responsibilities and concerns. Give yourself that 20 minutes each day.

From Syrjala, Danis, Abrams, and Keenan (1992). Copyright 1992 by Fred Hutchinson Cancer Research Center, Seattle, WA. Reprinted by permission.

Acknowledgments

This work was supported by the following grants from the National Cancer Institute: CA 68139, CA 78990, and CA63030.

References

Alman, B. M., & Carney, R. . E. (1980). Consequences of direct and indirect suggestions on success of posthypnotic behavior. *American Journal of Clinical Hypnosis, 23*, 112–118.

Barber, J. (1980). Hypnosis and the unhypnotizable. *American Journal of Clinical Hypnosis, 23*, 4–9.

Barber, T. X. (1969). *Hypnosis: A scientific approach*. New York: Van Nostrand Reinhold.

Barber, T. X., & Calverley, D. S. (1963). "Hypnotic-like" suggestibility in children. *Journal of Abnormal and Social Psychology, 66*, 589–597.

Bernstein, D. A., & Borkovec, T. D. (1973). *Progressive relaxation training: A manual for the helping professions*. Champaign, IL: Research Press.

Chapman, C. R., & Syrjala, K. L. (2001). Measurement of pain. In J. D. Loeser, S. D. Butler, C. R. Chapman, & D. C. Turk (Eds.), *Bonica's management of pain* (3rd ed., pp. 310–328). Baltimore: Williams & Wilkins.

Crasilneck, H. B. (1979). Hypnosis in control of chronic low back pain. *American Journal of Clinical Hypnosis, 22*, 71–78.

Danziger, N., Fournier, E., Bouhassira, D., Michaud, D., De Broucker, T., Santarcangelo, E., Carli, G., Chertock, L., & Willer, J. C. (1998). Different strategies of modulation can be operative during hypnotic analgesia: A neurophysiological study. *Pain, 75*, 85–92.

Diamond, M. (1984). It takes two to tango: The neglected importance of the hypnotic relationship. *American Journal of Clinical Hypnosis, 26*, 1–13.

Ellis, J. A., & Spanos, N. P. (1994). Cognitive-behavioral interventions for children's distress during bone marrow aspirations and lumbar puncture: A critical review. *Journal of Pain and Symptom Management, 9*, 96–108.

Erickson, M. H. (1959). Hypnosis in painful terminal illness. *American Journal of Clinical Hypnosis, 1*, 117–122.

Fernandez, E., & Turk, D. C. (1989). The utility of cognitive coping strategies for altering pain perception: A meta-analysis. *Pain, 38*, 123–135.

Fricton, J. R., & Roth, P. (1985). The effects of direct and indirect hypnotic suggestions for analgesia in high and low susceptible subjects. *American Journal of Clinical Hypnosis, 27*, 226–231

Frischholz, E. J., Spiegel, D., Spiegel, H., Balma, D. L., & Markell, C. S. (1981). Differential hypnotic responsivity of smokers, phobics, and chronic pain. *Journal of Abnormal Psychology, 91*, 269–272.

Hendler, C. S., & Redd, W. H. (1986). Fear of hypnosis: The role of labeling in patients' acceptance of behavioral interventions. *Behavior Therapy, 17*, 2–13.

Hilgard, E. R., & Hilgard, J. R. (1965). *Hypnotic susceptibility*. New York: Harcourt, Brace & World.

Hilgard, E. R., & Hilgard, J. R. (1983). *Hypnosis in the relief of pain* (Rev. ed.). Los Altos, CA: William Kaufman.

Hilgard, J., & LeBaron, S. (1984). *Hypnotherapy of pain in children with cancer*. Los Altos, CA: Kaufmann.

Holroyd, J. (1996). Hypnosis treatment of clinical pain: Understanding why hypnosis is useful. *The International Journal of Clinical and Experimental Hypnosis, 44*, 33–51.

Kabat-Zinn, J., Lipworth, L., & Burney, R. (1985). The clinical use of mindfulness meditation for the self-regulation of chronic pain. *Journal of Behavioral Medicine, 8*, 163–190.

Katz, E. R., Kellerman J., & Ellenberg, L. (1987). Hypnosis in the reduction of acute pain and distress in children with cancer. *Journal of Pediatric Psychology, 12*, 379–394.

Kiernan, B. D., Dane, J. R., Phillips, L. H., & Price, D. D. (1995). Hypnotic analgesia reduces R-III nociceptive reflex: Further evidence concerning the multifactorial nature of hypnotic analgesia. *Pain, 60,* 39–47.

Kohen, D. P., & Olness, K. (1993). Hypnotherapy with children. In J. W. Rhue, S. J. Lynn, & I. Kirsch (Eds.), *Handbook of clinical hypnosis* (pp. 357–381). Washington, DC: American Psychological Association.

Kuttner, L. (1988). Favorite stories: A hypnotic pain-reduction technique for children in acute pain. *American Journal of Clinical Hypnosis, 30,* 289–295.

Lang, E. V., Benotsch, E. G., Fick, L. J., Lutgendorf, S., Berbaum, M. L., Berbaum, K. S., Logan, H., & Spiegel, D. (2000). Adjunctive non-pharmacological analgesia for invasive medical procedures: A randomised trial. *Lancet, 355,* 1486–1490.

Liossi, C., & Hatira, P. (1999). Clinical hypnosis versus cognitive behavioral training for pain management with pediatric cancer patients undergoing bone marrow aspirations. *International Journal of Clinical and Experimental Hypnosis, 47,* 104–116.

Lynn, S. J., Neufeld, V., & Matyi, C. L. (1987). Inductions versus suggestions: Effects of direct and indirect wording on hypnotic responding and experience. *Journal of Abnormal Psychology, 96,* 76–79.

McCaul, K. D., & Malott, J. M. (1984). Distraction and coping with pain. *Psychological Bulletin, 95,* 516–533.

McGlashan, T. H., Evans, F. J., & Orne, M. T. (1969). The nature of hypnotic analgesia and the placebo response to experimental pain. *Psychosomatic Medicine, 31,* 227–246.

Melzack, R., & Wall, P. D. (1965). Pain mechanisms: A new theory. *Science, 50,* 971–979.

Montgomery, G. H., DuHamel, K. N., & Redd, W. H. (2000). A meta-analysis of hypnotically induced analgesia: How effective is hypnosis? *International Journal of Clinical and Experimental Hypnosis, 48,* 138–153.

Olness, K., & Gardner, G. G. (1988). *Hypnosis and hypnotherapy with children* (2nd ed.). New York: Grune & Stratton.

Olness, K., MacDonald, J., & Uden, D. (1987). Prospective study comparing propanolol, placebo, and hypnosis in the management of juvenile migraine. *Pediatrics, 79,* 593–597.

Patterson, D. R., Everett, J. J., Burns, G. L., & Marvin, J. A. (1992). Hypnosis for the treatment of burn pain. *Journal of Consulting and Clinical Psychology, 60,* 713–717.

Price, D. D., & Barber, J. (1987). An analysis of factors that contribute to the efficacy of hypnotic analgesia. *Journal of Abnormal Psychology, 96,* 46–51.

Rainville, P., Hofbauer, R. K., Paus, T., Duncan, G. H., Bushnell, M. C., & Price, D. D. (1999). Cerebral mechanisms of hypnotic induction and suggestion. *Journal of Cognitive Neuroscience, 11,* 110–125.

Sacerdote, P. (1965). Additional contributions to the hypnotherapy of the advanced cancer patient. *American Journal of Clinical Hypnosis, 7,* 308–319.

Sacerdote, P. (1970). Theory and practice of pain control in malignancy and other protracted or recurring painful illnesses. *International Journal of Clinical and Experimental Hypnosis, 18,* 160–180.

Schafer, D. W. (1976). Patients reactions to hypnosis on a burn unit. In F. H. Frankel & H. S. Zamansky (Eds.), *Hypnosis at its bicentennial: Selected papers* (pp. 229–235). New York: Plenum Press.

Shor, R. E., & Orne, E. C. (1962). *The Harvard Group Scale of Hypnotic Susceptibility, Form A.* Palo Alto, CA: Consulting Psychologists Press.

Smith, J. T., Barabasz, A., & Barabasz, M. (1996). Comparison of hypnosis and distraction in severely ill children undergoing painful medical procedures. *Journal of Counseling Psychology, 43,* 187–195.

Spanos, N. P., Kennedy, S. K., & Gwynn, M. I. (1984). Moderating effects of contextual variables on the relationship between hypnotic susceptibility and suggested analgesia. *Journal of Abnormal Psychology, 93,* 285–294.

Spanos, N. P., Radtke-Bodorik, H. L., Ferguson, J. D., & Jones, B. (1979). The effects of hypnotic susceptibility, suggestions for analgesia, and the utilization of cognitive strategies on the reduction of pain. *Journal of Abnormal Psychology, 88,* 282–292.

Spanos, N. P., Radtke, H. L., Hodgins, D. C., Stam, H. J., & Bertrand, L (1983). The Carleton University Responsiveness to Suggestion Scale: Normative data and psychometric properties. *Psychological Reports, 53,* 523–535.

Spanos, N. P., Robertson, L. A., Menary, E. P., & Brett, P. J. (1986). Component analysis of cognitive skill training for the enhancement of hypnotic susceptibility. *Journal of Abnormal Psychology, 95,* 350–357.

Spiegel, D. (1985). The use of hypnosis in controlling cancer pain. *CA: A Cancer Journal for Clinicians, 35,* 221–231.

Spiegel, D., & Bloom, J. R. (1983). Group therapy and hypnosis reduce metastatic breast carcinoma pain *Psychosomatic Medicine, 45,* 333–339.

Spiegel, H. (1997). Nocebo: The power of suggestibility. *Preventive Medicine, 26,* 616–621.

Spiegel, H., & Spiegel, D. (1978). *Trance and treatment: Clinical uses of hypnosis.* New York: Basic Books.

Sthalekar, H. A. (1993). Hypnosis for relief of chronic phantom pain in a paralysed limb: A case study. *Australian Journal of Clinical Hypnotherapy and Hypnosis, 14,* 75–80.

Suls, J., & Fletcher, B. (1985). The relative efficacy of avoidant and nonavoidant coping strategies: A meta-analysis. *Health Psychology, 4,* 249–288

Syrjala, K. L., Cummings, C., & Donaldson G. (1992). Hypnosis or cognitive behavioral training for the reduction of pain and nausea during cancer treatment: A controlled clinical trial. *Pain, 48,* 137–146.

Syrjala, K. L., Davis, B., Abrams, J. A., & Keenan, R. (1992). *Coping skills for bone marrow transplantation*. Seattle, WA: Fred Hutchinson Cancer Research Center.

Syrjala, K. L., Donaldson, G. W., Davis, M. W., Kippes, M. E., & Carr, J. E. (1995). Relaxation and imagery and cognitive-behavioral training reduce pain during cancer treatment: A controlled clinical trial. *Pain, 63,* 189–198.

Turk, D. C., & Melzack, R. (Eds.). (2001). *Handbook of pain assessment* (2nd ed.). New York: Guilford Press.

Turner, J., Deyo, R. A., Loeser, J. D., Von Korff, M.,

& Fordyce, W. E. (1994). The importance of placebo effects in pain treatment and research. *Journal of the American Medical Association, 271,* 1609–1614.

Turner, J. A., & Jensen, M. P. (1993). Efficacy of cognitive therapy for chronic low back pain. *Pain, 52,* 169–177.

Vandeman, G. E. (1973). *Psychic roulette*. Mountain View, CA: Pacific Press.

Weitzenhoffer, A. M., & Hilgard, E. R. (1959). *Stanford Hypnotic Susceptibility Scale, Forms A and B*. Palo Alto, CA: Consulting Psychologists Press.

10

Graded Exposure In Vivo for Pain-Related Fear

Johan W. S. Vlaeyen
Jeroen de Jong
Judith Sieben
Geert Crombez

Pain is a common and universal experience and leads to the urge to escape the situation from which pain has emerged. Thus pain can best be conceptualized as an emotional experience, as emotions are believed to be drives for action. Not surprisingly, the etymological meaning of the word "emotion" also comes from the Latin *movere,* which means "to act." In acute injury, the escape from the harmful situation and the associated withdrawal behavior promotes the healing process. In the majority of cases, healing occurs within a couple of weeks and the pain resolves quickly. However, for certain people with pain, the immediate withdrawal behaviors do not lead to the anticipated reduction of pain, which then is interpreted as a signal of a continuous threat to the integrity of the body. In fact, a mismatch occurs between what the patient expects (quick decrease of pain) and what actually happens (increasing or lasting pain). Such a negative interpretation may not always reflect the real threat, and in such cases catastrophic misinterpretations of benign physical sensations may occur. Sometimes, these misinterpretations may be fueled by external information, such as unfavorable pain histories of relatives or acquaintances and verbal and

visual information provided by health care providers, suggesting the probability of a serious illness causing the pain complaints. Catastrophic interpretations consequently lead to an increase of the individual distress level and fear reactions in particular.

In pain patients, interpretational errors such as catastrophizing inevitably result in pain-related fear: fear of pain, fear of injury, fear of physical activity, and so forth, depending on the anticipated source of threat. There is now accumulating evidence that these misinterpretations and the associated pain-related fear are likely to cause a cascade of psychological and physical events, including hypervigilance, muscular reactivity, avoidance and guarding behaviors, and physical disuse, which in turn are responsible for the maintenance of the pain problem.

Following this line of thought, and in an attempt to explain how and why some people develop a chronic pain syndrome, biopsychosocial models have been developed. These include the "fear–avoidance model of exaggerated pain perception" (Lethem, Slade, Troup, & Bentley, 1983) and, more recently, a cognitive-behavioral model of fear of movement/(re)injury (Vlaeyen, Kole-Snijders, Boeren, & van Eek,

1995; Vlaeyen, Kole-Snijders, Rotteveel, et al., 1995). The central concept of these models is "fear of pain," or the more specific "fear that physical activity will cause (re)injury." Two opposing behavioral responses to pain are postulated: "confrontation" and "avoidance" (Figure 10.1). In the absence of a serious somatic pathology, confrontation is conceptualized as an adaptive response that eventually may lead to the reduction of fear and the promotion of recovery of pain or function. In contrast, avoidance leads to the maintenance or exacerbation of fear, possibly resulting in a condition comparable to a phobia. The avoidance results in the reduction of both social and physical activities, which in turn leads to a number of physical and psychological consequences augmenting the disability (Philips, 1987). Prospective studies in acute low back pain patients (Klenerman et al., 1995) and healthy people (Linton, Buer, Vlaeyen, & Hellsing, 2000) have provided support for the idea that pain-related fear may be an important precursor of pain disability.

Characteristics of Pain-Related Fear

In 1990, Kori, Miller, and Todd introduced the term "kinesiophobia" (kinesis = move-

ment) for the condition in which a patient has "an excessive, irrational, and debilitating fear of physical movement and activity resulting from a feeling of vulnerability to painful injury or reinjury." Recent evidence revealed that during confrontation with feared movements, chronic low back pain patients who are fearful of movement/(re)injury typically show cognitive (worry), psychophysiological (muscle reactivity), and behavioral (escape and avoidance) responses, rendering support for the idea that chronic pain and chronic fear share important characteristics (Asmundson, Norton, & Norton, 1999; Philips, 1987; Vlaeyen & Linton, 2000). Indeed, when comparing the major features of specific phobia according to the fourth edition of *Diagnostic and Statistical Manual of Mental Disorders* (DSM-IV; American Psychiatric Association, 1994) and pain-related fear in chronic pain patients, there is much similarity between the two conditions (Kori et al., 1990). One point on which they differ is that people with a phobia are aware that the fear is excessive and irrational, whereas most pain patients reporting pain-related fear are convinced of the fact that avoidance has a protective function (Table 10.1).

There is evidence that pain-related fear is associated with specific worries, often referred to as pain catastrophizing. Pain cata-

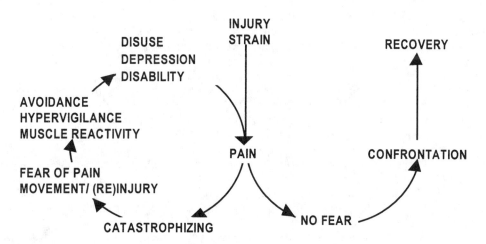

FIGURE 10.1. Cognitive-behavioral model of pain-related fear. From Vlaeyen and Linton (2000). Copyright 2000 by Elsevier. Adapted by permission.

TABLE 10.1. Differences and Similarities between Specific Phobia (According to DSM-IV) and Pain-Related Fear

Specific phobia	Pain-related fear
1. Marked and persistent fear that is excessive or unreasonable cued by the presence or anticipation of a specific object or situation.	1. Marked and persistent fear that is (often) excessive and unreasonable, cued by the presence or anticipation of a *pain-eliciting situation*.
2. Exposure to the phobic stimulus almost invariably provokes an immediate anxiety response, which may take the form of a situational predisposed panic attack.	2. Exposure to the pain-eliciting stimulus almost invariably provokes an immediate anxiety response, including *avoidance/escape behaviors, increased arousal levels, and hypervigilance*.
3. The person recognizes that the fear is excessive or unreasonable.	3. The person often *does not* recognize that the fear is excessive or unreasonable.
4. The phobic situation is avoided or else is endured with intense anxiety or distress.	4. The phobic situation is avoided or else is endured with intense anxiety or distress.
5. The avoidance, anxious anticipation, or distress in the feared situation(s) interferes significantly with the person's normal routine, occupational (or academic) functioning, or social activities or relationships, or there is marked distress about having the phobia.	5. The avoidance, anxious anticipation, or distress in the feared situation(s) interferes significantly with the person's normal routine, occupational (or academic) functioning, or social activities or relationships, or there is marked distress about having the *pain problem*.
6. In individuals under age 18 years, the duration is at least 6 months.	6. *Not considered relevant*
7. The anxiety, panic attacks, or phobic avoidance associated with the specific object or situation are not better accounted for by another mental disorder.	7. The anxiety, panic attacks, or phobic avoidance associated with the specific object or situation are not better accounted for by another mental or *physical* disorder.

strophizing is considered an exaggerated negative orientation toward noxious stimuli and has been shown to mediate distress reactions to painful stimulation (Sullivan, Bishop, & Pivik, 1995). Crombez, Eccleston, Baeyens, and Eelen (1998) found that pain-free volunteers with a high frequency of catastrophic thinking about pain became more fearful when threatened with the possibility of occurrence of intense pain than did students with a low frequency of catastrophic thinking. Chronic pain patients who catastrophize report more pain intensity, feel more disabled by their pain problem, and experience more psychological distress (Severeijns, Vlaeyen, van den Hout, & Weber, 2001). Also, a strong association has been found between pain catastrophizing and pain-related fear, and it has been suggested that pain catastrophizing is likely to be a precursor of pain-related fear (Mc-

Cracken & Gross, 1993; Vlaeyen, Kole-Snijders, Boeren, & van Eek, 1995). In addition, there is evidence that people who catastrophize about pain or are fearful do not respond well to pain-coping strategies training, such as attention diversion and applied relaxation (Heyneman, Fremouw, & Gano, 1990; Vlaeyen et al., 1997).

In line with the cognitive theory of anxiety, a number of studies have also shown that pain-related fear is associated with increased body awareness and attentional focus toward pain and noxious body stimuli. Indirect evidence on association between pain-related fear and body hypervigilance is found using a priming task paradigm in which chronic pain patients are requested to direct their attentional focus toward an attentionally demanding task. Degradation in task performance on the cognitive task can be taken as an index of attentional interference due to hypervigilance. A number of studies have demonstrated that disruption of performance to an attentionally demanding task was most pronounced in chronic pain patients who reported high negative affect, somatic awareness, and high pain intensity (Eccleston, Crombez, Aldrich, & Stannard, 1997) and fear of (re)injury (Crombez, Eccleston, Baeyens, van Houdenhove, & van den Broeck, 1999). Reactivity of lumbar musculature in fearful chronic low back pain patients was studied in an experiment in which the subjects were watching a neutral nature documentary, followed by a fear-eliciting video presentation displaying a person vigorously performing physical activity (Vlaeyen et al., 1999). Although self-reported tension increased from the nature documentary to the activity exposure in the fearful chronic low back pain patients, there was a general decrease in muscular reactivity in both subgroups, probably due to initial contextual fear. This decrement, however, was less in fearful patients who remained at about the same reactivity level.

It has repeatedly been shown that pain-related fear is associated with escape–avoidance behaviors. In a study in which chronic pain sufferers volunteered to undergo cold pressor pain, Cipher and Fernandez (1997) showed that expected danger significantly predicted avoidance of another cold pressor immersion. Chronic pain patients who associate pain with damage tend to avoid activities that produce pain. Other studies that used physical performance tests reported that poor behavioral performance appeared to be more strongly associated with pain-related fear than with pain severity (Crombez, Vlaeyen, Heuts, & Lysens, 1999) and biomedical findings (Vlaeyen, Kole-Snijders, Boeren, & van Eek, 1995). The effects of pain-related fear on behavioral performance also appear to generalize to restrictions in daily life situations. Waddell, Newton, Henderson, Somerville, and Main (1993) demonstrated that fear-avoidance beliefs about work are strongly related to disability of daily living and work lost in the past year, and more so than pain variables such as anatomical pattern of pain, time pattern, and pain severity, and concluded that "fear of pain and what we do

about it may be more disabling than pain itself" (p. 164).

Disconfirmations of Harm Beliefs

What are the clinical implications of aforementioned findings? Philips (1987) was one of the first to argue for the systematic application of graded exposure in order to produce disconfirmations between expectations of pain and harm, the actual pain, and the other consequences of the activity. She suggested further that "these disconfirmations can be made more obvious to the sufferer by helping to clarify the expectations he or she is working with, and by delineating the conditions or stimuli which he feels are likely to fulfill his expectations. Repeated, graded, and controlled exposures to such situations under optimal conditions are likely to produce the largest and most powerful disconfirmations" (Philips, 1987, p. 279). Experimental support for this idea is provided by the match–mismatch model of pain (Rachman, 1994) that states that people initially tend to overpredict how much pain they will experience, but after some exposures these predictions tend to be corrected to match with the actual experience. Crombez, Vervaet, Baeyens, Lysens, and Eelen (1996), in a sample of chronic low back pain patients who were requested to perform four exercise bouts (two with each leg) at maximal force, found a similar pattern. During each exercise bout the baseline pain, the expected pain, and the experienced pain were recorded. As predicted, the chronic low back pain patients initially overpredicted pain, but after repetition of the exercise bout the overprediction was readily corrected. The expectancy did not seem to generalize to the exercise episode with the other leg as a small increase in pain expectancy reemerged. Also here, expectancies were immediately corrected after another performance. Recently, these findings were replicated with two other physical activities: bending forward and straight leg raising (Goubert, Francken, Crombez, Vansteenwegen, & Lysens, 2002). In sum, it is quite plausible that, in analogy with the treatment of phobias, graded exposure to back-stressing movements may indeed be a successful treatment approach for back pain patients reporting substantial fear of movement/(re)injury, although special attention should be drawn to generalization issues.

Graded Exposure In Vivo versus Graded Activity

At first glance, graded exposure *in vivo* may appear quite similar to the usual graded activity programs (Fordyce, Brockway, Bergman, & Spengler, 1986; Lindström et al., 1992) in that it gradually increases activity levels despite pain. However, both conceptually and practically, exposure *in vivo* is quite different from graded activity. *First*, graded activity is based on instrumental learning principles, and selected health behaviors are shaped through positively reinforcing predefined quota of activities. Exposure *in vivo*, originally based on extinction of Pavlovian conditioning (Bouton, 1988), is currently viewed as a cognitive process during which fear is activated and catastrophic expectations are being challenged and disconfirmed, resulting in reductions of the threat value of the originally fearful stimuli. *Second*, during graded activity, special attention goes to the identification of positive reinforcers that can be provided when the individual quotas are met, whereas graded exposure pays special attention to the establishment of an individual hierarchy of the pain-related fear stimuli. *Third*, usual graded activity programs include individual exercises according to functional capacity and observed individual physical work demands graded, whereas graded exposure includes activities that are selected based on the fear hierarchy and the idiosyncratic aspects of the fear stimuli. For example, if the patient fears the repetitive spinal compression produced by riding a bicycle on a bumpy road, then the graded exposure should include an activity that mimics that specific activity and not just a stationary bicycle.

According to the suggestions made by Butler (1989) for the cognitive-behavioral treatment of phobic disorders, and Turner (1996) for the application of behavioral interventions of back pain in primary care, we suggest that the intervention generally be designed in three steps: cognitive-behavioral assessment, education, and exposure *in vivo* with behavioral experiments.

Cognitive-Behavioral Assessment

This section deals with specific questionnaires, the interview, the establishment of graded hierarchies, and behavioral tests that can be applied to gain sufficient information about the idiosyncratic aspects of pain-related fear responses in patients with chronic musculoskeletal pain.

Specific Questionnaires

A basic question that may be asked is, What is the patient afraid of? Or, in other words, What is the nature of the perceived threat? An answer to this question is not as simple as it seems. Patients may not view their problem as involving fear at all and may simply see difficulty in performing certain movements or activities. In addition, the specific nature of pain-related fear varies considerably, making an idiosyncratic approach almost indispensable. Most patients fear pain itself. Other patients may fear not so much current pain but pain that will be experienced at a later time, for example, the day after increased physical exercise. Finally, patients may not fear pain itself but the impending (re)injury that it is supposed to indicate, such as fear to become permanently handicapped. For these patients, pain is seen as a warning signal for a seriously threatening situation. The literature reflects this variety of fear stimuli by discussing measures for the assessment of fear of pain, fear of work and physical activity, and fear of (re)injury as a result of movement. Table 10.2 outlines several "pain-related fear" questionnaires, including sample items.

FEAR OF PAIN

An early attempt to assess fear of pain is the Pain and Impairment Relationship Scale (PAIRS) developed to study chronic pain patients' attitudes concerning activity and pain (Riley, Ahern, & Follick, 1988). The scale has 15 items rated on 7-point Likert scales and it has been found to have good psychometric characteristics. The original study demonstrated that beliefs that activity

TABLE 10.2. Examples of Items from Pain-Related Fear Questionnaires

Tampa Scale for Kinesiophobia (TSK)

Harm
I wouldn't have this much pain if there weren't something potentially dangerous going on in my body.
My body is telling me I have something dangerously wrong.

Fear of reinjury
I'm afraid that I might injure myself accidentally.
I'm afraid that I might injure myself if I exercise.

Exercise
It's really not safe for a person with a condition like mine to be physically active.
My pain would probably be relieved if I were to exercise [reverse scored].

Avoidance of activity
If I were to try to overcome it, my pain would increase.
Pain lets me know when to stop exercising so that I don't injure myself.

Pain and Impairment Relationship Scale (PAIRS)

An increase in pain is an indication that I should stop what I am doing until the pain decreases.
I have to be careful not to do anything that might make my pain worse.
I have come to accept that I am a disabled person, due to my chronic pain.
All of my problems would be solved if my pain would go away.

Fear–Avoidance Beliefs Questionnaire (FABQ)

Fear–avoidance beliefs about work
My pain was caused by my work or by an accident at work.
My work might harm my back.

Fear–avoidance beliefs about physical activity
My pain was caused by physical activity.
I cannot do physical activities which (might) make my pain worse.

Pain Anxiety Symptoms Scale (PASS)

Cognitive anxiety
I can't think straight when in pain.
During painful episodes it is difficult for me to think of anything besides the pain.

Escape/avoidance
I go immediately to bed when I feel severe pain.
I will stop any activity as soon as I sense pain coming on.

Fear
I think that if my pain gets too severe, it will never decrease.
When I feel pain I am afraid that something terrible will happen.

Physiological anxiety
I begin trembling when engaged in an activity that increases pain.
Pain seems to cause my heart of pound or race.

would increase pain were related to physical impairment. In 1992, the Pain Anxiety Symptoms Scale (PASS; McCracken, Zayfert, & Gross, 1992) was developed to measure cognitive anxiety symptoms, escape and avoidance responses, fearful appraisals of pain, and physiological anxiety symptoms related to pain. It is a 40-item questionnaire with internally consistent sub-scales. The validity of the PASS has been supported by positive correlations with measures of anxiety, cognitive errors, depression, and disability. A more recent exploratory factor analysis revealed five factors that could be labeled as catastrophic thoughts, physiological anxiety symptoms, escape/avoidance behaviors, cognitive interference, and coping strategies (Larsen, Taylor, & Asmundson, 1997). An abbreviated version of the PASS, consisting of only 20 items, is also available (McCracken & Dhingra, 2002).

FEAR OF WORK-RELATED ACTIVITIES

The Fear–Avoidance Beliefs Questionnaire (FABQ; Waddell et al., 1993) focuses on patients' beliefs about how work and physical activity affect their low back pain. The FABQ consists of two scales, fear–avoidance beliefs of physical activity and fear–avoidance beliefs of work, of which the latter was consistently the stronger. The authors found that fear–avoidance beliefs about work are strongly related with disability of daily living and work lost in the past year, and more so than biomedical variables such as anatomical pattern of pain, time pattern, and severity of pain. On the other hand, the FABQ physical subscale is much stronger in predicting behavioral performance tests (Crombez, Vlaeyen, et al., 1999).

FEAR OF MOVEMENT/(RE)INJURY

The Survey of Pain Attitudes (SOPA; Jensen & Karoly, 1992) was developed to assess patients attitudes toward five dimensions of the chronic pain experience: pain control, pain-related disability, medical cures for pain, solicitude of others, and medication for pain. Because of the authors' clinical observation of an association between chronic patients' hesitancy to exercise and the expressed fear of possible injury, a new scale (Harm) was added to the original instrument. As well as the Disability and Control scales, the Harm scale appeared to independently predict levels of dysfunction. The Tampa Scale for Kinesiophobia (TSK, Miller, Kori, & Todd, 1991) is a 17-item questionnaire aimed at the assessment of fear of (re)injury due to movement. Each item is provided with a Likert scale with scoring alternatives ranging from "strongly agree" to "strongly disagree." Most psychometric research has been carried out with the Dutch version of the TSK, which appears to be sufficiently reliable (alpha = .77) and valid (Vlaeyen, Kole-Snijders, Boeren, & van Eek, 1995). Modest but significant correlations were found with measures of pain intensity, catastrophizing, impact of

pain on daily life activities, and generalized fear. Regression analyses revealed that levels of disability were best predicted by pain-related fear, and that the latter was best predicted by catastrophizing. Pain intensity levels and biomedical findings were significantly less predictive of both pain-related fear and disability levels (Vlaeyen, Kole-Snijders, Boeren, & van Eek, 1995). Moreover, the TSK discriminated well between avoiders and confronters during a behavioral performance task (Crombez, Vlaeyen, et al., 1999; Vlaeyen et al., 1995). A factor analysis revealed four nonorthogonal factors, to which following labels were assigned: Harm, Fear of (re)injury, Importance of exercise, Avoidance of activity (Vlaeyen, Kole-Snijders, Boeren, & van Eek, 1995). Because of the relatively high intercorrelations among the subscales, the more favorable internal consistency, and construct validity of the TSK total score, the latter is preferable to the subscales.

In sum, questionnaires for the assessment of pain-related fear are now available, although the validity of some of them needs to be further explored. For clinical purposes, these questionnaires seem to be appropriate as a first screening to identify patients who suffer excessive pain-related fear. However, the questionnaires do not tell us what the individual is exactly fearful of.

Interview

In case of elevated scores, the aforementioned fear questionnaires only are indicative of the presence of pain-related fear. The assessment should be continued to further validate the hypothesis that the patient's disability is determined mainly by these fears. The semistructured interview is an additional and important tool to obtain information about the cognitive, behavioral, and psychophysiological aspects of the symptoms and to better estimate the role of pain-related fear in the maintenance of the pain problem. It also includes information about the antecedents (situational or internal) of the pain-related fear and about the direct and indirect consequences. This screening might also include other areas of life stresses, as they might increase arousal levels and indirectly also fuel pain-related fear. Phobogenic beliefs of fearful patients with chronic pain often take the form of conditional assumptions of the type "If P, then Q" whereby P the predictor is of catastrophic consequence (Q). For example, "If I do this particular movement, pain will increase" and "If I feel pain, it means that my injury is getting worse." Often these forms of reasoning follow a confirmation bias in the sense that the rule if P then Q is seldom falsified. Falsification would be to test if there are instances in which P is followed by non-Q. In case of dysfunctional assumptions, the selective search of confirming evidence and the lack of falisificative evidence reinforced the credibility of the false assumptions (Smeets, de Jong, & Mayer, 2000).

During the interview, it is essential to gather as much information as possible about logical assumptions about the relationships between physical activity, pain, and (re)injury. It has to be kept in mind that chronic pain patients do not always conceive of their problem as a phobia, and they may not talk about fear. We suggest the interview to be geared to the patient's perception of his or her pain problem. Looking back to first meetings with the patients to whom we have offered exposure treatment so far, we paraphrased their personal story in terms of harmfulness ("You feel that it might be better not to do these activities," "I understand that you think that these activities might further harm your back") rather than using the words "fear" and "anxiety." As often was the case, patients later in treatment spontaneously started reconceptualizing their pain problem as a fear problem.

Factors that often seem to be associated with the development of the fear are the characteristics of pain onset and the ambiguity around the presence or absence of positive findings on medico-diagnostics. For example, a person involved in a traffic accident may develop a fear of driving as a result of the traumatic experience. Likewise, a back pain patient may develop a fear of lifting after experiencing pain while lifting or after receiving information from a medical doctor that lifting can damage nerves in the spinal cord. Most chronic back pain patients who present with pain-related fear appear to found their conviction about vulnerability to (re)injury on the results of the diagnostics tests such as test such as X-rays

and MRI. The combination of (threatening) information conveyed by the medical specialist and the experience of pain and discomfort seem to strengthen that conviction. The visual confrontation with the X-rays and just hearing the diagnosis can be quite upsetting to some patients, as this information might be interpreted as being more threatening than meant by the specialist.

Although reports about misconceptions and misinterpretations of information can be used during the educational part of the intervention, it is more useful to identify the current level of severity and the maintaining factors of the pain problem and associated pain-related fear. The severity can often be estimated by inquiring about the extent to which the pain problem interferes with daily life, including the ability to carry on paid work, leisure activities, and normal relationships. Maintaining factors usually are negative thoughts about the danger of the physical activities, the avoidance of these activities, and hypervigilance to signals of threat. Negative thoughts can be elicited by inquiring about the patient's personal theory about his pain and associated functional incapacity. Expectations about the future are also worth inquiring about: "What do you think will happen if the pain is left untreated?" For example, the back and pelvic pain complaints of a female patient started during her first pregnancy and increased after the delivery. She started worrying about the future, because a relative who received the same diagnosis finally became wheelchair bound. Her main belief was that during certain movements, the tissue and nerves around the ridged symphysis pubis could be damaged or ruptured, possibly resulting in paralysis of the lower limbs. In most cases these thoughts make people alert to bodily sensations that may signal impending danger. Situations that provoke these sensations are fearfully avoided. To gain insight into avoidance behaviors, the therapist may ask questions such as the following: "What does the pain prevent you from doing?" and "If you no longer had this pain problem, what differences would it make to your daily life?" One can also ask directly about the situations that may worsen the pain problem. Finally, the assessment should also clarify whether other problems such as major depression, marital conflicts, or disability claims warrant specific attention before or after treatment. In some cases, when more complicated problems are expected to arise once the pain problem diminishes, it may also be warranted to leave the pain disability problem untreated as it is. Table 10.3 contains a summary of the topics covered during the interview.

Determining Treatment Goals

There are several reasons why it is wise to spend some time on the determination of treatment goals (Kirk, 1989). *First*, cognitive-behavioral treatments for pain, including exposure *in vivo*, never aim at the reduction of pain but at the restoration of functional abilities despite pain (see Turk, Chapter 7, this volume). It helps to make this general goal explicit, and both patient and therapist should agree on one or more realistic and specific goals that are formulated in positive terms. Typical examples are being able to go shopping to the supermar-

ket alone and go swimming twice a week for half an hour. In cases in which the goal is to return to work, it may be wise to consult with the occupational physician or vocational counselor. Often the exposure treatment can be run in synchrony with a graded resumption of work activities. *Second*, setting goals also helps to structure the treatment and to design the hierarchy of stimuli that will be introduced during the actual exposure *in vivo*. For example, if a patient wishes to resume his sports activities, the therapist will make sure that aspects of such activities will be included in the graded exposure activities. *Third*, setting functional goals also redirects the focus of attention from pain and physical symptoms toward daily life activities, with the emphasis on the possibility of change away from the disability status. *Finally*, as the patient is invited to formulate his or her own goals, goal setting inadvertently reinforces the notion that active participation is an essential part of the treatment.

Graded Hierarchies

Once it has become clear that pain-related fear is pivotal in the maintenance of a person's pain disability, it is useful to inquire about the essential stimuli: What is the patient actually afraid of? So far, there is a lack of standardized questionnaires for identifying these stimuli. In our experience, it is quite difficult for pain patients to verbally estimate the threat value of different situations. One of the problems is that the avoidance behaviors are not really acknowledged as consequences of fear but as a direct consequence of the pain and the experienced vulnerability for (re)injury. In addition to checklists of daily activities, the presentation of visual materials, such as pictures of back-stressing activities and movements, might be worthwhile. They can be quite helpful in the development of graded hierarchies, reflecting the full range of situations avoided by the patient, beginning with those that provoke only mild discomfort and ending with activities or situations that are beyond the patient's present abilities.

The Photograph Series of Daily Activities (PHODA; Kugler, Wijn, Geilen, de Jong, & Vlaeyen, 1999)[1] is a standardized method

---

TABLE 10.3. Summary of Topics Covered during the Interview

1. Description of the current pain problem
2. Detailed description when the pain problem first occurred:
   a. Situation: Where and when did it occur? What were you doing?
   b. Behavior: How did you respond to the pain? What did other people do?
   c. Cognitions: What did you think was going on?
   d. Information provided by others: What did other people say about the pain?
   e. Bodily reactions: How did you feel?
3. Current situations: List of situations the pain us most likely to occur or to be most severe
4. Avoidance: What are you not doing anymore because of the pain?
5. Modulators: What are the things that make it better or worse?
6. Current cognitions: What do you think is the cause of the pain problem
7. Attitudes and behaviors of others: What do other people (spouse/doctor/therapists) think is the cause of the pain problem?
8. Previous treatments
9. Personal strengths and assets
10. Social and financial circumstances
11. Medication use

that appears appropriate to design graded hierarchies. PHODA uses 98 photographs representing various physical daily life activities, including lifting, bending, walking, bicycling, and so forth, which are presented to the patients, who is requested to place each photograph along a fear thermometer. This scale consists of a vertical line with 11 anchor points (ranging from 0 to 100) printed on a 60 cm × 40 cm hardboard. The fear thermometer is placed on a table in front of the patient with the following instruction: "Please watch each photograph carefully, and try to imagine you performing the same movement. Place the photograph on the thermometer according to the extent in which you feel that this movement is harmful to your back." In our experiences, abrupt changes in movements (e.g., suddenly being hit) or activities consisting of repetitive spinal compressions (riding a bicycle on a bumpy road) are frequently mentioned stimuli in chronic back pain patients who score high on the pain-related fear measures. These situations are feared because of beliefs about the causes of pain, such as ruptured or severely damaged nerves. ("If I lift heavy weights, the nerves in my back might be damaged.") It is also interesting that the same activity can be rated differently depending on the context in which the activity is performed. For example, the activity "running" receives an 80 when performed in a wood and 50 when performed on an even terrain. It is therefore a good idea to expose patients to physical activities in a variety of contexts.

Behavioral Tests

Sometimes, patients find it hard to really estimate the harmfulness of an activity when they have avoided it extensively. In such cases, behavioral tests can be introduced. They consist of performing an activity that has been avoided previously while performance indices (such as time, distance, or number of repetitions) are measured. Target behaviors can be derived from PHODA items, and in most cases the behavioral tests can be considered as a variant of the exercise tolerance test described by Fordyce (1976). To assess the extent in which avoidance occurs, patients are asked to perform the activity "until pain, weakness, fatigue or any other rea-

son causes you to wish to stop" (p. 170). Behavioral tests have the advantage that anticipatory anxiety and the anxiety during exposure can be measured separately (Butler, 1989). In addition, they provide a more objective measure of avoidance behavior.

Education

Pain patients who are convinced that certain movement will harm their body will be reluctant to immediately start falsifying their basic assumptions about the sequence movement–pain–injury. Therefore, unambiguously educating the patient in a way that the patient views his or her pain as a common condition that can be self-managed rather than a serious disease or a condition that needs careful protection is a useful first step. One of the major goals of the educational part is to increase the willingness of patients to finally engage in activities they have been avoiding for a long time. The aim is to correct the misinterpretations and misconceptions that have occurred early on during the development of the pain-related fear.

The educational part is more than just reassuring the patient that there are no specific physical abnormalities. In the absence of an alternative explanation for the pain problem and the associated functional limitations, just reassurance can have paradoxical and opposite effects (McDonald, Daly, Jelinek, Panetta, & Gutman, 1996). Therefore, the patient is given a careful explanation of the fear–avoidance model, using the patient's individual symptoms, beliefs and behaviors to illustrate how vicious circles (pain → catastrophic thought → fear → avoidance → disability → pain) maintain the pain problem. In cases in which the pain-related fear appears fueled by the visual confrontation with (presumably "positive") diagnostic test, it may be useful to review these tests together with a physician. It can be explained to patients that they probably have overestimated the value of these tests, and that in symptom-free people similar abnormalities can also be found time (Jensen et al., 1994). In addition, the therapist can suggest one of the existing patient books and leaflets (e.g., the British *Back Book,* Burton, Waddell, Burtt, & Blair, 1996; the *New Zealand Acute Back Pain Patient* brochure, Kendall, Linton, & Main,

1997; and a recently developed Dutch brochure, *Het Rugboekje,* Goossens, Vlaeyen, Portegijs, de Vet, & Weber, 2000).

Exposure *In Vivo* with Behavioral Experiments

Exposure In Vivo

Current treatments of excessive fears and anxiety are based on the experimental psychological work of Wolpe (1958) on systematic desensitization. In this keystone treatment method, individuals progress through increasingly more anxiety-provoking encounters with phobic stimuli while using relaxation as a reciprocal inhibitor of rising anxiety. Because relaxation was intended to compete with the anxiety response, a graded format was chosen to keep anxiety levels as weak as possible. Later studies revealed that the exposure to the feared stimuli appeared to be the most essential component of the systematic desensitization and, applied without relaxation, produced comparable effects (Craske & Rowe, 1997). Because for fearful patients firsthand evidence of actually experiencing themselves behaving differently is far more convincing than rational argument, the most essential step consists of graded exposure to the situations the patients has identified as "dangerous" or "threatening." Subsequently, individually tailored practice tasks are developed based on the graded hierarchy of fear-eliciting situations. Further, the general principles for exposure are followed. The patient agrees to perform certain activities or movements that he or she used to avoid. Patients are also encouraged to engage in these fearful activities as much as possible until disconfirmation has occurred and anxiety levels have decreased. This decrease can be monitored by asking patients to predict the occurrence of harm and repeating the same question after the first exposure to that activity: "How would you rate the probability that you may experience a severe pain attack after doing this activity?" If the rating has decreased significantly, the therapist may consider moving on to the next item of the hierarchy. Alternatively, the therapist can ask the patient to report his or her subjective units of distress on a scale from 0 to 10 and repeat the exposure task

until the level of distress has substantially decreased. Each activity or movement is first modeled by the therapist, who demonstrates how the activity can be done in ergonomically the most efficient manner. The presence of the therapist, who may serve as an initial safety signal to promote more exposures, is gradually withdrawn to facilitate independence and to create contexts that mimic those of the home situation (Vlaeyen, de Jong, Geilen, Heuts, & van Breukelen, 2001).

Behavioral Experiments

Following from cognitive theory that assumes that cognitive "errors" can be corrected through conscious reasoning, behavioral experiments have been developed in which a collaborative empiricism is the bottom line. The essence of a behavioral experiment is that the patient performs an activity to challenge the validity of his catastrophic assumptions and misinterpretations. These assumptions take the form of "If P, then Q" statements and are empirically tested during a behavioral experiment. Three steps can be distinguished: First, the patient formulates a hypothesis. For example, a back pain patient may expect that jumping down from a stair will inevitably cause nerve damage in the spine and excruciating pain. Second, an experiment is designed. For example, if the patient is convinced that jumping down is harmful, the therapist can further inquire about the minimal height that is needed to cause nerve injury. Finally, the experiment is carried out and evaluated. The therapist invites the patient to jump down from the stair and the consequences are being evaluated (see Table 10.4). In practice, behavioral experiments are difficult to separate from mere exposure, and they can best be used simultaneously.

Although many patients with chronic musculoskeletal pain have similar fears (fear of physical activities that produce pain, or that are assumed to cause reinjury), the origin of their fears may be different. Rachman (1977) suggested three pathways of the acquisition of excessive fears: direct trauma (classical conditioning), vicarious observation (social learning), and informational transmission. Each of these can be recognized in the pain histories of fearful patients

TABLE 10.4. Dialogue between a Patient and the Therapist during a Behavioral Experiment

THERAPIST: OK, today we'll start with the next activity. Why don't we try lifting this shopping bag? What do you think?

PATIENT: (*Sighs.*) I don't think I can manage that.

THERAPIST: What do you think might happen?

PATIENT: I'm sure I'll get more pain, and I don't think it's good for my back.

THERAPIST: If you would do this lifting activity right now, what would be the worst thing that could happen?

PATIENT: I am afraid that my back will give away, hear one of those nasty cracks in my back. I told you before that I don't want to end up paralyzed.

THERAPIST: I fully understand. We both know that in principle it is safe to be more active, but because of the pain you remain concerned about harming your back. Is that right?

PATIENT: I guess so.

THERAPIST: How much pain do you feel right now on a scale of 0 to 100?

PATIENT: about 40.

THERAPIST: How much do you think it will hurt while lifting this shopping bag?

PATIENT: I am not sure, but certainly more than a 80.

THERAPIST: Well, the best way to find out is to try and see what happens. I'll do it first, and then it's your turn. [At this point the therapist models the lifting task, and invites the patient to do the same, and while the patient is holding the bag, the therapist goes on inquiring about what happens.] Great, how bad is the pain right now?

PATIENT: (*visibly sweating*) It is not that bad actually. Somewhat more, a 50 I would say.

THERAPIST: Good, how big a chance is there that you are going to become paralyzed?

PATIENT: This time, it seems OK. But there was no crack.

THERAPIST: Would the situation be different if you would have felt a crack?

Patient: Oh yes, definitely.

THERAPIST: How can you bring on such a crack?

PATIENT: When I was still working, I usually carried heavier weights than the one I just lifted.

THERAPIST: Shall we make this one a bit heavier?

PATIENT: I have started, I can as well continue now. (*Laughs nervously.*)

THERAPIST: OK, go ahead and add more weight. [After the patient has filled the bag, the therapist models the activity before the patient is exposed to it herself.] How much pain do you feel right now?

PATIENT: A little more pain now, almost a 60.

THERAPIST: Do you feel a crack?

Patient: Not really, but you know, suppose I would fall while lifting, that would make the situation much more dangerous.

THERAPIST: OK, is that worrying you more than lifting objects?

PATIENT: I think so, yes.

By doing this behavioral experiment, a new stimulus is identified: falling. At this point, the therapist invites the patient to go to the canvas where different "falling" exercises can be done, such as a forward and backwards somersault. Again, this is done in a graded and gentle fashion, always modeled by the therapist and with systematically challenging expected threat using behavioral experiments.

who seek treatment at our center. We describe two cases here in which fear has originated from direct trauma and informational transmission respectively.

Case Illustrations

Mr. A is a 50-year-old married man who was working as a plumber. His neck pain had started 8 years ago as a result of a car crash that had taken place a half year earlier. While reaching out above his head, he felt a "shooting" pain in his neck. Initially, he interpreted this pain as a normal muscle twist in his neck, but as his pain complaints increased, and he gradually became unable to carry out a number of daily activities, he became frightened that there was something seriously wrong in his neck, shoulders, and head. He did not understand what was going on. During the smallest movements he experienced, beside the pain, certain inexplicable body sensations. He started to interpret his sensations now as signs of muscle or nerve damage. He tried to avoid those movements as much as possible. In addition to the pain complaints, Mr. A had also experienced memory problems and difficulties concentrating. After 6 years of medical assessments Mr. A was told he had a whiplash-associated disorder (WAD). Following the advice of the neurologist, Mr. A attended an educational course to learn how to cope with WAD. However, this program did not diminish his fear of making the injury worse. His main assumption was that during certain movements, the tissue and nerves in and around his neck and shoulder could be damaged or ruptured, possibly resulting in paralysis of the upper and lower limbs. He finally was referred to the rehabilitation unit for a behavioral treatment program.

Mr. A started with a behavioral rehabilitation program following operant treatment principles (Fordyce, 1976; Lindström et al., 1992), including graded activity, pacing techniques, relaxation, and education about ergonomics. After 8 weeks the rehabilitation physician concluded that the actual treatment program was unsuccessful in reducing Mr. A's disability levels (Roland Disability Questionnaire [RDQ] score remained at 19) and associated pain-related fear (TSK score = 52; PHODA total score = 780). The consulting psychologist performed a cognitive-behavioral analysis of

the pain problem as described earlier and concluded that a graded exposure *in vivo* treatment was indicated. Following the cognitive analysis, a fear hierarchy was made (Table 10.5). During the first (educational) session, Mr. A was provided with a rationale explaining that painful body sensations can occur without signaling muscle and nerve damage, and how this catastrophic misinterpretation and avoidance behavior was maintaining the pain problem. The exposure *in vivo* part consisted of 18 sessions, 60 minutes each, spread over 6 weeks. One of the essential stimuli was reaching above shoulder level. It was decided to start the exposure with simple reaching tasks such as hanging a coat on a coat hook and clearing out kitchen cabinets. Initially, Mr. A was reluctant to pursue, and he wondered whether his pain problem was taken seriously enough. The therapist reassured Mr. A that there was no doubt that his pain complaints were real but explained to him that a behavioral experiment was set up to challenge the validity of his catastrophic expectations and misinterpretations. During the subsequent sessions, the activities became gradually physically more intense as the patient was ascending the fear hierarchy. Sometimes, safety behaviors were observed. For example, during jumping activities, Mr. A came down on one foot at a time, to absorb the shock. He reportedly was afraid that a landing on both feet could make a tremendous

TABLE 10.5. Fear Hierarchy of Mr. A

Pretreatment hierarchy	PHODA item	Posttreatment PHODA score (0–100)
100	Trampolining	20
90	Charge down the stairs	20
80	Cycling at an unpaved road	0
70	Playing table tennis	0
60	Put away a crate with 24 bottles on a rack above shoulder level	0
50	Rake the garden	0
40	Prune a tree	0
30	Drive a car	0
20	—	—
10	Hang something on a coat hook	0
0	Put down the dog's food in a kneeling position	0

impact in his neck, increasing risk for reinjury. This fear again was used in a subsequent behavioral experiment in which the consequences of jumping on both feet simultaneously were challenged.

During the last sessions, Mr. A played table tennis and performed all the daily household chores. After nine sessions of exposure therapy the TSK score decreased to 23, with a PHODA total score of 170, and an RDQ score of 6. At the end of the exposure therapy, Mr. A's disability and pain-related fear levels were significantly decreased (TSK: 19, PHODA: 160, RDQ: 4). Figure 10.2 shows daily measures of pain-related fear (fear of movement/reinjury) and pain measured with a visual analog scale at a 1-week baseline and the subsequent exposure treatment. Of interest is that pain levels decreased to a certain degree, but that despite existing pain, the level of pain-related fear gradually decreased and became almost nil.

Ms. B is a 45-year-old woman with two pain complaints of which she was quite fearful. She suffered both from back pain and from complex regional pain syndrome (CRPS) in the left wrist. The CRPS developed after surgery, during which an inflamed lump was removed. Over the years after the operation, Ms. B's pain complaints in the left forearm increased. The smallest movement and even a little touch were painful. Because of the hyperalgesia and dysesthesia, Ms. B became unable to carry out any activities with her left arm and decided to quit her job as a flower shopkeeper. She also avoided crowded places because she was afraid of pain resulting from unexpected physical contact with other people. Ms. B believed that the surgeon had unwittingly damaged or ruptured certain nerves during the operation, because she had never felt any pain before. The first 2 years following surgery, Ms. B. had numerous sessions of occupational and physical therapy, without improvement. Finally, the orthopedic surgeon prescribed a corset around the left forearm, which Ms. B started wearing daily. She avoids movements with her left arm as much as possible, because she fears that such movements could worsen the injury. Her belief that nerve injury is the cause of her arm pain also generalized to her chronic low back pain problem. She is convinced that her back pain also is the result of nerve damage and that too much physical exertion might cause reinjury.

Before starting the exposure, it was

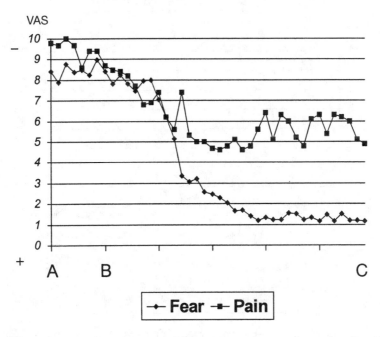

FIGURE 10.2. Daily measures of pain-related fear and pain of Mr. A during baseline (A-B) and exposure treatment (B-C).

agreed that the corset was no longer useful and Ms. B should not wear it anymore. The first two sessions consisted of lightly touching her left arm. Although pain initially increased, she discovered that it hurt less than expected and that the pain waned away more rapidly than anticipated. Subsequently, activities included in the exposure treatment ranged from light household activities (e.g., washing dishes and dusting cupboards) to those activities she used to do in the flower shop (e.g., making a Christmas bouquet) and ended with bicycling and falling on a mattress. Of interest, even though her arm pain remained at about the same level, Ms. B's worries that pain signaled further reinjury drastically decreased (see top part of Figure 10.3). Ms. B general-

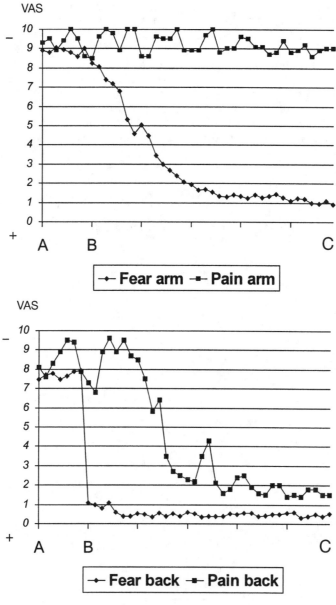

FIGURE 10.3. Daily measures of pain-related fear and pain of Ms. B for her arm and back pain problem during baseline (start A) and exposure treatment (start B). *Top part:* for the arm; *bottom part:* for the back.

ized this learning experience to her back pain problem and spontaneously started doing activities that she had thought had to be avoided. Only two exposure sessions were devoted to her back pain, which resulted in a significant reduction of her back pain complaints (see bottom part of Figure 10.3).

Complicating Factors

PAIN INCREASES

Although patients have agreed that the treatment is not primarily aimed at reducing pain levels, it may be frightening for them to experience a sudden pain attack during the exposure treatment. In most cases, increases in pain are temporary and wane after a couple of hours. In such cases, the following steps can be taken. First, the therapist should check whether there are medical reasons for the pain increase. Second, if not, the patient is provided with an acceptable rationale in which it is reiterated that although pain is bothersome, it does not a signal something dangerously. For example, pain can be explained as the possible result of disuse of the muscles, or as the reaction of the muscles to increased exertion during therapy. Third, and preferably directly following the second step, exposure to physical activity is continued. If patients are excessively reluctant, the therapist may decide to repeat some of the previous activities at a lower level on the fear hierarchy. Fourth, again a behavioral experiment can be set up to challenge the belief that something seriously might have happened that caused the pain increase. Our experience is that fear levels quickly go down again and that when encountering a similar pain increase in the future, patients are less worried and pain increases tend to interfere less with current activities. Actually, the occurrence of pain increase during the treatment can be beneficial, as it provides the possibility for both the patient and the therapist to prepare for the period after termination of the treatment during which pain increases are likely to reoccur, especially for musculoskeletal pain problems, which are recurrent by nature.

SAFETY BEHAVIORS

There are a number of behavioral reactions, more volitional in nature, that have to be considered important in the maintenance of pain-related fear, especially during the exposure procedure. For example, a chronic back pain patient who is exposed to a lifting task with his dominant arm may lift while holding his other arm on his back as to protect his back, or he may focus more attention on the precise lifting motion or try to relax before starting the lifting task. These subtle and sometimes covert responses constitute "safety behaviors" (Salkovskis, Clark, Hackmann, Wells, & Gelder, 1999) that are intended to avert feared events. Safety behaviors are known to play a significant role in the maintenance of anxiety. Although the behaviors may relieve anxiety in the short term, they unintentionally preserve the belief in the catastrophe, as they prevent exposure to disconfirmations. In other words, combining exposure *in vivo* treatment with coping strategies such as relaxation attention diversion techniques may actually weaken the impact of the exposure. Indeed, the nonoccurrence of the catastrophe may be attributed to the use of safety behaviors rather than being correctly attributed to the fact that catastrophe will not occur ("If I hadn't relaxed while lifting, I might have experienced a pain attack"). For example, coming down on one foot at once instead of both feet simultaneously during a jump was a typical safety behavior by Mr. A. Other safety behaviors include bracing, guarded walking, and seeking physical support. The therapist should be aware of these often subtle behaviors and closely observe patients during exposure sessions. When safety behaviors have been identified, we suggest that the therapist repeat the exposure session with the instruction to leave out that safety behavior (response prevention).

In this respect, firm ergonomic advice about lifting, carrying, and sitting, often provided in the so-called back schools, conveying the message that activities are safe only when performed in an ergonomically "justified" way, can best be omitted for fearful patients undergoing an exposure *in vivo* procedure. Indeed, they may be interpreted as evidence that if not followed as suggested, the feared catastrophe may occur. Of course, this does not mean that patients can be exposed to any kind of stimulus. All stimuli used in the exposure procedure should be reasonable and safe for anyone, always be modeled first by the therapist and negotiated with the patient.

Generalization and Maintenance of Change

What is actually learned during exposure? Although some researchers assume that exposure leads to a disconfirmation of overpredictions of the aversive characteristics of fear stimuli, there is growing evidence that exposure cannot simply be equated with unlearning. Studies have demonstrated that a competition occurs between the original threatening (excitatory) meaning of the stimuli and a new (inhibitory) meaning. In other words, during successful exposure, exceptions to the rule are learned rather than a fundamental change of that rule (Bouton, 1988). Goubert and colleagues (2002) showed that in chronic low back pain patients, exposure to one movement (bending forward) did not generalize toward another, dissimilar movement (straight leg raising). The conclusion that the authors made was that during exposure, patients appear to learn exceptions to the rule (if P, then Q) rather than a fundamental change of that rule, which is in line with animal studies on learning (Bouton, 2000). In other words, exposure to physical activities is not likely to result in a fundamental change in the belief of the pain patient that certain movements are harmful or painful. More likely, he or she will learn that the movements involved in the exposure treatment are less harmful or painful than anticipated.

Research findings on exposure in anxiety disorders suggest that generalization and maintenance can be enhanced by a number of measures. First is providing exposures to the full spectrum of contexts and natural settings in which fear has been experienced (e.g., Mineka, Mystkowski, Hladek, & Rodriguez, 1999). The PHODA might be a useful tool in eliciting information about these contexts in chronic pain patients. It is preferable to carry out an exposure session in the context in which the fear has been acquired. For example, for one patient (reported in Vlaeyen et al., 2001) the fear started at work, when she heard a "crack" in her lower back while lifting a trash bag and throwing it into a big container. A "shooting" pain immediately followed the crack, and the patient interpreted subsequent cracking sounds in the back as signs of tissue or nerve damage. For this patient, one of the final exposure sessions consisted of going back to that same place at the work site. Second is varying the stimuli during the exposure (Rowe & Craske, 1998b).

Activities to be included in the exposure procedure can best be extended from those derived from PHODA to other activities as well. For example, bicycling can be done in different ways: using a mountain bike rather than a city bike, biking uphill as well as downhill, biking on rough as well as even terrain, and so on. A third way to enhance generalization and maintenance is to use an expanded-spaced rather than a massed exposure schedule (Rowe & Craske, 1998a). It is preferable to spread the treatment over a longer period rather than concentrate the treatment in a limited number of weeks.

Exposure in Primary Care Settings

So far, we described exposure *in vivo* treatment as it has been carried out mostly in chronic pain patients at tertiary care settings. There is now increasing evidence that such an approach would be desirable in a much earlier stage. Klenerman and colleagues (1995) collected biopsychosocial measures from a sample of 300 acute low back pain patients within 1 week of presentation, and at 2 months as to predict 12-month outcome. Their data showed that most subjects who had not recovered by 2 months became chronic low back pain patients. Moreover, fear-avoidance beliefs turned out to be the most powerful predictor of chronic disability. Consistent with these results, Sieben, Vlaeyen, Tuerlinckx, and Portegijs (in press) following acute back pain patients in primary care found that fear of movement/(re)injury as measured with the TSK was the best predictor disability at 3-month and 1-year follow-up, even when controlling for pain severity. Given the serious consequences of chronic pain, and because sufficient evidence supporting primary prevention of acute low back pain is still lacking, it seems to be more appropriate to look for possibilities to prevent acute pain from becoming chronic (Linton, 1998). The easiest way to select patients at risk is *to wait and see* for some weeks. Most episodes of back pain resolve within days or a few weeks, often without work loss or health care. Patients who are still out of work after a month have a 20% risk of chronic disability (Waddell, 1998). This "self-selected" group requires special attention from health care providers to prevent long-term problems. This course of action is adopted, for example, by the Dutch General Practice Guideline for Low Back Pain (Faas, Chavannes, Koes, Romeijnders, & Van der Laan, 1996). However, a drawback of this approach is that it may be difficult to reverse the negative consequences of back pain once it has already existed for several weeks.

Another option is *early screening* of all acute back pain patients, in order to identify high-risk patients as soon as possible. For example, screening on "psychosocial yellow flags" has been proven to be an effective tool to early select patients with a poor prognosis (Kendall et al., 1997; Linton & Hallden, 1998). Pain-related fear is one of these yellow flags. Preventive intervention during the acute stage might be easier to do and more cost-effective than rehabilitation of subacute or chronic patients. For example, Moore, Von Korff, Cherkin, Saunders, and Lorig (2000) offered a two-session self-care group and an individual meeting and telephone conversation with the group leader, a psychologist experienced in chronic pain management. The intervention was supplemented by educational materials (book and videos) supporting active management of back pain. The control group received usual care supplemented by a book on back pain care. Interestingly, compared to the usual care, participants assigned to the self-care intervention showed significantly greater reductions in back-related worry and fear-avoidance beliefs than did the control group. In sum, the identification of acute patients "at risk" and the subsequent provision of cognitive-behavioral interventions appear applicable in primary care.

Therefore, we have begun to examine the effectiveness of an exposure *in vivo* treatment for acute back pain patients reporting substantial pain-related fear in a primary care setting. Although levels of pain-related fear may be comparable to those of patients seen in tertiary care, acute primary care patients generally show different patterns of avoidance. Their avoidance of physical activities is less typical than in chronic patients; it has not yet developed into generalized and structural habits. Besides, at the beginning of an episode or immediately following injury, avoidance strategies may be appropriate coping responses to reduce pain and facilitate tissue healing. Many patients report an active and confronting lifestyle when they are not suffering from back pain. Nevertheless, they do have high-risk cognitions about their back pain (concerning the cause of their pain, for example); they seem to be at risk of becoming avoiders in the future if their pain-related fear is not properly treated while it might be relatively easy to modify.

The intervention currently being evaluated in an experimental design consists basically of the same three components (screening, education, exposure) as the exposure treatment for chronic patients. However, the format is somewhat adjusted for its use in a primary care setting (see Table 10.6). For example, a shorter version of the PHODA is used to identify fear-eliciting movements and activities. Furthermore, the

---

TABLE 10.6. Exposure in Primary Care Format: Summary of Topics

Screening
- Assessment by the general practitioner: using brief pain-related fear questionnaire such as TSK
- Brief PHODA (modified) to identify fear-eliciting movements
- Structured interview, with special attention to current concerns about beliefs about back pain (causes, management)

Education
- Explanation of the fear-avoidance model
- Importance of physical activity and movement
- Possibilities and advantages of self-management

Exposure
- Tailored fear-reducing exercises in the home-context based on PHODA

Action plans
- Self-exposure: situations that will be practiced at home
- Self-management: how to prepare for future pain episodes

structured interview not only explores be-liefs about back pain but also addresses the patient's ideas and expectations about the care provided by the physician. The con-tents of the educational part of the interven-tion are largely similar, with a strong em-phasis on the fear-avoidance model and self-management of back pain. Also, the ex-posure exercises are designed and conduct-ed following the same principles as in chronic patients. In addition, action plans are developed and carried out in between treatment sessions to enhance self-exposure and resumption of normal daily activities.

This primary care exposure treatment is implemented in a stepped-care home-visit format. In an individualized stepped-care approach, care is modified based on the pa-tient's outcome (Von Korff, 1999). All pa-tients reporting acute low back pain and high levels of pain-related fear (TSK score > 42) receive an initial intervention of two home-visits as described previously. The home-visit format provides excellent oppor-tunities to observe the patient in his or her social context and to perform "real-life" ex-posure exercises in and around the house. It is assumed that for most patients these two sessions will be sufficient to initiate other-wise spontaneous recovery mechanisms. Presuming a positive vicious cycle, (self-)ex-posure will increasingly readjust incorrect cognitions toward pain and physical activity and change the avoidance behavior into more adaptive habits, with better physical fitness and decreasing disability as a result.

After the first step, progress is evaluated. The subgroup of patients who maintain high levels of pain-related fear after the first two sessions will move on to the second step, consisting of two additional home vis-its. These sessions will be more intensively aimed at identifying and solving the prob-lems that inhibit successful (self-)exposure and reduction of pain-related fear (e.g., lacking motivation, skills, social support, or self-efficacy). In this way the duration of treatment is adjusted to the patient's needs, and resources are distributed efficiently.

Other Forms of Exposure

The *in vivo* form of graded exposure de-scribed earlier is specifically developed for patients with chronic musculoskeletal pain,

and back pain in particular, who are severe-ly disabled and who report substantial pain-related fear. Nevertheless, one has to bear in mind that the literature on the cognitive-behavioral treatment of phobias described several variations in the way exposure can be conducted, most of which have not been systematically evaluated. For example, one could consider imagined exposure or expo-sure using virtual reality instead of *in vivo*. Patients with an ability to create vivid im-ages may be asked to imagine performing the "harmful" physical activities they tend to avoid. Instead of the massed version we described (once every day for several weeks), a spaced form (one every week for several months) might also be an option. Rather than approaching the fearful stimuli in a graded fashion, an interesting question would be to what extent the process of change would be accelerated by directly ex-posing patients to the most intensely feared stimuli. Finally, the treatment would be made more accessible to a larger group of patients if self-exposure, with a manual, would be as effective as the therapist guided exposure we described here. The reason we have chosen graded exposure with the aid of the therapist is that based on our experi-ence, we felt it would provide the most cred-ible, safe, and effective treatment approach.

Therapist Characteristics

As mentioned earlier, graded exposure *in vivo* may appear quite similar to the usual graded activity programs, in that it gradual-ly increases activity levels despite pain, but it is quite different, conceptually and as well as practically. This means that this type of treatment requires specific therapist charac-teristics. As exposure *in vivo* with behav-ioral experiments is a cognitive-behavioral intervention, training in cognitive-behav-ioral principles is a necessary prerequisite, and supervision by psychologist experi-enced in working in the field of behavioral medicine and the area of chronic pain in particular is a sine qua non. In addition, the treatment will work best when delivered by therapists who feel quite comfortable in ex-posing patients to movements, and who are not fearful themselves that too much physi-cal activity might harm the patients' physi-cal condition. Rainville, Bagnall, and Phalen

(1995) conjectured that "patients' attitudes and beliefs (and thereby patients disability levels) may be derived from the projected attitudes and beliefs of health care providers" (p. 288). In line with this, a recent study on health care providers attitudes (Houben et al., 2002) reported that therapists who hold a more biomedical or biomechanical view on chronic pain rate daily physical activities as more harmful for patients with common back pain than do their colleagues whose attitudes toward pain are more behaviorally oriented.

Effectiveness

We recently conducted a number of empirical studies to examine the effectiveness of a graded exposure *in vivo* treatment with behavioral experiments as compared to usual graded activity in reducing pain-related fears, catastrophizing, and pain disability in chronic low back pain patients reporting substantial fear of movement/(re)injury (Vlaeyen et al., 2001; Vlaeyen, de Jong, Geilen, Heuts, & van Breukelen, in press; Vlaeyen, de Jong, Onghena, Kerckhoffs-Hanssen, & Kole-Snijders, in press). In two studies, a replicated single case crossover design was applied with four and six consecutive chronic low back pain patients each. Only patients who reported substantial fear of movement/(re)injury (TSK score > 40), and who were referred for outpatient behavioral rehabilitation, were included. After a no-treatment baseline measurement period, the patients were randomly assigned to one of two interventions. In intervention A, patients received the exposure first, followed by graded activity. In intervention B, the sequence of treatment modules was reversed. Daily measures of pain-related cognitions and fears were recorded with visual analog scales. Before and after the treatment, the following measures were taken: pain-related fear, pain catastrophizing, pain control, and pain disability.

Although the supplemental value of this "background" treatment program cannot be ruled out in this study, the remarkable improvements that are observed whenever the graded exposure was initiated suggests that the therapeutic power of the graded exposure is much stronger. Not only were improvements found on the self-report measures of pain-related fear, pain catastrophizing, and pain disability (Vlaeyen et al., 2001), but they were also generalized to increases in physical acitivity in the home situation as measured with ambulatory activity monitors (Vlaeyen, de Jong, Geilen, et al., in press). The crossover design gave us the opportunity to examine the differential effects of graded exposure and graded activity and the additional treatment effect of the second treatment module. As the order of treatment modules did not make any difference to the final outcome, no such effect was found in this study. On the other hand, carryover effects were clearly observed when graded exposure was followed by graded activity. The third study revealed similar effects in two low back pain patients (Vlaeyen, de Jong, Onghena, et al., in press). In this study, exposure *in vivo* was delivered as the only treatment, and without the background rehabilitation program that seems to suggest that it is the exposure treatment that is responsible for the results. The external validity of the exposure treatment is also supported by Swedish study in which two patients were given treatment in a different hospital setting (Linton, Overmeer, Janson, Vlaeyen, & de Jong, in press).

What can be said about the possible mediators of treatment effects? The treatment duration was much too short to produce significant increases in muscle strength. The abrupt change in the daily measures is suggestive of cognitive changes. Although the exposure was provided during a period of 3 weeks, the reduction of catastrophizing and fear was achieved within 7 days or three exposure sessions. Rachman and Whittal (1989) proposed that such abrupt changes are more characteristic of insight learning, rather than the usual gradual progression of trial-and-error learning. In our study, the presentation of the rationale at the start of the exposure might have contributed to this insight. Many patients reported that for the first time, they received a credible rationale for their current level of disability.

Although these initial results are quite promising, there are a number of caveats to be considered. The preliminary evidence reported here is limited in that it included a small number of patients. On the other hand, a single-case experimental design was chosen with appropriate time series statistical analyses. Because in the crossover design all patients received both interventions, long-term differential effects could not be established. Replication studies in the form of randomized controlled trial using larger samples and long-term follow-up measurements are warranted.

Summary

"Fear of pain and what we do about it may be more disabling than pain itself" (Waddell et al., 1993, p. 164). With this statement, the intuitively appealing idea—that the lowered ability to accomplish tasks of daily living in chronic pain patients is merely the consequence of pain severity—is refuted. The recent literature supports the early conjecture that chronic pain and phobia share important characteristics. Indeed, studies have shown that during the confrontation with feared movements, chronic low back pain patients who are fearful of movement/(re)injury typically show psychophysiological (muscle reactivity), behavioral (escape and avoidance), and cognitive (worry) responses. It was not until recently that this line of thought was extended to the behavioral assessment and management of chronic pain. Specific pain-related fear measures, for pain patients whose level of disability is likely to be controlled by pain-related fears, have been developed. For its use in primary care, a screening questionnaire aiming at the identification of acute back pain patients at risk has been developed which includes several items on fear and avoidance (Kendall et al., 1997; Linton & Hallden, 1998). In addition, the cognitive-behavioral assessment also includes the semistructured interview, the development of graded hierarchies, and the application of behavioral tests. In this chapter we described an exposure *in vivo* treatment for the reduction of pain-related fear in chronic low back pain patients. An exposure *in vivo* consist of individually tailored practice tasks based on a graded hierarchy of fear-eliciting situations and not just a physical training program or usual graded activity that does not take into account these essential and idiosyncratic fear stimuli. Preliminary outcome data show that such exposure *in vivo* may help the patient to confront rather than avoid physical movement, and that a reduction in self-reported disability levels follows. Although cognitive-behavioral treatments for chronic pain are quite favorable (Morley, Eccleston, & Williams, 1999), there is an urgent need for further refinement of our treatments, including a better match between treatment modalities and patient characteristics. We hope that our chapter will contribute to the process of customization of cognitive-behavioral treatments in the care of chronic pain patients.

Acknowledgments

We wish to thank Peter Heuts, Mario Geilen, Maria Kerckhoffs-Hanssen, Herman Mulder, Noel Dortu, the staff of the Department of Pain Rehabilitation of the Hoensbroeck Rehabilitation Center and the staff of the Department of Rehabilitation of the University Hospital Maastricht for their contribution in making the application of the exposure treatment possible. This contribution is supported by Grant No. 904-65-090 of the Council for Medical and Health Research of the Netherlands (NWO-MW) to Johan W. S. Vlaeyen.

Note

1. A CD-ROM version of PHODA including the 98 pictures and a brief manual, is available and can be requested from PHODA@ HSZUYD.NL.

References

American Psychiatric Association. (1994). *Diagnostic and statistical manual of mental disorders* (4th ed.). Washington, DC: Author.

Asmundson, G. J., Norton, P. J., & Norton, G. R. (1999). Beyond pain: The role of fear and avoidance in chronicity. *Clinical Psychology Review, 19*, 97–119.

Bouton, M. E. (1988). Context and ambiguity in the extinction of emotional learning: Implications for exposure therapy. *Behaviour Research and Therapy, 26*, 137–149.

Bouton, M. E. (2000). A learning theory perspective on lapse, relapse, and the maintenance of behavior change. *Health Psychology, 19*(1 Suppl.), 57–63.

Burton, A. K., Waddell, G., Burtt, R., & Blair, S. (1996). Patient educational material in the management of low back pain in primary care. *Bulletin of the Hospital for Joint Diseases, 55*, 138–141.

Butler, G. (1989). Phobic disorders. In K. Hawton, P. M. Salkovskis, J. Kirk, & D. M. Clark (Eds.), *Cognitive behaviour therapy for psychiatric problems: A practical guide* (pp. 97–128). Oxford, UK: Oxford University Press.

Cipher, D. J., & Fernandez, E. (1997). Expectancy variables predicting tolerance and avoidance of pain in chronic pain patients. *Behaviour Research and Therapy, 35*, 437–444.

Craske, M. G., & Rowe, M. K. (1997). A comparison of behavioral and cognitive treatments of phobias. In G. C. L. Davey (Ed.), *Phobias: A handbook of theory, research and treatment.* (pp. 247–280). Chichester, UK: Wiley.

Crombez, G., Eccleston, C., Baeyens, F., & Eelen, P. (1998). When somatic information threatens, catastrophic thinking enhances attentional interference. *Pain, 75*, 187–198.

Crombez, G., Eccleston, C., Baeyens, F., van Houdenhove, B., & van den Broeck, A. (1999). Attention to chronic pain is dependent upon pain-related fear. *Journal of Psychosomatic Research, 47*, 403–410.

Crombez, G., Vervaet, L., Baeyens, F., Lysens, R., & Eelen, P. (1996). Do pain expectancies cause pain in chronic low back patients? A clinical investigation. *Behavior Research and Therapy, 34*, 919–925.

Crombez, G., Vlaeyen, J. W., Heuts, P. H., & Lysens, R. (1999). Pain-related fear is more disabling than pain itself: Evidence on the role of pain-related fear in chronic back pain disability. *Pain, 80*, 329–339.

Eccleston, C., Crombez, G., Aldrich, S., & Stannard, C. (1997). Attention and somatic awareness in chronic pain. *Pain, 72*, 209–215.

Faas, A., Chavannes, A. W., Koes, B., Romeijnders, A.C.M., R., & Van der Laan, J. R. (1996). *NHG-standaard lage-rugpijn* [Practice Guideline "Low Back Pain"]. *Huisarts & Wetenschap, 39*, 18–31.

Fordyce, W. E. (1976). *Behavioral methods for chronic pain and illness.* St. Louis, MO: Mosby.

Fordyce, W. E., Brockway, J. A., Bergman, J. A., & Spengler, D. (1986). Acute back pain: A control-group comparison of behavioral vs traditional management methods. *Journal of Behavioral Medicine, 9*, 127–140.

Goossens, M. E. J. B., Vlaeyen, J. W. S., Portegijs, P., de Vet, H. C. W., & Weber, W. (2000). *Het rugboekje: patiëntenbrochure "omgaan met lage rugpijn" [The little back book: brochure "How to deal with low back pain"].* Maastricht: Pijn Kennis Centrum.

Goubert, L., Francken, G., Crombez, G., Vansteenwegen, D., & Lysens, R. (2002). Exposure to physical movement in chronic back pain patients: no evidence for generalization across different movements. *Behaviour Research and Therapy, 40*, 415–419.

Heyneman, N. E., Fremouw, W. J., & Gano, D. (1990). Individual differences and the effectiveness of different coping strategies for pain. *Cognitive Therapy and Research, 14*, 63–77.

Houben, R., Vlaeyen, J. W. S., Ostelo, R., Stomp, S., Wolters, P., & Peters, M. L. (2002). *Health care providers' attitudes back pain. The case of physical therapy.* Manuscript submitted for publication, Maastricht University.

Jensen, M. C., Brant-Zawadzki, M. N., Obuchowski, N., Modic, M. T., Malkasian, D., & Ross, J. S. (1994). Magnetic resonance imaging of the lumbar spine in people without back pain. *New England Journal of Medicine, 33*, 69–73.

Jensen, M. P., & Karoly, P. (1992). Pain-specific beliefs, perceived symptom severity, and adjustment to chronic pain. *Clinical Journal of Pain, 8*, 123–130.

Kendall, N. A. S., Linton, S. J., & Main, C. J. (1997). *Guide to assessing psychosocial yellow flags in acute low back pain: Risk factors for long-term disability and work loss.* Wellington, New Zealand: Accident Compensation Corporation.

Kirk, J. (1989). Cognitive-behavioural assessment. In K. Hawton, P. M. Salkovskis, J. Kirk, & D. M. Clark (Eds.), *Cognitive behaviour therapy for psychiatric problems. A practical guide* (pp. 13–51). Oxford, UK: Oxford University Press.

Klenerman, L., Slade, P. D., Stanley, I. M., Pennie, B., Reilly, J. P., Atchison, L. E., Troup, J. D., & Rose, M. J. (1995). The prediction of chronicity in patients with an acute attack of low back pain in a general practice setting. *Spine, 20*, 478–484.

Kori, S. H., Miller, R. P., & Todd, D. D. (1990, January/February). Kinesiophobia: A new view of chronic pain behavior. *Pain Management*, 35–43.

Kugler, K., Wijn, J., Geilen, M., de Jong, J., & Vlaeyen, J. W. S. (1999). *The Photograph series of Daily Activities (PHODA)* [CD-ROM version 1.0]. Heerlen, The Netherlands: Institute for Rehabilitation Research and School for Physiotherapy.

Larsen, D. K., Taylor, S., & Asmundson, G. J. (1997). Exploratory factor analysis of the Pain Anxiety Symptoms Scale in patients with chronic pain complaints. *Pain, 69*, 27–34.

Lethem, J., Slade, P. D., Troup, J. D., & Bentley, G. (1983). Outline of a fear-avoidance model of exaggerated pain perception: I. *Behaviour Research and Therapy 21*, 401–408.

Lindström, I., Ohlund, C., Eek, C., Wallin, L., Peterson, L. E., Fordyce, W. E., & Nachemson, A. L. (1992). The effect of graded activity on patients with subacute low back pain: A randomized prospective clinical study with an operant-conditioning behavioral approach. *Physical Therapy, 72*, 279–290.

Linton, S. J. (1998). The socioeconomic impact of chronic back pain: Is anyone benefiting? [Editorial]. *Pain, 75*, 163–168.

Linton, S. J., Buer, N., Vlaeyen, J. W. S., & Hellsing, A.-L. (2000). Are fear-avoidance beliefs related to the inception of an episode of back pain? A prospective study. *Psychology and Health, 14*, 1051–1059.

Linton, S. J., & Hallden, K. (1998). Can we screen for problematic back pain? A screening questionnaire for predicting outcome in acute and subacute back pain. *Clinical Journal of Pain, 14*, 209–215.

Linton, S.J., Overmeer, T., Janson, M., Vlaeyen, J.W.S., de Jong, J.R. (in press) Graded *in-vivo* exposure treatment for fear-avoidant pain patients with functional disability: A case study. *Cognitive Behavioural Therapy.*

McCracken, L. M., & Dhingra, L. (2002). A short version of the Pain Anxiety Symptoms Scale (Pass-20): Preliminary development and validity. *Pain Research and Management, 7*, 45–50.

McCracken, L. M., & Gross, R. T. (1993). Does anxiety affect coping with chronic pain? *Clinical Journal of Pain, 9*, 253–259.

McCracken, L. M., Zayfert, C., & Gross, R. T. (1992). The Pain Anxiety Symptoms Scale: Development and validation of a scale to measure fear of pain. *Pain, 50*, 67–73.

McDonald, I. G., Daly, J., Jelinek, V. M., Panetta, F., & Gutman, J. M. (1996). Opening Pandora's box: The unpredictability of reassurance by a normal test result. *British Medical Journal, 313*(7053), 329–332.

Miller, R. P., Kori, S. H., & Todd, D.D. (1991). *The Tampa Scale for Kinisophobia.* Unpublished report, Tampa, FL.

Mineka, S., Mystkowski, J. L., Hladek, D., & Rodriguez, B. I. (1999). The effects of changing contexts on return of fear following exposure therapy for spider fear. *Journal of Consulting and Clinical Psychology, 67*, 599–604.

Moore, J. E., Von Korff, M., Cherkin, D., Saunders, K., & Lorig, K. (2000). A randomized trial of a cognitive-behavioral program for enhancing back pain self-care in a primary care setting. *Pain, 88*, 145–153.

Morley, S., Eccleston, C., & Williams, A. (1999). Systematic review and meta-analysis of randomized controlled trials of cognitive behaviour therapy and behaviour therapy for chronic pain in adults, excluding headache. *Pain, 80*, 1–13.

Philips, H. C. (1987). Avoidance behaviour and its role in sustaining chronic pain. *Behavior Research and Therapy, 25*, 273–279.

Rachman, S. (1977). The conditioning theory of fear-acquisition: A critical examination. *Behavior Resarch and Therapy, 15*, 375–387.

Rachman, S., & Whittal, M. (1989). Fast, slow and sudden reductions in fear. *Behavior Research and Therapy, 27*, 613–620.

Rainville, J., Bagnall, D., & Phalen, L. (1995). Health care providers' attitudes and beliefs about functional impairments and chronic back pain. *Clinical Journal of Pain, 11*, 287–295.

Riley, J. F., Ahern, D. K., & Follick, M. J. (1988). Chronic pain and functional impairment: Assessing beliefs about their relationship. *Archives of Physical Medicine and Rehabilitation, 69*, 579–582.

Rowe, M. K., & Craske, M. G. (1998a). Effects of an expanding-spaced vs massed exposure schedule on fear reduction and return of fear. *Behavior Research and Therapy, 36*, 701–717.

Rowe, M. K., & Craske, M. G. (1998b). Effects of varied-stimulus exposure training on fear reduction and return of fear. *Behavior Research and Therapy, 36*, 719–734.

Salkovskis, P. M., Clark, D. M., Hackmann, A., Wells, A., & Gelder, M. G. (1999). An experimental investigation of the role of safety-seeking behaviours in the maintenance of panic disorder with agoraphobia. *Behavior Research and Therapy, 37*, 559–574.

Severeijns, R., Vlaeyen, J. W., van den Hout, M. A., & Weber, W. E. (2001). Pain catastrophizing predicts pain intensity, disability, and psychological distress independent of the level of physical impairment. *Clinical Journal of Pain, 17*, 165–172.

Sieben, J. M., Vlaeyen, J. W. S., Tuerlinckx, S., & Portegijs, P. (in press). Pain-related fear in acute low back pain: The first two weeks of a new episode. *European Journal of Pain.*

Smeets, G., de Jong, P. J., & Mayer, B. (2000). If you suffer from a headache, then you have a brain tumour: Domain-specific reasoning "bias" and hypochondriasis. *Behavior Research and Therapy, 38*, 763–776.

Sullivan, M. J. L., Bishop, S. R., & Pivik, J. (1995). The Pain Catastrophizing Scale: Development and validation. *Psychological Assessment, 7*, 524–532.

Turner, J. A. (1996). Educational and behavioral interventions for back pain in primary care. *Spine, 21*, 2851–2857.

Vlaeyen, J. W. S., de Jong, J., Geilen, M., Heuts, P. H., & van Breukelen, G. (in press). The treatment of fear of movement/(re)injury in chronic low back pain: Further evidence for the effectiveness of exposure *in vivo. Clinical Journal of Pain.*

Vlaeyen, J. W. S., de Jong, J., Geilen, M., Heuts, P. H., & van Breukelen, G. (2001). Graded exposure *in vivo* in the treatment of pain-related fear: A replicated single-case experimental design in four patients with chronic low back pain. *Behavior Research and Therapy, 39*, 151–166.

Vlaeyen, J. W. S., de Jong, J., Onghena, P., Kerckhoffs-Hanssen, M., Kole-Snijders, A. M. J. (in press). Can pain-related fear be reduced? The application of cognitive-behavioural exposure *in vivo* in chronic low back pain. *Pain Research and Management.*

Vlaeyen, J. W., Kole-Snijders, A. M., Boeren, R. G., & van Eek, H. (1995). Fear of movement/(re)injury in chronic low back pain and its relation to behavioral performance. *Pain, 62*, 363–372.

Vlaeyen, J. W. S., Kole-Snijders, A. M. J., Rotteveel, A. M., Ruesink, R., & Heuts, P. H. T. G. (1995). The role of fear of movement/(re)injury in pain disability. *Journal of Occupational Rehabilitation, 5*, 235–252.

Vlaeyen, J. W., & Linton, S. J. (2000). Fear-avoidance and its consequences in chronic musculoskeletal pain: A state of the art. *Pain, 85*, 317–332.

Vlaeyen, J. W. S., Nooyen-Haazen, I. W. C. J., Goossens, M. E. J. B., van Breukelen, G., Heuts,

P. H. T. G., & Goei The, H. (1997). The role of fear in the cognitive-educational treatment of fibromyalgia. In T. S. Jensen, J. A. Turner, & Z. Wiesenfeld-Hallin (Eds.), *Proceedings of the 8th World Congress on Pain* (Vol. 8, pp. 693–704). Seattle, WA: IASP Press.

Vlaeyen, J. W., Seelen, H. A., Peters, M., de Jong, P., Aretz, E., Beisiegel, E., & Weber, W. E. (1999). Fear of movement/(re)injury and muscular reactivity in chronic low back pain patients: An experimental investigation. *Pain, 82,* 297–304.

Waddell, G. (1998). *The back pain revolution.* Edinburgh: Churchill Livingstone.

Waddell, G., Newton, M., Henderson, I., Somerville, D., & Main, C. J. (1993). A Fear-Avoidance Beliefs Questionnaire (FABQ) and the role of fear- avoidance beliefs in chronic low back pain and disability. *Pain, 52,* 157–168.

Wolpe, J. (1958). *Psychotherapy by reciprocal inhibition.* Stanford, CA: Stanford University Press.

11

Group Therapy for Patients with Chronic Pain

Francis J. Keefe
Pat M. Beaupre
Karen M. Gil
Meredith E. Rumble
Ann K. Aspnes

Pain is a private experience that has important social consequences. Knowing that someone is experiencing pain changes the way we treat and respond to that person. The social responses to pain, in turn, can affect how the individual copes with pain. People who receive support and encouragement for their attempts to remain active and involved in life, despite persistent pain, often have less severe pain and a better ability to tolerate pain. Individuals, however, whose access to support and attention is limited only to the times they are having difficulty coping with pain often have high levels of pain and are much more disabled.

Given that pain occurs in a social context, it is not surprising that psychologists have emphasized the utility of group therapy approaches in helping patients learn to cope with persistent and disabling pain. Group therapy approaches have many advantages. First, a group provides a setting in which chronic pain patients can be exposed to other individuals having similar problems and learn that they are not alone in experiencing behavioral and psychological problems. Second, group therapy can help patients gain a much better understanding of pain and the role that their own behavior, thoughts, and feelings can play in influencing pain. Third, group therapy can teach patients specific and effective coping skills and provide concrete demonstrations of how one can use these skills to deal with difficult situations such as pain flare-ups. Finally, group therapy enables one to treat a larger number of patients in a more cost-effective fashion than individual therapy.

Over the past decade, group therapy has emerged as one of the major forms of psychological treatment for persistent pain. Controlled research studies evaluating the efficacy of group therapy interventions have been conducted with patients suffering from low back pain (Basler, Jaekle, & Kroener-Herwig, 1997; Newton-John, Spence, & Schotte, 1995; Nicholas, Wilson, & Goyen, 1991; Turner & Jensen, 1993), rheumatoid arthritis (Bradley et al., 1987; Parker et al., 1988), osteoarthritis (Keefe et al., 1990), and facial pain (Harrison, Watson, & Feinmann, 1997). These studies have demonstrated that group therapy can significantly reduce pain and improve the psychological and physical functioning of many patients with chronic pain.

Although there is an emerging research literature on the efficacy of group therapy for pain patients, practical information on how one conducts such groups is not widely available. The purpose of this chapter is to address such a need. We divided the chapter into three sections. The first section discusses three types of group therapy used in the management of chronic pain: coping skills training groups, patient education groups, and social support groups. The second section provides an overview of the methods used in a cognitive-behavioral pain management group, including such practical topics as providing a rationale for group therapy, training in pain coping skills, and introducing methods for helping patients maintain treatment gains. The third section of this chapter focuses on important clinical issues in conducting group therapy with patients who have chronic pain.

Basic Approaches to Group Therapy for Chronic Pain

Group therapy approaches for chronic pain typically focus on one of three major goals: (1) teaching pain coping skills, (2) educating patients about their pain or disease, or (3) providing social support. The specific goal is important in determining the basic format and structure of the group, the types of patients treated, and the level of training required by the group therapist.

Cognitive-Behavioral Therapy Pain Coping Skills Groups

Pain coping skills groups are based on the assumption that, with instruction and practice, patients will be able to acquire and maintain a new set of coping skills that will help them reduce pain and improve day-to-day functioning. The groups are structured to facilitate the learning of cognitive and behavioral pain coping skills. They are typically small (six to nine patients) and provide patients with many opportunities for practice and feedback. Coping skills training groups are usually closed (i.e., scheduled so that all patients start and end treatment together). Treatment is short term (8–10 weeks) and focuses on the acquisition of a variety of behavioral and cognitive pain coping skills. The format is structured and emphasizes instruction, rehearsal, and prac-

tice with pain coping skills. Although patients are provided with a common core of training experiences, the need to tailor these training experiences to address the unique problems experienced by the patient is emphasized. Therapists usually follow a treatment manual that provides details on the methods to be used in each session. Many of these manuals are available by contacting researchers who have conducted randomized clinical trials of pain coping skills.

Patients who are most appropriate for therapy groups focused on pain coping skills are those who accept the fact that their pain is likely to persist and who are open and willing to learn new pain management skills. Because most groups use written materials and require patients to keep home diary records of practice, an ability to read and write is necessary. Patients who lack formal education can also benefit from these groups if arrangements are made to assist them with written assignments. Pain coping skills groups often are made up of individuals having a similar duration of pain (e.g., chronic) and a similar type of pain problem (e.g., back pain or headaches). This similarity increases the likelihood that patients will share common problems and issues in managing pain.

Pain coping skills interventions are typically led by doctoral-level psychologists who have a background in pain management. This high level of training is helpful because of the fact that many of the interventions focus on changing long-standing behaviors and beliefs that may be tied to complex and emotionally difficult issues. Pain coping skills interventions led by individuals with lower levels of formal training in psychology are also becoming popular, though these intervention programs typically either screen out patients with complex emotional problems or focus primarily on basic coping skills and avoid training techniques that are targeted on changing more challenging cognitions and emotions.

Evidence for the effectiveness of cognitive-behavioral and behavioral group therapy interventions for chronic pain is strong. Studies have shown that these group therapy approaches can significantly reduce pain and improve functional status when compared to control conditions (Cole, 1998; Keefe et al., 1990; Linton & Andersson,

2000; Linton & Ryberg, 2001). Studies suggest that patients who show the greatest increases in the use and perceived effectiveness of cognitive and behavioral pain coping skills over the course of group therapy are likely to have the best short- and long-term outcomes (Keefe et al., 1990; Parker et al., 1989).

Patient Education Groups

Group therapy interventions also can focus primarily on educating patients about their pain or disease. The basic assumption underlying this approach is that information can lead to improved knowledge and a much better adjustment to persistent pain. A good example of group therapy approaches to patient education is Kate Lorig's early research on arthritis pain (Lorig, Lubeck, Kraines, Seleznick, & Holman, 1985). Lorig developed a six-session educational course, entitled the Arthritis Self-Help Group, designed to provide basic information about arthritis and its treatment. The course used a small-group format. Each session included a didactic lecture presentation and opportunities for group discussion. Visual aids and handouts were used to supplement the lecture material. The course leaders included not only nurses and other health professionals but also laypeople who themselves suffered from arthritis. Topics covered in the course included the nature of arthritis, methods of diagnosis, medical and surgical treatments, and home remedies. Participants were given tests before and after the completion of the group sessions to evaluate improvements in their knowledge about arthritis. The Arthritis Self-Help group materials are available through the Arthritis Foundation and have been widely used to set up educational groups in community settings.

Patient education groups are currently used with a wide range of patients. Patient education interventions are often used with patients whose pain is related to a disease such as arthritis or cancer. Because the focus is on information rather than change in coping skills, a lower level of patient motivation may be required. Patients must, however, be willing to attend sessions on a regular basis.

Patient education interventions traditionally have been conducted by nurses. As noted previously, Lorig and colleagues (1985) have successfully used laypeople suffering from arthritis as educational group therapists. Research is needed to assess the relative effectiveness of trained nurses and laypersons as therapists leading patient education groups.

Patient education groups are widely employed in medical settings. Evidence for the efficacy of these groups is limited. Most studies show that while they are effective in increasing patient knowledge, the improvements in knowledge that are achieved often fail to correspond to improvements in pain and functional status (Daltroy & Liang, 1988; Goeppinger, Arthur, Baglioni, Brunk, & Brunner, 1989). Based on these findings, Lorig and her colleagues began incorporating behavioral and cognitive-behavioral coping skills training interventions into their patient education courses (Holman, Mazonson, & Lorig, 1989). These more comprehensive group therapy protocols appear to be more effective than patient information group sessions alone.

Social Support Groups

Group therapy interventions for chronic pain may also have as their primary goal increasing social support. Social support groups are based on the idea that many people who have chronic pain feel isolated and alone in coping with pain and may benefit from the support and encouragement of others in the same situation.

Informal social support groups for chronic pain sufferers are available in many communities.[1] The format for these groups varies widely, but typically it is much less structured than for cognitive-behavioral or educational group therapy approaches. Although there may be a brief didactic component, most of each group session is devoted to discussion of participants' experiences in coping with pain. Group leaders are typically people having chronic pain. Their role is often intentionally limited to administrative issues (identifying a meeting place, scheduling session) so that they can still participate as regular group members. Leadership of the group may change from session to session to avoid one individual having primary responsibility for the group. Support group sessions may be scheduled weekly or monthly, with the number of sessions varying widely across groups. The group sessions are typically open with patients free to participate in as many or as few sessions as they like.

The research literature on social support groups for chronic pain is sparse. One of the few studies that have included a social support therapy condition in a controlled treatment outcome study noted that this group did reduce psychological distress in chronic pain patients (Bradley et al., 1987). In a study of osteoarthritis patients conducted in our lab, we found that a group focused on education and spousal social support produced no significant improvements in pain and disability (Keefe et al., 1996, 1999). The efficacy of social support groups in reducing pain and disability in chronic pain patients, however, has yet to be determined.

A Practical Guide to Cognitive-Behavioral Group Therapy for Pain Management

A number of practical issues need to be addressed in carrying out group therapy for patients with persistent pain. These issues include getting the group started, helping patients cope with their pain, and developing a plan to help patients maintain progress once group therapy has ended. In this section we draw on our experience with cognitive-behavioral therapy groups for training in pain coping skills, to address these practical issues (see also Turk, Chapter 7, this volume).

Screening Patients for Group Therapy

Patients who have chronic pain differ in terms of their ability to benefit from group therapy. It is important to interview patients first to determine whether they are appropriate candidates for group therapy. Patients who do best in pain coping skills training groups are those who are willing to attend group sessions regularly and to take an active role in their own pain management. Those who have behavioral problems (e.g., inactivity and excessive dependence on others), cognitive problems (e.g., overly negative thoughts about themselves, others,

or the future), or emotional problems (e.g., anxiety and depression) that can serve as targets for group therapy efforts also tend to respond well. Patients who are extremely angry and hostile may be inappropriate for group therapy. These patients often ruminate about their negative experiences with medical personnel and can monopolize group sessions. They often fail to respond to corrective feedback from therapists or group members. Severely depressed patients are also poor candidates for group therapy. These individuals are often so withdrawn that they are unable to interact in the group setting. Some chronic pain patients have extreme fears of social situations, particularly groups, and are thus better treated through individual therapy. Patients with low levels of intelligence may have difficulty with the cognitive therapy components of group therapy. Nevertheless, we have found that many people who have limited formal education benefit substantially from cognitive-behavioral group therapy. These individuals sometimes require additional assistance during and after the group sessions to maximize their response, but when provided with such assistance they often respond quite positively.

During the initial screening interview, a careful behavioral assessment of the patient's pain problems should be carried out. We have previously discussed the basic elements of cognitive-behavioral interviewing for patients who have persistent pain (Keefe, 1988). These elements include (1) an assessment of the intensity, location, and quality of the patient's pain; (2) identification of factors that increase or decrease pain; (3) a review of the patient's family and work activities to examine patterns of pain and well behavior; (4) an assessment of cognitive factors such as beliefs about pain (e.g., my pain is a punishment for my actions), irrational cognitions (e.g., because I have pain, I am a worthless individual), and negative expectations (e.g., the future is hopeless); and (5) an analysis of emotional responses that may be contributing to pain (e.g. depression, anxiety, or guilt). The interview provides the group therapist with an indication of the cognitive and behavioral problems experienced by the patient. These problems can then be targeted for intervention in group therapy.

As part of the screening process, each patient should be provided with a basic description of the group. Information should be given on the number of participants, frequency of sessions, and basic goals of the group. In addition, the therapist should highlight how the group can help the patient with his or her specific problems in coping with pain.

Structure of the Group

Pain coping skills sessions can be structured in a variety of ways. When setting up a group, one is faced with decisions as the number, length, and timing of sessions; the size of the group; whether the group is to be open to new members or closed; and the training of therapists.

Most group therapy pain coping skills programs are relatively short in duration (e.g., 6 to 12 sessions). Sessions are usually 1½ to 2 hours in duration. We typically schedule sessions once a week for outpatients and on a daily basis for inpatients or outpatients who are enrolled in intensive daily treatment programs. We recommend running the sessions late in the day (e.g., 4:00–6:00 P.M.) because it provides group leaders with an opportunity to review how patients applied learned pain coping methods earlier in the day. We typically conduct groups of four to eight patients. When fewer than four patients are enrolled the cohesiveness of the group may be threatened if a patient misses a session. When there are more than eight patients in a group, it is usually difficult to provide enough time for individualized skills rehearsal and feedback.

Pain coping skills groups typically use a closed-group format in which all patients start and complete the group together. The description of group therapy methods that follow is based on such a format. However, we have also found that these groups can be carried out using an open format in which each participant may start and complete the group at different time points. An open-group format is particularly well suited to an inpatient setting in which patients may have varying lengths of stay. In an open group, pain coping skills are taught using modules that can be introduced at any point in treatment. In these groups we typically begin each session by reviewing each patients status in order to target particular cognitive problems (e.g., excessive worry) or behavioral problems (e.g., excessive tension evident in pain avoidant posturing) that need intervention. We then introduce a module (e.g., relaxation training) designed to address a problem shared by several group members. Invariably in an open group there are some patients who have been in the group for a while who have been exposed to a particular module previously. These veteran participants are asked to describe how the methods worked for them. The modeling provided by these more experienced patients can play a key role in prompting newer group members to get involved in treatment.

We usually use two co-therapists to run group therapy sessions. We prefer that at least one of the therapists is a doctoral-level clinical psychologist with thorough training and experience in cognitive-behavioral approaches to pain management. A psychology trainee or other mental health specialist (e.g., social worker or psychiatric nurse) can serve as a co-therapist.

The First Group Session

The first session of pain coping skills training is focused on establishing the basic structure and rationale for treatment. An effort is made to help group members become acquainted and ground rules for the group are discussed. Patients are also given a chance to discuss their adaptations to persistent pain. Finally, a rationale for group therapy is presented that emphasizes how coping skills training can be used to control and decrease pain.

WARMUP AND GROUND RULES OF GROUP

The first therapy session begins with the therapists introducing themselves and describing their roles in the group. To help group members get acquainted, it is often helpful to use a warmup exercise. We usually ask each patient to pair off with another patient and spend 10 minutes becoming acquainted (i.e., learning something about the each other's pain), family situation, and general interests. At the end of 10 minutes, each patient returns to the group and introduces his or her partner rather than him- or herself. After everyone is introduced, the participants' reactions to the warmup exercise are discussed. The warmup exercise is a good way to get participants to talk and helps them realize that they share much with other group members. The exercise also invariably engenders some good-natured joking when participants are making introductions and find that they have forgotten some information about their partner.

Basic information about the group and general group rules and expectations are also discussed with patients. The patients are told that each group session deals with a different topic and a list of each of the topics is typically reviewed. The therapists start and end each group session on time so it is important that patients come to every group session and be on time. In the event a patient knows he or she will miss a session, the patient is asked to announce this absence in the group session the week preceding his or her absence. Patients are given phone numbers where therapists may be reached in case of an emergency or if they unexpectedly need to miss a group session. To protect confidentiality, the participants are also requested not to discuss personal matters raised during the group sessions outside the group.

ADAPTATION TO PAIN

To help group members understand how pain has changed their lives we use an adaptation model. Figure 11.1 is a simple diagram that can be drawn on the board to illustrate this model. The model starts with the basic assumption that every group member has a pain problem that has gone on for some time. As pain has persisted, patients' lives have changed in some important ways.

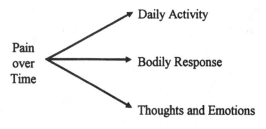

FIGURE 11.1. Adaptation model.

Some of these adjustments to pain have been helpful; others have not been. To focus the discussion on issues relevant to pain coping skills training, group members are asked to discuss life changes they have noted in three major areas: (1) daily activities (e.g., how active they are overall and what they are able to do and not able to do), (2) bodily responses (e.g., sleep disruption and muscle weakness), and (3) thoughts and emotions (e.g., negative thoughts about themselves or others and feelings of depression, anger, or guilt). This discussion gives patients a chance to talk about their pain history and learn that they have much in common with other group members. It also increases patients' level of comfort about talking in a group setting.

We begin the discussion of the adaptation model by having group members talk about how their activities have changed in response to persistent pain. This is a good topic to start with because it is relatively nonthreatening and a problem area for most patients. Group members can easily identify specific changes that have occurred in their lives, such as a decrease in time spent up and out of bed, an inability to work or carry our household chores, and an increase in pain-related behaviors such as taking medications, going to the doctor, or talking about pain. Typically, there are patients in the group who are able to recognize that the changes they have made to avoid pain (e.g., reclining in bed) can in turn have long-term negative consequences for pain coping (e.g., a decreased tolerance for activity).

After discussing changes in activity, the group members are asked to discuss changes in bodily responses that have developed as pain has persisted. Group members often report being bothered by a low energy level and difficulty sleeping. This may be due to the physical deconditioning that occurs when patients spend excessive time in bed. The group therapist tries to help patients become aware of how adaptations to pain in one area (e.g., activities) can affect other major areas (e.g., bodily responses).

We typically delay a discussion of the impact of chronic pain on thoughts and emotions until the latter part of the discussion about adjustment to pain. Some patients are reluctant to share their negative feelings and thoughts with others. They may fear that they will be seen as emotionally disturbed or that their pain will not be taken seriously. Delaying discussion of this topic helps overcome this problem by giving patients an opportunity to become more comfortable with each other. In addition, reports of changes in feelings and thoughts often emerge spontaneously during discussion of changes in activities and bodily responses. We have found that once one or two group members open up and discuss changes in their thoughts and feelings, other group members are usually willing to share their own experiences. Occasionally, a few patients have difficulty identifying changes in their thoughts and feelings. To deal with this problem we typically prompt the participants to review the changes in their daily activities that have occurred and ask them to reflect on what they think and feel about these changes.

In closing the discussion of the adaptation model, the group leader points out that a major goal of pain coping skills training is to alter how patients adapt to pain. Patients will learn new coping strategies to help them better adapt to pain.

RATIONALE FOR COPING SKILLS TRAINING

Helping patients reconceptualize their pain and their own ability to control pain is one of the most important goals of pain coping skills training (Turk, Meichenbaum, & Genest, 1983). To accomplish this goal, we typically use a simplified version of the gate control theory (Melzack & Wall, 1965). Figure 11.2 illustrates this model. The diagram includes a representation of the basic elements of the traditional pain pathway, including (1) special nerves that pick up pain signals in the periphery at the site of injury, (2) spinal nerves that carry pain signals to the brain, and (3) sensory areas of the brain where pain is experienced. Not only is the traditional pain pathway described, but its limitations are also discussed. For example, the pain pathway concept fails to explain phenomena such as the presence of pain following limb amputation (phantom limb pain) and the surprising lack of pain that

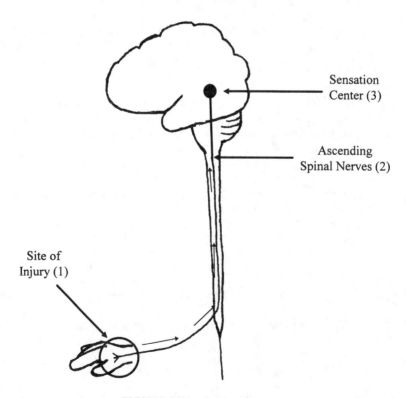

FIGURE 11.2. Pain pathway.

has been evident in some soldiers injured in battle. Group members are encouraged to share puzzling experiences that they or others have had with pain. Many patients, for example, report having been surprised in the past when they had little or no pain following a sports injury suffered during an important game. Other patients have friends or family members who have suffered from phantom limb pain or other unusual pain phenomena.

The gate control model is presented as an alternative to the pain pathway model. To illustrate this model a schematic depiction of a gate is added to the pain pathway diagram, as shown in Figure 11.3. Patients are told that the gate can be fully or partially opened or closed, determining the intensity of pain that is experienced. The role that thoughts and emotions can play in opening and closing the gate is described. Group members are asked to identify specific thoughts and emotions that they have noticed which influence their pain and may affect the gate-control mechanism. Patients often mention guilt, anger, depression, and anxiety as emotions that might open the gate, and happiness and feeling calm as emotions that might close the gate. Negative thoughts that might increase pain often include "I can't deal with this anymore" or "No one really cares about or understands my pain." Patients often recognize that distracting activities (e.g., reading a favorite book and listening to music) can change their negative thinking and reduce pain. If group members have difficulty identifying factors that influence pain, it is often helpful to prompt them by referring back to the thoughts and feelings that were identified in the earlier group discussion of adaptations to pain.

Patients are told that the purpose of group therapy is to help them learn skills for

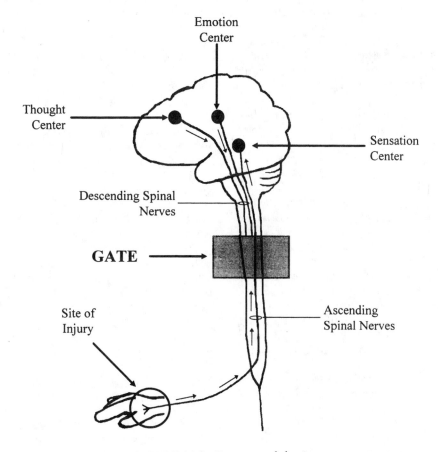

FIGURE 11.3. Gate control theory.

controlling pain by changing the thoughts and emotions that affect pain. Patients are told that they will be exposed in subsequent group sessions to a menu of pain coping skills. The coping skills menu is compared to a menu in any fine restaurant. Each skill item on the menu is designed to be consistently high in quality and on certain days, or in specific situations, one skill from the menu may be preferred over the others. Emphasizing that group members have choices and control over coping is important because research has shown that these factors can influence perceived pain (Litt, 1988). The importance of regular home practice in the development of effective coping skills is also emphasized and patients are told that they will be given home assignments that will be reviewed at the start of each group therapy session.

It is important to discuss patients' reactions to the aforementioned rationale. Often, the gate control model validates an experience with pain that a group member has had (e.g., increased pain when feeling depressed or angry) but has been reluctant to discuss with others. Group members generally respond quite favorably to this rationale. After the rationale is presented, group members often report that this is the first time they feel like someone has understood their pain and that they now believe they might be able to develop some control over their pain.

COMMENT

Getting a group started is, in many ways, the most important phase of group therapy. If the group leaders are perceived as competent and willing to help the patients, patients are more apt to develop positive expectations and to be motivated to actively participate in treatment. The first therapy session provides an opportunity for each of the group members to discuss their pain in a nonthreatening environment. In hearing other's stories, the participants develop a realization that they are not alone in their pain experiences. Because of the importance of the first session, we usually spend considerable time training new therapists in how to present this session.

The first session of coping skills training also gives many patients their first exposure to an alternative to the medical model of pain management. Conceptualizing pain using Melzack and Wall's (1965) model assists patients in seeing their pain differently. It also helps focus them on the importance of learning new pain coping skills.

Pain Coping Skills Education

The second phase of cognitive-behavioral group therapy is devoted to teaching pain coping skills. To illustrate this phase of treatment, we discuss the basic format of pain coping skills sessions and the methods used for teaching patients relaxation, activity–rest cycling, and attention diversion strategies.

BASIC FORMAT OF COPING SKILLS SESSIONS

The coping skills training phase typically begins with the second group therapy session and continues for 6 to 10 sessions. Each session begins with a review of group members' home practice over the past week. We ask participants to keep home diary records of practice. The therapist reviews the records and reinforces those patients who have been able to practice regularly. Problem-solving methods are used to assist patients who have had difficulty with their practice. Specific obstacles to practice (e.g., lack of free time and frequent interruptions during relaxation practice) are identified and the patient with help from the group is asked to identify potential ways to overcome these obstacles. Group members often have innovative solutions to problems in practicing. Having patients share these solutions with each other is a good way to model problem-solving skills.

During the review of home practice, group members are asked to discuss how they have applied pain coping skills in real-life situations in which pain is likely to be a problem. In particular, patients are asked to share information about any situations in which they were able to use pain coping skills to control or decrease their pain. A key emphasis is on having people who have experienced successes in coping model adaptive coping for others. This sharing is beneficial in two ways. First, the patient who has experienced success has an opportunity to get encouragement and positive feedback from other group members. Second, reports of success often motivate other group members to continue with their practice.

Behavioral rehearsal is one of the most effective ways to teach pain coping skills practice sessions in group therapy. Behavioral rehearsal involves therapist instruction in a coping skill, patient rehearsal, and therapist feedback. Before beginning behavioral rehearsal we assess baseline pain level by having patients perform an activity for 15 to 30 seconds that will increase their pain somewhat (e.g., walking and transferring from a sitting to a standing position). Care is taken to ensure that each group member is able to perform the activity they have chosen without causing too much of an increase in pain. At the end of the activity, each group member rates the pain they experienced using a 0- to 100-point scale on which 0 = no pain and 100 = pain as bad as it can be. The therapist then teaches the group members a specific pain coping skill (e.g., relaxation) and models how this skill might be applied during the specific activities chosen by group members. The group members are then asked to apply the coping skill while they perform the pain-inducing activity. During rehearsal, the therapist provides feedback on performance along with suggestions about how to best use the coping skill. After the group discusses their reactions, each group member is asked to rehearse using the pain coping skill on his or her own while engaging in the pain-inducing activity. Each group member then rates his or her pain on a 0 to 100 scale and these pain ratings are compared to those taken at baseline. Many patients are surprised to find that when they apply the pain coping skill they are able to reduce their pain by 25% to 40%. Reasons for reductions in pain (e.g., distraction from pain and relaxation of tense muscles) are discussed in the group. The therapist also encourages patients who failed to achieve pain relief to discuss their reactions to the exercise. Possible explanations for a lack of change in pain include individual differences in responsiveness to different coping skills and the need for additional practice to achieve mastery of the skill. Most patients report an increased sense of self-efficacy after going through the behavioral rehearsal exercise. Behavioral rehearsal can even be helpful for those patients who do not experience immediate pain relief. These patients benefit from the positive modeling provided by other patients and often report being more optimistic about the outcome of coping skills training.

Home practice assignments are reviewed at the end of each coping skills training session. The assignments are written down and are very specific (e.g., listening to the relaxation tape once a day). They are also graduated in terms of difficulty, with earlier assignments being easier and later assignments requiring more time and skill. This graduated approach to home practice is important for two reasons. First, it helps patients more easily phase the coping skills into their daily routine. Second, it challenges patients to gradually extend the application of coping skills to a much broader range of daily activities and events.

Readings and handouts can provide useful adjuncts to group therapy. For each coping skills session, we typically give patients a one- to two-page handout that provides a brief review of the rationale and recommended home practice procedures. Patients are encouraged to read the information on the handout between sessions. The handouts also serve as reference material after the group ends.

RELAXATION TRAINING

Relaxation training is one of the most widely used and effective pain coping skills (see also Syrjala & Abrams, Chapter 9, this volume). Relaxation training can be easily carried out in group therapy sessions. Because patients respond so readily to relaxation training, we usually introduce it early in the course of pain coping skills training.

Conceptual Background. From a conceptual standpoint, there are a variety of reasons that relaxation training is helpful in pain control. First, relaxation methods can help break the link between stressful events and pain. Severe stressors can produce autonomic arousal and emotional reactions that can exacerbate pain (Keefe & Gil, 1986). Research has shown that stressors such as family conflict and job disruption are related to increased pain in chronic low back pain patients (Feuerstein, Sult, & Houle, 1985). Second, relaxation methods can reduce muscle spasm and tension, which have long been thought to be an important cause of chronic pain (Travell, Rinzler, & Herman, 1943). Through relaxation training, patients can learn to control spasm and excessive tension in specific muscle groups that are contributing to their pain (e.g., the upper trapezius muscles for a patient having neck pain following a whiplash injury). Third, relaxation training may be useful in altering abnormal patterns of muscle activity that contribute to pain. Patients who engage in abnormal pain avoidant posturing when walking or transferring from one position to another often report increased pain and fatigue. By applying relaxation methods such as biofeedback training, these patients can learn to reduce pain by decreasing excessive tension and normalizing their movements (Wolf, Nacht, & Kelly, 1982). Finally, relaxation training can reduce emotional responding during pain episodes. The gate control theory (Melzack & Wall, 1965) highlights the role that emotional responses such as depression and anger can play in exacerbating pain. After going through relaxation training, patients often report that they can maintain a calmer emotional disposition during episodes of increased pain. As a result, the intensity and duration of the pain are reduced.

Before beginning relaxation training, it is important to discuss patients' beliefs and concerns about relaxation methods. Most patients readily grasp the role that relaxation training can play in pain control. Some patients, however, may be worried about using relaxation methods. A common concern is that the therapist, not the patient, will be in control during relaxation. It is important to acknowledge such fears and to point out that they are common (Bernstein & Borkovec, 1973). Patients can be reassured that they will be in control of both the timing and level of tension and relaxation during the relaxation practice sessions. Allowing patients to keep their eyes open during relaxation practice can be helpful in overcoming many concerns about loss of control.

Progressive Relaxation Training. When teaching relaxation training in group thera-

py, we use a protocol developed by Surwit (1979) that is a modified version of Jacobson's (1938) original progressive muscle relaxation method. This protocol consists of a series of exercises in which the individual tenses and slowly relaxes muscle groups starting with muscles in the feet and legs and progressing to muscles in the face and head. The group therapist briefly demonstrates each of the relaxation exercises and then has the patients repeat these exercises. This demonstration and rehearsal of the tense–relax exercises helps the therapist identify patients who may misunderstand the instructions or who may have increased pain or difficulty with particular exercises. To prevent increased pain, patients are urged to use caution when tensing muscle groups surrounding a painful area. If patients are unable because of physical limitations to tense a muscle group, they are simply told to eliminate this particular tense–relax exercise.

After demonstrating the exercises, the therapist guides the group members through a 20-minute relaxation session. During the session, patients are instructed to systematically focus on sensations of muscle tension as they tense and relax their muscles. The therapist emphasizes the importance of gradually building up and then slowly releasing tension. Patients are asked to pay particular attention to the way their muscles feel when they are tense and, by contrast, when they are relaxed.

At the end of the relaxation session, group members are asked to discuss their reactions. Patients often report that they have less pain and feel much more calm and relaxed. The therapist encourages patients to share any problems that they may have had during the relaxation sessions such as muscle cramping, sleepiness, or difficulty concentrating. Bernstein and Borkovec (1973) have identified a number practical suggestions for overcoming such problems. Cramping, for example, can be avoided by using lower levels of tension during the exercises and holding the tension for shorter periods. Difficulty falling asleep can be minimized by having patients keep their eyes open during the session or by reducing the length of practice periods. Concentration typically becomes less of a problem as patients develop a regular practice schedule.

Involving the group members in identifying and solving problems with relaxation training is a useful way to overcome obstacles to practice and prevent setbacks in coping (Keefe & Van Horn, 1993).

To facilitate home practice, each member of the group can be provided with a relaxation audiotape. The tape we use was developed by Richard Surwit (1979). Patients are instructed to practice with the tape twice a day. It is important that practice be done in a quiet, comfortable place, with no interruptions or time pressures.

Brief Relaxation Methods: The Mini-Practice Technique. We also use the group therapy setting to teach a brief relaxation method (the "mini-practice"). This training is introduced after patients have practiced with progressive relaxation training for one or more weeks and have developed an ability to relax when in a reclining or seated position. Brief relaxation can provide a means of reducing tension or pain when one is unable to go to a quiet area and do a full progressive relaxation practice session.

We use the mini-practice because it takes a short time (20–30 seconds). The therapist initially models the mini-practice while the group members observe. The therapist then guides the patients through a mini-practice with the following instructions: (1) stop whatever activity you are doing, (2) take a deep breath, (3) think the word "relax," (4) as you exhale allow sensations to flow downward from muscles of the face and neck, to those of the arms, trunk, legs, and feet, and (5) hold that feeling of relaxation for 10 to 15 seconds before returning to your activity.

Using behavioral rehearsal, patients are taught to apply mini-practices in a wide variety of situations. Patients are initially taught to use the mini-practices when they are in a quiet, seated position with their eyes closed. Later they are taught to apply this skill during more demanding situations such as while standing, sitting, walking, or conversing. The importance of using mini-practices to achieve differential relaxation is stressed. That is, patients are taught to relax unnecessary tension while maintaining the tension needed to engage in the activity. For example, it is necessary to have some tension in the leg muscles while standing, but

muscles in the neck, shoulders, lower back, and face can be relaxed.

The group setting is an ideal one for training in brief relaxation methods. Patients often serve as effective models for each other, pointing out the situations in which they have been able to use a mini-practice to reduce their pain or tension. Patients are encouraged to identify a variety of real-life situations in which they might have difficulty using mini-practices such as during meetings at work, while bending down to pick something from the floor, or standing in line at the grocery store. The group is then given the task of developing a strategy for using the mini-practice in these situations and then rehearsing that strategy in the group itself.

Patients are initially given the goal of doing five mini-practices a day as part of their home practice. This goal is gradually increased until patients reach 20 mini-practices per day. Given that the mini-practice takes so little time, the goal of 20 mini-practices per day is realistic for most patients. Patients are encouraged to use physiological cues (e.g., increase in pain or tension) and environmental cues (e.g., sitting at a stop light and waiting for an elevator) as reminders to do a mini-practice. In the group sessions, a list of potential cues for doing mini-practices is compiled weekly. This list is helpful in that it provides concrete examples of situations where brief relaxation techniques might be helpful.

ACTIVITY–REST CYCLING

Activity–rest cycling (Gil, Ross, & Keefe, 1988) is a method to help patients control pain by learning to pace their activities to decrease pain and enable them to gradually increase their activity level.

Conceptual Background. As people in pain attempt to perform activities, they often persist until severe pain forces them to stop and rest. Activities that formerly could be performed thus become associated with severe pain. We typically use a simple figure such as that in Figure 11.4 to illustrate the pain cycle. With repetition, the pain cycle (i.e., overactivity leading to extreme pain leading to prolonged rest) becomes an entrenched and maladaptive habit. The nega-

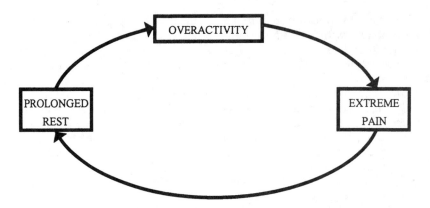

FIGURE 11.4. Pain cycle.

tive consequences of this pain cycle include increased fear of activity, fatigue, muscle tension, decreased tolerance of specific activities (e.g., sitting, standing, or walking), and avoidance of activity (Fordyce, 1976; Gil et al., 1988). Ultimately, patients in this pain cycle adopt an overly sedentary lifestyle in which they spend only minimal amounts of time up and out of the reclining position.

Training in Activity–Rest Cycling. The activity–rest cycle represents an adaptive alternative to the pain cycle. To introduce the activity–rest cycle we draw a simple diagram of the pain cycle and ask group members to discuss the relevance of this cycle for their own pain. Figure 11.5 displays this dia-

gram. Most patients who have chronic pain readily recognize that this cycle has been a major influence on their lives. We usually ask patients to identify the reasons for getting stuck at different points in the cycle (e.g., overdoing activity or resting excessively). Many patients report that external factors (e.g., financial problems and the need to care for young children) are important. Internal factors (e.g., depression, anger, or guilt) also can play a role. Group members also frequently report that they have made unsuccessful attempts to break out of the cycle. Patients also are able to identify the negative impact that the pain cycle has had on their own lives and the lives of their family and friends.

The activity–rest cycle works by making activity levels contingent upon time and not pain (Fordyce, 1976; Gil et al., 1988). Patients set a goal to engage in a period of moderate activity followed by limited rest. Specific time periods for moderate activity (e.g., 30 minutes walking) and limited rest (e.g., 10 minutes sitting) are set. As patients repeat this activity–rest cycle throughout the day, they often their find that their pain is reduced and their tolerance for activity is increased. Over the course of weeks, patients are able to gradually increase their level of activity and decrease the amount of time they spend resting.

Group members are asked to use brainstorming to generate a list of the potential benefits and limitations of activity–rest cycling. Benefits of activity–rest cycling that are often mentioned include the avoidance of extreme pain, fewer and shorter pain

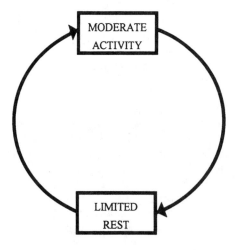

FIGURE 11.5. Activity–rest cycle.

episodes, an increase in productivity, a more stable level of activity, and less tension and fatigue. Limitations of the activity–rest cycle are that it requires recordkeeping, tends to structure the day, and can interrupt ongoing activities. Before implementing the activity–rest cycle, group members are asked to weigh the potential benefits of activity–rest cycle against the limitations. Typically, most patients agree that the benefits are worth the costs involved in acquiring and maintaining this behavioral coping skill.

To implement the activity–rest cycle, a baseline record of current activity patterns is needed. Patients are given a home practice assignment of keeping daily records of the time they spend up and out of a reclining position. Reviewing these records in group sessions can be revealing. Patients are often surprised to find that they are more active than they thought or more active than many other group members. Patients also are usually able to identify pain cycling patterns as they review their own records. It is particularly helpful for patients to realize that, while the specifics may vary, pain cycling is a common pattern. Some patients, for example, are active during the day and then spend almost all their time in the evening reclining. Other patients may have 2 or 3 days of overactivity followed by 4 or 5 days of rest.

The activity–rest cycle involves four basic steps. First, patients set a goal in minutes or hours, for engaging in a moderate amount of activity. Moderate activity is defined as a level of activity that patients can maintain without increasing their pain to a high level. For some patients moderate activity might be spending 30 minutes up and out of bed. For other patients, moderate activity might be working at a word processor for 60 minutes. Second, patients set a goal for a limited rest period that they will take after completing their moderate activity goal. This rest period should be sufficient to enable them to have some pain relief but not so long that their total rest each day exceeds their average rest time during baseline recording. A limited rest period for a sedentary patient might be 30 minutes in bed, whereas for an active patient it might be 5 minutes sitting in a relaxed position. Third, patients are instructed to repeat the cycle of moderate activity followed by limited rest (e.g., 45 minutes up and out of bed, 15 minutes of rest) frequently throughout the day. The goal is to use the cycle at least 70% of the waking day. Patients keep a daily record of the number of repetitions of the activity–rest cycle they are able to achieve. This monitoring helps increase awareness of how to use this skill in a variety of situations and helps reinforce patients for adherence. Fourth, over a period of days to weeks, patients are instructed to gradually increase their goal for moderate activity and decrease their goal for limited rest. The ultimate goal of activity–rest cycling is to enable patients to be able to tolerate up to 1½ to 2 hours of activity followed by a 5- to 10-minute relaxation break.

At the start of each group therapy session, patients' home practice with the activity–rest cycling is reviewed. It is useful initially to have patients who are adhering to the cycle and experiencing success to talk about their experiences. A number of patients may have practical problems implementing this cycle. Group members are asked to identify obstacles to the use of activity–rest cycling and then generate ideas about ways to overcome these obstacles. Obstacles frequently mentioned include simply forgetting about the time limit and feeling embarrassed about the need to rest. Ideas for solving problems are discussed in the group setting and patients are encouraged to think of creative strategies to overcome these problems. For example, several years ago one of our group members who had difficulty following through with the activity–rest cycle brought a digital kitchen timer to one of our group sessions and told group members about how helpful it was in prompting him about when to start and stop activity periods. Since then, we have regularly advised patients about this strategy. Another strategy we use is role playing. Role playing is used to help patients become more comfortable about explaining the activity–rest cycle to family, friends, and coworkers. Role playing helps with feelings of embarrassment and in getting support from others during periods of stress.

In working on activity–rest cycling in group therapy, it may be important to discuss patients' thoughts and feelings about resting. Problems arise when patients fear stopping their activity because of the belief that they will not be able to resume the activity. In addition, some patients view changing their activity levels as "giving in" to their pain and subsequently fight to maintain control by continuing or even increasing their activities. Other patients may believe that resting is a sign of laziness. Reiterating how the pain cycle works, as well as giving these patients permission to rest during their activity, often alleviates these problems.

ATTENTION DIVERSION STRATEGIES

Patients vary in their response to attention diversion strategies (see also Syrjala & Abrams, Chapter 9, this volume). Patients may find one attention diversion strategy (e.g., pleasant imagery) to be quite helpful but report little benefit from another strategy (e.g., counting backwards). Group therapy provides a good setting for training in attention diversion strategies because it gives patients an opportunity to sample different strategies and to be exposed to modeling influences. Patients who have persistent pain often become much more interested in learning specific attention diversion strategies when they observe that these methods work for other patients.

Conceptual Background. There is a large research literature supporting the effectiveness of attention diversion strategies for pain control (McCaul & Malott, 1984). Diverting attention from pain by distraction and refocusing attention on something other than pain, in particular, appear to be effective in pain management (Turk et al., 1983).

Training Methods. To introduce attention diversion strategies, it is helpful to once again review the gate control model (Melzack & Wall, 1965) and emphasize the role that shifting concentration can play in modulating pain perception. We typically instruct patients in three attention diversion techniques: pleasant imagery, focal point, and counting backwards. Patients are reminded that they are in control when using these strategies, which require alertness and concentration. The attention diversion tech-

niques can be used to enhance relaxation, and patients are encouraged to use them either after listening to the relaxation tape or a doing mini-practice. Attention diversion training is usually introduced after patients have practiced with relaxation for several weeks.

Pleasant imagery is one of the most common and effective attention diversion strategies (Turk et al., 1983). It involves shifting attention from an unpleasant situation (e.g., increased pain during prolonged sitting) to an imagined pleasant scene (e.g., reclining on a beach on a warm, sunny day). In teaching pleasant imagery in group therapy, we ask patients to identify and share with the group members pleasant or enjoyable experiences that they have had or would like to have. These experiences might include watching the sun set over a lake, sitting by a brook, walking through a field of flowers on a spring day, or watching a movie with a special friend. Patients are then asked to close their eyes, do a mini-practice, focus on particular pleasant scene, and try to involve all their senses in the imagery. The group therapist cues patients when to start and stop the pleasant imagery with practice periods varying between 2 and 10 minutes. After practicing with imagery, patients are encouraged to discuss their reactions. Patients often report that they find pleasant imagery to be very relaxing. We have found that patients vary greatly in the amount of pain relief they initially experience using imagery. Some patients have substantial decreases in pain, while others report little or no change in pain. Although individual differences are evident in response to imagery, with regular practice most patients are able to develop an ability to control pain using pleasant imagery.

The use of a focal point is a second attention diversion strategy that can be helpful in pain control (Turk et al., 1983). Focal point distraction involves deliberately directing one's attention to objects in the immediate environment (e.g., a picture of a loved one or a floral arrangement) for a 1- to 2-minute period. The focal point has long been used to assist women in coping with labor pain and has been extended to management of chronic pain (Turk et al., 1983).

Counting techniques represent a third attention diversion strategy that can be used to enhance pain control (Turk et al., 1983). We usually ask patients to count backwards slowly by ones from 100 to 1. It is often helpful to think the word "relax" between numbers. Some patients also imagine the numbers by seeing white numbers superimposed on a black screen and having each number melt away or flip over to the next number.

We typically introduce attention diversion over the course of several group sessions. Patients are initially guided through use of the strategies by the therapist and then learn to practice on their own. Behavioral rehearsal, outlined earlier, is used to teach patients how to apply these techniques during activities that increase pain. For problem situations that cannot be rehearsed in group, one can use cognitive rehearsal in which patients imagine themselves applying the strategies in a step-by-step fashion.

After patients have been exposed to each of the attention diversion strategies, they are encouraged to combine them to cope with particularly difficult pain situations. For example, to reduce pain during a flare-up in disease activity, a rheumatoid arthritis patient might use counting techniques while walking and imagery or focal point distraction techniques while resting.

Preparing Patients for Maintenance of Coping Skills

Regular and continued practice of pain coping skills is essential if patients are to achieve effective control over their pain. To help patients maintain treatment gains, it is important that group therapists plan ahead instead of expecting maintenance to occur automatically. Marlatt and Gordon (1985) developed a relapse prevention model during their work with patients who were addicted to alcohol and other drugs. They examine the situational, interpersonal, and emotional factors as well as patients' thought processes surrounding relapse. We have modified this model for use with patients having chronic pain and outlined a number of relapse prevention methods (Keefe & Van Horn, 1993). These methods can be integrated into cognitive-behavioral group therapy sessions.

A discussion of maintenance of pain coping skills should not be left until the last group session. Maintenance issues should be addressed in the initial session and in every group therapy. One way to begin a discussion of maintenance issues is to have group members identify obstacles and high-risk situations that might interfere with their practicing and applying pain coping skills on a daily basis. Group discussion often helps patients identify problem situations that they have not considered. To help patients assess their confidence in their ability to cope with these situations, they are asked to provide ratings on a 0 to 10 scale of their current ability to cope with the situation and the likelihood that the situation might cause them to stop practicing pain coping skills. The ratings are reviewed in the group and similarities and differences in ratings across patients and situations are discussed.

To help patients better cope with setbacks in coping and ensure that these setbacks are minor and temporary, group training is provided in a four-step relapse prevention method (Marlatt & Gordon, 1985). The first step involves stopping and paying attention to the cues that a setback is occurring. The second step is to keep calm, using relaxation or other strategies to prevent overly emotional responding. The third step is to review the situation leading up to the setback. The final step is to make an immediate plan for implementing coping.

Patients have an opportunity in the group therapy session to role-play how they might cope with setbacks and relapse situations. With rehearsal and therapist feedback, patients are often able to develop a higher level of confidence in their ability to cope with high-risk situations.

Clinical Issues in Group Therapy

Although the application of group therapy approaches to chronic pain may seem straightforward, it can raise a number of potentially difficult clinical issues. These clinical issues can be divided into three groups: (1) problems related to conducting group therapy itself, (2) issues regarding the involvement of the spouse and family members, (3) issues relating to integrating group therapy with other pain treatment modalities, and (4) telephone-based group therapy.

Problems in Conducting Group Therapy with Chronic Pain Patients

Group therapists encounter a number of problems when leading groups of chronic pain patients. Two of the most common and important problems are a mismatch between patient expectations and the goals of therapy and dealing with anger and high levels of emotional distress. To illustrate these problems we present a clinical vignette followed by a discussion of strategies for managing the problem.

DEALING WITH PATIENT EXPECTATIONS

Mr. Jones came to the group therapy session but was visibly annoyed. The session focused on learning how to cope with pain. Mr. Jones was quiet during the group, speaking up only when asked to do so. When approached by the therapist after the group session, Mr. Jones explained that he was not interested in learning how to cope but only in getting rid of his pain. He stated, "If you can't do anything to take my pain away, I'd rather not waste my time with the sessions."

One of the most important issues in group therapy is dealing with patients' expectations about treatment. These expectations can vary greatly. Some chronic pain patients expect group psychological therapy to fail because they view their pain as a medical problem that can only be addressed through medical treatment. Other patients unrealistically expect that group therapy will give them unique insights or powerful techniques that will permanently eliminate their pain. In either case, patients are likely to be dissatisfied when treatment fails to meet their expectations. These patients may fail to become involved in treatment or may prematurely drop out of group therapy.

Several methods can be used before and during group therapy to deal with problems related to patient expectations. First, a screening interview should be carried out with all patients before they start group therapy. In the interview, patients should be encouraged to discuss their thoughts and beliefs about pain and its treatment. The interviewer should take a supportive, nonjudgmental approach in order to gather as much information as possible about patient expectations. Patients may have fears or concerns based on their own or others' experiences with group therapy. At the end of the screening interview patients should be provided with basic information about the group therapy. Patients often benefit from a discussion that focuses on the nature of pain problems typically experienced by patients undergoing group therapy, the goals of the group, intervention methods, and typical outcomes in terms of pain relief and functional status.

Second, it is important that group therapists directly address patient expectations early in the course of the group itself. One way of doing this is to conduct a brief group exercise in which each patient briefly discusses what he or she hopes to accomplish in the group. Patients are encouraged to discuss both their hopes and their doubts about treatment outcome. This exercise is particularly effective when a new patient is entering an established group. The veterans of the group often frankly discuss their own initial skepticism and concerns about the effectiveness of the group. These veteran patients also can convincingly convey that group therapy is not only helpful in terms of pain relief but also in terms of increased activity and improved mood.

Third, therapists can meet individually with patients outside the group to discuss and deal with such problems. As noted previously, one of the most common and difficult problems is that chronic pain patients often consider pain relief to be the only meaningful index of their improvement. When they fail to achieve substantial reductions in pain, their motivation for treatment may drop. Diary records can be used to help patients shift their focus from pain relief, per se, toward a broader conceptualization of treatment outcome. For example, patients can keep daily diary records in which they monitor not only their pain level but also their exercise and activity level, participation in pleasant activities, and mood. The records can be reviewed daily, and simple graphs can be used to display changes in pain and improvements in activity and mood measures. By reviewing the graphs, patients are able to see that moderate reductions in pain may be accompanied by substantial increases in the level and range of pleasant activities.

DEALING WITH ANGER AND EMOTIONAL DISTRESS

During a group session focusing on negative thinking and pain, Mrs. Edwards vented her angry feelings toward her doctors. "It is all Dr. Smith's fault. He told me the operation would take care of the pain. Now the pain is worse than ever. If he hadn't operated and cut that nerve this never would have happened." Other group members joined in and shared their anger toward physicians and other health professionals. As the group went on, the level of anger escalated, with some members crying and visibly shaking as they made statements such as "The doctors are useless," "None of the people who have treated me understand or believe me," and "I wish they could walk in my shoes for just one day, then they would know what pain is like."

Anger is one of the most common and difficult emotions that chronic pain patients experience. Some psychodynamic pain theorists such as Engel (1959) believe that unresolved anger is a key factor in the maintenance of chronic pain. Anger and resentment can certainly interfere with group treatment. We have found that, for some patients, engaging in a prolonged discussion of their feelings of anger or resentment is not fruitful. These patients often report that they remain emotionally upset long after these sessions and that they gain little insight or improvement in coping from a persistent focus on these feelings.

Several strategies can be used to handle high levels of anger and emotional distress in group therapy. First, therapists can help group members calm themselves to the point that they can cope with anger more rationally. One way of doing this is to interrupt discussion for a relaxation break. Patients can be guided through a relaxation exercise designed to help reduce emotional arousal and enable them to cope more effectively. Another method is to intentionally limit the amount of time devoted to discussing anger and postpone the discussion to a later session in which the issues can be handling more productively.

Second, therapists can help group members identify the underlying source of their anger. For many patients, anger is related to issues of loss. The loss of the ability to work, in particular, can be associated with high levels of anger and resentment. Losses in the ability to engage in valued recreational or family activities also can fuel angry feelings. For other patients, anger is related to a sense that life has been unfair to them. Identifying sources of anger is an important first step in problem solving. Once the sources of anger have been identified, problem-solving methods can be used to help group members better cope with their feelings. In problem solving, patients develop a plan for coping with anger and then implement it. Problem solving is particularly effective in a group setting where some patients may have learned to cope with anger while others have not. Patients often suggest coping methods to each other. For example, a patient who is angry with her doctor might be encouraged by group members to talk to her doctor. Role playing could be used to teach the patient how to effectively communicate. Patients often encourage group members to focus on acceptance rather than on their anger. This focus involves shifting their attention from blaming others for losses to emphasizing what they can do to replace losses.

Third, we have used a time-out strategy with patients whose angry feelings are so strong that they are unable to get much out of group and actually disrupt the group. We typically meet with these patients individually and suggest that they try a time-out approach in which they will attend group but remain silent for two to three group sessions. These patients are encouraged to simply listen to what other group members are saying. The therapist meets individually with such patients after each group to review their reactions. With use of the time-out method, angry patients often report feeling less resentful, more comfortable with the group, and more optimistic about how it might help them. After several sessions with this time-out procedure, most patients are able to resume a normal role in group and to work on learning new pain coping methods.

We have found that a combination of the strategies discussed previously works most of the time in dealing with patients who are angry. In some instances, however, patients seem "stuck" and do not respond to these interventions. In these cases, we work individually with the patient until he or she is ready for group therapy.

Involving Spouse and Family in Group Therapy

Chronic pain is not only a problem for the patient but for the spouse and family members. There is growing recognition that the responses of spouse and family members to pain can influence the patient's ability to cope (Keefe, Dunsmore, & Burnett, 1992). There is also heightened interest in involving the patient's spouse and other family members in pain treatment programs.

Group therapy provides an excellent setting in which to work with patients and their families. We often have spouse and family members sit in on regular group therapy sessions with the patient. Sitting in provides family members with exposure to other individuals having pain and helps them better understand the patient's own problems in coping. We also conduct special multifamily group therapy sessions that are attended by two or three patients and their families. The multifamily groups have two major goals: (1) reviewing how the patients difficulties in coping have affected the family and (2) identifying one or more specific ways that family members can become involved in the patient's pain management program.

We have recently developed a comprehensive spouse training intervention designed to be used in the context of a 10-week couples group therapy program for managing osteoarthritic knee pain (Keefe et al., 1996, 1999). The intervention integrates spouse training with training in patient pain coping skills. The intervention has three key components. The first component, *patient-spouse behavioral rehearsal*, is used to teach spouses how to prompt and reinforce pain coping skills in problem situations. Patient-spouse rehearsal is particularly useful in teaching spouses to prompt pain control techniques (e.g., relaxation methods) in public situations where patients may be reluctant to use them (e.g. while talking with a store clerk in a mall or conversing with friends at a party). The second component of spouse training, *joint practice*, teaches couples how to practice together with relax-ation, imagery, and other cognitive coping skills in practice sessions at home or during demanding physical activities (e.g., stair climbing and transferring from a sitting to a standing position). This joint practice not only familiarizes the spouse with the specifics of coping skills but also enhance the spouses' confidence in the patient's ability to cope with problem situations. The third component of spouse training, *maintenance enhancement training*, teaches couples strategies for maintaining frequent practice of pain coping skills. The couple learns how to identify high-risk situations that may set back coping efforts, how to develop a plan for dealing with pain flares, and how to identify natural cues that may serve to maintain coping efforts.

We have found that most spouses of chronic pain patients are eager to participate and benefit substantially from involvement in group therapy. In some cases, however, there are impediments to involving spouse or family members. Some patients are resistant to the idea of having their spouses attend group sessions. In addition, some spouses may be unwilling to participate in treatment. Often these problems can be overcome by meeting with the patients, their spouses, and/or their family members for a preliminary interview before the group therapy sessions. The meeting can be used to elicit and address concerns about group treatment and to provide basic information on the structure and nature of the group sessions. Most spouses are reassured by the information provided and agree to participate fully in treatment. A continued refusal to participate is almost invariably a negative prognostic sign.

Integrating Group Therapy with Other Treatments

Group therapy approaches need not, and in most cases should not, be the sole treatment modality for chronic pain. The methods outlined in this chapter are typically one component of a comprehensive treatment program that also involves the use of exercise, medications, and other pain management modalities.

Combining group therapy with other pain treatments does raise a number of important clinical issues. The first issue is confidentiality. If patients are to open up in group, they need to feel comfortable that there are limits on what will be communicated to other members of the treatment team. Typically, therapists provide feedback on the specific treatment provided and the patient's progress. Therapists often use a need-to-know rule in determining when to share more confidential information with other treatment team members. That is, detailed information on emotionally sensitive topics is not shared with other team members unless it is likely to have a significant impact on the patients' treatment course.

A second issue is the need for other treatment team members to support and reinforce the goals of group therapy. Patients are more likely to view group treatment as important if the goals and methods used are viewed as valuable by other treatment specialists. Educational efforts are sometimes needed to teach these specialists about group therapy and to identify how they might assist the patient in progressing through treatment.

A third issue is how the goals of group therapy fit with those of other treatment modalities. A group therapy program that encourages patients to become active might be seen by a patient as being incompatible with a physical therapy regimen that emphasizes the use of rest, hot packs, and ultrasound. Ideally, treatment team members need to communicate and agree as to the goals of therapy before treatment begins. If inconsistencies arise over the course of treatment, a brief telephone call can often address the problems. Treatments that seem inconsistent may not be so. In the example given previously, the physical therapist had instructed the patient to use hot packs and rest after a period of moderate activity and exercise. The therapist agreed that activating the patient was important and felt that the hot packs and rest might serve as effective reinforcers for increased activity.

Telephone-Based Group Therapy

A factor that has limited the use of group therapy is that it is primarily offered through special centers located in major tertiary medical centers. Thus, the group usually requires patients to attend multiple treatment sessions at a center that is often quite distant from their homes. The need to travel to receive treatment prohibits the participation of many patients having persistent pain whose symptoms make traveling difficult. In fact, travel problems have been cited as a major obstacle preventing many patients with persistent pain conditions from enrolling in treatment (Turk & Rudy, 1991). Given this limitation, there is a clear need to develop new strategies for delivering group therapy to patients in a way that not only produce beneficial outcomes but also can be implemented in a pragmatic, feasible, and cost-effective manner.

Over the past decade, researchers have developed telephone-based group therapy protocols. Although no studies have examined the efficacy of telephone-based interventions for patients having chronic pain, several studies have demonstrated the feasibility and efficacy of telephone group therapy for other populations. Telephone support groups have been used in several studies of HIV/AIDS patients and their caregivers (Meier, Galinsky, & Rounds, 1995; Rounds & Galinsky, 1995; Rounds, Galinsky, & Stevens, 1991; Wiener, Spencer, Davidson, & Fair, 1993). Telephone-based cognitive therapy and cognitive-behavioral therapy also have been used to treat depression in multiple sclerosis patients (Mohr et al., 2000) and visually impaired older adults (Evans & Jaureguy, 1982; Evans, Werkhoven, & Fox, 1982).

Telephone-based group interventions are a promising method for treating patients having persistent pain. Despite the potential benefits of using a telephone-based group format for teaching coping skills to patients having pain, this training has not yet been evaluated. Indeed, as Turk and Rudy's (1991) critical review of treatment studies points out, the development of home-based, practical strategies for training in coping skills is one of the most neglected topics in the pain management literature.

There are several reasons that telephone-based group therapy might be particularly helpful for patients having persistent pain. First, telephone-administered group intervention is more accessible than clinic-based treatment. Patients who live in remote areas or whose symptoms interfere with their ability to travel, thus, can participate in treatment sessions. Second, telephone-based treatment is less costly. Telephone-based group therapy circumvents the costs associated with travel and lodging and the costs of providing adequate meeting space in which groups convene. In the current era of managed care, the costs of face-to-face group therapy are often considered to be prohibitive, particularly when patients need to travel to a tertiary care medical center for treatment. Finally, telephone-based group interventions are easier to integrate into busy general medical practice settings than are face-to-face therapist-administered treatments.

Final Comments

Although further research is needed to evaluate its effectiveness, group therapy does appear to represent a viable treatment option for many patients who have chronic pain. As pointed out in this chapter, successful group therapy requires attention to a number of important practical and therapeutic issues. It is our hope that this chapter will stimulate a broader use of group therapy and lead to heightened recognition of the benefits of this psychological treatment approach.

Acknowlegments

Preparation of this chapter was supported in part by the following grants from the National Institutes of Health: Grant Nos. NIAMS AR 46305, NHLBI HL 65503, and NIMH MH 63429; National Cancer Institute Grant Nos. R21-CA88049-01 and R01 CA91946, and by support from the Arthritis Foundation and Fetzer Institute.

Note

1. Two national self-help organizations provide materials to people who wish to start their own chronic pain support group: (1) the American Chronic Pain Association (P.O. Box 850, Rocklin, CA 95677) and (2) the National Chronic Pain Outreach Association (7979 Old Georgetown Road, Suite 100, Bethesda, MD 20814).

References

Basler, H., Jaekle, C., & Kroener-Herwig, B. (1997). Incorporation of cognitive-behavioral treatment into the medical care of chronic low back patients: A controlled randomized study in German pain treatment centers. *Patient Education and Counseling, 31,* 113–124.

Bernstein, & Borkovec, T. D. (1973). *Progressive relaxation training: A manual for the helping professions.* Champaign, IL: Research Press.

Bradley, L. A., Young, L. D., Anderson, J. O., Turner, R. A., Agudelo, C. A., McDaniel, L. K., Pisko, E. J., Semble, E. J., & Morgan, T. M. (1987). Effects of psychological therapy on pain behavior of rheumatoid arthritis patients: Treatment outcome and six-month follow-up. *Arthritis and Rheumatism, 30,* 1105–1114.

Cole, J. (1998). Psychotherapy with chronic pain patients using coping skills development outcome study. *Journal of Occupational Health Psychology, 3,* 217–226.

Daltroy, L. H., & Liang, M. H. (1988). Patient education in the rheumatic diseases: A research agenda. *Arthritis Care and Research, 1,* 161–169.

Engel, G. (1959). Psychogenic pain and the pain-prone patient. *American Journal of Medicine, 26,* 899–918.

Evans, R. L., & Jaureguy, B. M. (1982). Phone therapy outreach for blind elderly. *The Gerontologist, 22,* 32–35.

Evans, R. L., Werkhoven, W., & Fox, H. R. (1982). Treatment of social isolation and loneliness in a sample of visually impaired elderly persons. *Psychological Reports, 51,* 103–108.

Feuerstein, M., Sult, S., & Houle, M. (1985). Environmental stressors and chronic low back pain: Life events, family, and work environment. *Pain, 22,* 295–307.

Fordyce, W. E. (1976). *Behavioral methods for chronic pain and illness.* St. Louis, MO: Mosby.

Gil, K. M., Ross, S. L., & Keefe, F. J. (1988). Behavioral treatment of chronic pain: Four pain management protocols. In R. D. France & K. R. Krishnan (Eds.), *Chronic pain* (pp. 376–414). New York: American Psychiatric Association.

Goeppinger, J., Arthur, M. W., Baglioni, A. J., Jr., Brunk, S. E., & Brunner, C. M. (1989). A reexamination of the effectiveness of self-care education for persons with arthritis. *Arthritis and Rheumatism, 32,* 706–717.

Harrison, S., Watson, M., & Feinmann, C. (1997). Does short-term group therapy affect unexplained medical symptoms? *Journal of Psychosomatic Research, 43,* 399–404.

Holman, H., Mazonson, P., & Lorig, K. (1989). Health education for self-management has significant early and sustained benefits in chronic arthritis. Transactions of the *Association of American Physicians, 102,* 204–208.

Jacobson, E. (1938). *Progressive relaxation.* Chicago: University of Chicago Press.

Keefe, F. J. (1988). Behavioral assessment methods for chronic pain. In R. D. France & K. R. R. Krishnan (Eds.), *Chronic pain* (pp. 299–320). Washington, DC: American Psychiatric Press.

Keefe, F. J., Caldwell, D. S., Baucom, D., Salley, A., Robinson, E., Timmons, K., Beaupre, P., Weisberg, J., & Helms, M. (1996). Spouse-assisted coping skills training in the management of osteoarthritis knee pain. *Arthritis Care and Research, 9,* 279–291.

Keefe, F. J., Caldwell, D. S, Baucom, D., Salley, A., Robinson, E., Timmons, K., Beaupre, P., Weisberg, J., & Helms, M. (1999). Spouse-assisted coping skills training in the management of knee pain in osteoarthritis: Long-term followup results. *Arthritis Care and Research, 12,* 101–111.

Keefe, F. J., Caldwell, D. S., Williams, D. A., Gil, K. M., Mitchell, D., Robertson, D., Robertson, C., Martinez, S., Nunley, J., Beckham, J. C., & Helms, M. (1990). Pain coping skills training in the management of osteoarthritic knee pain: A comparative study. *Behavior Therapy, 21,* 49–62.

Keefe, F. J., Dunsmore, J., & Burnett, R. (1992). Behavioral and cognitive-behavioral approaches to chronic pain: Recent advances and future directions. *Journal of Consulting and Clinical Psychology, 60,* 528–536.

Keefe, F. J., & Gil, K. M. (1986). Behavioral concepts in the analysis of chronic pain syndromes. *Journal of Consulting and Clinical Psychology, 54,* 776–783.

Keefe, F. J., & Van Horn, Y. V. (1993). Cognitive-behavioral treatment of rheumatoid arthritis pain: Maintaining treatment gains. *Arthritis Care and Research, 6,* 213–222.

Linton, S., & Andersson, T. (2000). Can chronic disability be prevented? A randomized trial of a cognitive-behavior intervention and two forms of information for patients with spinal pain. *Spine, 25*(21), 2825–2831.

Linton, S., & Ryberg, M. (2001). A cognitive-behavioral group intervention as prevention for persistent neck and back pain in a non-patient population: A randomized controlled trial. *Pain, 90,* 83–90.

Litt, M. D. (1988). Self-efficacy and perceived control: Cognitive mediators of pain tolerance. *Journal of Personality and Social Psychology, 54,* 149–160.

Lorig, K., Lubeck, D., Kraines, R. G., Seleznick, M., & Holman, H. R. (1985). Outcomes of self-help education for patients with arthritis. *Arthritis and Rheumatism, 28,* 680–685.

Marlatt, G. A., & Gordon, J. R. (1985). *Relapse prevention: Maintenance strategies in the treatment of addictive behaviors.* New York: Guilford Press.

McCaul, D., & Malott, J. M. (1984). Distraction and coping with pain. *Psychological Bulletin, 95,* 516–533.

Meier, A., Galinsky, M. J., & Rounds, K. A. (1995). Telephone support groups for caregivers of persons with AIDS. *Social Work with Groups, 18,* 99–108.

Melzack, R., & Wall, P. (1965). Pain mechanisms: A new theory. *Science, 50,* 971–979.

Mohr, D. C., Likosky, W., Bertagnolli, A., Goodkin, D. E., Van Der Wende, J., Dwyer, P., & Dick, L. P. (2000). Telephone-administered cognitive-behavioral therapy for the treatment of depressive symptoms in Multiple Sclerosis. *Journal of Consulting and Clinical Psychology, 68,* 356–361.

Newton-John, T., Spence, S., & Schotte, D. (1995). Cognitive-behavioral therapy versus EMG biofeedback in the treatment of chronic low back pain. *Behaviour Research and Therapy, 33,* 691–697.

Nicholas, M. K., Wilson, P. H., & Goyen, J. (1991). Comparison of operant-behavioral and cognitive-behavioral group treatment, with and without relaxation training for chronic low back pain. *Behaviour Research and Therapy, 29,* 225–238.

Parker, J. C., Frank, R. G., Beck, N. C., Smarr, K. L., Buescher K. L., Phillips, L. R., Smith, E. I., Anderson, S. K., & Walker, S. E. (1988). Pain management in rheumatoid arthritis patients: A cognitive-behavioral approach. *Arthritis and Rheumatism, 31,* 591–601.

Parker, J. C., Smarr, K. L., Buescher, K. L., Phillips, L. R., Frank, R. G., Beck, N. C., Anderson, S. K., & Walker, S. E. (1989). Pain control and rational thinking: Implications for rheumatoid arthritis. *Arthritis and Rheumatism, 32,* 984–990.

Rounds, K. A., & Galinsky, M. J. (1995). Evaluation of telephone support groups for persons with HIV disease. *Research on Social Work Practice, 5,* 442–459.

Rounds, K. A., Galinsky, M. J., & Stevens, L. S. (1991). Linking people with AIDS in rural communities: The telephone group. *Social Work, 36,* 13–18.

Surwit, R. S. (1979). *Progressive relaxation training manual* [Videotape]. (Available from the Behavioral Physiology Laboratory, Duke University Medical Center, P.O. Box 3842, Durham, NC 27710)

Travell, J., Rinzler, S., & Herman, M. (1943). Pain and disability of the shoulder and arm: Treatment by intramuscular infiltration with procaine hydrochloride. *Journal of the American Medical Association, 120,* 209–233.

Turk, D. C., Meichenbaum, D., & Genest, M. (1983). *Pain and behavioral medicine: A cognitive-behavioral perspective.* New York: Guilford Press.

Turk, D. C., & Rudy, T. E. (1991). Neglected topics in the treatment of chronic pain—relapse, non-compliance, and adherence enhancement. *Pain, 44,* 5–28.

Turner, J. A., & Jensen M. P. (1993). Efficacy of cognitive therapy for chronic low back pain. *Pain, 52,* 169–177.

Wiener, L. S., Spencer, E. D., Davidson, R., & Fair, C. (1993). National telephone support groups: A new avenue toward psychosocial support for HIV-infected children and their families. *Social Work with Groups, 16,* 55–71.

Wolf, S. L., Nacht, M., & Kelly, J. L. (1982). EMG feedback training during dynamic movement for low back pain patients. *Behavior Therapy, 13,* 395–406.

12

Treating Families of Chronic Pain Patients: Application of a Cognitive-Behavioral Transactional Model

Robert D. Kerns
John D. Otis
Emily A. Wise

Health care providers are increasingly recognizing the significant role of the family in the initiation and maintenance of a variety of health-related behaviors and medical conditions. Studies suggest that the family can be an influential learning environment across the entire lifespan. Recent research has shown that family interactions can play an influential role in shaping the course of childhood illness and disorders (Johnson, 1998), as well as the adaptation and adjustment of adults to medical procedures and diagnoses (Marriott, Donaldson, Tarrier, & Burns, 2000; Rodrigue, Pearman, & Moreb, 1999). Within the chronic pain literature there has been a persistent call to attend to the social context and the role of the family in patient adaptation and adjustment to chronic pain (e.g., Roy, 1992, 2001). This perspective is informed and encouraged by specific calls for attention to the role of the family in chronic illness (Schmaling & Sher, 2000; Turk & Kerns, 1985a), systems perspectives on health and illness (Ramsey, 1989; Schwartz, 1982), and multidimensional theoretical models of chronic pain (Fordyce, 1976; Kerns & Jacob, 1995; Turk,

Meichenbaum, & Genest, 1983). Further, this approach is supported by reports of clinical observations and a growing empirical base that describes the interactions between the experience of chronic pain and the family.

The family perspective on the adaptation and adjustment of individuals with chronic pain has led to the development of clinical assessment strategies with a family or couple focus (Romano & Schmaling, 2001). Using these assessment techniques, numerous studies have shown that interactions between the spouse and the patient can contribute to the development and maintenance of dimensions of the chronic pain experience, including pain, disability, and emotional distress (e.g., Goldberg, Kerns & Rosenberg, 1993; Kerns & Rosenberg, 2001). However, there have been relatively few empirical investigations of the efficacy of couple-based treatment approaches to pain management (Keefe et al., 1996; Moore & Chaney, 1985; Radojevic, Nicassio, & Weisman, 1992; Saarijarvi, 1991), and no controlled empirical studies of family therapy for pain management. The lack of activity in this area of pain research is unfortunate because such studies would have the potential to significantly advance theory development and improve treatment efficacy.

Our primary aim in this chapter is to illustrate the potential theoretical and clinical utility of a cognitive-behavioral transactional model of family functioning to better understand the reciprocal interactions between the family and the person with a chronic pain condition. We begin with a presentation of several integrative theoretical perspectives that attempt to organize information about ways the family can influence a patient's experience of chronic pain. We then propose the cognitive-behavioral transactional model as a testable framework that provides an integrative model of the role of family functioning for people with chronic pain. We then describe the relevant empirical literature that supports this model. In the last section of the chapter, we present two case illustrations to highlight ways in which the cognitive-behavioral transactional model for family treatment can be applied to chronic pain patients and their families. We close with a brief discussion of future directions for theory building, a call for continued research, and suggestions for directions in the clinical arena.

Theoretical Perspectives

Biopsychosocial Perspective

In contrast to the traditional biomedical model, which assumed that all illness was a function of biological malfunctions, the biopsychosocial model emphasizes the dynamic and reciprocal relationships between the social, biological, and psychological domains of physical health problems. Consistent with more general systems theory (von Bertanlanffy, 1968), the model notes that a change in one domain (e.g., the biological domain in the case of a chronic painful condition) necessarily results in changes in the other domains (e.g., psychological and social domains). Ultimately, the biopsychosocial system is driven to restore homeostasis within the system. Based on this model, effective treatment would necessarily involve all three domains (biological, psychological,

and social) at different levels depending on the person's needs.

The biopsychosocial model has been commended for emphasizing that the social domain should be attended to in terms of its impact on the experience of chronic pain (Kerns & Jacob, 1995; see also Turk & Monarch, Chapter 1, this volume). For example, changes such as shifting family roles, loss of income, and increased family and marital distress can have negative effects on pain and disability. However, the model's specific influence on the chronic pain field has been limited. The model has failed to contribute to specific theoretical refinements about mechanisms of transaction, particularly the potential influence of the social (and family) domain on the development and perpetuation of the chronic pain condition or its associated problems.

Family Systems Models

The role of the family in the onset and maintenance of maladaptive thoughts and behaviors associated with chronic illness has been an important topic of theory and investigation (Burg & Seeman, 1994). Family systems and family stress models have emerged as potentially influential frameworks for understanding the role of the family with a chronically ill individual (Olson, 1989; Patterson & Garwick, 1994a; Reiss, 1989). Central to these models is the assumption that change in one part of the system leads to change in other parts as well (von Bertanlanffy, 1968). These perspectives have been important in hypothesizing mechanisms (or at least factors) that may influence the response of the family to the person with chronic pain and, via circular and continuous feedback, may influence the adjustment and adaptation of the family member with the chronic pain condition.

One particularly informative family systems model for understanding the role of the family in chronic illness is the "family adjustment and adaptation response" (FAAR) model (Patterson & Garwick, 1994a, 1994b). According to this model, the degree of stress experienced by a family is a function of the interaction between potentially stressful events (e.g., functional loss associated with a chronic pain condition) and the family's resources and coping abilities. There are two phases to the FAAR model, adjustment and adaptation, separated by a family crisis. The adjustment phase is a relatively stable period during which the family resists change in response to the demands of an acute illness. The crisis emerges as the demands of the illness exceed their existing coping resources. Adaptation occurs as a family attempts to restore homeostasis by developing new coping resources, by reducing the challenges of the condition, and by altering its appraisals of the situation and the family.

The FAAR model appears to have important strengths that enhance its potential utility in the field of chronic pain. First, the specification of the hypothesized constructs of the model (i.e., stress, coping, adaptation, and adjustment) and the articulation of the critical mediating role of cognitive appraisal are advances of the FAAR model over the more general biopsychosocial perspective and other family systems-stress theories. Second, psychometrically sound measures have been developed for many of the central constructs of the FAAR model. Finally, the model is important to the extent that it emphasizes that the family system, rather than the individual, should be the primary target of clinical analysis and intervention. There are several noted weaknesses to the FAAR model. First, the model's scope and complexity may be too cumbersome to be practically applied in empirical research, and considerable overlap has been noted among the definitions of some key constructs. Second, although there have been important advances in the assessment of key constructs, the implications of the model for family intervention have not yet been well articulated. Finally, the model has not yet been specifically refined or elaborated for the problem of chronic pain.

Operant Behavioral Perspective

Wilbert Fordyce (1976) is credited with the elaboration of a specific operant behavioral formulation of the development and maintenance of chronic pain, and with the further refinement of a learning-theory-based perspective on this complex clinical problem (see Sanders, Chapter 6, this volume). Central to the model is the notion that observable "pain behaviors" (complaining, grimacing, bracing,) may be maintained via contingent social reinforcement (e.g., the sympathetic response of significant others), even in the absence of continued nociception. Family members, as well as health care providers, have been specifically noted to play potentially critical roles as primary sources of social reinforcement for pain behaviors, to the detriment of alternative "well behaviors" such as continued productive activity, exercise, and other health-promoting behaviors.

Interest in testing the model with clinical samples contributed to the development of intensive inpatient treatment environments. Such controlled environments were viewed as necessary to alter these contingencies and improve outcomes. Although these inpatient programs were successful, enthusiasm for them was tempered by their high costs and questionable maintenance of improved outcomes once the patients returned to their home environments. Unfortunately, more detailed elaboration of the hypothesized role of the family, empirical examinations of the importance of pain-related family interactions, and the development of family-based outpatient interventions consistent with the model have been slow in coming.

Cognitive-Behavioral Transactional Model

Building on cognitive-social learning theory and behaviorism, a cognitive-behavioral transactional model (CBTM) of the role of families in the course of chronic illness has been described (Kerns, 1999; Kerns & Weiss, 1994; Turk & Kerns, 1985b). The model shares important features with the FAAR model, Reiss's (1989) family paradigm model, and contemporary models of stress and coping (Friedman, 1992; Lazarus & Folkman, 1984). In addition, this model for understanding the role of the family in chronic pain can be viewed as a specific extension of a diathesis–stress model of chronic pain (Kerns & Jacob, 1995). Central to this model is the emphasis on the social context in general, and the family context in particular, as the key environment in which adaptation or maladaptation occurs in the face of a chronically painful condition. Figure 12.1 displays this diathesis–stress framework.

As can be seen in Figure 12.1, the family context is highlighted as the central environ-

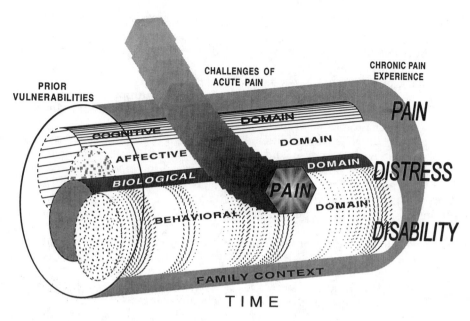

FIGURE 12.1. Diathesis–stress model of chronic pain. From Kerns and Jacob (1995). Copyright 1995 by Plenum Publishing Corp. Adapted by permission.

ment in which complex interactions occur between the individual's prior vulnerabilities in biological (i.e., central nervous system neurobiological), behavioral, cognitive, and affective domains and the specific challenges or stresses of the painful condition. The model suggests that these interactions take place within a social (family) learning environment that selectively reinforces coping attempts and outcomes in terms of optimal pain management, continued constructive activity, and emotional well-being, or, conversely, heightened pain, unnecessary impairment and disability, and affective distress. As such, the model has advantages over previous models by specifying a salient role of social and particularly family interactions as important influences on the course of the chronic pain condition. Consistent with a C-B perspective on chronic pain (Turk et al., 1983), this CBTM transactional family model hypothesizes that the family plays an active role in seeking out and evaluating information about the painful condition itself and the specific challenges it poses, as well as in making judgments about the family's (and its members') capacities and vulnerabilities in meeting the challenges. It is on the basis of these ap-

praisals that the family and its members make active decisions about alternative responses, act upon their decisions, and evaluate the adequacy of the response.

Also consistent with cognitive theory and with Reiss's (1989) description of family paradigms is the notion that the family and its members develop "schema" or a relatively fixed set of beliefs about the world, and, even more directly relevant, about concepts such as illness, pain, disability, and emotional responding. The family's more specific appraisals of its ongoing experiences in living with the individual with the painful condition are based in part on these more enduring schemas. These more specific appraisals of its present experiences are hypothesized to influence both the individual's and the family's responses to the challenges perceived, and ultimately to determine their level of adaptation. The family also maintains beliefs about its available resources to cope with the challenges posed by the painful condition. The family's flexibility versus rigidity in adopting new strategies for coping with the challenges of chronic pain, together with its more characteristic patterns of responding to stress and challenges, further mediates the response.

Finally, the family's appraisals of its success in mastering the challenges and in promoting optimal outcomes contribute to future responding. This later step in the appraisal-coping process—that is, the family and its members' evaluations of the success of the response—will determine whether the response is repeated or not.

Central to the CBTM is the additional notion that the family's response and its perceived effects in turn shape future appraisals of stress and challenge in a dynamic and reciprocal fashion. Perceptions of failed efforts to manage the painful condition will probably enhance the intensity of the perceived threat of the condition, perhaps contributing to a heightened level of perceived pain, increased disability, and affective distress. Conversely, perceptions of success in coping will probably moderate the experience of pain, increase confidence in the family's ability to respond effectively in the future, and reinforce the repeated use of similar strategies.

One final point should be emphasized with regard to the integrative diathesis–stress and CBTM models. The diathesis–stress model represented in Figure 12.1 emphasizes the importance of several domains of the chronic pain condition—namely, the condition itself, and the experiences of pain, disability, and emotional distress. Consistent with Fordyce's (1976) operant analysis of chronic pain, the cognitive-behavioral transaction model emphasizes the family's appraisals of discrete observable behaviors. As such, the family's response to behaviors representing one domain may be quite different than its response to behaviors representing another. Furthermore, the family's response to one set of behaviors, such as the person's report of pain, may have unexpected direct and indirect effects on another aspect of the individual's overall experience. This specification of the model may help to explain observations that a family's response may have positive effects on one domain but negative effects on another—for example, the observation that positive support from the spouse for the person's expressions of pain may buffer the individual from depression while inadvertently contributing to reports of heightened pain and increased pain behavior frequency (Kerns, Haythornthwaite, Southwick, & Giller,

1990). The CBTM argues for behavioral specificity in the family's influence on the course of the chronic pain experience.

Empirical Support for the Cognitive-Behavioral Transactional Model

Although the model as described previously is important in attempting to explain the reciprocal interactions between the chronic pain patient and the family, its empirical support is relatively limited. Evidence is mounting that challenges the widespread assumption that chronic pain has a predictable, even inevitable, negative effect on family functioning. Although investigators have offered evidence of marital and sexual dysfunction, increased prevalence of psychophysiological disorders, and elevated emotional distress (particularly depression) among the partners of individuals with chronic pain (e.g., Saarijaervi, Hyyppae, Lahtinen, & Alanen, 1990; Schwartz, Slater, Birchler, & Atkinson, 1991), these studies have generally been poorly controlled, and have been largely descriptive, in nature. On the other hand, there is considerable evidence of substantial adjustment and adaptation among families of chronic pain patients. Despite evidence of relative dysfunction on some dimensions of family functioning as measured by the Family Environment Scale (Moos, 1978), several studies have failed to find reliable differences between pain groups and healthy groups on important dimensions of family functioning (e.g., Kopp et al., 1995; Romano, Turner, & Jensen, 1997). Theory-driven research based on either family systems or CB perspectives is beginning to be reported, as investigators attempt to identify patterns of family beliefs or coping that account for variance in negative functioning or distress (Elliot, Trief, & Stein, 1986; Kopp et al., 1995). Such research will be valuable in informing future refinements of the theoretical model, as well as clinical assessment and intervention planning.

Research on the influence of the family on the person's adaptation to the chronic pain experience has received more attention, particularly the examination of the validity of operant formulations of chronic pain. Fordyce and others have indicated that spouses may play particularly influential roles because they serve as a primary source of social reinforcement. Consistent with these claims, investigators have focused much of their attention on this dyadic relationship. Research has generally supported the hypothesis that positive attention from a spouse contingent upon a patient's expressions of pain is associated with higher reported levels of pain and pain behaviors (Block, Kremer, & Gaylor, 1980; Kerns et al., 1990), higher frequency of observed pain behaviors (Romano et al., 1992), and reports of greater disability and interference (Flor, Turk, & Rudy, 1989; Turk, Kerns, & Rosenberg, 1992). In addition, there is evidence that a high frequency of negative responding to pain is reliably associated with depressive symptom severity and other demonstrations of affective distress (Kerns et al., 1990; Kerns, Southwick, et al., 1991). There is also emerging evidence that level of global marital satisfaction and gender may moderate these findings (Flor et al., 1989; Turk et al., 1992).

Recent research supports the notion of the complexity of these relationships, specifically the previously noted behavioral interactions between chronic pain patients and their spouses (Romano et al., 1995; Schwartz, Slater, & Birchler, 1996). For example, Romano and colleagues (1995) found that the relationship between solicitous responses from spouses to observed pain behaviors and physical dysfunction held strictly for pain patients who had higher depression scores. In addition, this study revealed that rates of observed pain behaviors were associated with spouses' solicitous responses exclusively for subjects with higher pain ratings (Romano et al., 1995). Furthermore, an examination of relationships between pain behaviors and marital conflict in chronic pain couples revealed that when compared to solicitous spouse behaviors (in response to patients' pain behaviors), negative spouse behaviors were better predictors of patient impairment. Specifically, significant positive relationships emerged for punitive spouse responses and patient psychosocial and functional impairment, as well as patient pain intensity (Schwartz et al., 1996).

Investigators (Romano et al., 1995; Schwartz et al., 1996) have offered hypotheses regarding these differential findings and the complexity of the interrelationships between chronic pain patients and their spouses, including the notion that different subgroups may exist within such dyads. Kerns and his colleagues have begun to examine these more complex patterns of pain-relevant interactions (Kerns & Rosenberg, 2001; Weiss & Kerns, 1995) and the role of cognitive appraisal in these interactions, in an effort to improve the prediction of pain and disability. Recently, Kerns and Rosenberg (2001), in examining couples' patterns of pain-relevant interactions, identified reliable subgroups of pain couples differentiated by five patterns of responding. These subgroups, labeled High Responders, High Negative, High Solicitous, Low Solicitous, and Mean Responders were shown to be differentially associated with several salient aspects of the chronic pain experience. Clinical implications of such findings may translate into treatment planning that is prescriptive in nature and more specifically aimed at addressing the pain-relevant communications revealed during assessment (Kerns & Rosenberg, 2001).

Despite extensive encouragement in the literature for the application of family therapy for chronic pain and the availability of relatively detailed descriptions of family therapy approaches (Roy, 1986, 1989), there have been no reports to date of controlled empirical evaluations of family therapy for chronic pain. There have been a few published reports documenting the efficacy of couple's therapy for chronic pain (Moore & Chaney, 1985; Radojevic et al., 1992; Saarijarvi, 1991). Unfortunately, descriptions of the treatment in these published reports were generally not detailed enough to permit an evaluation of their consistency with any specific theoretical framework that could be applied to the idiosyncrasies of the chronic pain experience. In addition, demonstrations of the effectiveness of the treatments relative to control conditions were weak and inconclusive.

More recently, there has been some empirical support for an intervention with chronic pain couples grounded in C-B theory, specifically, spouse-assisted pain coping skills training for patients with chronic pain (Keefe et al., 1996). Results of this study indicated that spouse-assisted coping skills training (CST) when compared to a control condition (i.e., arthritis education-spousal support) was significantly more effective, such that posttreatment, patients in the spouse-assisted CST group reported lower levels of pain and psychological disability and demonstrated less pain behavior. The authors acknowledge that the spouse-assisted CST group did not reveal significant differences on outcome measures when compared to a CST group without spouse involvement. However, after examination of the overall pattern of results, Keefe and colleagues (1996) conclude that spouse-assisted CST potentially may serve as a method for decreasing disability and pain in individuals with osteoarthritic knee pain and is an intervention warranting further research.

Taken together, the studies reviewed offer preliminary support and encouragement for the continued investigation of the utility of the CBTM. Future studies investigating this model would contribute to this literature by adopting a family systems perspective to treatment and using appropriate assessment instruments to evaluate treatment efficacy.

Family Therapy for Chronic Pain

Clinical Implications of the Cognitive-Behavioral Transactional Model

Both the FAAR model and the CBTM encourage a view of the family system as the primary unit of analysis and intervention. This approach has been promoted as the appropriate perspective for health care problems in general (Litman, 1974), and for chronic pain in particular (e.g., Kerns, 1999).

Consistent with the view of the family as the primary unit of analysis, the cognitive-behavioral transactional model emphasizes on the active, reciprocal transactions among family members, including the person with the chronic pain condition. Although the clinician may, for the sake of parsimony and clarity, focus primarily on one "direction" of the transaction relative to the other at times (e.g., focusing on ways in which a spouse reinforces behaviors of a patient with chronic pain), or on one dyadic pair (e.g., the marital relationship), the model encourages ongoing reframing of these interactions within a family context.

A family systems perspective encourages a hypothesis-generating and hypothesis-testing approach to clinical assessment, treatment planning, and intervention. The cognitive-behavioral transactional model can be used to inform and to guide the development of integrative conceptualizations of the problems experienced by the patient and the family. Ongoing assessment is critical for refining specific hypotheses about a patient's problems and the factors maintaining them. Ultimately, such a hypothesis-testing approach will begin to shape revisions in the treatment plan and delivery of services.

The cognitive-behavioral transactional model emphasizes the importance of a comprehensive approach to pain assessment. The model identifies several specific targets for assessment, such as (1) the domains of the chronic pain experience (e.g., pain, disability, and emotional distress); (2) pain associated challenges or problems for the family and its members; and (3) historical information about the available resources and supports for coping with or solving these problems or challenges. The model encourages efforts to develop a "time line" of information that evaluates dynamic interactions between the challenges of the pain problem and the person's and family's efforts to master the challenges. Finally, the model highlights the importance of assessing the family's attitudes, beliefs, and attributions concerning the pain experience, as well as the family's behavioral and affective responses to the patient's pain. On the basis of a comprehensive assessment, the clinician should be able to generate specific hypotheses about the nature of the problems being experienced and the mechanisms or factors that may be contributing to their maintenance over time. It is on the basis of this conceptualization that a multidimensional plan for treatment can be developed.

According to a cognitive-behavioral perspective (Turk et al., 1983, see also Turk, Chapter 7, this volume), treatment should be time-limited, goal-oriented, and learning-based. Broadly, family therapy should first encourage the development of an adaptive problem-solving perspective to the problems of chronic pain. Increasing the effective use of available family resources, teaching family members new skills, and helping them to draw on available external resources are important areas of intervention. Efforts to help family members reduce the stress and challenges of the painful condition and/or reconceptualize the problems and challenges as less threatening constitute a second general goal. Reduction of the negative impact of the pain problem on the family and its members (including the individual with the chronic pain condition) and promotion of adaptive family functioning and well-being are the overarching or higher-order goals of the therapeutic approach.

It is important to note that the structure of a family system is likely to vary across people and over the course of a single individual's life. Just as siblings, parents, and teachers can reinforce pain behaviors and disability in children (see McGrath & Hillier, Chapter 27, this volume), spouses and adult children and residential caregivers can influence the experience of pain in older adults (Kerns, Stein, & Otis, 2001). Treatment providers using a family systems perspective are encouraged to be flexible in their definition of "family," as they may find it necessary at times to expand the borders of the family system to include people outside the nuclear family who possess high reinforcement potential. This is an especially important consideration when treating patients from different cultures who may reside with extended family members or in multifamily dwellings. For such patients, it may be clinically useful to incorporate an extended family member (e.g., aunt or grandparent) or close friend to maximize treatment efficacy.

Despite a paucity of empirical research evaluating the effectiveness of family treatment for chronic pain, the models presented can be used to guide relatively "prescriptive" treatment planning (Kerns, 1994). Ultimately, the clinician, in collaboration with the family, can develop a plan for treatment that specifically targets identified problems and hypothesized contributing mechanisms. For example, treatment of one family may focus primarily on patterns of solicitous pain-relevant communication, whereas treatment of a second family may specifically target the family's pervasive depressionogenic cognitions. Given the complexity of the experience of chronic pain, the intervention plan commonly incorporates multiple treatment targets and strategies. Optimally,

the clinician's treatment plan and its implementation will remain integrative and internally consistent with the model and with family's treatment goals.

In the following sections, we describe two case examples of family therapy for chronic pain. In each instance, we briefly introduce the case and follow with a more detailed discussion of the assessment and treatment of the family.

Case Examples

Mr. H

Mr. H was a 54-year-old married Caucasian male who was originally referred by the Neurosurgery Service for a clinical neuropsychological evaluation of his competence to have his left arm amputated, in order to relieve severe chronic pain. He reported that the pain, although having increased in severity in recent years, had been present for 16 years. He attributed his present pain to a series of surgeries, and only through extensive interviewing was the original organic cause of his pain uncovered—a fractured bone in his wrist that had occurred nearly 30 years earlier. Clearly, by the very nature of the referral question, one can assume the severe distress of a man who would literally "give an arm" to experience relief from pain. At the time of the evaluation, the only medical treatments were occasional nerve blocks and 5 mg Valium three times a day, which the patient described as only minimally effective in reducing pain.

ASSESSMENT

In response to the referral, an initial screening appointment with the patient and his wife was scheduled. It was in this meeting that the couple acknowledged that they were concerned about the psychological impact of the pain problem on their two adolescent sons, and that their own relationship was threatened. We decided to include the two sons (an older married daughter who did not live with them was not included) in subsequent assessment meetings. The clinician planned a comprehensive evaluation. Several strategies were used in the assessment process, including a semistructured pain assessment interview involving the family during three 1-hour meetings; the administration of several questionnaires, inventories, and psychological tests (described later); the patient's self-monitoring of his daily pain intensity, as well as situational antecedents and consequences of periods of peak pain; and daily "pain diaries" kept by the spouse and sons. A similar assessment format was conducted immediately after treatment and at 3- and 6-month follow-up intervals.

Beginning with the initial visit, the clinician took care to establish expectations that the family members were "in this together" and that the assessment and treatment process would best involve each of the family members as equally important participants. The family members were encouraged to take a "family view" of the problems they were experiencing, and to accept the idea that solutions would necessarily require a family effort. All members were reassured that each of their concerns and views about the problems would be heard, and that efforts would be made to help each of them feel better about the current situation and the future.

The clinician began the interview by discovering the family members' views of the pain problem, including a description of the problem (e.g., site, changes over time, medical history, intensity, and fluctuations), attributions of causality, and expectations for recovery or rehabilitation. The clinician made a concerted effort to involve each family member in the discussion and to reflect when there appeared to be a shared "family view" and when there appeared to be individual differences in perspectives. For example, it was clear that the patient and his children generally held a medical view of the cause of the pain problem and believed that doctors should be able to do something about it. The sons believed that their father was experiencing an extremely high level of pain, and they reported a high level of worry and sadness about their father. On the other hand, it was clear that Mrs. H believed that her husband exaggerated his pain and should be able to be more active around the home, despite his pain. She verbalized a high degree of frustration, irritability, and frank anger toward her husband and a high level of worry about her sons. All felt relatively helpless and hopeless about finding a solution to the problem.

A second major focus of the interview related to perceived impact of the pain problem on the patient's and the family's functioning. In this area, there was a strong consensus that the pain condition was associated with a significant decline in family-related activities, in other activities around the home, and in social and recreational activities on the part of Mr. H. He did, however, continue to work full time as an accounting assistant, although he was frequently absent or left work early secondary to complaints of pain. Mr. H expressed dissatisfaction with his level of employment, independent of his pain condition. The family reported that Mr. H typically withdrew into his bedroom or lay on the couch upon returning from work. He was reported to do few household chores, rarely participated in any activities with his sons, and even less frequently left home for any family-related activity. Mr. H became tearful when describing his limited involvement with his sons. His younger son, in particular, acknowledged his disappointment that his father was not involved in activities. His wife acknowledged that she and her husband were never sexual with each other and that he rarely showed any affection toward her. Mr. H believed that he was unable to do any more than he was already doing, given his current pain condition. His sons generally agreed. As already noted, Mrs. H thought that he was unnecessarily restricting his activities, and that his major problems were that he was depressed and avoidant of responsibility.

Mr. H demonstrated markedly depressed mood and frequently became tearful during the interview and remained generally quiet and withdrawn throughout. His wife's affect was notably angry. The younger son appeared to be quite sad and also frequently became tearful, whereas the older son remained generally tense and reserved. The family reported that their current distress had been building over a few years. Overall, the family evidenced a high level of affective distress throughout the interview process. They agreed that each of the family members was depressed and that they all wanted help to feel better.

The clinician interviewed the family members regarding their views of the family's and Mr. H's functioning prior to the onset of pain, the challenges represented by the pain problem, and their efforts to cope with the pain condition and to help Mr. H. All agreed that there had been a time when the family had been very happy and "did a lot together." Mrs. H reported that her husband was a good provider for her and her family but that she had always "been the strong one" when it came to coping with problems or challenges. She also said that he had never been involved with household chores or in parenting roles. The family members agreed that pain had always been an issue, but thought that Mr. H had "given up" over the last 3 years. Mrs. H was outspoken in her criticism of Mr. H's inability to "live with the pain" and stated that she thought that he was "weak." This conflict in views between Mr. and Mrs. H was clearly a source of considerable distress for the children. The sons stated that they were "tired of the fighting" and "wished that Dad could get well."

In addition to the interview, questionnaires and diaries were used to gather information and to engage the family in the therapeutic process outside the formal sessions with the clinician. The cornerstones of the questionnaire battery were Patient and Significant Other versions of the West Haven–Yale Multidimensional Pain Inventory (WHYMPI; Kerns & Rosenberg, 1995; Kerns, Turk, & Rudy, 1985). These measures are based in C-B theory, are brief, and together provide a comprehensive view of the experience of chronic pain. The first section of the Patient version of the WHYMPI has several subscales that provide a view of the patient's pain experience as well his or her own affective and behavioral responses. The second section is a set of three subscales reporting on the significant other's frequency of responding to the patient's pain with either solicitous (e.g., expressing sympathy), distracting (e.g., cuing adaptive coping), or negative (e.g., expressing irritation) responses. Two nearly identical sets of items make up the Significant Other version of the WHYMPI. Table 12.1 presents the items of the second section of the Significant Other version. A third section of the Patient version provides indices of the patient's activity level.

On the Patient version of the WHYMPI, Mr. H reported a high level of pain, a high

TABLE 12.1. Item Content of the Significant Other Version of the Pain-Relevant Response Scales of the WHYMPI

Solicitous responses
Ask what I can do to help.
Express sympathy.
Give him/her a massage.
Take over his/her jobs or duties.
Try to get him/her to rest.
Get him/her some medication.
Get him/her something to eat or drink.
Try to comfort him/her by listening to his/her complaints.
Tell him/her not to exert himself/herself.
Turn on the T. V. to take his/her mind off the pain.

Distracting responses
Talk to him/her about something else to take his/her mind off the pain.
Try to involve him/her in some activity.
Encourage him/her to work on a hobby.

Negative responses
Leave the room.
Express irritation at him/her.
Express my frustration at him/her.
Express anger at him/her

Note. From Kerns and Rosenberg (1995). Copyright 1995 by the International Association for the Study of Pain. Reprinted by permission of Elsevier Science.

degree of interference of pain in his life, a low level of activity, a low level of self-control in relation to his pain, a high level of depressed mood, and a low level of support from significant others. He also reported a high level of responses from significant others, including each of the categories of solicitous, distracting, and negative responses. Mrs. H and their children generally corroborated his report. However, Mrs. H reported a significantly lower level of positive responses to her husband's pain, whereas the children reported few negative responses. Mrs. H and their younger son reported high levels of personal distress in response to Mr. H's pain. Not surprisingly, Mrs. H and both the children viewed Mr. H as highly dependent on others.

Several other questionnaires were administered, including the Beck Depression Inventory (BDI; Beck, Ward, Mendelsohn, Mock, & Erbaugh, 1961), the State–Trait Anxiety Inventory (STAI; Spielberger, Gorsuch, & Luschene, 1976), the Locke–

Wallace Marital Adjustment Scale (MAS; Locke & Wallace, 1959), the Problem Solving Inventory (PSI; Heppner & Peterson, 1982), the Pain Behavior Checklist (PBCL; Kerns, Haythornthwaite, et al., 1991), and the McGill Pain Questionnaire (Melzack, 1975). These questionnaires revealed Mr. H to experience a severe level of depressive symptoms and anxiety and a moderately low level of marital satisfaction. He also acknowledged poor perceptions of personal control and problem-solving abilities. Mrs. H reported a mild level of depression and a high level of marital dysfunction. Both sons acknowledged a mild level of depressive symptoms.

Mr. H also completed a pain intensity self-monitoring procedure (Kerns, Finn, & Haythornthwaite, 1988), which demonstrated an overall high level of pain intensity with nearly daily exacerbations in the late afternoon and evening. Mrs. H and her sons were trained in a diary procedure that is displayed in Figure 12.2 (Flor, Kerns, & Turk, 1987). Each was trained to make entries in the diary when they observed Mr. H to be exhibiting pain (e.g., rubbing his forearm or grimacing). They were to record the behavior indicating pain, what they thought, what they felt, what they tried to do to help (if anything), and a rating of how effective they felt that they had been. These recordings were discussed extensively during the assessment process and continued to be a focus of discussion throughout the treatment phase. In particular, a pattern of solicitousness on the part of the sons, and frequently Mrs. H, in response to the patient's displays of pain was noted to be associated with feelings of helplessness and frustration and with ratings of limited effectiveness. There was little evidence of efforts to cue adaptive coping, activity, or verbal interaction. Figure 12.2 displays examples of Mrs. H's diary entries.

CONCEPTUALIZATION

By the end of the third assessment session, a more focused discussion took place that articulated several specific problem domains and hypothesized contributors to these problems. The clinician highlighted Mr. H's low level of pleasurable and constructive activity, which included a very low level of pleasurable interaction among the family members and an associated high level of affective distress experienced by each of the family members. Contributors to these difficulties included the family's beliefs that it

Name: _____   Date: _____

Time	Location	How you recognized spouse's pain	What you thought	How you felt	How you tried to help	Your effectiveness 0–5
2:00 P.M.	At home, in living room	He was lying down, face looked drawn, heard him breathing, moaning.	"It seems hopeless."	Frustrated Angry at doctors	I asked him if I could get him some painkillers or make some tea.	0
					I rubbed his shoulder.	4
					I made some tea.	4
11:00 P.M.	In bed, at home	Husband got out of bed, was pacing the floor and took some medicine.		Frustrated Helpless	I didn't know what to do so I turned over and cried myself to sleep.	0

FIGURE 12.2. Spouse Diary.

was helpless to do anything to promote positive change and that withdrawal/avoidance was an effective strategy in lowering Mr. H's pain and suffering.

TREATMENT

After this conceptual framework was discussed, the family agreed to remain involved in treatment. A plan was established that called for both individual and family therapy. Weekly individual sessions were planned. These sessions were intended to help Mr. H develop improved pain coping strategies and reduce his depressive cognitions. The clinician and Mr. H established goals for increasing physical activity and exercising and decreasing absenteeism from work, and these became additional targets in the individual therapy sessions. Monthly family therapy sessions were also scheduled. Primary goals of the family work included altering patterns of pain-relevant communication within the family, increasing time spent in non-pain-related conversation among the family members, and increasing pleasurable activities with the children and pleasurable spousal activities. In addition, Mr. H agreed to a referral for vocational/educational counseling related to his interest in improving his vocational skills in order to increase his marketability for higher-level positions.

Ultimately, active treatment lasted for 3 months and involved 12 individual and 3 family sessions. The clinician employed a didactic/problem-solving orientation in each session. For example, the clinician taught Mr. H and the family to distinguish the experiences of pain, disability, and distress and to consider discrete ways to reduce pain, increase functioning, and improve mood. In this context, for example, the family was encouraged to set activity goals and to work toward them, regardless of Mr. H's reports of pain or other members perceptions' of his pain. Family activities that had previously been viewed as pleasurable were particularly encouraged. Obstacles to goal accomplishment were specifically discussed, and the family discovered ways to continue to work toward the goals despite pain or other perceived barriers. Again, a collaborative process that placed value on each family member's input was employed.

Therapeutic efforts consistently attempted to reinforce the patient's sense of control or mastery of his pain and to reduce his feelings of helplessness and depression. Similarly, the family members were encouraged to appreciate that there were important ways to change their patterns of interaction with Mr. H that would be effective in helping him in his efforts to improve his management of pain and to improve his functioning. The clinician emphasized the important role of thoughts as mediators of each family member's behavior and emotional response. All members were made aware that their beliefs that they were helpless with regard to Mr. H's pain problem were inaccurate, and that maintenance of such beliefs was contributing to their own distress and to the family's generally inactive, passive, or avoidant approach to the problem. For example, diaries were used throughout the treatment process to reinforce the idea that one's appraisals (e.g., the wife's belief that her husband was using his pain as an excuse for avoiding doing the dishes) of another's behavior (e.g., Mr. H lying on the couch and moaning) contribute to the person's emotional and behavioral response (e.g., Mrs. H's expressing irritation). The clinician encouraged and consistently reinforced alternative ways of framing the situation (e.g., viewing it as an opportunity to cue adaptive behavior, such as an activity with the children).

Specific skills (i.e., autogenic relaxation and other attention diversion strategies) were presented, and practice of the skills was expected to occur at home. Although Mr. H was taught a relaxation exercise in his individual sessions, he agreed to teach his sons the exercise, and together they practiced at home throughout the remainder of the therapy. In the family sessions, the clinician engaged the family in discussions about alternative strategies. It was in this context that Mr. H's older son related that his father was particularly good at mental arithmetic and other mathematical manipulations. Mr. H became enthusiastic about the idea of using mental arithmetic (in fact, performing mathematical proofs in his head!) as an effective attention diversion strategy.

The clinician taught the family to encourage and reward Mr. H's involvement in pleasurable activities; weekly activity goals were established and progress was monitored. The family also chose to institute a family exercise program at home, and the patient decided to stop smoking as a function of family and individual discussions about increasing "well behaviors." Through his vocational counseling, Mr. H was able to obtain financial assistance to take college courses to improve his employability.

POSTTREATMENT ASSESSMENT

At the time of termination of treatment, all goals that the clinician had established prior to treatment and many other positive behavioral changes had been achieved. Mr. H's self-report of pain intensity had dramatically decreased. Quantifiable indices of depression, somatization, anxiety, and overall psychological distress had returned to levels within the normal range. The family reported a high level of satisfaction with the patient's changes. However, a mild degree of marital dissatisfaction reported at the initial assessment was still present. No change in Mr. H's vocational status had yet occurred, although he had made substantial progress toward enrollment at an area college. Maintenance of most of these positive changes was reported at both the 3-month and 6-month follow-up intervals. The only concern was a linear and mild increase in depressed mood over this period. The mild level of depression reported was not judged to be a significant problem at the 6-month follow-up, but the clinician encouraged Mr. H to recontact the clinic should he so desire.

Mr. F

Mr. F, a 64-year-old widowed male with a 12-year history of chronic neck pain, was referred by Oncology for a chronic pain evaluation. Mr. F was interviewed with his adult daughter with whom he lived.

ASSESSMENT

As in the case of Mr. H, a comprehensive evaluation was conducted, which included a semistructured pain assessment interview, administration of several questionnaires, and self-monitoring of daily pain intensity and situational antecedents and consequences of periods of peak pain. In the first assessment session, the clinician encouraged Mr. F and his daughter to adopt a perspective of a shared responsibility for the pain problem and for finding solutions for it. Consistent with this view, the clinician attempted to involve Mr. F and his daughter equally in all aspects of the assessment and treatment process and emphasized the importance of each of their perspectives.

As the assessment process started, it was clear that Mr. F and his daughter had different beliefs about the nature of the pain experience. Mr. F generally held a medical or biological perspective of the cause of the pain problem, and stated, "The doctors should be able to figure out why I have pain." In contrast, Mr. F's daughter believed that the situational events in the last 2 years (i.e., Mr. F's wife's death and the loss of his employment) were playing a significant role in the current pain experience. Both agreed they felt helpless in their attempts to reduce pain and hopeless about potential treatment efficacy.

Both Mr. F and his daughter described significant changes in their lives because of the pain experience. Mr. F described reductions in his activity level because "I am worried that something else is going to happen to me if I am not careful about what I do." Mr. F avoided most of his previously enjoyed activities such as golf, walking, yardwork, woodworking, and remodeling; he believed these activities might increase the damage to his neck and limit his abilities "even more." He also noted that he did not participate in social activities (visiting friends, going to the senior citizen center's activities, etc.), because "I don't feel like it" and "I don't want people feeling sorry for me because of my pain." Mr. F's daughter confirmed that her father's social and physical activities had decreased and added that she was concerned about his lack of activity.

Besides changes in his physical and social activities, Mr. F described changes in his mood and thoughts. He stated that he had been feeling depressed and frustrated when he thought about his pain. Mr. F reported that he felt "like an old decrepit man" when he couldn't perform household chores. He described getting down on himself and saying things like "I'm useless" and "I am a burden to my daughter." Mr. F and his daughter both noted that when Mr. F was "in a bad mood" he often reported that his pain was more severe and he stayed in bed. He also expressed feelings of uselessness and dependency, which may have contributed to his depressed mood. Despite Mr. F's depressed mood, his daughter denied symptoms of depressed mood and noted, "I have to be strong enough for both of us."

On further evaluation, Mr. F and his daughter completed 1 week of hourly pain ratings with a structured rating system (Kerns et al., 1988). Mr. F's ratings were varied, ranging (on a scale of 0 to 5) from 1 to 4, with higher ratings (e.g., 3 to 4) in the morning and late afternoon and lower ratings (e.g., 1 to 2) at midday and evening. These ratings tended to correspond with Mr. F's medication use. Mr. F's daughter rated the patient's pain as showing little variability across or within days, and she consistently rated his pain higher than he did.

Mr. F and his daughter also completed questionnaire packets for patients and family members that were similar to those administered to Mr. F. and his family. To evaluate pain severity, Mr. F's WHYMPI (Kerns et al., 1985) scores and McGill Pain Questionnaire (Melzack, 1975) ratings revealed a low level of reported pain severity when compared with levels in a clinical sample (i.e., other pain patients). In contrast, Mr. F's daughter reported on the Significant Other Version of the WHYMPI (Kerns & Rosenberg, 1995) that she rated Mr. F's pain severity higher than he did, and her ratings were in the average range compared with ratings in other clinical samples. Mr. F's WHYMPI subscales revealed a high level of solicitous responding by his daughter; this was consistent with the daughter's rating. Mr. F's and his daughter's scores were relatively low for punishing and distracting responses.

On the PBCL (Kerns, Haythornthwaite, et al., 1991), Mr. F reported few pain behaviors (e.g., affect, distorted ambulation, and facial distortion). In contrast, his daughter reported that she frequently noticed pain behaviors exhibited by her father. The daughter's reports were consistent with the clinician's ratings of pain behavior on the PBCL. Both the daughter and the clinician reported high levels of overt pain behavior, while Mr. F reported lower levels.

Mr. F completed several measures of affective distress, including the BDI (Beck et al., 1961) and the STAI (Spielberger et al., 1976). Most striking was Mr. F's acknowledgement of a mild level of depressive symptoms. Mr. F's daughter denied significant depressive symptoms for herself.

Mr. F and his daughter established four specific behavioral goals for Mr. F in treatment: (1) to attend activities at the senior center more often, (2) to golf with his brother, (3) to return to woodworking as a hobby, and (4) to assist the daughter with light housework. These goals were developed with the patient's physical limitations and current medical status in mind. He and his daughter negotiated a step-by-step process for completing these goals and decided which of these steps were realistically attainable.

CONCEPTUALIZATION

Conceptualization of the pain experience was an important next step. During the assessment, Mr. F and his daughter provided information about the pain experience based on their previous attempts to understand the pain and to figure out what to do about it. These preconceived beliefs and expectations about the pain experience affected how Mr. F and his daughter viewed potential treatments, and during the conceptualization phase they addressed these beliefs and expectations.

Mr. F described a 12-year history of chronic neck pain, but neither he nor his daughter could identify an event that corresponded with the onset of his pain. However, Mr. F stated that he believed his neck pain might have been caused by "overuse" of his neck and upper back muscles over the course of his vocational career. He also reported that 2 years ago "something happened in my neck." He reported that probably "getting older" was also contributing to his pain. However, Mr. F's daughter stated that prior to 2 years ago, she had known relatively little about her father's pain complaints and in fact had not realized the extent of his chronic pain problem. She stated her belief that Mr. F's neck pain was related to the death of her mother (the patient's wife). She stated that Mr. F's pain began after his wife (her mother) was diagnosed with breast cancer and had markedly increased since Mrs. F's death 14 months earlier. She believed that Mr. F had "not dealt with" the loss of his wife, and she wondered if this failure may have contributed to or caused his difficulties with pain.

During conceptualization, the clinician developed a clear understanding of both the patient's and his daughter's beliefs and expectations about the chronic pain problem. Once these beliefs and expectations had been outlined, the next step involved assisting Mr. F. and his daughter in reconceptualizing the chronic pain problem. Specifically, the clinician redefined it as a series of specific problems that had potential solutions (i.e., treatment), rather than as a generalized and vague problem.

Mr. F and his daughter agreed that there might well be other ways to view the pain problem, and they agreed to discuss some of these. After some discussion, Mr. F and his daughter agreed that anxiety and fear about injury, rather than actual physical limitation, were major contributors to Mr. F's inactivity. Mr. F had described, "not being able" to perform activities in the past, but he concluded that both his and his daughter's concern about injury currently kept him inactive. Because this was one of Mr. F's primary concerns, anxiety and fear about injury were viewed as one area targeted within his treatment.

Mr. F's daughter encouraged Mr. F to think about the impact of his wife's death and how it related to pain. Previously, Mr. F denied any significant relationship between his wife's death and his increased pain reports. The patient was encouraged to think broadly about depressed mood, anxiety, and anger, and about the impact of these emotions on his pain. Mr. F and his daughter decided that anxiety and depressed mood played a big role in how the patient described his pain, and that strategies to manage his mood might reduce his experience of pain.

Through discussion of Mr. F's day-to-day activities, a pattern of increased pain appeared. Because of chronic pain, Mr. F rested for long periods. This lack of activity caused Mr. F to lose strength and flexibility; thus, he felt as though he could not do anything. This lack of activity made him feel frustrated and depressed, as if he was not productive or living up to expectations. Thus, when he experienced lower pain he tended to push himself too hard, and then his pain symptoms returned and he could not finish what he started. Mr. F and his daughter described this as a common cycle of pain, depressed mood, and inactivity. This cycle of overexertion and inactivity was agreed on as a target for treatment.

Finally, Mr. F and his daughter were involved in a pattern of communication that actually reinforced Mr. F's pain complaints. Mr. F's daughter clearly wanted to "help" her father and often asked him how he was feeling and what she could do for him. In fact, she stated that she tried to do everything she could for him so that he would not have to be in pain. However, Mr. F stated that the more she did for him the less he did, and he actually felt less active and more depressed as a result. So, in performing most of the housework and routinely asking about Mr. F's pain, Mr. F's daughter inadvertently increased his pain. This pattern of communication between them was also targeted for treatment.

TREATMENT

Treatment for Mr. F's chronic pain focused on several areas. First, there were specific skills the patient and his daughter could learn, such as relaxation training, identification of distorted cognitive and behavioral patterns, distraction techniques, and problem solving. Second, cognitive and behavioral practice of these skills was incorporated into the patient's repertoire via out-of-session homework assignments. Treatment goals primarily focused on increasing activity (i.e., social activities) and altering distorted thinking and behavioral patterns. Third, the patient and his daughter were encouraged to play an active role in this process of developing strategies for pain management. This process of active involvement increased their confidence that they would learn strategies to manage Mr. F's pain effectively.

A strategy for altering distorted thinking patterns was addressed first. Mr. F and his daughter monitored thoughts, behaviors, feelings, situations, and reports of pain. Mr. F's and his daughter's diaries revealed a pattern of "all-or-nothing" or "black-and-white" thinking that dominated the way Mr. F thought and behaved in multiple situations and responded to pain. For example, Mr. F decided he would perform some light housework (e.g., dusting the living room). However, shortly after he started to dust, Mr. F noticed he was thinking, "I can't do anything important around the house" and "I'm useless." Once Mr. F started having these thoughts, he decided to quit dusting because "it isn't really going to help anyway." During treatment, the clinician encouraged Mr. F and his daughter to discuss the negative thought patterns and to develop alternative thoughts Mr. F would use while performing housework, such as "I am doing something to help" and "I am glad I can help around the house." In conjunction with these different thoughts, Mr. F's daughter stated she would reinforce these thoughts by making positive comments on her father's work, such as "the dusting looks great." Over time, Mr. F and his daughter concluded that his assisting with chores in the house was helpful, no matter how small the chores appeared, and that altering Mr. F's thought patterns made him feel like he was contributing to the household.

Mr. F and his daughter also wanted to increase activity in several areas of Mr. F's life. After some discussion, it became clear that one reason Mr. F had decreased his activities was that his wife was the person who planned activities for him; after she died, no one planned activities for him, so he did not have things to do. Mr. F and his daughter discussed how this problem could be addressed for multiple activities.

Mr. F had significantly decreased how often he went to the senior center in his town, despite the fact that he had many friends who routinely attended the center. He expressed a strong interest in increasing his attendance and participation in activities at the center. Mr. F started by calling a friend from the center and asking the friend to give him a ride to several chosen activities during the course of the week. Mr. F stated that this "forced me to go," and that once he got there, he had a good time and was glad he went. Mr. F's daughter agreed to ask routinely about the activities her father participated in at the center and support his attendance there.

Furthermore, Mr. F used to golf regularly with his brother but had stopped going with him. During goal setting, Mr. F decided to contact his physician to determine whether he could resume golfing safely to some extent. His physician stated that Mr. F could play golf but should limit himself to nine holes a day, take frequent breaks, and stop if he felt any "new" pain, discomfort, or weakness. Mr. F started to golf by riding in the cart and then putting only; eventually, he moved up to playing several holes a day. Mr. F reported feeling pleased with himself for golfing and "figuring out" how to accomplish this goal.

Also, Mr. F had been involved with woodworking and carpentry around the house, but in the past years had gotten away from this work. He stated that he wanted to increase his involvement with such activities and decided to make projects for people in the neighborhood (e.g., wooden reindeers for neighbors' yards at Christmas). He scheduled 30 minutes a day to work on projects in three 10-minute blocks of time during the day.

As Mr. F discussed some of his goals, his daughter said that she was nervous about his increasing his activity because he might get hurt; she thought Mr. F should spend more time resting. She also stated that she was performing much of the housework so that the patient would not have to "do things that could hurt him." As the discussion continued, it became clear that the daughter's concerns played a large role in supporting the patient's inactivity. After reassurance from the patient's primary physician, Mr. F's daughter agreed to support and encourage her father with his increased activity goals.

One of the specific skills Mr. F and his daughter focused on learning was a relaxation exercise. Although Mr. F and his daughter stated that Mr. F already used relaxation training, this use was described as listening to "one of those tapes" and repeating to himself, "You should relax more." During the assessment, both Mr. F and his daughter described themselves as having a high level of general arousal, "feeling worried and nervous most of the time." Mr. F and his daughter decided that relaxation training would be helpful for both of them, so they would perform the training together. During the treatment, a relaxation training session was audiotaped, and they used these tapes at home several times a week. Interestingly, Mr. F's daughter reported that the tapes assisted her in developing a "more relaxed attitude" toward many everyday issues, including the pain experience.

Finally, Mr. F and his daughter were involved in a pattern of communication that actually reinforced Mr. F's pain complaints. Mr. F and his daughter agreed that both of them knew that Mr. F had chronic pain and that his daughter would like to help him, so she did not need to ask questions about how he was feeling or whether he was in pain. In fact, when Mr. F exhibited pain behavior (e.g., grimacing, moaning, and taking pain medications), his daughter would not comment. Instead, she would focus comments on what activities he was performing and would provide support and encouragement for his "well behaviors."

POSTTREATMENT ASSESSMENT

Two weeks after treatment was concluded, Mr. F and his daughter returned for a follow-up session. Both Mr. F and his daughter reported that each had completed the behavioral, social, and personal goals set prior to treatment. Furthermore, Mr. F stated that he wanted to continue setting goals for himself to support the changes he had accomplished. Mr. F was particularly pleased with his daughter's efforts to support his increased activity and openly shared his feelings with her. Mr. F's daughter reported that the relationship between her and her father had greatly improved in quality over the course of treatment, and that one future goal for her was to do something with her father once a week. In describing pain reports, Mr. F and his daughter reported a decreased level of pain intensity and episodes of flare-ups. Overall, posttreatment questionnaires revealed a general decrease in psychological distress; specifically, Mr. F's depression ratings were significantly lowered.

Comments on the Cases

These two cases provide clinical details of how the transactional model for family

treatment for chronic pain may be applied. The first example of a couple and their children exemplifies how the chronic pain experience can have an impact on everyone in a family and how multiple areas of functioning for a family can be affected. Conversely, it exemplifies how other family members' beliefs contribute to patterns of interaction with patients that may serve to reinforce pain, disability, and distress. Treatment in this case was focused on involvement of the whole family in discussing, understanding, and developing strategies for the pain problem. With this emphasis on the family context, and specific engagement of the family in a process of reinforcing changes that the "patient" was making during treatment, multiple outcomes were enhanced. Ultimately, all family members experienced important benefits associated with their perceptions of contributing to a solution to the problem. The family's overall experience of helplessness and discouragement was replaced by one of accomplishment and optimism. The second case, a dyad, is probably more typical of those seen in clinical practice. Usually this dyad consists of a patient and significant other (e.g., spouse). However, the impact of the pain problem upon a dyad is similar to its impact on a family, as can be seen in the case summary.

Conclusions and Future Directions

The CBTM of family functioning has important implications for understanding the complexities of functioning within the family of a person with a chronic painful condition. The model, and the empirical data available to support it, offers a specific, testable framework for assessing family functioning—specifically, for examining the role of the family's influence on the ongoing adaptation and adjustment of the person with chronic pain. Particularly important is the development of methodologies that encourage examination of illness-specific family interactions in the context of more general patterns of family exchanges. Using these methods allows tests of specific learning-based hypotheses—an approach that has largely been lacking in literatures based on family systems perspectives or more traditional models of family functioning.

Critical to empirical efforts to evaluate the relevance of the CBTM is the continued development of reliable measures of family cognition, particularly the beliefs, attributions, and meanings concerning both the individual with the painful condition and pain-related interactions among family members. It is important to continue to respect the relatively independent domains of the experience of chronic pain (i.e., pain, disability, and emotional distress) and the patterns of verbal and nonverbal interaction that are specific to these domains. To complement available measures of spousal interaction, measures relevant to interactions with younger children, as well as adult children, or with others not living with the patient, should be evaluated. Efforts should be directed toward evaluating the predictive validity of aggregated scores versus individual family member's scores for behavioral and cognitive measures of pain-relevant interaction. Finally, given the obvious difficulties and limitations inherent in conducting longitudinal, naturalistic studies of family interactions that could test the model, treatment outcome studies that examine the efficacy of specific theory-driven family interventions are strongly encouraged.

Future directions in the clinical domain are similar to those outlined for research efforts. Of primary importance is the continued elaboration of family-focused models of clinical assessment and intervention with families of people experiencing chronic pain. This means equal attention to each member of the family, as well as attention to their composite family functioning. Increased use of available measures (such as several of those used in the case examples presented in this chapter) as well as of newly developed family-oriented measures consistent with the FAAR model is encouraged. Theory-driven conceptualization of the functioning of the family and the development of a family treatment plan should be based on a hypothesis-testing approach to assessment. Further specification of truly family-focused treatment strategies that are consistent with the CBTM is the ultimate goal. Such strategies will require creativity and probably some risk taking in order to break from the present tradition of individually oriented clinical efforts.

Acknowledgments

This chapter was supported by a Merit Review grant awarded to Robert D. Kerns from the Department of Veterans Affairs Office of Research and Development Medical Research Service.

References

Beck, A. T., Ward, C. H., Mendelsohn, M., Mock, J., & Erbaugh, J. (1961). An inventory for measuring depression. *Archives of General Psychiatry, 4*, 561–571.

Block, A., Kremer, E., & Gaylor, M. (1980). Behavioral treatment of chronic pain: The spouse as a discriminative cue for pain behavior. *Pain, 9*, 243–252.

Elliot, D. J., Trief, P. M., & Stein, N. (1986). Mastery, stress, and coping in marriage among chronic pain patients. *Journal of Behavioral Medicine, 9*, 549–558.

Flor, H., Kerns, R. D., & Turk, D. C. (1987). The role of spouse reinforcement, perceived pain, and activity levels of chronic pain patients. *Journal of Psychosomatic Research, 31*, 251–259.

Flor, H., Turk, D. C., & Rudy, T. E. (1989). Relationship of pain impact and significant other reinforcement of pain behaviors: The mediating role of gender, marital status and marital satisfaction. *Pain, 38*, 45–50.

Fordyce, W. E. (1976). *Behavioral methods for chronic pain and illness*. St. Louis, MO: Mosby.

Friedman, H. (1992). *Hostility, coping and health*. Washington, DC: American Psychological Association.

Goldberg, G. M., Kerns, R. D., & Rosenberg, R. (1993). Pain-relevant support as a buffer from depression among chronic pain patients low in instrumental activity. *Clinical Journal of Pain, 9*, 34–40.

Heppner, P. P., & Peterson, C. H. (1982). The development and implications of a personal problem solving inventory. *Journal of Counseling Psychology, 29*, 66–75.

Johnson, S. B. (1998). Family management of childhood diabetes. *Journal of Clinical Psychology in Medical Settings, 1*, 309–315.

Keefe, F. J., & Caldwell, D. S., Baucom, D., Salley, A., Robinson, E., Timmons, K., Beaupre, P., Weisberg, J., & Helms, M. (1996). Spouse-assisted coping skills training in the management of osteoarthritic knee pain. *Arthritis Care and Research, 9*, 279–291.

Kerns, R. D. (1994). Pain management. In M. Hersen & R. T. Ammerman (Eds.), *Handbook of prescriptive treatments for adults* (pp. 443–462). New York: Plenum Press.

Kerns, R. D. (1999). Family therapy for adults with chronic pain. In R. J. Gatchel & D. C. Turk (Eds.), *Psychosocial factors in pain: Critical perspectives* (pp. 445–456). New York: Guilford Press.

Kerns, R. D., Finn, P. E., & Haythornthwaite, J. (1988). Self-monitored pain intensity: Psychometric properties and clinical utility. *Journal of Behavioral Medicine, 11,* 71–72.

Kerns, R. D., Haythornthwaite, J., Rosenberg, R., Southwick, S., Giller, E. L., & Jacob, M. C. (1991). The Pain Behavior Check List (PBCL): Factor structure and psychometric properties. *Journal of Behavioral Medicine, 14,* 155–167.

Kerns, R. D., Haythornthwaite, J., Southwick, S., & Giller, E. L. (1990). The role of marital interaction in chronic pain and depressive symptom severity. *Journal of Psychosomatic Research, 34,* 401–408.

Kerns, R. D., & Jacob, M. C. (1995). Toward and integrative diathesis–stress model of chronic pain. In A. J. Goreczny (Ed.), *Handbook of health and rehabilitation psychology* (pp. 325–340). New York: Plenum Press.

Kerns, R. D., & Rosenberg, R. (1995). Pain-relevant responses from significant others: Development of a significant other version of the WHYMPI Scales. *Pain, 61,* 245–249.

Kerns, R. D., & Rosenberg, R. (2001). *Couples' patterns of pain-relevant communication and dimensions of the chronic pain experience.* Manuscript submitted for publication.

Kerns, R. D., Stein, K., & Otis, J. D. (2001). Cognitive-behavioral approaches to pain management for older adults. *Topics in Geriatric Rehabilitation, 16,* 24–33.

Kerns, R. D., Southwick, S., Giller, E. L., Haythornthwaite, J., Jacob, M. C., & Rosenberg, R. (1991). The relationship between reports of pain-related social interactions and expressions of pain and affective distress. *Behavior Therapy, 22,* 101–111.

Kerns, R. D., Turk, D. C., & Rudy, T. E. (1985). The West Haven–Yale Multidimensional Pain Inventory (WHYMPI). *Pain, 23,* 345–356.

Kerns, R. D., & Weiss, L. H. (1994). Family influences on the course of chronic illness: A cognitive-behavioral transactional model. *Annals of Behavioral Medicine, 16,* 116–130.

Kopp, M., Richter, R., Rainer, J., Kopp-Wilfling, P., Rumpold, G., & Walter, M. H. (1995). Differences in family functioning between patients with chronic headache and patients with chronic low back pain. *Pain, 63,* 219–224.

Lazarus, R. S., & Folkman, S. (1984). *Stress, appraisal and coping.* New York: Springer.

Litman, T. J. (1974). The family as basic unit in health and medical care: A social–behavioral overview. *Social Science and Medicine, 8,* 495–519.

Locke, H. J., & Wallace, K. M. (1959). Short marital-adjustment and prediction tests: Their reliability and validity. *Marriage and Family Living, 21,* 251–255.

Marriott, A., Donaldson, C., Tarrier, N., & Burns, A. (2000). Effectiveness of cognitive-behavioral family intervention in reducing the burden of care in carers of patients with Alzheimer's disease. *British Journal of Psychiatry, 176,* 557–562.

Melzack, R. (1975). The McGill Pain Questionnaire: Major properties and scoring methods. *Pain, 1,* 277–299.

Moore, J. E., & Chaney, E. F. (1985). Outpatient group treatment of chronic pain: Effects of spouse involvement. *Journal of Consulting and Clinical Psychology, 53,* 326–334.

Moos, R. (1978). *Family Environmant Scale.* Palo Alto, CA: Consulting Psychologist Press.

Olson, D. H. (1989). Circumflex model and family health. In C. N. Ramsey (Ed.), *Family systems in medicine* (pp. 75–94). New York: Guilford Press.

Patterson, J. M., & Garwick, A. W. (1994a). The impact of chronic illness on families: A family systems perspective. *Annals of Behavioral Medicine, 16,* 131–142.

Patterson, J. M., & Garwick, A. W. (1994b). Levels of family meaning in family stress theory. *Family Process, 33,* 287–304.

Radojevic, V., Nicassio, P. M., & Weisman, M. H. (1992). Behavioral intervention with and without family support for rheumatoid arthritis. *Behavior Therapy, 23,* 13–30.

Ramsey, C. N. (1989). *Family systems in medicine.* New York: Guilford Press.

Reiss, D. (1989). Families and their paradigms: An ecologic approach to understanding the family and its social world. In C. N. Ramsey (Ed.), *Family systems in medicine* (pp. 119–134). New York: Guilford Press.

Rodrigue, J. R., Pearman, T. P., & Moreb, J. (1999). Morbidity and mortality following bone marrow transplantation: Predictive utility of pre-BMT affective functioning, compliance, and social support stability. *International Journal of Behavioral Medicine, 6,* 241–254.

Romano J. M., & Schmaling KB. (2001). Assessment of couples and families with chronic pain. In D. C. Turk & R. Melzack (Eds.), *Handbook of pain assessment* (2nd ed., pp. 346–361). New York: Guilford Press.

Romano, J. M., Turner, J. A., Friedman, L. S., Bulcroft, R. A., Jensen, M. P., Hops, H., & Wright, S. F. (1992). Sequential analysis of chronic pain behaviors and spouse responses. *Journal of Consulting and Clinical Psychology, 60,* 777–782.

Romano, J., Turner, J., & Jensen, M. (1997). The family environment in chronic pain patients: Comparison to controls and relationship to family functioning. *Journal of Clinical Psychology in Medical Settings, 4,* 383–395.

Romano, J. M., Turner, J. A., Jensen, M. P., Friedman, L. S., Bulcroft, R. A., Hops, H., & Wright, S. F. (1995). Chronic pain patient-spouse behavioral interactions predict patient disability. *Pain, 63,* 353–360.

Roy, R. (1986). A problem-centered family systems approach in treating intractable pain. In A. D. Holzman & D. C. Turk (Eds.), *Pain management: A handbook of psychological treatment approaches* (pp. 113–130). Elmsford, NY: Pergamon Press.

Roy, R. (1989). *Chronic pain and the family: A problem-centered perspective.* New York: Human Sciences Press.

Roy, R. (1992). *The social context of the chronic pain sufferer.* Toronto: University of Toronto Press.

Roy, R. (2001). *Social relations and chronic pain.* New York: Plenum Press.

Saarijarvi, S. (1991). A controlled study of couple therapy in chronic low back pain patients. Effects on marital satisfaction, psychological distress and health attitudes. *Journal of Psychosomatic Research, 35,* 265–272.

Saarijaervi, S., Hyyppae, M., Lehtinen, V., & Alanen, E. (1990). Chronic low back pain patient and spouse. *Journal of Psychosomatic Research, 34,* 117–122.

Schmaling, K. B., & Sher, T. G. (2000). *The psychology of couples and illness: Theory research and practice.* Washington, DC: American Psychological Association.

Schwartz, G. E. (1982). Testing the biopsychosocial model: The ultimate challenge facing behavioral medicine. *Journal of Consulting and Clinical Psychology, 50,* 1040–1053.

Schwartz, L., Slater, M. A., & Birchler, G. R. (1996). The role of pain behaviors in the modulation of marital conflict in chronic pain couples. *Pain, 65,* 227–233.

Schwartz, L., Slater, M. A., Birchler, G. R., & Atkinson, J. (1991). Depression in spouses of chronic pain patients and the role of patients' pain, anger, and marital satisfaction. *Pain, 44,* 61–67.

Spielberger, C., Gorsuch, R., & Luschene, N. (1976). *Manual for the State–Trait Anxiety Inventory.* Palo Alto, CA: Consulting Psychologists Press.

Turk, D. C., & Kerns, R. D. (1985a). *Health, illness and families: A life span perspective.* New York: Wiley.

Turk, D. C., & Kerns, R. D. (1985b). The family in health and illness. In D. C. Turk & R. D. Kerns (Eds.), *Health, illness and families: A life span perspective* (pp. 1–22). New York: Wiley.

Turk, D. C., Kerns, R. D., & Rosenberg, R. (1992). Effects of marital interaction on chronic pain and disability: Examining the down side of social support. *Rehabilitation Psychology, 37,* 259–274.

Turk, D. C., Meichenbaum, D., & Genest, M. (1983). *Pain and behavioral medicine: A cognitive- behavioral perspective.* New York: Guilford Press.

von Bertalanffy, L. (1968). *General systems theory.* New York: Braziller.

Weiss, L. H., & Kerns, R. D. (1995). Patterns of pain-relevant social interactions. *International Journal of Behavioral Medicine, 2,* 157–171.

13

Integration of Pharmacotherapy with Psychological Treatment of Chronic Pain

Peter B. Polatin
Noor M. Gajraj

Pain is a dramatic symptom and one of the easiest and most successful ways of relieving it is by using medications or by performing an injection. In medicine today, many classes of drugs have documented efficacy in alleviating pain (Table 13.1). Early, or acute, pain is treated aggressively with agents that act directly on either the anatomic pain generator or the central receptors. The initial focus is on reducing the intensity of the primary nociceptive symptom.

The longer the pain lasts, the more complicated the treatment process becomes because of changes in anatomical pain pathways, receptors, and neurotransmitters. This is certainly true in the pharmacological approach to pain. As the pain process continues, other pharmacological agents may be used that act on the transmission or augmentation of the nociceptive signal in the nervous system, and on the secondary symptoms that may develop with chronicity. The psychotropic agents, particularly the antidepressants, have a well-documented role in the management of chronic pain, although it is sometimes unclear whether their primary effects are on the nociception or on the emotional distress.

Issues of tolerance, dependence, addic-

tion, and abuse are a concern, with some pharmacological agents used to treat pain, particularly the opioids, the stimulants, and the minor tranquilizers (anxiolytics). *Tolerance* is a physiological adaptive process and refers to the need to increase the dose of a drug over time to achieve the same effects. Tolerance is usually not a significant clinical problem except in addiction-prone patients, who can be identified by psychosocial assessment and in initial clinical monitoring. The need to increase doses of opiate in chronic pain patients is usually the result of disease progression. *Dependence* refers to the syndrome of symptoms precipitated by the cessation of a particular drug and ranges from mild restlessness to severe manifestations such as seizures or coma. *Addiction* is a behavioral term, which refers to the aberrant use of a substance in a manner characterized by loss of control, by preoccupation with procurement and usage (obsession and compulsion), and with consequent social and occupational impairment. *Abuse* refers to a maladaptive pattern of psychoactive substance usage outside sociocultural conventions or when there are no therapeutic indications. By definition, all use of illicit drugs is abuse, as is use of drugs not accord-

TABLE 13.1. Medications Used to Treat Chronic Pain

Acetaminophen	Antidepressants
Nonsteroidal anti-inflammatory drugs (NSAIDs)	Tramadol
	Alpha-2-adrenergic agonists
Opioids	Topical agents (EMLA cream, lidocaine 5%,
Muscle relaxants	capsaicin cream)
Anticonvulsants	

ing to a physician's orders. Regulatory measures from outside the medical profession, instituted to minimize such risks, exercise an influence on prescribing practices. In addition to these serious physiological and behavioral syndromes, other side effects of a particular agent, such as central nervous system depression, toxicity to liver or kidney function, or bone marrow suppression, may limit its usefulness for the long-term control of chronic pain.

Pharmacotherapy is an important treatment approach for chronic pain, but it is best used in a multidisciplinary context along with other biobehavioral interventions aimed at decreasing suffering and increasing functional and personal autonomy. This team effort requires interdisciplinary planning, communication, monitoring, and feedback. To assume that medication alone will resolve the complex psychosocioeconomic stressors with which the chronic pain patient is attempting to cope is both naive and simplistic. Therefore, because the treatment of chronic pain is a collaborative process between health care disciplines, it is important for not only physicians but also allied health professionals to be knowledgeable about choices of medication to control pain, efficacy of specific drugs in various chronic pain syndromes, dosage ranges, and side effects. Later in this chapter, we provide examples of this interdisciplinary approach in the treatment of some common chronic pain profiles.

Nociceptive and Psychological Symptoms in Chronic Pain

In chronic pain states, the experience of pain may differ depending on the site and nature of the pathology. Cluster headaches are descriptively different than migraine or muscle tension headaches. Low back pain secondary to degenerative disc disease is different than low back pain secondary to a herniated disc with nerve root irritation. This primary nociceptive difference is associated with variations in efficacy of different drugs. The opioids, while the most universally effective pain medication, are less successful with neuropathic syndromes and bone pain (Twycross, 1994). Neuropathic pain tends to be relatively opioid resistant and responds better to antidepressant and anticonvulsant medications. Bone pain responds better to nonsteroidal anti-inflammatory drugs (NSAIDs). Psychotropic agents, which do not have any recognized analgesic properties, nevertheless dramatically alleviate certain pain syndromes. For example, lithium carbonate, used to treat bipolar affective disorder, controls pain in some cases of migraine and cluster headaches (Mathew, 1978). Tegretol (carbamazepine), an antiepileptic and psychotropic, is the drug of choice to relieve the pain of trigeminal neuralgia (Delfino, 1983).

Secondary symptoms of emotional distress are frequently seen in patients with chronic pain (Burton, Polatin, & Gatchel, 1997; Kinney, Gatchel, Polatin, Fogarty, & Mayer, 1993; Polatin, Kinney, Gatchel, Lillo, & Mayer, 1993) and will worsen the prognosis unless adequately treated. In some cases, the onset follows and is a result of the pain. In other instances, emotional symptoms may have preceded pain onset but either resolved or became less troublesome and were exacerbated by the duration of the pain syndrome. Maladaptive coping styles, commonly associated with personality disorders or previous experiences of physical and psychic trauma, may become more clinically evident as a result of chronic pain. Studies have repeatedly documented high prevalence rates of major depression, anxiety syndromes, substance and alcohol abuse, and personality disorders in this group of patients (e.g., Brandt, Celentano, Stewart, Linet, & Polstein, 1990; Burton et al., 1997; Polatin et al., 1993). In addition, the worsening of preexisting biological illnesses such as schizophrenia and bipolar affective disorder, or increasing psychotic or dysfunctional symptoms in borderline or antisocial personality disorders, may require management with psychotropic medication. Therefore, the full range of clinical psychopharmacology is required to treat secondary symptoms of emotional distress in the chronic pain population.

Pharmacological Agents Used to Treat Chronic Pain

Opioids

The opioids are unquestionably the most useful agents for the relief of pain, because of their primary agonistic effects on μ opioidal receptors in the brain and spinal cord. Peripheral opioid receptors in primary afferent nociceptive neurons, when stimulated, may raise the pain threshold and inhibit the release of pain producing inflammatory substances from these neurons. There are mediating receptors in the spinal cord, midbrain, brainstem, and thalamus, as well as in the limbic system and cortex, all of which may be affected by both endogenous and exogenous opiates.

Concerns about psychological dependence including aberrant drug-seeking behavior have greatly restricted the use of the opioids, except in treating that group of patients with the worse prognosis, namely, cancer pain. The short-acting opioids such as hydrocodone (Vicodin, Lortab) and oxycodone (Percocet) are generally more abused than long-acting opioids such as methadone. Longer-acting opioids do not tend to cause the central nervous system "high" that the addict desires. However, recently there has been concern about the abuse potential and recreational diversion of one of these agents ("U.S. asks painkiller maker," 2001; "Shipment of potent pain pills," 2001).

Even in acute pain patients, surveys have shown that physicians underprescribe the opioids (Cooper, Czechowicz, Petersen, & Molinan, 1992; Gourlay & Cousins, 1984), with doses that are suboptimal, too infre-

quent, or for inadequate periods of time. Studies on the use of long-term opioids to treat chronic pain have demonstrated that the risk of addiction to a patient with opioid-responsive pain is low in the absence of factors such as a past history of substance abuse, severe personality disorder, or experience of childhood traumatic events (Portnoy & Foley, 1986; Taub, 1982).

Concern about respiratory depression has also limited the use of opioids in chronic pain. However, experience and research have demonstrated that pain physiologically antagonizes the central depressant effects of the opioids (Twycross, 1994; Walsh, Baxter, & Bowman, 1981), while this side effect is readily seen in the addict or control subject without clinical pain. Even high doses of potent narcotics may be used in chronic pain patients, with careful medical monitoring, without risk of respiratory depression.

Guidelines have been proposed for providing opioid maintenance therapy to patients with chronic, noncancer pain. These guidelines include prior trials of alternate analgesia (covered later in this chapter), exclusion of patients with risk factors for addiction, and primary medication responsibility by a single physician. The pain syndrome must be documented as responsive to opioids by clinical trial. Goals for functional improvement should be stipulated and agreed on to justify the regimen. Careful monitoring and documentation of degree of analgesia, side effects, functional status, and evidence of aberrant drug-related behavior should be performed on a regular basis (Portnoy, 1994).

These guidelines are primarily empirical and not supported by large clinical trials. For example, it has not been unequivocally established that prior addiction or personality disorder is always contraindicative for opioid treatment of chronic nonmalignant pain. Such patients have been successfully treated with opioids, although long-acting opioids such as methadone are recommended. Conversely, following all the guidelines does not protect the practitioner from exposing some patients to addiction. However, in spite of the tentative nature of the concept of long-term opioid maintenance for noncancer pain, guidelines are becoming institutionalized. In 1994 the state of California drafted a position paper addressing the treatment of chronic pain with opioids according to "principles of responsible professional practice." Physicians are expected to document a history, physical examination, formulated treatment plan, informed consent from the patient, periodic review of treatment, consultation as necessary, accurate recordkeeping, and compliance with controlled substance regulations (Medical Board of California, 1994). Similar guidelines have been set up in other states.

The most convenient route of administration is oral, but delivery per rectum, parenterally (subcutaneously, intramuscularly, or intravenously), and by interspinal injection is also described. Recently, fentanyl has been delivered by the oral transmucosal route in the form of a "lollipop" for breakthrough pain (Lichtor et al., 1999). The oral and rectal dose is generally two to three times higher than that by the parenteral routes. For maximum comfort, dosing intervals should not be "as needed" because by the time pain reemerges, the patient would have an interval of discomfort prior to the therapeutic onset of the next dose. Rather, patients should be dosed on a time-contingent basis according to the half-life of the particular medication, which may range from 2 hours for demerol to 8 hours for methadone (France & Krishnan, 1988).

Opioids with shorter half-lives, such as demerol and pentazocine, require more frequent dosing and are less desirable for the treatment of chronic pain.

The choice of particular medication should proceed from a weaker to a stronger agent, depending on the clinical response. Clearly, an increase in dose or potency proceeds from the need to control the pain but may be reflective of tolerance. In opioid responsive pain, patients will typically plateau at a particular dose, beyond which further increases will not be required to control pain. Thus, an initial trial with an NSAID with poor response would proceed to a weak opioid such as codeine or hydrocodone, and then—if necessary—to a strong opioid such as morphine, oxycodone, or methadone (Twycross, 1994) (see Table 13.2). The fentanyl patch allows transdermal administration of opioid and may be associated with less side effects than other opiates, high patient satisfaction, and less abuse potential (Simpson, Edmonson, Constant, & Collier, 1997). Kadian is a capsule formulation of morphine designed for 12- or 24-hourly dosing (Broomhead, Kerr, Tester, O'Meara, & Maccarrone, 1997).

Side effects of opioids are monitored carefully (see Table 13.3). Constipation is quite common, but can be controlled easily with laxatives. Respiratory depression is

TABLE 13.2. Opioid and Centrally Acting Analgesic Dosages (Compared to Morphine)

Drug	Dose (mg), oral	Dose (mg), i.m.	Duration (hr)
Morphine	30	10	4
Codeine	200	130	4–6
Hydrocodone (Lortab)	5–10	—	4–8
Hydromorphone (Dilaudid)	2–4	1–4	4–8
Levo-Dromoran	2	—	6–8
Methadone	20	10	6–8
Oxycodone	30	15	4
Meperidine	300	75	1–3
Pentazocine	180	60	2–3
Tramadol (Ultram)	50–100		4–6

Special preparations of long-acting opioids for treatment of chronic pain			
Drug	Dose, oral	Dose, s.c.	Duration
Oxycontin	10–40 mg		8–12 hr
MS Contin	15–60 mg		8–12 hr
Duragesic patch (fentanyl)		25–100 μg	3 days

TABLE 13.3. Side Effect of Opioids

CNS	Gastrointestinal
Mental clouding	Constipation
Mood changes	Abdominal pain
Drowsiness	Nausea, vomiting
Miosis	
Respiratory depression	*Other*
Suppressed cough	Urinary retention
	Sweating, itching, flushing
Cardiovascular	Tolerance, addiction, withdrawal
Orthostatic hypotension	

seen rarely in chronic pain patients, and only when pain is relieved, for example, after surgery or a neural ablative procedure, and the opioid dosage is not adjusted downward thereafter (Hanks, Twyercross, & Lloyd, 1981). Geriatric patients are at greater risk for oversedation, hypotension, and urinary retention but with careful monitoring of dosage and side effects may still be effectively managed for chronic pain complaints.

Non-Narcotic Analgesics

This group of medications includes aspirin, acetaminophen (Tylenol), and the NSAIDs. The major analgesic effect of the non-narcotic analgesics is at the tissue site of the pain, although there may be centrally mediated analgesic effects as well (Dubas & Parker, 1971; Malmberg & Yaksh, 1992). Although used quite frequently for chronic pain, their efficacy is proven only in those syndromes associated with inflammatory processes such as rheumatoid arthritis and osteoarthritis. They may also be useful for the short-term management of musculoskeletal pain and headaches and are a good initial choice for the control of mild to moderate acute pain. In chronic pain syndromes of central or peripheral origin, their utility is far more controversial, and they are not effective in chronic pain syndromes with secondary symptoms of emotional distress.

Dosage varies, depending on the agent, and is listed in Table 13.4. Certain of these medications may be given once a day, making them more convenient for responsive patients. Because these drugs have a ceiling effect, increasing the dosage beyond a certain threshold does not increase analgesia,

although it may increase duration of pain relief. Analgesia results from the blocking of stimulation of primary afferent nociceptors (Fields, 1987) through inhibition of the cyclo-oxygenase (COX) enzyme, thereby preventing prostaglandin biosynthesis and inflammatory response. Other, less prominent peripheral effects include direct spinal blockade of hyperalgesia (Malmberg & Yaksh, 1992) and prevention of release of certain inflammatory secretions from white blood cells (Abramson, 1991).

Side effects are frequent, and particularly in the gastrointestinal tract. Irritation of the stomach, lower esophagus, and colon may cause symptoms of indigestion, heartburn, and diarrhea progressing to passage of blood in vomitus or stool. With prolonged therapy, elevation of liver function tests may occur, although rarely does this elevation progress to tissue damage. Impaired kidney function, prolonged bleeding time, easy bruising, bronchospasm, worsening asthma, skin rashes, photosensitivity, and occasional central nervous system (CNS) effects (tinnitus, hearing loss, headache) may be seen with these drugs. Therefore, careful medical monitoring is essential. One side effect not seen, however, is dependence or addiction, making these agents more popular for the treatment of chronic pain than their documented clinical efficacy would justify.

There is no good way of choosing which NSAID to use, but if one drug does not work, the next choice should be from a different chemical group (see Table 13.4). Before the NSAIDs are rejected, trials of at least four different agents should be attempted, with 2 weeks on each drug and administration on a regularly scheduled basis (time contingent dosage). While these agents are being used, patients should be pe-

TABLE 13.4. NSAIDs: Chemical Group and Dosage

Group/drug	Dose (mg)	Times per day	Maximum daily dose (mg)
Proprionic acids			
Fenoprofen (Nalfon)	200–600	2–4	3,200
Flurbiprofen (Ansaid)	100	2–3	300
Ibuprofen (Motrin)	400–800	2–6	3,200
Ketoprofen (Orudis, Oruvail)	50–200	1–3	300
Naproxen sodium (Anaprox, Naprelan)	275–550	2–4	1,375
Naproxen (Naprosyn)	350–500	2–3	1,500
Oxaprozin (Daypro)	600–1,200	1–2	1,200
Ketorolac (Toradol)	10	2–4	40
Acetic acids			
Diclofenac (Voltaren, Cataflam)	50–75	2–3	200
Etodolac (Lodine)	300–600	2–3	1,200
Indomethacin (Indocin)	25–75	2–4	200
Sulindac (Clinoril)	200	2	400
Tolmetin (Tolectin)	200–600	2–4	2,000
Fenamates (anthranilic acids)			
Meclofenamate (Meclomen)	50–100	2–6	400
Mefenamic acid (Ponstel)	250	4	100
Oxicams			
Piroxicam (Feldene)	10–20	1–2	20
Meloxicam (Mobic)	7.5	1	15
Salicylic acids			
Salsalate (Disalcid)	500–750	2	1,500
Diflunisal (Dolobid)	250–500	2	1,000
Trisalicylate (Trilisate)	500–1,000	2	3,000
Naphthylalkanones			
Nabumetone (Relafen)	500–750	1–2	1,500
Coxibs			
Celecoxib (Celebrex)	100–200	1–2	800
Rofecoxib (Vioxx)	12.5–50	1–2	50

riodically questioned about side effects and have their bleeding time and liver and kidney function tests performed at some regular interval.

COX exists in two isoforms. COX-1 is involved in blood clotting and gastrointestinal protection while COX-2 mediates pain and inflammation. Selective COX-2 inhibitors such as celecoxib and rofecoxib are as efficacious as traditional NSAIDs but have a lower incidence of gastrointestinal side effects and no effect on blood clotting (Silverstein et al., 2000). These new agents are particularly useful for high-risk patients such as the elderly or patients with a previous history of gastrointestinal bleeding. However, because of the costs and constraints of many prescription plans, these agents are considered "second line" agents, and may only be used after two conventional NSAIDs have been tried.

Antidepressants

There is a documented role for the antidepressants in the treatment of chronic pain syndromes, particularly headache and neuropathic pain, less so in arthritis and low back pain, where they are most commonly employed (Monks, 1994; Onghena & van Houdenhove, 1992). It is frequently not clear whether these agents promote improvement in chronic pain by direct antinociceptive effect or by mitigation of the secondary symptom of depression, so commonly seen in these patients (France & Krishnan, 1988). However, several studies have documented the direct analgesic prop-

TABLE 13.5. Categories of Antidepressants

Heterocyclics		MAO inhibitors
Imipramine (Tofranil)	Amoxapine (Asendin)	Phenelzine (Nardil)
Amitriptyline (Elavil)	Fluoxetine (Prozac)	Isocarboxazid (Marplan)
Nortriptyline (Pamelor)	Sertraline (Zoloft)	Tranylcypromine (Parnate)
Despiramine (Norpramine)	Paroxetine (Paxil)	
Clomipramine (Anafranil)	Citalopram (Celexa)	
Doxepin (Sinequan)	Bupropion (Wellbutrin)	
Maprotiline (Ludiomil)	Venlafaxine (Effexor)	
Trazodone (Desyrel)	Mirtazepine (Remeron)	

erties of these agents (Spiegel, Kalb, & Pasternak, 1983). Clinical trials in groups of chronic arthritis and migraine patients without clinical depression have documented pain relief (Gomersall & Stewart, 1973; Gringas, 1976). Other research has been able to differentiate pain relief without improvement of depression in chronic pain patients treated with antidepressants (Couch, Zigler, & Hassanein, 1976; Watson, Evans, & Reed, 1982). It should be noted that although the use of antidepressants for chronic pain syndromes has been clinically recognized, Goodkin and Gullion (1989) have suggested that most clinical studies are unsatisfactory secondary to inadequate design and protocol criteria. However, a more recent critical review has focused on antidepressant efficacy in chronic neuropathic pain (Max, 1995).

Antidepressants may be divided into two general categories, as illustrated in Table 13.5. The heterocyclics exert their therapeutic effect by blockading the reuptake of biogenic amines at interneuronal synaptic junctions in the CNS and spinal cord. The amines most critically involved in depression and chronic pain are norepinephrine and serotonin, and the heterocyclics vary in their specificity for one or both of these amines (see Table 13.6).

The monoamine oxidase (MAO) inhibitors act on a different metabolic pathway. They inhibit the enzyme monoamine oxidase in the brain and, therefore, block degradation of the biogenic amines. In clinical practice, these agents are less desirable than the heterocyclics because of the risk of potentially severe hypertension caused by the effect of certain foods and pharmacological agents on the monoamine oxidase-inhibited patient. People on MAO inhibitors must be on a tyramine-free diet and also avoid a number of prescription and over-the-counter medications. The MAO inhibitors have, nevertheless, been demonstrated to relieve migraine headache and atypical facial pain (Anthony & Lance, 1969; Lascelles, 1966), as well as the symptoms of depression.

HETEROCYCLIC ANTIDEPRESSANTS

Table 13.7 notes dosages of the various heterocyclic agents. These drugs have two different dosage ranges, depending on whether

TABLE 13.6. Specificity of Serotonin versus Norepinephrine Reuptake Blockade of the Heterocyclics

Serotonin only	Serotonin and norepinephrine equally	Norepinephrine only
Trazodone (Desyrel)	Doxepin (Sinequan)	Maprotiline (Ludiomil)
Fluoxetine (Prozac)	Imipramine (Tofranil)	Despramine(Norpramin)
Paroxetine (Paxil)	Venlafaxine (Effexor)	Nortriptyline (Pamelor)
Sertraline (Zoloft)	Bupropion (Wellbutrin)	
Nefazodone (Serzone)	Amoxapine (Asendin)	
Fluvoxamine (Luvox)	Clomipramine (Anafranil)	
Citalopram (Celexa)	Amitriptyline (Elavil)	
	Mirtazapine (Remeron)	

TABLE 13.7. Dosages of Heterocyclic Antidpressants

Drug	Dose for pain (mg)	Dose for depression (mg)
Desipramine (Norpramine)	75	75–200
Nortriptyline (Pamelor)	50–100	75–150
Maprotiline (Ludiomil)	?	75–300
Doxepin (Sinequan)	50–100	150–300
Imipramine (Tofranil)	50–75	150–300
Amitriptyline (Elavil)	75–150	150–300
Trazodone (Desyrel)	?	150–400
Fluoxetine (Prozac)	?	20–80
Sertraline (Zoloft)	?	50–200
Paroxetine (Paxil)	40–60	20–80
Venlafaxine (Effexor)	?	75–375
Clomipramine (Anafranil)	?	100–250
Bupropion (Wellbutrin)	?	200–450
Amoxapine (Asendin)	?	200–300
Nefazodone (Serzone)	?	300–600
Fluvoxamine (Luvox)	?	100–300
Mirtazepine (Remeron)	?	15–60

pain or depression is the symptom being treated. Pain responds at a lower dose and at a shorter time after initiation of therapy than does depression. This is particularly important when treating a chronic pain patient without depression, where the lower dose will be used. It is less relevant when both symptoms are present, because the antidepressant dosage will be used.

It follows that evaluation for depression should occur before antidepressant therapy is initiated. All heterocyclics have demonstrated antidepressant effects, but some more than others have a mitigating effect on chronic pain, particularly syndromes of neuropathic etiology. These include amitriptyline, desipramine, doxepin, imipramine, and clomipramine (see, e.g., France, Houpt, & Ellinwood, 1984; France & Krishnan, 1988; Onghena & Van Houdenhove, 1992). There is also increasing documentation of a primary analgesic affect with newer agents such as trazodone, fluoxetine, paroxetine, citalopram, mirtazepine, and sertraline (Anderberg, Marteinsdottir, & von Knorring, 2000; Ansari, 2000, Brannon & Stone, 1999).

The choice of heterocyclic agent will be based on degree of sedation desired, side effect profile, and specificity of biogenic amine reuptake blockade. Patients with agitation, anxiety, and insomnia will benefit from a more sedating heterocyclic such as doxepin, amitriptyline, trazodone, or mirtazepine. Those with anergia and psychomotor retardation would do better on a drug with a more energizing profile, such as nortriptyline, fluoxetine, sertraline, or citalopram.

The issue of which biogenic amine is primarily affected by the heterocyclic agent has both conceptual and clinical application. Heterocyclic agents with the best-documented nociceptive effects appear to be those agents with the ability for both serotonin and norepinephrine reuptake blockade, although primary serotonin and primary norepinephrine reuptake blockers have also demonstrated analgesia in chronic pain (Ansari, 2000; Ward, Bloom, & Friedel, 1979).

Beyond this conceptual consideration, the degree of norepinephrine versus serotonin reuptake blockade of any individual heterocyclic will influence its side effect profile (see Table 13.5). Heterocyclics with a high degree of noradrenergic activity are associated with primary autonomic, cardiac, and ocular side effects, which may be particularly problematic for the older patient with heart disease, glaucoma, prostatic hypertrophy, or cognitive impairment. Primarily serotonergic agents may be preferable in this age group, and in patients who have had a particularly refractory reaction to a previously tried heterocyclic, such as increased appetite, sedation, or intolerable dry mouth. However, the serotonergic agents are more frequently associated with headaches, gastric symptoms, and agitation and may not be helpful in patients with a high level of anxiety.

Side effects of the heterocyclic antidepressants are common, and require careful clinical monitoring (Table 13.8). Doses of all heterocyclics are started low and titrated upward, guided by improvement in pain or depression and by emergence of side effects. With several of the older tricyclics (elavil, sinequan, tofranil), a therapeutic blood level is associated with some dry mouth or morning "hangover." However, any side effect that is associated with distress or impaired functioning will require dosage modification or a change of medication.

The drawing of blood levels to monitor clinical response is useful when (1) an agent with a "therapeutic window" is being prescribed such as imipramine; (2) the clinical response is ambiguous, raising the questions of absorption and compliance; (3) an older or more medically complicated patient is be-ing treated. The routine use of blood levels is, however, not essential for a safe and effective administration of these antidepressant medications.

The heterocyclic antidepressants have also been used as adjuncts to narcotic analgesics in the treatment of chronic pain (France, Urban, & Keefe, 1984; Urban, France, & Sternberger, 1986). Patients on this combined regimen tend to tolerate a lower narcotic maintenance dosage without dependence or abuse. Pain syndromes previously refractory to narcotics alone may be more responsive to combined therapy.

MAO INHIBITORS

The use of the MAO inhibitors to treat chronic pain with or without depression has documented efficacy (Anthony & Lance, 1969; Lascelles, 1966), but the precautions required by this group of agents makes it a less desirable choice than the heterocyclic an-

---

TABLE 13.8. Side Effects of Heterocyclic Antidepressants

Autonomic
  *Dry mouth
  *Blurred vision
  Retarded ejaculation
  *Decreased intestinal mobility
  *Urinary retention
  Pathological sweating
  Anorexia
  Insomnia
  Psychomotor stimulation

CNS
  *Sedation, psychomotor slowing
  Muscle weakness, nervousness
  *Headaches
  *Agitation
  Vertigo
  Tremor, ataxia
  Dysarthria
  Nystagmus
  Lowered seizure threshold
  Toxic delerium (central anticholinergic syndrome)
  *Withdrawal syndrome

Cardiac
  *Postural hypotension
  Tachycardia
  Arrhythmia
  EKG changes (flattened T waves, prolonged QT
    intervals, depressed ST segments)

Ocular
  Blurred vision
  Worsening of narrow angle, glaucoma

Gastric
  Constipation
  Heartburn
  *Nausea

Hematologic
  Leukocytic effects
  Purpura
  Agranulocytosis

Skin
  Rash, petechiae
  Photosensitivity
  Urticaria

Miscellaneous
  Priapism (trazodone)
  Tinnitus
  Increased appetite
  Edema
  Alopecia

---

*Commonly seen.

TABLE 13.9. MAO Inhibitors and Their Dosages

Drug	Dose for pain (mg)	Dose for depression (mg)
Phenelzine (Nardil)	15–45	15–60
Isocarboxazid (Marplan)	10–20	10–40
Tranylcypromine (Parnate)	10–40	10–40

tidepressants. Before an MAO inhibitor is initiated, the patient must be fully educated about a tyramine-free diet and the avoidance of certain medications (meperidine, sympathomimetic amines, and heterocyclic antidepressants). Pretreatment evaluation includes a blood count, liver function tests, and an electrocardiogram and blood pressure determination, particularly in the elderly.

Table 13.9 lists available MAO inhibitors and their dosage ranges. Phenelzine (Nardil) is the most commonly used, starting at a low dose and titrated up gradually while monitoring side effects and clinical response. Periodic blood assessment of degree of platelet MAO inhibition gives information about adequacy of therapeutic level. Pain inhibition has been found with platelet MAO inhibition of 80% (Raft & Davidson, 1981).

The difference between an antinociceptive and an antidepressant dosage is not as striking as with the heterocyclics. Maintenance dose should be at the same level as the initial dose. Side effects include dizziness, nausea, drowsiness, orthostatic hypotension, headache, difficulty urinating, inhibition of ejaculation, weakness, fatigue, dry mouth, blurred vision, and skin rashes. Some patients report tremor, insomnia, and increased sweating. There is some risk of liver toxicity.

The most serious toxic effect is hypertensive crisis, caused by the interaction of ingested tyramine, sympathomimetic amines, or certain drugs in a patient on an MAO inhibitor. This abrupt and severe elevation of blood pressure is a medical emergency. Because of this high-toxicity profile, these agents, in spite of significant antidepressant and antinociceptive effect, are used only if there have been previous trials of heterocyclics with documented poor response.

Anticonvulsants

Certain anticonvulsive agents have documented efficacy in mitigating chronic pain syndromes of *neurogenic* origin. The pathophysiologic etiology of epilepsy and deafferentation pain are similar (Loeser & Ward, 1967). These agents stabilize the hyperexcitable neural membranes of pain transmitting cells (Glaser, Penry, & Woodbury, 1980; Hisbani, Pincus, & Lee, 1974) and reduce repetitive discharge of stimulated second order neurons (Fromm & Killiam, 1967).

The anticonvulsants that have been found to be most helpful in chronic pain, and Table 13.10 records their therapeutic dosages. The responsive pain syndromes in-

TABLE 13.10. Dosages of Anticonvulsants for Chronic Pain

Drug	Dosage (mg/day)
Diphenyldantoin (Dilantin)	150–400 (avg. 300)
Carbamazepine (Tegretol)	100–1,600 (avg. 400–600)
Clonazepam (Klonopin)	1.5–6.0
Valproic Acid (Depakene)	250–1,000
Gabapentin (Neurontin)	300–3,600
Topiramate (Topamax)	25–400
Levitiracetam (Keppra)	500–3,000
Tiagabine (Gabatril)	2–16
Oxcarbazepine (Trileptol)	600–2,400
Lamotrigine (Lamictal)	50–250
Felbamate (Felbatol)	400–3,600
Zonisamide (Zonergran)	100–600

clude trigeminal neuralgia, diabetic neuropathy, central thalamic pain syndrome, migraine headaches, postherpetic neuralgia, and postsympathectomy neuralgia. Carbamazepine and diphenylhydantoin were until recently the first-line anticonvulsants used with neuropathic pain syndromes, either alone or adjunctively with antidepressants. Valproic acid has also been found to be useful in some clinical trials (Hering & Kuritzky, 1989, 1992). Clonazepam, a benzodiazepine with anticonvulsant properties, may also be useful for neuropathic pain (Smirne & Scarlato, 1977) and has a lower side effect profile.

Patients are started at a low dose and titrated upward at set intervals with monitoring of therapeutic response and emergence of side effects. Blood levels are checked periodically. The total daily dose depends on therapeutic response or intolerable side effects. Side effects can be severe and limit the usefulness of these agents. CNS symptoms such as nystagmus, ataxia, slurred speech, confusion, and drowsiness are common and dose related. Gastrointestinal effects include nausea, vomiting, and constipation. There is a risk of hepatitis or liver damage, particularly with Dilantin. The most severe side effects may be on the hematopoietic system and include anemia and bone marrow suppression. Therefore, patients need to be monitored carefully, with full medical evaluation prior to the initiation of therapy and interval assessment of blood count and liver functions. Clonazepam, while more benign in its side effect profile, does have the potential for dependence and addiction.

However, the newer antiepileptic agents, including gabapentin (Neurontin), lamotrigine (Lamictal), and topiramate (Topamax), are rapidly becoming the initial agents of choice for neuropathic pain syndromes (Attal, 2000). Gabapentin has a favorable side effect profile and does not require blood levels (Mao & Chen, 2000). Lamotrigine and topiramate have less favorable side effect profiles but have also been found to be clinically effective (Attal, 2000). Newer and promising agents include levitiracetam (Keppra), tiagabine (Gabitril), oxcarbazepine (Trileptol), felbamate (Felbatol), and zonisamide (Zonegran) (Ipponi, Lamberti, Medica, Bartolini, & Malmberg-Aiello,

1999; Tremont-Lukats, Megeff, & Backonja, 2000).

Lithium

Lithium, a psychotropic agent used to treat bipolar affective disorder, has been found to mitigate pain in some cases of cluster headache (see, e.g., Domasio & Lyon, 1980; Ekbom, 1981) and migraine (Medina & Diamond, 1981). Although its exact mechanism of action is unknown, lithium appears to affect serotonin and dopamine and to have a particular benefit in cyclical disorders. However, given the fact that controlled trials are lacking and that relapse and lack of response are also documented in the few current studies, lithium should be considered a second-order agent in the treatment of these chronic pain syndromes.

Lithium is commonly administered on a two- or three-times-a-day dosage schedule, with initial regular monitoring of serum blood level. The dosage range for pain control is between 300 mg and 1,200 mg per day, which is significantly lower than its psychiatric dosage (900–2,400 mg per day). The desirable blood level is within the range of 0.4–0.8 mEq per liter.

Pretreatment patient evaluation should include a cardiovascular history, an electrocardiogram, blood count, electrolytes, and kidney and thyroid function tests. Common side effects include diarrhea, nausea, fine motor tremor, and somnolence. Patients should be monitored for more severe toxic reaction such as polyurea, polydipsia, edema, hypothyroidism, rigidity, tremor, and electrocardiogram (EKG) changes. Lithium toxicity, which may occur even with a moderate lithium blood level, manifests itself as vomiting, diarrhea, tremor, weakness, vertigo, ataxia, hyperreflexia, and somnolence. Lithium has adverse interactions with certain NSAIDs, sedatives, and diuretics. However, with careful medical monitoring, lithium is an effective and safe psychotropic agent and may be a reasonable choice for cluster headaches or migraine syndromes, which have not responded to other measures.

Muscle Relaxants

The term "muscle relaxants" (see Table 13.11) is a misnomer, because these drugs

TABLE 13.11. Muscle Relaxants

Cyclobenzaprine (Flexeril)	Chlorzoxazone (Parafon forte)
Carisoprodol (Soma)	Orphenadrine (Norflex)
Baclofen (Lioresal)	Diazepam (Valium)
Methocarbamol (Robaxin)	Tizanidine (Zanaflex)
Metaxolone (Skelaxine)	

have no peripheral action on "tight muscles" but rather act on the CNS, as do the benzodiazepines such as diazepam which are also prescribed for "muscle spasm." They are sedating, have addictive potential and a withdrawal syndrome, with little therapeutic benefit for chronic pain (Schoefferman, 1994). They may, however, be useful in the early treatment of acute musculoskeletal pain (Gross, 1998). Baclofen, however, has been found to be effective in relieving the pain of trigeminal neuralgia (Fromm & Killian, 1967), and it may have usefulness in the control of other chronic neuropathic pain syndromes (Steardo & Leo, 1984), primarily through central facilitation of gamma-aminobutyric acid (GABA) transmission. Baclofen is initiated at a low dose and titrated upward to a range of 50–60 mg per day, in divided doses. Side effects include drowsiness, dizziness, ataxia, confusion, and epigastric distress. After prolonged use, it should be tapered slowly, to avoid hallucinations, anxiety, and tachycardia. Carisoprodol (Soma) is metabolized to meprobamate and has a significant association with dependence and abuse (Littrell, Hayes, & Stillner, 1993). Metaxolone (Skelaxine) acts centrally by suppressing polysynaptic spinal cord reflexes and thereby reduces skeletal muscle spasm (Gross, 1998). Tizanidine (Zanaflex) is a central alpha-2-adrenergic agonist and has numerous pharmacological properties, including reduction in the release of excitatory neurotransmitters and inhibition of spinal reflexes. It has been used to treat headache, musculoskeletal pain, and neuropathic pain (Berry & Hutchinson, 1988; Semenchuk & Sherman, 2000).

Antianxiety and Sedative Agents

A number of pharmacological agents are useful to control core symptoms of anxiety and insomnia (see Tables 13.12 and 13.13). To treat these secondary symptoms in chron-

ic pain patients, physicians will certainly use antianxiety and sedative medications. Although some clinical studies have suggested an antinociceptive effect in acute pain due to decreased emotional response (Chapman & Feather, 1973; Gracely, McGrath, & Dubner, 1978), there has been only equivocal documentation of such an effect in chronic pain states (Lance & Curran, 1965; Yosselson-Superstine & Lipman, 1985). Clonazepam (Klonopin) is an exception and is mentioned under anticonvulsants.

The benzodiazepines are the major class of psychotropics employed for the control of anxiety and insomnia in chronic pain. They are used frequently in acute pain to decrease muscle spasm or to reduce anticipatory anxiety prior to a procedure. Their mechanism of action is through alteration of metabolism of biogenic amines in the brain, particularly by increasing release of the inhibitory neurotransmitter GABA (Polatin, 1991). There are a variety of benzodiazepines (see Table 13.14) useful for the short-term treatment of anxiety. They are best used over a period of a few weeks or months to control initial symptoms, in conjunction with other biobehavioral interventions, and then tapered slowly as the patient stabilizes with nonpharmacological cognitive-behavioral techniques. Side effects such as drowsiness or ataxia are common. Less frequently seen are psychomotor impairment, short-term memory loss, and behavioral disinhibition. These agents do have addictive potential, with risk for tolerance or dependence, and should be used carefully in patients with a history of drug abuse or predisposing psychopathology. In addition,

TABLE 13.12. Antianxiety Agents

Benzodiazepines	Barbiturates
Buspirone (Buspar)	Meprobamate (Equanil)
Propranolol (Inderal)	Antihistamines

TABLE 13.13. Sedatives

Benzodiazepines	Zolpidem (Ambien)
Flurazepam (Dalmane)	Zaleplon (Sonata)
Temazepam (Restoril)	Not recommended
Triazolam (Halcion)	Glutethimide (Doriden)
Barbiturates	Methyprylon (Noludar)
Chloral derivatives	Methaqualone (Quaalude)
Antihistamines	Ethchlorvyne (Placidyl)

there is a withdrawal syndrome, requiring a tapering dosage under medical supervision. This is particularly true with alprazolam, where symptoms of "delayed withdrawal" such as irritability or increased anxiety may develop 3 or 4 weeks after the medication has been discontinued.

Certain benzodiazepines are considered to be primarily sedatives, and there are several other useful classes of medication for this purpose (see Table 13.12). Choosing an agent to treat insomnia should take into consideration any primary etiological diagnoses. A patient with chronic pain and insomnia, with or without depression, should be treated with a sedating antidepressant, because these agents may mitigate the sleep-disruptive pain as well as improve sleep patterns even if depression is not present. In chronic pain, primary sedatives should be reserved for those patients whose insomnia has been refractory to a trial of several antidepressants, or for those who are unable to tolerate any antidepressants secondary to side effects. Many of the primary sedatives do have potential for oversedation, addiction, dependence, and withdrawal and should be used cautiously, particularly in patients with risk factors for drug abuse.

Neuroleptics

The neuroleptics are also called "major tranquilizers" or "antipsychotic agents." Table 13.15 lists the pharmacological groups with equivalent doses as compared to chlorpro-mazine, which was the first of these agents used in clinical psychopharmacology. These medications have a potent effect on psychotic behavior and agitation, primarily by the blockade of dopamine receptors in various brain pathways. However, there is little evidence for a primary analgesic affect, although the neuroleptics have been used to potentiate opioid analgesia postoperatively (Minuck, 1972) and to control some chronic pain syndromes (Maltbie, Cavener, Sullivan, Hammett, & Zung, 1979), with some positive results.

These agents do have significant side effects, including various movement disorders, sedation, cardiac toxicity, and bone marrow suppression. The higher potency agents are less sedative but do have more potential for extrapyramidal reactions. Tardive dyskinesia, which is often irreversible, poses a significant risk with long-term continuous use of the neuroleptics. Given the lack of evidence for significant benefit in chronic pain states, their side effect profile limits the use of neuroleptics in chronic pain unless a psychosis or a volatile personality disorder necessitates their usage by traditional psychopharmacological guidelines. Such a situation may include the concomitant use of an antiparkinsonian agent to prevent or control extrapyramidal side effects.

Adjuvant Agents

Several types of medications have been found to enhance the analgesic affect of the

TABLE 13.14. Bendodiazepine Anxiolytics

Lorazepam (Ativan)	Chlorazepate (Tranxene)
Oxazepam (Serax)	Diazepam (Valium)
Alprazolam (Xanax)	Prazepam (Centrax)
Chlordiazepoxide (Librium)	

TABLE 13.15. Antipsychotic Agents

Drug	Equivalent dosage (mg)
Chlorpromazine (Thorazine)	100
Thioridazine (Mellaril)	100
Loxapine (Loxitane)	15
Perphenazine (Trilafon)	10
Molindone (Moban)	10
Trifluoperazine (Stelazine)	5
Haloperidol (Haldol)	2–5
Thiothixene (Navane)	5
Fluphenazine (Prolixin)	2–5
Respiridone (Risperdal)	4–8
Clozapine (Clozaril)	50
Quetiapine (Seroquel)	25
Olanzapine (Zyprexa)	5
Ziprasidone (Geodon)	20–40

non-narcotic analgesics and the opioids (see Table 13.16) in chronic pain states. The antidepressants, neuroleptics, and anticonvulsants have primary application in chronic pain as described previously but may also be used as adjuvants.

Caffeine has been used to enhance NSAID analgesia and shortens the time to onset of effect (Schactel & Fillingim, 1991; Ward & Whitney, 1991). The usage of antihistamines along with opioids in chronic pain states allows the use of a lower dose of narcotic and provides additional sedation (Sunshine & Olsen, 1994). Both of these categories of drugs are relatively nontoxic, with minimal side effect profiles. Neuroleptics may have some enhancing effects on opioid analgesia but at the very least reduce the nausea commonly seen with use of the narcotics.

Psychostimulants such as dextroamphetamine and ritalin augment narcotic analgesia and also counteract sedation seen with the opioids. However, the risk of CNS toxicity

TABLE 13.16. Adjuvant Agents to Enhance Analgesia

With NSAIDs	With opioids
Caffeine	Heterocyclic antidepressants
	Neuroleptics
	Anticonvulsants
	Antihistamines (hydroxyzine)
	Amphetamines

and addiction is significant in these agents and must be monitored carefully.

Topical Agents

EMLA cream, a mixture of lidocaine and prilocaine, can be used to treat postherpetic neuralgia and scar pain (Gajraj, Pennant, & Watcha, 1994). A new formulation of topical 5% lidocaine has also been shown to relieve the pain of postherpetic neuralgia (Galer, Rowbotham, Perander, & Friedman, 1999). Capsaicin cream is derived from the pepper and acts by depleting neurotransmitters such as substance P (Wachtel, 1999). It has been used to treat neuropathic pain conditions, including painful diabetic neuropathy, although it is limited by side effects such as burning, localized itching, and rash.

Integration of Pharmocotherapy and Psychological Treatments of Chronic Pain

General Comments

Physicians evaluating chronic pain patients for pharmacotherapeutic management do not make decisions in a vacuum. Integral to the process is a good medical history, including an inquiry of previous psychiatric or psychological treatment and prior response to medications. A comprehensive physical examination should be performed, including an assessment of general health, cardiovascular, pulmonary, gastrointestinal, genitourinary, and neuromuscular function. Psychological assessment, including behavioral observations and the results of initial psychometric testing, such as the Beck Depressive Inventory (BDI; Beck, Steer, & Garbin, 1988), Hamilton Rating Scale for Depression (HRSD; Rush, Becks, Kovacs, & Hollon, 1977), and Minnesota Multiphasic Personality Inventory (MMPI) indicates severity of depression, somatization, and other relevant psychopathology (see Gatchel, Chapter 21, this volume). Clinically, the BDI to screen for depression is useful, but the HRSD, which is a clinically administered questionnaire, can confirm the diagnosis. Symptoms requiring medication control and contraindications to certain pharmacotherapeutic approaches such as long-term opiate maintenance will be delineated on psychological assessment. Socioeconomic stressors affecting the patients' presentation may be provided to the treatment team by a social worker or disability case manager.

Symptoms and behaviors initially observed by the physical and occupational therapists in the rehabilitation setting, such as noncompliance with exercise routines, lack of attendance, pain sensitivity, functional and physical capacity deficits, decreased level of alertness, inability to retain instruction, or poor interpersonal skills, are important pieces of information for the managing physician in monitoring clinical response to medications and detecting side effects such as oversedation or obtundation. The most effective form in which such an exchange of information can take place is an interdisciplinary staff meeting, which should occur at least on a weekly basis while a patient is in rehabilitation.

Chronic pain remains a clinical challenge. Because pain is a subjective symptom, it is frequently difficult to assess and monitor, and the clinician must depend on the self-report of patients whose complex psychosociodemographic issues may unpredictably augment their pain complaint. Therefore, there is no single way to treat chronic pain, and the most successful therapies integrate the best efforts of many disciplines.

The following cases illustrate the importance of an interdisciplinary approach to chronic pain. Each example illustrates a particular patient profile. None of these could be adequately treated solely with pharmacotherapy. As emphasized earlier (see also Turk, Chapter 7, and Gatchel, Chapter 21, this volume), chronic pain is associated with a complex array of psychosocioeconomic stressors that need to be appropriately managed by behavioral-psychological methods.

The Somatic Patient

A 50-year-old, married female was seeking treatment because of a recent flare-up of intense neck and shoulder pain, which initially occurred following an automobile accident 10 years earlier. There were no litigation issues outstanding on this case. The patient described this pain as "paralyzing" to her during the day while doing house-

work. She also had a history of chronic headaches, as well as joint pain, which she attributed to arthritis. Her reports of intense pain did not appear to be congruent with her actual observed movement and impairment during therapy. She regularly reported pain but would often complete a required task, although it was a struggle and the therapist had to constantly urge her on. She would also often request rest breaks and passive means of pain relief (medication, massage, ice, etc.).

Her initial injury 10 years previously had caused severe neck and shoulder pain that lasted for 3 years and resolved over a period of 6 months after the case was litigated successfully. Six months ago, her husband had sustained a back injury at work and had been disabled since that time. On initial psychological testing, she presented with a BDI score of 16, an HRSD score of 15, and an MMPI presenting with elevations above 70 on Scales 1 and 3. She was reluctant to discuss psychological issues but did not demonstrate marked elevations on indices of depression.

This patient was currently being treated in an interdisciplinary setting and was presented in a staff meeting. Physical therapists working with her were instructed to take a supportive approach with her pain complaints but to emphasize the importance of adequate stretching and strengthening exercises, using passive modalities as a reinforcement for hard work in rehabilitation exercises. In addition, she was given instruction on the interrelationship between pain and emotional distress, and in psychological counseling she was encouraged to discuss her feelings about her husband's recent disability and the demands placed on her because of this disability. She was also evaluated by the physician on the team, who recommended, in spite of the absence of significant depression, a trial of a somewhat sedating antidepressant at a low dose because of complaints of ongoing pain, some increased anxiety, and a primary and secondary sleep disturbance.

The patient was placed on Elavil, starting at 25 mg before bedtime, and reported some dry mouth and slight morning hangover which resolved after the first 2 days such that she was able to increase the dose further up to 50 mg at bedtime. At this dosage, she noted that she was sleeping through the night, with some dry mouth, which decreased after an additional week on this dose. She began to voice somewhat lesser intensity of her pain, which allowed her to continue to work more easily in the pain management setting. After 2 weeks on this medication, she was perceived as significantly improved, more easily participating in the physical rehabilitation exercises, and beginning to demonstrate an interest in some of the educational interpretations offered to her. She continued on the Elavil, at a dose of 50 mg at bedtime. She noted, on one occasion when she ran out of the medication over a weekend that she had an immediate recurrence of sleep disturbance and increased perception of pain, which resolved after 2 days back on the medication.

The patient completed rehabilitation after 4 weeks but was maintained on the Elavil for an additional 4 months, after which it was discontinued. She noticed some transitory sleep disturbance and increased irritability for 1 week after stopping the Elavil but then improved, and continued to do well without medication.

The Depressed Patient

A 45-year-old assembly-line worker and divorced mother of two developed neck and shoulder pain after falling at work. She was referred for physical therapy after this pain continued for 6 weeks. She had had an orthopedic evaluation with negative workup for cervical disc herniation, radiculopathy, or shoulder impingement. She had some initial response to nonsteroidal anti-inflammatory medication but continued with ongoing pain. She had been unable to return to work and there had been some concern about progressive physical deconditioning. In initial rehabilitation, she was quite passive and lethargic and had to be constantly pushed to exert maximal effort during therapy. She did not seem to be following through with recommended home exercises and complained that she could never find the time or energy to do the exercises. She admitted to difficulty with sleep and loss of appetite, low energy, and reported recent headaches. Whenever she was confronted by her physi-

cal therapist, she became tearful and depressed and promised to try to do better in the future.

On further questioning, she admitted to a feeling of sadness most of the day every day for the past month. She had had thoughts of death, but no suicidal ideation, had lost interest in things that previously engaged her in her life, was socially isolating herself, and had a triphasic sleep disturbance and anergia. She had been divorced 3 years previously. At that time she had been hospitalized for 3 weeks with depression and was treated with Desyrel. She had stayed on that medication for 6 months and then tapered it with no recurrence of depression.

She currently had a BDI score of 30 and an HRSD score of 26. MMPI demonstrated elevations above 70 on Scales 1, 2, and 3. On interview, she presented as a somewhat disheveled, downcast, middle-age woman. Her mood was clearly depressed, with some tearfulness during the interview and blunting of her affect. She was oriented to time, place, and person, with an adequate fund of knowledge suggestive of average intelligence. She demonstrated no pressured speech, flight of ideas, ideas of reference, loosening of association, or any other abnormality of thought process. She did seem somewhat ruminative and pessimistic.

This patient was discussed in an interdisciplinary staffing conference. It was decided to continue her physical therapy with additional supportive encouragement to be provided by her therapist. She was referred to a psychologist for implementation of brief cognitive therapy for her depression, education about the interrelation of pain and emotional distress, and relaxation training to assist her in decreasing severity of pain experience. A vocational specialist was called in to interface with her employer and to help her construct a return-to-work plan, with a transitional part-time, light-duty "phase-in" period while she was still in treatment. She was placed back on Desyrel, because of her previous good response, initially at a dose of 50 mg before bedtime and progressed over a 1-week period up to 150 mg before bedtime. She slept much better almost immediately and also reported lessening of her pain within 1 week after starting the Desyrel. Although she had some initial morning hangover at the 150-mg dose, when she took the medication 2 hours earlier, this side effect diminished.

After a period of 3 weeks, she began to note a lessening of her depression and was visibly brighter. She returned to work with light-duty restrictions for limited hours but continued in interdisciplinary treatment. Over the next 4 weeks, she progressed to full-time, full-duty work. Although she still had pain, she was more comfortable applying specific learned techniques to reduce it and was able to continue working. However, she became more depressed when the Desyrel was tapered at 6 months but improved when it was restarted at the same dose. We decided to continue the Desyrel at the full antidepressant dose, with periodic medical follow-up over the next 12 months.

The Psychotic Patient

A 32-year-old woman was referred for hand therapy 4 weeks after a right carpal tunnel release. She had developed symptoms in her right wrist while at work as an assembler and was fearful that she would not be able to return to that job. She reported that the pain had not improved at all since surgery. She had been compliant with initial postsurgical treatment. She demonstrated residual tenderness over the operated wrist but no evidence of nerve compression. Her pinch and grip strength were markedly decreased bilaterally. She attended therapy regularly, appeared compliant, and actually demonstrated gradual improvement but still suboptimal functional capacity after another 3 weeks of therapy. Pain complaint continued unchanged. She was noted to be tearful at times, and expressed discouragement.

She admitted to a suicide attempt 5 years previously, followed by a 1-month hospitalization. At that time, she was treated with an antidepressant and a neuroleptic and reported that she had been hearing voices prior to her suicide attempt. Twelve years earlier, she had had a prior brief psychiatric hospitalization but did not recall much about it.

The patient's BDI score was 40, HRSD score was 30, and MMPI demonstrated elevations on Scales 1, 2, 3, and 8. On interview, she presented as a somewhat unkempt, agitated middle-age woman. Her mood was clearly anxious. She was oriented but demonstrated some pressured speech and paranoid ideation and admitted to hearing voices again. She also reported that she was isolating herself at home, staying in bed most of the day when she was not in therapy.

The patient was presented at an interdisciplinary staff meeting where staff identified problems of compliance, motivation, somatization, depression, and psychosis. She was placed in a structured tertiary care setting. Attendance and compliance with prescribed routines were closely monitored by the physical and occupational therapists. A psychologist encouraged her to acknowledge her depression and to understand that she was experiencing hallucinations related to depression. She was also given education about the effects of her current emotional distress on her pain levels.

The patient was seen by the physician and Effexor XR, a new antidepressant, was prescribed, as well as Risperidal, a neuroleptic. She progressed slowly from 37.5 mg of Effexor XR once a day up to 75 mg once a day, increasing the dose by 37.5 mg after 1 week. At the initial dose, she had some nausea and jitteriness but could tolerate these side effects. After an additional week, the dose of Effexor XR was titrated up to 150 mg per day. The Navane was begun at 1 mg twice a day, and she was closely observed for any extrapyramidal and other side effects but tolerated this medication. Within 2 days of being placed on the neuroleptic, she reported significant diminution of the auditory hallucinations, and within 1 week she was no longer hearing the voices at all. She had a visible brightening of affect and decrease in her agitation by the end of the first week and by the end of the second week was clearly less depressed and working more easily in rehabilitation. At that time, a vocational specialist became involved to interface with her employer and to implement a return-to-work plan. She completed rehabilitation after 6 weeks and returned to work. She continued in once-a-week psychotherapy for 3 more months. After 1 month, her Risperidal was discontinued with no recurrent psychosis. However, she was kept on Effexor XR at a dose of 150 mg once a day with bimonthly medical monitoring for an additional extended period.

The Anxious Patient

A 40-year-old man was referred for physical therapy with complaint of neck pain, which developed after a motor vehicle accident 3 weeks previously. He had marked tenderness in the paracervical areas bilaterally with tightness and some spasm and with marked restriction of cervical mobility. On initial presentation, he spent some time describing his symptoms and was fearful of being examined. He attended physical therapy regularly but continued to complain of pain and muscle tension. He practiced his exercises at home, expressed motivation to recover, but was not progressing. He admitted to previously being treated for "nerves" with Xanax, but was not taking it now. On careful questioning, he admitted to having panic attacks every other day. He had a BDI score of 20, an HRSD score of 24, and an MMPI demonstrating elevations of Scales 1, 2, and 3.

He was presented at interdisciplinary staffing, at which it was decided to continue physical therapy for mobilization and strengthening but to also initiate psychological consultation. The patient was educated on the interrelationship of muscle tension, anxiety, and pain severity, and relaxation training was initiated, with dramatic relief of neck pain. He was additionally seen in consultation by a physician, who started him on Paxil at a dose of 10 mg once a day, progressing up to a dose of 20 mg once a day. Initially, the patient noticed increased sweating and jitteriness, which gradually resolved. After an additional 2 weeks the Paxil was increased to 40 mg per day. At the same time, he was placed back on Xanax at a dose of 0.5 mg twice a day. Panic attacks were immediately relieved. After a period of 10 days, when the Paxil was up to a dose of 20 mg a day, the patient was able to taper his Xanax with no worsening of panic attacks. He was visibly more relaxed and began to improve significantly in physical therapy, with decrease in his pain complaint, improved range of motion of the cervical spine, and markedly decreased spasm. After a period of 1 month, he was essentially pain free. He continued on the Paxil but was able to discontinue his physical therapy; he continues with home stretching, strengthening, and relaxation exercises. The Paxil was tapered after 6 months by 10 mg per week, with no recurrence of panic attacks or pain.

The Intellectually Disadvantaged Patient

A 32-year-old man presented with low back pain after a work-related injury. He had been disabled since his injury and was referred for work hardening. On initial testing, he demonstrated low functional capacity, with poor effort on testing and some inconsistency in the test results. On physical examination, there was marked superficial tenderness, stocking anesthesia, and exclamations of pain, suggestive of symptom magnification. He subsequently demonstrated poor attendance in therapy and failed to progress. The therapist noted some confusion in his ability to follow directions, with mistakes being made each time, even after explanation. He moved slowly, hardly spoke, and did not appear to establish any relationships with either therapists or peers. Other patients ignored or avoided him because of his poor personal hygiene. He did not talk about his work and did not even know if his job was available.

He had dropped out of school in the 8th grade, had held a number of manual labor jobs, and was unmarried. He lived in a trailer in his mother's backyard. He had a Wechsler Adult Intelligence Scale (WAIS) demonstrating a Full Scale IQ of 70, with a BDI score of 20 and an HRSD score of 15. MMPI was invalid with many incomplete items. He did admit to a sleep disturbance, primarily because of pain at night.

This patient was presented at interdisciplinary staffing, at which time it was decided to transfer him to a tertiary functional restoration program. He was assigned physical and occupational therapists, who spent extra time monitoring compliance, with positive reinforcement of praise for regular attendance and good performance. His exercise progression was closely supervised and he was repeatedly instructed as necessary on use of the exercise equipment. A case manager was assigned to establish a return-to-work plan, with some involvement of vocational retraining facility, as it was found that his job would not be available. Relaxation training to improve sleep and to assist in decreasing reactivity to pain was initiated, as well as basic education on pain and stress. He was assessed by a physician, and started on Prozac 20 mg per day. There was some visible brightening of affect within a period of 10 days. He began to speak with other patients and was more appropriate in social situations, with less frequent complaints of pain. He was given some basic social and hygiene instructional information, to which he responded, and he gradually began to progress in therapy. Upon completion of the program, he entered job retraining which he completed in 3 more months and had a trial placement. His Prozac was continued for 4 months and then discontinued, with no adverse affect.

The Highly Stressed Patient

This 45-year-old man presented with pain in the right upper extremity. He had been injured at work as a press operator when he sustained a crush injury to the index and middle finger of his right hand. He was initially treated with reconstructive surgery to the hand but thereafter had progressive increase in pain extending up the entire extremity into the neck. He subsequently had several decompressive procedures, including a right carpal tunnel release and a right cubital tunnel release, with some temporary relief of pain but recurrence within a period of 2 months and progressive worsening of the extremity pain. On presentation, he had almost no function of his right upper extremity, with some generalized wasting of the musculature and a coolness and dryness of the limb. A diagnosis of reflex sympathetic dystrophy (complex regional pain syndrome, Type 1) had been made. He had been referred for rehabilitation therapy in the past but had not been able to progress because of worsening of his pain. In addition, he reported that he had become more irritable at home and was fearful of harming his wife or one of his children because of temper outbursts. He had a prominent sleep disturbance, admitted to feeling hopeless, and had thoughts of suicide.

This patient had been on military combat duty 20 years ago. He reported that he had not been wounded but did witness a number of violent events. When he returned to the United States, and after discharge he did receive therapy at the Veterans Administration for what was then diagnosed as "stress syndrome." He reported that although he was markedly improved after a number of years, he still had occasional "flashbacks" and nightmares. However, he had been able to hold a job and to lead a fairly normal life. His symptoms had gotten worse after his current injury. He had a BDI score of 40, and an HRSD score of 28. His MMPI demonstrated elevations on Scales 1, 2, 3, 4, 7, and 8.

This patient was discussed in an interdisciplinary staff meeting. Identified problems appeared to be extreme pain sensitivity, refusal to use his right upper extremity, emotional lability, insomnia, and depression. Because of his outbursts, he was a management problem in the rehabilitation milieu, and the therapists were afraid of him. In addition, his residual deficits would limit employability, and although he had indicated a preference to continue working, he had also applied for long-term disability.

He was placed in a tertiary interdisciplinary functional restoration program. A psychologist immediately initiated a suicide contract and began supportive psychotherapy in which coping strategies were emphasized. Relaxation training helped to reduce anxiety and decrease emotional outbursts, and the patient was receptive to education about the relationship between emotional distress and pain. At the same time, the psychologist emphasized the importance of regular attendance and participation in the rehabilitation program and was "on call" for the physical and occupational therapists if irritability became problematic in the rehabilitation setting.

Concurrently, this patient was evaluated by a physician who placed him on Asendin, a sedating antidepressant with additional dopamine receptor selectivity, and Klonopin, a benzodiazepine and anticonvulsant. He progressed on the Asendin from 25 mg before bedtime up to 150 mg over a period of 2 weeks, raising the dose by 25 mg every other day. Initially, he experienced lightheadedness, dry mouth, and constipation. Because of his underlying anxiety and suspiciousness, he initially refused to continue the medication, but after the physician spent additional time explaining the rationale for treatment and the side effects he agreed to continue. Although dry mouth and postural hypotension persisted, the patient accepted these side effects, and did note improved sleep, decreased irritability, and decreasing depressed mood.

He became easier to work with in the rehabilitation program, following through on his exercises and progressing well. He underwent vocational evaluation and was referred for job retraining after he completed functional restoration.

The Asendin was continued for 6 months at full dosage. The Klonopin was tapered from 0.5 mg three times a day after 1 month, with no increase in irritability or anxiety but with some increase in pain, so that it was reinstituted at 0.5 mg twice a day. After 6 months, the Asendin was tapered by 25 mg every other day with no adverse affect.

A Patient for Narcotic Maintenance

A 60-year-old man presented with chronic low back pain radiating to his right foot. He had been aware of this pain for the past 10 years. He had had a lumbar discectomy and then a posterior lumbar interbody fusion with some initial relief of pain but subsequent recurrence. Lumbar MRI scan demonstrated lumbar epidural fibrosis, which is fibrous adhesions around the spinal nerve roots. He had been through intensive rehabilitation with improvement after his last surgery. He reported that although he had severe pain, he continued to work full time as an attorney, sometimes putting in as many as 70 or 80 hours a week. He remained active, playing racquetball and working out regularly at his health club. His pain sometimes was so severe that he had to spend a day or two in bed, and occasionally he had gone to a hospital emergency room for a "pain shot." He had used NSAIDs intermittently with some control of the pain. His BDI score was 15, and his HRSD score was 10. His MMPI demonstrated no abnormal scales. He appeared younger than his stated age, well conditioned, and in no acute distress. He was focused on the problem of intermittent pain that interfered with his ability to perform his daily activities.

This patient was referred to a pain program. He indicated, however, that he did not wish rehabilitation or pain management therapy but wanted to have medication available to him when his pain became unbearable. His case was reviewed in a staff meeting. He did not demonstrate significant psychopathology. He was active and oriented toward function. He appeared to be coping well with his pain and was clear about his needs. He was placed on a low dose of Sinequan (25 mg at bedtime) and reported that at this low dose he had some lessening of his pain but continued to be symptomatic. He intermittently used Naprosyn, an NSAID, but still requested some "backup" pain medication. After careful discussion with him, his managing physician agreed to prescribe a low-dose narcotic, Hydrocodone 5 mg, not to exceed three pills a day and with careful monitoring of the refillable prescription. After a week, the dose was increased up to 7.5 mg three times a day, which provided him with better pain relief. He was also referred to a psychologist for biofeedback to reduce muscle tension and thereby more effectively control pain. Over a period of 2 months, he reported that he was able to further limit his usage of Hydrocodone, although he still found it useful to have some available for particularly severe pain episodes.

Summary

Pharmacological treatment of chronic pain has as its goals analgesia and the relief of emotional distress, and it uses medications at doses and for applications that may not be always readily recognized by the medical community. This is particularly true for the antidepressants, the anticonvulsants, lithium, and baclofen. In addition, the use of opioids for the long-term treatment of chronic noncancer pain is still considered controversial. It is, therefore, important that clinicians treating chronic pain patients be familiar with these pharmacological approaches and be prepared to educate colleagues, who may challenge some of these prescriptions.

Because of the clinical complexities of these syndromes, it is not uncommon to see patients on a number of different pharmacological agents. Progressing from the most directly analgesic agent to psychotropics for control of emotional distress, the utilization of an NSAID, an opioid, an antidepressant, and an anticonvulsant concomitantly is not uncommon. Optimal communication between treatment disciplines is essential and may only be achieved by frequent interdisciplinary staff meetings in which clinical and behavioral observations, medical assessment, and treatment planning are shared responsibilities.

References

Abramson, S. (1991). Therapy and mechanisms of nonsteroidal anti-inflammatory drugs. *Current Opinion in Rheumatology, 3*, 336–340.

Anderberg, U., Marteinsdottir, I., & von Knorring, L. (2000). Citalopram in patients with fibromyalgia: A randomized, double-blind, placebo controlled study. *European Journal of Pain, 4*, 27–35.

Ansari, A. (2000). The efficacy of newer antidepressants in the treatment of chronic pain: A review of current literature. *Harvard Review of Psychiatry, 7*, 257–277.

Anthony, M., & Lance, J. (1969). Monoamine oxidase inhibition in the treatment of migraine. *Archives of Neurology, 21*, 263–268.

Attal, N. (2000). Chronic neuropathic pain: Mechanisms and treatment. *Clinical Journal of Pain, 16*, S118–S130.

Beck, A., Steer, R., & Garbin. M (1988). Psychometric properties of the Beck Depression Inventory: Twenty-five years of evaluation. *Clinical Psychology Reviews, 8*, 77–100.

Berry, H., & Hutchinson, D. (1988). Tizanidine and ibuprofen in acute low back pain: Results of a double-blind multicentre study in general practice. *Journal of International Medical Research, 16*, 83–91.

Brandt, J., Celentano, D., Stewart, W., Linet, M., & Polstein, M. (1990, March). Personality and emotional disorder in a community sample of migraine headache sufferers. *American Journal of Psychology, 147*, 303.

Brannon, G., & Stone, K. (1999). The use of mirtazapine in a patient with chronic pain. *Journal of Pain and Symptom Management, 18*, 382–385.

Broomhead, A., Kerr, R., Tester, W., O'Meara, P., & Maccarrone, C. (1997). Comparison of a once-a-day sustained-release morphine formulation with standard oral morphine treatment for cancer pain. *Journal of Pain and Symptom Management, 14*, 63–73.

Burton, K., Polatin, P., & Gatchel, R. (1997). Psychosocial factors and the rehabilitation of patients with chronic work-related upper extremity disorders. *Journal of Occupational Rehabilitation, 7*, 139–153.

Chapman, C., & Feather, B. (1973). Effects of diazepam on human pain tolerance and pain sensitivity. *Psychosomatics Medicine, 35*, 330–340.

Cooper, J., Czechowicz, D., Petersen, R., & Molinan, S. (1992). Prescription drug diversion control and medical practice. *Journal of the American Medical Association, 268*, 1306–1310.

Couch, J., Ziegler, D., & Hassanein, R. (1976). Amitriptyline in the prophylaxis of migraine. *Neurology, 26*, 121–127.

Delfino, U. (1983). An advance in trigeminal therapy. In S. Lipton & J. Miles (Eds.), *Persistent pain, IV-Modern methods of treatment* (pp. 67–83). London: Grune & Stratton.

Domasio, H., & Lyon, L. (1980). Lithium carbonate in the treatment of cluster headaches. *Journal of Neurology, 224*, 1–8.

Dubas, T., & Parker, J. (1971). A central component in the analgesic action of sodium salicylate. *Archives of Internal Pharmacodynamic Therapeutics, 194*, 117–122.

Ekbom, K. (1981). Lithium for cluster headache: Review of the literature and preliminary results of long-term treatment. *Headache, 21*, 132–139.

Fields, H. (1987). *Pain*. New York: McGraw-Hill.

France, R., Houpt, J., & Ellinwood, E. (1984). Therapeutic effects of antidepressants in chronic pain. *General Hospital of Psychiatry, 6*, 55–63.

France, R., & Krishnan, K. (Eds.). (1988). *Chronic pain*. Washington, DC: American Psychiatric Press.

France R., Urban, B., & Keefe, F. (1984). Long-term use of narcotic analgesics and chronic pain. *Social Science and Medicine, 19*, 1379–1382.

Fromm, G. H., & Killian, J. M. (1967). Effect of some anticonvulsant drugs on the spinal trigeminal nucleus. *Neurology, 17*, 275–280.

Gajraj, N., Pennant, J., & Watcha, M. (1994). Eutectic mixture of local anesthetics (EMLA) cream. *Anesthesia and Analgesia, 78*, 574–583.

Galer, B., Rowbotham, M., Perander, J., & Friedman, E. (1999). Topical lidocaine patch relieves postherpetic neuralgia more effectively than a vehicle topical patch: Results of an enriched enrollment study. *Pain, 80*, 533–538.

Glaser, G., Penry, J., & Woodbury, D. (1980). *Antiepileptic drugs: Mechanism of action*. New York: Raven Press.

Gomersall, J., & Stewart, A. (1973). Amitriptyline in migraine prophylaxis. *Journal of Neurosurgical Psychiatry, 36*, 684–690.

Goodkin, K., & Gullion, C. (1989). A critical review of clinical trials using heterocyclic antidepressants for the relief of chronic pain syndromes with a focus on chronic low back pain. *Annals of Behavioral Medicine, 11*, 83–101.

Gourlay, G. K., & Cousins, M. J. (1984). Strong analgesics in severe pain. *Drugs, 28*, 79–91.

Gracely, R., McGrath, P., & Dubner, R. (1978). Validity and sensitivity of sensory and affective verbal pain descriptors: Manipulation of affect by diazepam. *Pain, 5*, 19–29.

Gringas, M. (1976). A clinical trial of tofranil in rheumatic pain in general practice. *Journal of Internal Medicine Research, 4,* 41–49.

Gross, L. (1998). Metaxalone: A review of clinical experience. *Journal of Neurological and Orthopedic Medical Surgery, 18,* 76–79

Hanks, G., Twycross, R., & Lloyd, J. (1981). Unexpected complication of successful nerve block. *Anesthesia, 36,* 37–39.

Hering, R., & Kuritzky, A. (1989). Sodium valproate in the treatment of cluster headache: An open clinical study. *Cephalalgia, 9,* 195–198.

Hering, R., & Kuritzky, A. (1992). Sodium valproate in the prophylactic treatment of migraine: A double blind study versus placebo. *Cephalalgia, 12,* 81–84.

Hisbani, M., Pincus, J., & Lee, S. (1974). Diphenylhydantoin and calcium movement in lobster nerves. *Archives of Neurology, 31,* 250–254.

Ipponi, A., Lamberti, C., Medica, A., Bartolini, A., & Malmberg-Aiello P. (1999). Tiagabine antinociception in rodents depends on $GABA_B$ receptor activation: Parallel antinociception testing and medial thalamus GABA microdialysis. *European Journal of Pharmacology, 368,* 205–211.

Kinney, R., Gatchel, R., Polatin, P., Fogarty W., & Mayer, T. (1993). Prevalence of psychopathology in acute and chronic low back pain patients. *Journal of Occupational Rehabilitation, 3,* 95–103.

Lance, J., & Curran, D. (1965). Investigations into the mechanism and treatment of chronic headaches. *Medical Journal of Australia, 2,* 909–914.

Lascelles, R. (1966). Atypical facial pain and depression. *British Journal of Psychiatry, 112,* 651–659.

Lichtor, J., Sevarino, F., Joshi, G., Busch, M., Nordbrock, E., & Ginsberg, B. (1999). The relative potency of oral transmucosal fentanyl citrate compared with intravenous morphine in the treatment of moderate to severe postoperative pain. *Anesthesia and Analgesia, 89,* 732–738.

Littrell, R., Hayes, L., & Stillner, V. (1987). Carisoprodol (Soma): A new cautious perspective on an old agent. *Southern Medical Journal, 86,* 753–756.

Loeser, J., & Ward, A. (1967). Some effects of deafferentation on neurons of the cut spinal cord. *Archives of Neurology, 17,* 629–636.

Malmberg, A., & Yaksh, T. (1992). Hyperalgesia mediated by spinal glutemate or substance receptor blocked by spinal cyclo-oxygenase inhibition. *Science, 257,* 1277–1280.

Maltbie, A. A., Cavener, J. O., Jr., Sullivan, J. L., Hammett, E. B., & Zung, W. W. (1979). Analgesia and haloperidol: A hypothesis. *Journal of Clinical Psychiatry, 40,* 323–326.

Mao, J., & Chen, L. (2000). Gabapentin in pain management. *Anesthesia and Analgesia, 91,* 680–687.

Mathew, N. (1978). Clinical subtypes of cluster headaches and response to lithium therapy. *Headache, 18,* 26–30.

Max, M. (1995). Thirteen consecutive well-designed randomized trials show that antidepressants reduce pain in diabetic neuropathy and postherpetic neuralgia. *Pain Forum, 4,* 248–253

Medical Board of California. (1994). *Guidelines for prescribing controlled substances for intractable pain.* Sacramento, CA: Author.

Medina, J., & Diamond, S. (1981). Cyclical migraine. *Archives of Neurology, 38,* 343–344.

Minuck, R. (1972). Postoperative analgesia-comparison of methotrimeprazine and meperidine as postoperative analgesia agents. *Canadian Anesthesiological Society Journal, 19,* 87–96.

Monks, R. (1994). Psychotropic drugs. In P. Wall & R. Melzack (Eds.), *Textbook of pain* (3rd ed., pp. 963–989). New York: Churchill Livingstone.

Onghena, P., & Van Houdenhove, B. (1992). Antidepressant-induced analgesia in chronic non- malignant pain: A meta-analysis of 39 placebo-controlled studies. *Pain, 40,* 205–219.

Polatin, P. (1991). Psychoactive medications as adjuncts in functional restoration. In T. Mayer, V. Mooney, & R. Gatchel (Eds.), *Contemporary conservative care for painful spinal disorders* (pp. 465–472). Philadelphia: Lea & Febiger.

Polatin, P., Kinney, R., Gatchel, R., Lillo, E., & Mayer, T. (1993). Psychiatric illness and chronic low back pain: The mind and the spine-which goes first? *Spine, 18,* 66–71.

Portnoy, R. (1994). Opioid therapy for chronic nonmalignant pain: Current status. In H. Fields & J. Liebeskind (Eds.), *Progress in pain research and management* (Vol. I, pp. 104–116), Seattle, WA: IASP Press.

Portnoy, R., & Foley, K. (1986). Chronic use of opioid analgesics in nonmalignant pain: Report of 38 cases. *Pain, 25,* 171–186.

Raft, D., & Davidson, J. (1981). Relationship between response to phenelzine and MAO inhibition in a clinical trial of phenelzine, amitriptyline, and placebo. *Neuropsychobiology, 7,* 122–126.

Rush, J., Beck, A., Kovacs, M., & Hollon, S. (1977). Comparative efficacy of cognitive therapy and imipramine in the treatment of depressed outpatients. *Cognitive Therapy and Research, 1,* 17–37.

Schactel, B., & Fillingim, J. (1991). Caffeine as an analgesic adjuvant. A double-blind study comparing aspirin with caffeine to aspirin and placebo in patients with sore throat. *Archives of Internal Medicine, 151,* 733–737.

Schoefferman, J. (1994, February). *The use of medications for pain of spinal origin.* Paper presented at "The Final Link to Therapeutic Success" course, San Francisco.

Semenchuk, M., & Sherman, S. (2000). Effectiveness of tizanidine in neuropathic pain: An open-label study. *Journal of Pain, 4,* 285–292

"Shipment of potent pain pills suspended." (2001, May 1). *Washington Post,* p. 16.

Silverstein, F., Faich, G., Goldstein, J., Simon, L., Pincus, T., Whelton, R., Makuch, R., Eisen, G., Agraval, N., Stenson, W., Burr, A., Zhao, W., Kent, J., Lefkowith, J., Verburg, K., & Geis, G.

(2000). Gastrointestinal toxicity with celecoxib vs nonsteroidal anti-inflammatory drugs for osteoarthritis and rheumatoid arthritis. The CLASS study: A randomized controlled trial. *Journal of the American Medical Association, 284,* 1247–1255.

Simpson, R., Edmonson, E., Constant, C., & Collier, C. (1997). Transdermal fentanyl as treatment for chronic low back pain. *Journal of Pain and Symptom Management, 14,* 218–224.

Smirne, S., & Scarlato, G. (1977). Clonazepam in cranial neuralgias. *Medical Journal of Australia, 1,* 93–94.

Spiegel, K., Kalb, R., & Pasternak, G. (1983). Analgesic activity of tricyclic antidepressants. *Annals of Neurology, 13,* 462–465.

Steardo, L., & Leo, A. (1984). Efficacy of baclofen in trigeminal neuralgia and some other painful conditions: A clinical trial. *European Neurology, 23,* 51–55.

Sunshine, A., & Olson, N. (1994). Non-narcotic analgesics. In P. Wall & R. Melzack (Eds.), *Textbook of pain* (3rd ed., pp. 923–942). New York: Churchill Livingstone.

Taub, A. (1982). Opioid analgesics in the treatment of chronic intractable pain of non-neoplastic origin. In L. Kitahata & J. Collins (Eds.), *Narcotics, analgesics in anesthesiology* (pp. 199–208). Baltimore: Williams & Wilkins.

Tremont-Lukats, I., Megeff, C., & Backonja M. M.

(2000). Anticonvulsants for neuropathic pain syndromes: Mechanism of action and place in therapy. *Drugs, 60,* 1029–1052.

Twycross, R. (1994). Opioids. In P. Wall & R. Melzack (Eds.), *Textbook of pain* (3rd ed., pp. 943–962). New York: Churchill Livingstone.

"U.S. asks painkiller maker to help curb wide abuse." (2001, May 1). *New York Times,* p. A8.

Urban, B., France, R., & Sternberger, E. (1986). Long-term use of narcotic/antidepressant edication in the management of phantom limb pain. *Pain, 24,* 191–196.

Wachtel, R. (1999). Capsaicin. *Regional Anesthesia and Pain Medicine, 24,* 361–363

Walsh, T., Baxter, R., & Bowman, K. (1981). High dose morphine and respiratory function in chronic cancer pain. *Pain, 3*(Suppl. 1), 39.

Ward, N., Bloom, V., & Friedel, R. (1979). The effectiveness of tricyclic antidepressants in the reatment of coexisting pain and depression. *Pain, 7,* 331–341.

Ward, N., & Whitney, C. (1991). The analgesic effects of caffeine in headache. *Pain, 44,* 151–155.

Watson, C., Evans, R., & Reed, K. (1982). Amitriptyline versus placebo in postherpetic neuralgia. *Neurology, 32,* 671–673.

Yosselson-Superstine, S., & Lipman, A. (1985). Adjunctive antianxiety agents in the management of chronic pain. *Israel Journal of Medical Science, 21,* 113–117.

III

SPECIFIC SYNDROMES
AND POPULATIONS

14

Improving the Management of Low Back Pain: A Paradigm Shift for Primary Care

Sheri D. Pruitt
Michael Von Korff

The Scope of the Back Pain Problem

Addressing patients' pain reports is a daily, if not hourly, undertaking in the practice of a primary care provider. In fact, in the United States, only upper respiratory symptoms prompt more office visits (Hart, Deyo, & Cherkin, 1995). Although the assortment of pain complaints can be as varied as areas in the body (e.g., head, abdominal, chest, neck, and shoulder), back pain is the most frequently described pain problem in the primary care setting (Andersson, 1999; Cherkin, Deyo, Wheeler, & Ciol, 1994).

Given epidemiological patterns suggesting that back pain is almost ubiquitous, the high frequency of reports in primary care is not surprising. Up to 80% of adults experience low back problems at some point in their lives (Clinical Standards Advisory Group, 1994), and back pain is the most common cause of work-related disability in people under 45 years of age (Agency for Health Care Policy and Research [AHCPR], 1994). Back pain is expensive; the combined medical and disability compensation costs reach an estimated $50 billion annually in the United States (Deyo, 1998).

Guidelines Failed to Improve Care and Control Costs

Despite the availability of clinical practice guidelines for more than a decade (AHCPR, 1994; Spitzer et al., 1987), physicians' management and diagnostic strategies for back pain continue to vary widely (Di Iorio, Henley, & Doughty, 2000; Freeborn, Shye, Mullooly, Eraker, & Romero, 1997). Radiographic imaging and surgery rates in the United States diverge from guideline recommendations and are excessive when compared to rates in other countries (Carey & Garrett, 1996; Swedlow, Johnson, Smithline, & Milstein, 1992). The Institute of Medicine (1987) recognized this excess even before guidelines were published and called surgery for chronic back pain "overused" and "misused." Similarly, the clinical management of back pain has been criticized as being "overly specialized, invasive, and expensive," prompting Waddell

(1996) to deem the problem a "health care disaster."

The distribution of evidence-based guidelines was expected to change physicians' clinical practices, presuming that a knowledge deficit was the principal reason for variability in practice, but this single method approach has failed (Lomas, 1991; Lomas et al., 1989). Because a predominantly educational intervention was not effective in changing physician behavior, a variety of explanations for primary care providers' lack of compliance in implementing back pain guidelines have been proposed. Experience (Frost, Lamb, Moffett, Fairbank, & Moser, 1998), habits (Mittman, Tonesk, & Jacobson, 1992), beliefs and attitudes (Rainville, Carlson, Polatin, Gatchel, & Indahl, 2000), community norms (Conroy & Shannon, 1995), and social factors (Dixon, 1990) have all been implicated and are purported to have greater influence over providers than does the scientific literature. Greater specificity in the back pain guidelines may be necessary to improve implementation (Shekelle et al., 2000). Finally, some propose that the missing link between guidelines and practice for low back pain is the lack of practical tools to assist physicians in operationalizing the guideline recommendations (Rossignol et al., 2000).

Back Pain Guidelines Are Unique

Back pain guidelines may not be comparable to other clinical practice recommendations. For example, the guidelines developed and disseminated for asthma management have been effective in altering providers' behavior (Dennis, Vickers, Frost, Price, & Barnes, 1997). The disparity in implementation may be due to the fact that the new provider behavior required for adherence to the asthma guidelines is within the same functional class as the existing behavior; that is, prescribing medications for managing a medical condition is a familiar behavior for physicians. The back pain guidelines (AHCPR, 1994) are different in that they require an expanded set of provider behaviors that fall outside their well-practiced repertoire. For instance, physicians are guided to reassure patients about their symptoms, to encourage patients to return to usual activities, and to continue to make these suggestions even when patients are "slow to recover." Adherence to these guidelines requires a set of skills that goes beyond writing a medication prescription.

Moreover, pain is distinct from other chronic conditions and their management because of the medications that commonly are prescribed. Unlike other chronic conditions such as chronic obstructive pulmonary disease (COPD), hypertension, and diabetes, highly reinforcing and sedating medications often are initiated with acute back pain and continued over the long term. In addition to their sedating side effects, the pain-contingent administration and long-term use of opioids and muscle relaxants are an ideal recipe for iatrogenic disability. Essentially, the still too frequently used "tools of the trade" of medicine actually interfere with high-quality back pain management, diminish patient health outcomes, and often serve to frustrate primary care providers.

Variability in clinical practice, prevalence rates, and high costs combined with alarming rates of associated disability make back pain particularly intriguing to researchers. Subsequently, a substantial amount of information has accumulated over previous decades regarding evaluation and treatment. Although far from complete, our understanding of low back problems is relatively advanced compared to other pain complaints. For this reason, in the current chapter we focus primarily on nonspecific, chronic recurrent pain problems involving the low back and review effective interventions, promising primary care strategies, and the need for a paradigm shift in primary care. Although back pain is highlighted, the general model for services and the conceptual framework for the delivery of care apply to other ongoing pain problems (e.g., neck pain, tension type headache, and osteoarthritis).

A Significant Challenge for Primary Care Providers

When patients decide to pursue medical care for common pain problems, they turn to their primary care physician for advice

(American Academy of Family Physicians, 1987). However, because back pain rarely is associated with anatomical findings, providers are challenged with the task of evaluating and planning treatment for a symptom. Moreover, in the case of back pain, the symptom is episodic and variable in terms of severity and the time since onset. The solution is not as simple as finding and repairing a lesion in the spine that is presumed to be causal.

Provider Dissatisfaction

When back pain becomes chronic, physiological findings (if present, at all) become less important than the role of patient's attitudes, beliefs, behaviors, coping abilities, and other and psychosocial factors in management and outcome predictions (Clinical Standards Advisory Group, 1994; Linton, 1999; Waddell, 1992). Without a physical etiology to direct familiar biomedical interventions, primary care providers are challenged with complex biopsychosocial problems that they are ill prepared to handle (Cherkin, MacCornack, & Berg, 1988). They acknowledge their difficulties in managing patients with chronic problems and express uncertainty about what to do (Van Tulder, Koes, & Bouter, 1997; Von Korff, 1999). The failure of the biomedical model becomes increasingly obvious, and, as a result, physicians feel frustrated, helpless and that they have little to offer patients with ongoing back problems (Klein, Najman, Kohrman, & Munro, 1982). Consequently, they stereotype patients as difficult, dependent, and unmotivated (Cherkin et al., 1988). Patients report similar negative emotions, expressing frustration and dissatisfaction with back care (Cherkin & MacCornack, 1989).

On top of the vexation that primary care providers experience in trying to manage patients with chronic pain symptoms, physicians have been criticized for providing less than optimal back pain care. Physicians have been charged with discouraging self-care and behavioral management, inadvertently endorsing disability, and facilitating the misuse of pain medications by implicitly promising medical cures for chronic pain problems (Fordyce, 1976; Osterweis, Kleinman, & Mechanic, 1987).

Office Visits: What Really Happens

Examples of primary care practice insufficiencies have been observed in an audiotape analysis of the content and organization of primary care visits for back pain (Turner, LeResche, Von Korff, & Ehrlich, 1998; Von Korff, 1999). In general, back pain visits revolved around discussions about diagnosis, medications, and pain history with unfocused advice about patient self-management. These conclusions prompted the authors to suggest the need for improvements in providers' behavior for most aspects of the primary care visit. They recommended enhancing assessment procedures and reassuring common patient worries regarding exercise and future disability during the primary care office visit. Additional strategies for improving back pain visits included physicians' encouraging self-care, relating realistic and reassuring prognostic statements, and clarifying and setting goals. Finally, physicians could better assess pain's interference with daily activities and allot more time for relating specific advice for symptom control and self-care.

Insufficient preparation in medical school combined with time-pressured office visits in which intertwined biopsychosocial factors (Turk & Rudy, 1987) and unrealistic patient expectations must be met (Moffett, Newbronner, Waddell, Croucher, & Spear, 2000) render back problems among the conditions most disliked by primary care physicians (Klein et al., 1982; Najman, Klein, & Munro, 1982). Rectifying these multiple hindrances to quality back care requires careful thought and strategic planning about primary care services for back pain. Indeed, a restructuring of the primary care team and the services provided is indicated.

Services Are Not Organized to Address the Problem

When evaluating back pain care, the organization of primary care services deserves closer examination. As they currently are organized, services are far from solving the prevalent problem of back pain, and in fact, some have charged that pain problems have been exacerbated as a result of current management approaches (Waddell, 1996). Possible explanations for care that is less than optimal include the historical assumption that back pain is, in most cases, an acute problem with a clear physiological etiology and an anticipated favorable outcome. In contrast, studies have demonstrated that a recurrent course of back pain is typical, and that chronic back pain problems are common (Von Korff, Deyo, Cherkin, & Barlow, 1993; Von Korff & Saunders, 1996). In fact, approximately 30% of patients seen in primary care for back pain have persistent problems 12 months later, and approximately 20% continue to experience moderate to severe activity limitations attributed to back problems (Von Korff & Saunders, 1996).

As back pain conceptualizations shift from an acute, rapidly resolving problem to a chronic problem with anticipated, episodic symptoms, primary care services need to shift as well. Patients need accurate prognostic information reflective of the expected course of their problem. For many patients, explicit reassurance, information, and education during an initial visit may be adequate. In fact, most patients will not desire or need additional primary care services if sufficiently educated during the early phase of their back pain course. Unfortunately, reassurance and education are routinely not provided in primary care settings (Turner et al., 1998) even though this verbal intervention has the potential to be highly effective for preventing future problems for a great number of patients.

A Team Approach

Ongoing pain and activity limitations are reported by a subset of patients a month or more following an initial back pain visit, and for this group, services that augment a primary care office visit may be indicated. These patients who experience continued symptoms and limitations will have more favorable outcomes with active participation in self-care activities (e.g., exercise, continuation of routine activities, and medication management) than they will with "usual care" that likely includes additional diagnostics and physician initiated interventions (Von Korff, 1999). Thus, augmented primary care services that promote self-care

and behavior change need to be available. When it comes to recurrent back pain, patient behavior is recognized as the cornerstone of treatment.

Integrating nonphysician providers who have expertise in the science of behavior change is essential when contemplating better care for back pain. A primary care team comprised of providers from disciplines outside medicine (e.g., psychologists and nurses) may prove to be optimal for managing this patient group. In fact, for a number of chronic conditions, evidence exists to support the effectiveness of innovative, modified health care teams over traditional, independent physician practices and minimally structured systems (DeBusk et al., 1994; Peters, Davidson, & Ossorio, 1995). Effective multidisciplinary care teams for chronic conditions have the following elements: support for self-management, informed patients, and prepared, proactive practice teams (Davis, Wagner, & Groves, 2000). It is difficult to argue that the chronic condition of recurrent back pain should be considered any differently.

Overwhelming Demands

The need for better back pain care presents against a backdrop of growing demands on primary care services to provide preventive, coordinated, and comprehensive care for a defined population (Von Korff, 1999). In this context, providers are expected to address psychological and social factors of illness in addition to diagnosis and treatment of both chronic and acute problems. Primary care providers also serve a gatekeeping function that includes making decisions regarding which patients will benefit from specialty care. The expectation seems to be that primary care services will be clinically effective, evidence-based, cost-effective, and delivered in the span of intermittent 15-minute office visits throughout a patient's lifetime.

Expectations of primary care services are arguably daunting. These expansive demands, in conjunction with the sole reliance on primary care physicians to manage the problem of back pain, have yielded disappointing results. Unfortunately, primary care physicians have not proven able to alter their practices to improve the management of back pain problems. Efforts to change provider behavior using continuing medical education formats, while effective in increasing physicians' knowledge and confidence in managing pain, have not been effective in improving patient outcomes (Cherkin, Deyo, & Berg, 1991; Cherkin, Deyo, Berg, Bergman, & Lishner, 1991). Neither, as noted previously, has the act of practice guideline dissemination been effective in altering provider behavior to improve back pain management (Barnett, Underwood, & Vickers, 1999; Di Iorio et al., 2000; Schers, Braspenning, Drijver, Wensing, & Grol, 2000).

Although today's primary care providers are expected to attend to psychological, behavioral, and social factors that extend far beyond pathophysiology, evidence suggests that physicians struggle with identifying behavioral problems in their patients, and when they do, they experience frustration with trying to change patients' behaviors (Alto, 1995). These findings are especially concerning when organizing primary care for back pain, as it is increasingly accepted that patients' beliefs, attitudes, and daily behaviors about back pain need to be addressed (Burton, Tillotson, Main, & Hollis, 1995; Crombez, Vlaeyen, Heuts, & Lysens, 1999; Linton, 1999). Unfortunately, the cognitive and behavioral skills necessary to assess and impact these factors are not part of traditional medical education. Moreover, interventions that would be helpful in altering patients' attitudes, beliefs, and coping abilities are not available in most primary care settings (Von Korff, 1999). To expect physicians to provide such interventions at the level that is necessary is unrealistic (Schroth, 1996). They may be able to deliver basic cognitive and behavioral interventions, but their time limits and skill sophistication are exceeded by patients' needs.

The mismatch between what patients with back pain need and what they receive in primary care has been acknowledged (Waddell, 1996). The challenge is to reorganize primary care services to incorporate prepared providers who can prevent the development of chronic problems in some patients and assist those with ongoing symptoms in self-management.

Is Primary Care the Optimal Setting for Back Pain Management?

Primary care is accepted as the most appropriate venue for the management of nonspecific back problems (Freeborn et al., 1997; Waddell, 1996), and though currently less than optimal, with some sensible restructuring, primary care has the potential to revolutionize care for back pain. Those who have recognized the potential have apportioned several responsibilities to primary care settings. Secondary to identifying serious disease that may be the cause of pain, primary care is charged with prevention of chronicity (Van Tulder, Koes, Metsemakers, & Bouter, 1998), the reduction of iatrogenic disability (Frank et al., 1996), the control of costs (Engel, Von Korff, & Katon, 1996), the appropriate use of specialty care (Carey et al., 1995; Cherkin et al., 1994; Waddell, 1996), and the effective management of the chronic condition of back pain (Von Korff, 1999). These tasks can be accomplished by integrating what we know about back pain management into primary care services.

First Visit Opportunities

Most patients never visit a physician for back pain, but for those who do, the initial primary care visit can be pivotal in directing the course of treatment (Malmivaara et al., 1995). Physicians absolutely can influence a patient's future with back pain by what they do and say at an initial visit. For example, their initial diagnoses are predictive of chronic disability (Abenhaim et al., 1995). Consider that during a first visit, patients can receive reassurance, advice, and recommendations that can potentially reduce their risk of developing chronic problems. Alternatively, patients can be misguided and mismanaged to the point that they experience iatrogenic problems (e.g., inadvertent physician-caused disability) (Deyo, 1993; Nachemson, 1992). Chronic disability consistently is reported to be 5–10% of patients with nonspecific back pain (Frank et al., 1996). It is worth considering how much of this chronicity could be prevented with a reduction in overtreatment, excessive investigation, labeling, and attention during the early phase of back care (Abenhaim et al., 1995).

Setting patients on the correct course is the key to better outcomes, and primary care is an ideal location in which such direction can occur.

Costs from a Population Perspective

In addition to providing quality care at pain onset, well-organized primary care services can potentially affect health care costs from a population standpoint. Because of the high volume of back pain visits, small reductions in the costs associated with an episode of pain can have significant economic impact on health care costs. It is now understood that a minority of primary care patients account for the majority of health care costs for pain-related services (Engel et al., 1996). For instance, 21% of patients with back pain account for 66% of the costs of back pain care. The predictors of high costs in this group of patients suggest that interventions designed to address psychosocial and behavioral issues (e.g., depression, ongoing pain complaints, and associated dysfunction) likely could reduce the use of health care services. Providing these services seems a reasonable strategy for cost control.

More Is Not Better

Quality back pain care in the primary care setting has the potential to reduce the number of specialty referrals. When patients see orthopedic surgeons, neurosurgeons, or chiropractors instead of primary care physicians for back pain problems, the cost of care is greater even though the outcomes do not differ (Carey et al., 1995). As a result of this finding, Waddell (1996) suggested that resources be reallocated from specialty to primary care services. Primary care services are less costly, and reassigning resources could enhance the quality of care that currently is provided. For example, interprovider practice variability is an area ripe for improvement as cost differences have been observed among the practice styles of primary care physicians. Those who prescribe bed rest and pain medications have significantly higher costs than those who prescribe these two strategies less frequently (Von Korff, Barlow, Cherkin, & Deyo, 1994). This is another example in which more intensive care does not improve back

pain outcomes. Ensuring a consistently less medicalized approach is a reasonable first target when resources are reallocated.

Primary Care Can Be Optimal

Back pain is the most common chronic pain problem, yet primary care services are not structured to address back pain as a chronic condition. To do so would involve significant changes in delivery systems, such as those called for in the management of other chronic conditions including asthma, diabetes, and arthritis (Davis et al., 2000). However, reorganization of care may not be as overwhelming as it initially appears. There is increasing recognition that management strategies for chronic conditions share common themes that make differences among specific chronic conditions inconsequential. Self-care tasks, shared by all chronic conditions including pain, consist of engaging in health-promoting activities, minimizing impact on daily activities, monitoring and adapting to changes, collaborating with health care providers, and adhering to the management plan (Lorig, 1993; Von Korff, Gruman, Schaefer, Curry, & Wagner, 1997).

The multiple tasks ascribed to primary care settings in relation to back pain will not be accomplished without a reorganization of services. It will be necessary for administrators, physicians, and patients to adjust their paradigms if back care is to be improved. The focus must shift from frustrated efforts to cure the pain in the back to effective management of the patient who complains about it. Fortunately, much is known about helping patients manage back pain problems.

What Works for Back Pain

Activating Interventions

Level of activation and fears related to physical activity are emerging as primary determinants of functional outcomes in patients with chronic recurrent back pain (see, e.g., Abenhaim et al., 2000; Frost et al., 1998; Mannion, Muntener, Taimela, & Dvorak, 1999; Moffett et al., 1999). Interventions have been developed to address these factors. Activating interventions usually include giving advice to patients about the importance of moving and staying active, often in the form of suggesting exercise and/or the return to normal activities as quickly as possible following back pain onset. Such straightforward advice clearly is effective. A review of randomized controlled trials comparing advice for activity versus bed rest found that primary care physicians' advice to stay active resulted in reduced chronicity, quicker return to work, and fewer recurrent pain problems (Waddell, Feder, & Lewis, 1997).

Communicating Advice for Activity

The message to remain active appears simplistic; however, its delivery merits consideration. In managing chronic conditions, a patient-centered approach is thought to be more effective than a direct tactic when promoting self-care behaviors (Anderson, 1995). Yet, when physicians advise patients with recurrent back pain about the importance of exercise, it is uncommon for them to use a patient-focused perspective. For example, physicians rarely inquire about patients' preferences or interests related to exercise or provide a menu of options for activity. Moreover, when patients spontaneously relate that they already participate in some form of exercise, physicians do not consistently offer verbal praise or support for such efforts (Turner et al., 1998; Von Korff, 1999). Physicians' encouragement of exercise in those patients who are active would increase the likelihood that patients would continue this behavior and improve their back pain course.

Exercise Programs

Structured exercise programs also can be considered activating interventions, and there is evidence that exercise is efficacious for the treatment of low back pain (Koes, Bouter, & van der Heijden, 1995; Van Tulder et al., 1997). Fitness programs with aerobics, stretching, and strengthening components have been evaluated and found effective for patients with "slow to recover" (4–6 months' duration) and chronic back pain problems (Frost et al., 1998; Mannion et al., 1999; Moffett et al., 1999).

A recent comparison of activating interventions (i.e., active physical therapy, muscle reconditioning using training equipment, and aerobics) suggested that clinical improvements were not due to changes in physical status as a result of specific treatments but, rather, to a change in patients' beliefs or perceptions of pain and disability (Mannion et al., 1999). The crucial point seems to be that patients alter the way they think about pain and their perceptions of their physical abilities when they become physically active. These findings are encouraging as exercise programs are relatively inexpensive and can easily be administered, and the type of exercise may not be so critical. However, adherence to activity recommendations becomes a concern as it may be difficult for patients with pain problems to incorporate an exercise regimen into daily routines (Deyo & Weinstein, 2001). Adherence to any medical recommendation is increasingly more difficult as patients are asked to learn new behaviors, alter their daily patterns, and maintain the changes over time (see, e.g., Marlatt & Gordon, 1985; Meichenbaum & Turk, 1987). Future investigations of exercise for long-term back pain management will have to address relapse prevention and maintenance issues.

Whether advised to remain active or to participate in a structured exercise program, a key feature of the activation concept is to avoid giving patients the message that they need bed rest to promote recovery from back pain. Although there is evidence of increased awareness in clinical practice about the importance of exercise and avoidance of prolonged bed rest, a recent survey of family physicians identified continued problems with physicians' advice. Physicians' recommendations for ongoing back problems frequently restricted patients' work and activities (Rainville et al., 2000) rather than encouraged exercise. Some have suggested that a straightforward but fundamental change in physicians' advice could significantly improve outcomes and reduce costs associated with back pain (Waddell et al., 1997).

Changing Patients' Beliefs

Activity interventions often overlap with those designed to address patients' beliefs because misperceptions about back pain are tied to concerns about physical activity. Beliefs that have emerged as determinants of disability are that (1) movement and activity cause pain (i.e., avoidance) and (2) the worry that pain will return (i.e., fear). Patients who endorse these beliefs tend to have reduced activity levels and increased disability. Interventions designed specifically to address patients' fear and avoidance behaviors during acute back pain episodes have demonstrated better functional outcomes when compared to bed rest or to back exercises (Malmivaara et al., 1995). Table 14.1 lists common fears endorsed by primary care patients with back pain.

Successful fear–avoidance interventions have included addressing the fear of physical activity by providing reassurance about the safety of movement and stressing the importance of normal walking and personal goal setting (Indahl, Velund, & Reikeraas, 1995). Multiple sessions of cognitive-behavioral therapy designed to alter patients' behaviors, beliefs, and coping abilities also have been efficacious in reducing fear–avoidance beliefs, health care use, and absenteeism (Linton & Andersson, 2000). Moreover, interventions designed to increase activation resulted in reduced functional limitations, in addition to reduced worry and fear–avoidance beliefs (Moore, Von Korff, Cherkin, Saunders, & Lorig, 2000; Von Korff et al., 1998).

Patient beliefs about back pain also have been shifted using judiciously selected information provided in written educational materials. Burton, Waddell, Tillotson, & Summerton (1999) implemented a low-cost,

low-intensity intervention that consisted of giving patients information and advice in a booklet format at the end of a physician visit for back pain. The written material emphasized strength of the spine, the lack of serious disease, the association between recovery and activity, and the importance of positive attitudes about getting better. Contrast this presentation with traditional educational approaches that have been biomedical in focus with an overemphasis on anatomy, pathophysiology, and movement restriction. This minimal intervention resulted in positive changes in beliefs and reductions in self-reported disability among primary care patients with back pain.

Shifting the Paradigm: Promising Strategies for Reorganization

A shift from an acute care paradigm to an expanded model appropriate for chronic conditions is necessary before the management of low back pain will be noticeably improved in primary care. Current back pain care is conducted with an acute emphasis, protracted diagnostics, medications, and vague suggestions about activity and self-management. When symptoms fail to improve or when providers become frustrated with attempts to cure chronic pain problems, patients typically are referred to specialty clinics (e.g., orthopedics) that in many cases reflect an even stronger acute care model and biomedical focus. These continued health care practices are unfortunate as low back pain no longer is consid-

TABLE 14.1. Percentage of Patients Reporting Specific Fear–Avoidance Beliefs 2 Months Following a Primary Care Visit for Back Pain

	% of patients
Fear ($n = 250$)	
The wrong movement could lead to a serious problem.	64
I wouldn't have this much pain if there weren't something dangerously wrong.	45
Avoidance (n 226)	
Avoiding unnecessary movements is the safest way to prevent pain from worsening.	51
I might injure myself if I exercise.	31
It's not safe to be physically active.	13

ered acute and self-limiting but has a typical course that is manifested by episodic symptoms over time. As a result, back pain care needs to be organized around the concept of pain management, not pain amelioration.

Shifting the emphasis from cure of an acute malady that solicits patients' passivity to management of a chronic problem that requires patients to make behavioral changes necessitates a shuffling of the primary care team members. Integrating cognitive and behavioral expertise to assist patients in changing their beliefs and to initiate and maintain behavior changes seems ever more prudent given our current knowledge. Behavioral experts can provide direct clinical services to primary care patients, in addition to training primary care providers in the basics of cognitive and behavioral management techniques that can enhance the implementation of and adherence to practice guidelines. As highlighted earlier, interventions that alter patients' beliefs, attitudes, and coping abilities are imperative for improving outcomes associated with back pain, but these are not available in primary care clinics. Following a shift from an acute to a chronic care model in which behavioral expertise is incorporated, back pain care can be delivered according to an algorithm or pathway that matches patients' care needs to the intensity of services they receive.

Shifting the paradigm from acute care to chronic disease management is a significant challenge for primary care settings. Providers must implement effective back pain care to patients who vary widely in severity and chronicity of back pain symptoms (Von Korff, Ormel, Keefe, & Dworkin, 1992). For example, patients visit their primary care provider at different stages along their course of back pain. Some are experiencing an initial episode, others are in the so-called slow to recover or subacute period, and many are encountering periodic back pain flare-ups. A smaller, but not insignificant group of patients with back pain problems (approximately 8%) are unable to work because of pain (Von Korff, 1999).

The heterogeneity of the back pain population has made research difficult. Although the number of randomized trials in primary care settings is beginning to accumulate, effective strategies for integrating efficacious interventions into routine primary care practice remain unclear.

The Stepped-Care Algorithm

Stepped care is a framework for organizing services based on the intensity of patients' needs. It has been described as a useful strategy for organizing primary care services for behaviorally based problems (Pruitt, Klapow, Epping-Jordan, & Dresselhaus, 1998). In addition, hypertension (SHEP Cooperative Research Group, 1991), cholesterol (Oster et al., 1995), nicotine dependence (Hurt, 1993), and alcohol dependence (Donovan & Marlatt, 1993) are problems that have been managed effectively using this progressive strategy.

In general, a stepped approach initially provides the least intensive, and often least expensive, intervention as a first step in improving outcomes. If patients do not experience a favorable result, services are intensified or "stepped up" to the next level of intervention that typically is more costly and more complex. The obvious benefit of a stepped-care approach is that services are better matched to patients' needs, and excessive or unnecessary services are minimized resulting in greater efficiency and cost savings. Furthermore, low-cost, low-intensity interventions have been effective for a variety of problems ranging from fevers in pediatric populations to somatizing adults (Ritvo et al., 1997; Robinson, Schwartz, Magwene, Krengel, & Tamburello, 1989; Smith, Rost, & Kashner, 1995). As noted, in the case of back pain, a low-cost intervention (i.e., advice) delivered during a primary care office visit at the time of an initial back pain onset can prevent chronicity (Waddell et al., 1997).

Von Korff (1999; Von Korff & Moore, 2001) has outlined a stepped-care framework for managing back pain in primary care (see Table 14.2 for an outline). Step 1, the lowest-intensity intervention, consists of addressing patients' fear–avoidance beliefs through education and information, and through advice about the importance of returning to usual activities as quickly as possible. This level of intervention is brief and

TABLE 14.2. Stepped Care for Back Pain in Primary Care

Intensity of care	Focus of intervention	Provider	Format
Step 1	Reassurance	Physician	Office visit
Step 2	Activity increase	Behaviorist	Group/individual
Step 3	Rehabilitation	Behaviorist/case manager	Group/individual

can occur during an office visit with a primary care provider. Moreover, it may be all that is necessary for a number of patients with nonspecific low back pain. Step 2, an increased intensity intervention, is reserved for patients who continue to report back pain 6 to 8 weeks following the onset of an episode and demonstrate persistent limitations in physical activity. An intervention at the Step 2 level could include a structured exercise program or additional cognitive and behavioral strategies to address fears and help patients resume their usual work and leisure activities. Intervention at this level requires more than can be offered in a single, 15-minute office visit. An extended visit or multiple visits can produce improved outcomes for patients who need this level of intensity; however, interventions could be efficiently provided in a group format. The incorporation of providers from other disciplines (e.g., behaviorists, physical therapists, health educators, or nurses) will be important for providing the more intensive interventions at Step 2.

For patients who have failed to improve with either Step 1 or Step 2 interventions, Step 3 intensity should be available. Step 3 is reserved for patients who are experiencing significant work disability and are at risk for becoming permanently work disabled. Intervention at this level is more costly and complex than interventions provided at Steps 1 and 2. It should address psychiatric comorbidities (e.g., major depression) and target role responsibilities in work, home, and social arenas. Step 3 interventions can be provided in primary care if personnel, time, and space are available. Using a group format can increase efficiency. Alternatively, patients who require this level of intensity could be referred to specialty services that might include multidisciplinary pain clinics, psychiatry, or physical rehabilitation for patients with persistent pain problems.

The stepped-care approach need not be applied only in a progressive fashion. Patients may come to the attention of the primary care provider already in need of intensive intervention for an ongoing pain problem that has failed to resolve, is associated with physical limitations, and is placing the patient at risk of work disability. In these cases, a stratified approach is advised in which steps can be "skipped" and patients can be immediately matched to the level of care appropriate for their needs.

A stepped-care approach has advantages beyond those outlined above if it is routinely integrated into primary care. If Step 1 care is regularly provided for every patient who reports back pain, there is significant potential to reduce the chances of chronicity, minimize disability, and limit excessive use of health care services (Indahl et al., 1995; Malmivaara et al., 1995; Waddell et al., 1997). Perhaps more important, the failure of primary care providers to address beliefs and activation (the Step 1 intervention) may, at best, do little to benefit the patient and, at worst, lead to unnecessary chronicity and disability.

Fundamental changes in the conceptualization of back pain and how it is managed in primary care are essential; otherwise, the number of patients with persistent back pain problems will continue to expand. These numbers can be controlled to the point that they eventually can be diminished, but primary care services must incorporate fear–avoidance and activity recommendations to such an extent that these recommendations become "usual care." Table 14.3 contrasts current approaches with a stepped-care framework.

Integrating Back Pain Expertise

Incorporating informed providers (i.e., physicians, nurses, and/or psychologists with

TABLE 14.3. Back Pain: Current Primary Care Services versus Stepped-Care Approach

	Current primary care services	Stepped-care approach
Model of care	Acute	Expanded, chronic
Provider	Physician	Physician plus providers from other disciplines
Focus of visits	Diagnosis and pain history	Altering beliefs and increasing activities
Basis for intervention	Familiarity, social/community standards, peers	Evidence-based
Care strategy	Unplanned, PRN	Stepwise progression based on patient response and need
Educational materials	Not systematic	Routine dissemination of materials that reinforce verbal information
Role of physician	Directive, "repairman" mentality	"Coach," supportive of team members' efforts
Cost	Variable, expensive	Controlled

advanced pain knowledge) into primary care settings is a practical approach for integrating appropriate education, information, and behavioral interventions for back pain management. A recent study (Rossignol et al., 2000) found that adding expertise into regular care enhanced the implementation of back pain guidelines and resulted in positive outcomes for patients with subacute low back pain. In this randomized controlled trial, supplemental providers worked with treating physicians to determine appropriate use of diagnostic tests, optimal interventions, and a management plan for each patient according to the current practice guidelines. Although the experimental group did not return to work more quickly than did the usual care group, significant differences were demonstrated between the two groups on exercise participation, pain, functional status, and health care costs. The authors attributed the success of the intervention to the confidence instilled in the patients as a result of receiving a thorough pain assessment, including medical, psychosocial, and occupational elements even though all evaluations stayed within the economical guideline recommendations. However, noteworthy is the fact that patients in the experimental group were followed in weekly phone calls from a nurse who encouraged function, return to usual activities, and problem solving.

Other interventions of integrated exper-

tise have been described. A brief, multicomponent intervention provided by a psychologist was determined to be moderately successful in reducing worries, self-care attitudes, pain intensity, fear–avoidance, and functional outcomes in primary care patients at least 2 months after their office visit for back pain (Moore et al., 2000). The intervention included two cognitive-behavioral group meetings, an individual self-care plan meeting, book and videotape, and telephone follow-up calls. Skills for back pain self-management, accurate information, and reassurance messages were imparted according to a structured and standardized protocol. The results of this intervention were similar to an 8-week progressive exercise program described earlier (Moffett et al., 1999).

Stepped care as a framework for back pain service delivery is flexible. It can support the inclusion of guideline-based educational material, the addition of expert providers from other disciplines, and the incorporation of structured interventions for increasing activation and reducing fear–avoidance beliefs. Turner (1996) recommended the integration of educational and behavioral interventions into primary care settings subsequent to her review of randomized clinical trials that showed that these two elements are the most promising for improving long-term outcomes. At present, the number of randomized controlled trials evaluating these interventions in primary care settings is increasing, leaving little argument over the efficacy of behavioral (i.e., activating) interventions for back pain problems in primary care.

The next research questions to be answered must consider the feasibility, practicality, and efficiency of educational and activating interventions in primary care settings using a stepped-care approach. Can primary care providers more effectively address fear–avoidance beliefs in a brief office visit? How intensive do interventions need to be at each level of care? What is the most effective way to deliver fear-reducing information? What types of providers most effectively and efficiently intervene with patients with back pain, and does provider type differ with level of care?

Challenges to Change: Costs and Organizational Barriers

There are challenges to restructuring primary care services for back pain. First, reimbursement systems are not in place to support the integration of nonmedical providers into mainstream primary care clinics even though these providers are the most skilled in delivering services or designing programs for altering patients' beliefs and daily behaviors to promote back pain self-management. Academic institutions that value innovation in educating future health care providers and staff model health maintenance organizations that support teams of providers to manage patients and contain costs are most likely to embrace the concept of primary care teams to address chronic health problems. Even in these cases, health care administrators have to recognize the need to invest in expertise and program development that may not have immediately realized savings. There is a need for administrators to shift their paradigms in the same direction as physicians because short-term cost accountability continues to drive most budget decisions. The problem of low back pain may provide a convincing argument for change. Well-organized primary care services for pain have the potential to reduce costs across a system of care (i.e., from primary to specialty services), to improve patients' health status,

and to serve as a model for organizing services for other chronic conditions.

Conclusion

Effective interventions can be integrated into primary care services to improve care for the vast number of patients reporting back pain. Benefits of enhancing care for this population include the reduction of the number of patients who develop long-term physical limitations often associated with work disability, fewer iatrogenic problems, and controls on excessive health care use. Back pain care can be advanced by making straightforward, yet fundamental changes in the manner in which primary care providers attend to their patients with pain problems. The essential changes include requiring providers to address patients' beliefs and fears by providing reassurance and normalization of back pain while offering focused advice about exercise and other physical activities. Although the verbiage appears easy to impart, the conveyed message will be a striking departure from current clinical practice that continues to "medicalize" a problem with few, and increasingly irrelevant physiological findings.

The delivery of back pain care can take advantage of stepped care as a framework for organizing services in graduated intensity based on patients' needs. "Stepped" services reserve the most costly and intensive interventions only for patients who need them and provide least costly and least intensive interventions to all patients experiencing the problem. Despite evidence that the relatively low-cost intervention of physicians' advice or carefully selected written information (Step 1) can be powerful in limiting chronicity in many patients, some patients will have persistent problems. For this smaller group, more intensive interventions that target activity limitations and self-management (Step 2) can be followed by increasingly intensive interventions for an even smaller group of patients who need help with rehabilitation, work-role disability, and psychological comorbidities (Step 3).

Steps 2 and 3 interventions extend beyond the time parameters of a regular primary care visit and augment services provided by physicians. In these steps, repeated visits, typically within a structured program, are necessary. Because of the increasingly recommended emphasis on behavior change, self-management, and adherence (Fordyce, 1976; Von Korff, Wagner, Dworkin, & Saunders, 1991; Waddell, 1991), behavioral experts or other non-physician providers may best provide interventions at Steps 2 and 3. Providers with expertise in the science of behavior change and self-management may prove to be efficient and effective in this regard.

With the integration of additional health care providers, it is imperative that the entire clinical team express a clear and consistent approach to patients regarding information and strategies for managing back pain. Contradictory advice contributes to patients' fear and pessimism about recovery (May, Rose, & Johnstone, 2000; Nordin, 1995). Moreover, as team members, primary care physicians could use their credibility to create accurate and positive expectations for self-management and group interventions, thereby enhancing participation rates of patients referred to self-care interventions (cf. Winkler, Underwood, Fatovich, James, & Gray, 1989).

Physician education strategies need to be more effective as current efforts have not been sufficient to significantly change clinical practice (Cherkin, Deyo, Wheeler, & Ciol, 1995; Moffett et al., 2000). At Kaiser Permanente in Sacramento, California, physicians observe Step 2 interventions prior to having access to Step 2 or Step 3 interventions for their patients experiencing ongoing pain problems. The purpose of this contingency is to ensure that providers give a consistent message to patients at every "step." It is an opportunity for physicians to observe a competent model demonstrating effective reassurance and activation communication strategies that the physician can reproduce during office visits. After all, patients will continue to be cared for by their primary physician following participation in intensive interventions even if these occur in a specialty clinic. At future primary care visits, physicians can reiterate information imparted in the Step 2 interventions and encourage patients' maintenance of self-care activities.

Effective treatment for back pain requires a transformation of primary care services that move away from an acute care paradigm to one that is expanded to include early intervention and self-management over the long term. This shift requires physicians to alter their practices to address patient worries and concerns, initially, and to actively support patients' self-management efforts over time. In turn, patients are required to adopt self-care strategies such as exercise and self-management of episodic flare-ups. And, finally, health care systems and administrators must support the transformation from our current "quick fix" system to one that is broader and more thoughtful by allocating resources for comprehensive back care services. Effective back pain patient care benefits everyone.

References

Abenhaim, L., Rossignol, M., Gobeille, D., Bonvalot, Y., Fines, P., & Scott, S. (1995). The prognostic consequences in the making of the initial medical diagnosis of work-related back injuries. *Spine, 20,* 791–795.

Abenhaim, L., Rossignol, M., Valat, J. P., Nordin, M., Avouac, B., Blotman, F., Charlot, J., Dreiser, R., Legrand, E., Rozenberg, S., & Vautravers, P. (2000). The role of activity in the therapeutic management of back pain. Report of the International Paris Task Force on Back Pain. *Spine, 25*(Suppl. 4), 1S–33S.

Agency for Health Care Policy and Research. (1994). *Acute low back problems in adults.* Rockville, MD: U.S. Department of Health and Human Services.

Alto, W. A. (1995). Prevention in practice. *Primary Care, 22,* 543–544.

American Academy of Family Physicians. (1987). *Facts about: Family practice.* Kansas City, MO: Author.

Anderson, R. M. (1995). Patient empowerment and the traditional medical model: A case of irreconcilable differences? *Diabetes Care, 18,* 412–415

Andersson, G. B. J. (1999). Epidemiologic features of chronic low-back pain. *Lancet, 354,* 581–585.

Barnett, A. G., Underwood, M. R., & Vickers, M. R. (1999). Effect of UK national guidelines on services to treat patients with acute low back pain: Follow up questionnaire survey. *British Medical Journal, 318,* 919–920.

Burton, A. K., Tillotson, K. M., Main, C. J., & Hollis, S. (1995). Psychosocial predictors of outcome in acute and subchronic low back trouble. *Spine, 20,* 722–728.

Burton, A. K., Waddell, G., Tillotson, K. M., & Summerton, N. (1999). Information and advice to patients with back pain can have a positive effect. A randomized controlled trial of a novel educational booklet in primary care. *Spine, 24,* 2484–2491.

Carey, T. S., & Garrett, J. (1996). North Carolina Back Pain Project. Patterns of ordering diagnostic tests for patients with acute low back pain. *Annals of Internal Medicine, 125,* 807–814.

Carey, T. S., Garrett, J., Jackman, A., McLaughlin, C., Fryer, J., & Smucker, D. R. (1995). The outcomes and costs of care for acute low back pain among patients seen by primary care practitioners, chiropractors and orthopaedic sugeons. *New England Journal of Medicine, 333,* 913–917.

Cherkin, D. C., Deyo, R. A., & Berg, A. O. (1991). Evaluation of a physician education intervention to improve primary care for low-back pain II: Impact on patients. *Spine 16,* 1173–1178.

Cherkin, D. C., Deyo, R. A., Berg, A. O., Bergman, J. J., & Lishner, D. M. (1991). Evaluation of a physician education intervention to improve primary care for low-back pain I: Impact on physicians. *Spine, 16,* 1168–1172.

Cherkin, D. C., Deyo, R. A., Wheeler, K., & Ciol, M. A. (1994). Physician variation in diagnostic testing for low back pain: Who you see is what you get. *Arthritis and Rheumatism, 37,* 15–22.

Cherkin, D. C., Deyo, R. A., Wheeler, K., & Ciol, M. A. (1995). Physician views about treating low back pain. The results of a national survey. *Spine, 20,* 1–9.

Cherkin, D. C., & MacCornack, F. A. (1989). Patient evaluations of low back pain care from family physicians and from chriopractors. *Western Journal of Medicine, 150,* 351–355.

Cherkin, D. C., MacCornack, F. A., & Berg, A. O. (1988). The management of low back pain: A comparison of the beliefs and behaviors of family physicians and chiropractors. *Western Journal of Medicine, 149,* 475–480.

Clinical Standards Advisory Group. (1994). *Report of a CSAG Committee on Back Pain.* London: HMSO.

Conroy, M., & Shannon, W. (1995) Clinical guidelines: Their implementation in general practice. *British Journal of General Practice, 45,* 317–375.

Crombez, G., Vlaeyen, J. W., Heuts, P. H., & Lysens, R. (1999). Pain-related fear is more disabling than pain itself: Evidence on the role of pain-related fear in chronic back pain disability. *Pain, 80,* 329–339.

Davis, R. M., Wagner, E. G., & Groves, T. (2000). Advances in managing chronic disease. *British Medical Journal, 320,* 525–526.

DeBusk R. F., Miller, N. H., Superko, H. R., Dennis, C. A., Thomas, R. J., Lew, H. T., Berger, W. E III, Heller, R. S. Rompf J., Gee, D., Kraemer, H. C., Bandura A., Ghandour, F., Clark M., Shah, R. V., Fisher, L., & Taylor, C. B. (1994). A case-management system for coronary risk factor modification after acute myocardial infarction. *Annals of Internal Medicine, 120,* 721–729.

Dennis, S. M., Vickers, M. R., Frost, C. D., Price, J. F., & Barnes, P. J. (1997). Effect of the asthma management guidelines on recruitment to a RCT of early introduction of inhaled steroids in asthma. *Thorax, 52*(Suppl. 6), A18.

Deyo, R. A. (1993). Practice variations, treatment fads, rising disability. Do we need new clinical research paradigm? *Spine, 18,* 2153–2162.

Deyo, R. A. (1998, August). Low-back pain. *Scientific American,* 49–53.

Deyo, R. A., & Weinstein, J. N. (2001). Low back pain. *New England Journal of Medicine, 344,* 363–370.

Di Iorio, D., Henley, E., & Doughty, A. (2000). A survey of primary care physician practice patterns and adherence to acute low back problem guidelines. *Archives of Family Medicine, 9,* 1015–1021.

Dixon, A. S. (1990). The evolution of clinical policies. *Medical Care, 28,* 201–220.

Donovan, D. M., & Marlatt, G. A. (1993). Recent developments in alcoholism behavioral treatment. *Recent Developments in Alcoholism, 11,* 397–411.

Engel, C. C., von Korff, M., & Katon, W. J. (1996). Back pain in primary care: Predictors of high health-care costs. *Pain, 65,* 197–204.

Fordyce, W. E. (1976). *Behavioral methods in chronic pain and illness.* St. Louis, MO: Mosby.

Frank, J. W., Brooker, A. S., DeMaio, S. E., Kerr, M. S., Maetzel, A., Shannon, H. S., Sullivan, T. J., Norman, R. W., & Wells, R. P. (1996). Disability resulting form occupational low back pain. Part II: What do we know about secondary prevention? A review of the scientific evidence on prevention after disability begins. *Spine, 15,* 2918–2929.

Freeborn, D. K., Shye, D., Mullooly, J. P., Eraker, S., & Romero, J. (1997). Primary care physicians use of lumbar spine imaging tests. Effects of guidelines and practice pattern feedback. *Journal of General Internal Medicine, 12,* 619–625.

Frost, H., Lamb, S. E., Moffett, J. A., Fairbank, J. C. T., & Moser, J. S. (1998). A fitness programme for patients with chronic low back pain: 2-year follow-up of a randomised controlled trial. *Pain, 75,* 273–279.

Hart, L. G., Deyo, R. A., & Cherkin, D. C. (1995). Physician office visits for low back pain frequency, clinical evaluation, and treatment patterns frmm a U.S. national survey. *Spine, 20,* 11–19.

Hurt, R. D. (1993). Nicotine dependence-treatment for the 1990's [Editorial]. *Journal of Internal Medicine, 233,* 307–310.

Indahl, A., Velund, L., & Reikeraas, O. (1995). Good prognosis for low back pain when left untampered. A randomized clinical trial. *Spine, 20,* 473–477.

Institute of Medicine. (1987). Overuse of surgery in chronic back pain. In M. Osterweis, A. Kleinman, & D. Mechanic (Eds.), *Pain and disability: Clinical, behavioral and public policy perspectives* (p. 204). Washington DC: National Academy Press.

Klein, D., Najman, J., Kohrman, A. F., & Munro, C. (1982). Patient characteristics that elicit negative responses from family physicians. *Journal of Family Practice, 5,* 881–888.

Koes, B. W., Bouter, L. M., & van der Heijden G. J. M. G. (1995). Methodological quality of randomised clinical trials on treatment efficacy in low back pain. *Spine, 20,* 228–235.

Linton, S. J. (1999). Prevention with special reference to chronic musculoskeletal disorders. In R. J. Gatchel & D. C. Turk (Eds.), *Psychosocial factors in pain: Critical perspectives* (pp. 374–389). New York: Guilford Press.

Linton, S. J., & Andersson, T. (2000). Can chronic disability be prevented? A randomized trial of a cognitive-behavior intervention and two forms of information for patients with spinal pain. *Spine, 25,* 2825–2831.

Lomas, J. (1991) Words without action? The production, dissemination, and impact of consensus recommendations. *Annual Review of Public Health, 12,* 41–65.

Lomas, J., Anderson, G. M., Domnick-Peirre, K., Vayda, E., Enkin, M. W., & Hannah, W. J. (1989). Do practice guidelines guide practice? The effect of a consensus statement on the practice of physicians. *New England Journal of Medicine, 321,* 1306–1311.

Lorig, K. (1993). Self-management of chronic illness: A model for the future. *Generations,* 11–14.

Malmivaara, A., Hakkinen, U., Aro, T., Heinrichs, M., Koskenniemi, L., Kuosma, E., Lappi, S., Paloheimo, R., Servo, C. Vaaranen, V., & Hernberg, S. (1995). The treatment of acute low back pain—bed rest, exercises, or ordinary activity? *New England Journal of Medicine, 332,* 351–355.

Mannion, A. F., Muntener, M., Taimela, S., & Dvorak, J. (1999). A randomized clinical trial of three active therapies for chronic back pain. *Spine, 24,* 2435–2448.

Marlatt, G. A., & Gordon, W. H. (1985). Relapse prevention: Introduction and overview of the model. *British Journal of Addiction, 79,* 261–273.

May, C. R., Rose, M. J., & Johnstone F. C. (2000). Dealing with doubt: How patients account for chronic low back pain. *Journal of Psychosomatic Research, 49,* 223–225.

Meichenbaum, D., & Turk, D. C. (1987). *Facilitating treatment adherence: A practitioner's guidebook.* New York: Plenum Press.

Mittman, B. S., Tonesk, X., & Jacobson, P. D. (1992). Implementing clinical guidelines: Social influence strategies and practitioner behavior change. *Quality Review Bulletin, 18,* 413–422.

Moffett, J. K., Newbronner, E., Waddell, G., Croucher, K., & Spear, S. (2000). Public perceptions about low back pain and its management: A gap between expectations and reality? *Health Expectations, 3,*161–168.

Moffett, J. K., Torgerson, D., Bell-Syer, S., Jackson, D., Llewlyn-Phillips, H., Farrin, A., & Barber, J. (1999). Randomised controlled trial of exercise for low back pain: Clinical outcome, costs, and

preferences. *British Medical Journal, 319,* 279–283.

Moore, J. E., Von Korff, M., Cherkin, D., Saunders, K., & Lorig, K. (2000). A randomized trial of a cognitive-behavioral program for enhancing back pain self-care in a primary care setting. *Pain, 88,* 145–153.

Nachemson, A. L. (1992). Newest knowledge of low back pain. *Clinical Orthopaedics and Related Research, 279,* 8–20.

Najman, J. M., Klein, D., & Munro, C. (1982). Patient characteristics negatively stereotyped by doctors. *Social Science in Medicine, 16,* 1781–1789.

Nordin, M. (1995). Back pain: Lessons from patient education. *Patient Education and Counseling, 26,* 67–70.

Oster, G., Borok, G. M., Menzin, J., Heys, J. F., Epstein, R. S., Quinn, V., Benson, V. V., Dudl, R. J., & Epstein, A. (1995). A randomized trial to assess effectiveness and cost in clinical practice: Rationale and design of the Cholesterol Reduction Intervention Study. *Controlled Clinical Trials, 16,* 3–16.

Osterweis, M., Kleinman, A., & Mechanic, D. (1987). *Pain and disability: Clinical, behavioral and public policy perspectives.* Washington, DC: National Academy Press.

Peters, A. L, Davidson, M. B., & Ossorio, R. C. (1995). Management of patients with diabetes by nurses with support of subspecialists. *HMO Practice, 9,* 8–12.

Pruitt, S. D., Klapow, J. C., Epping-Jordan, J. E., & Dresselhaus, T. R. (1998). Moving behavioral medicine to the front line: A model for the integration of behavioral and medical sciences in primary care. *Professional Psychology: Research and Practice, 29,* 230–236.

Rainville, J., Carlson, N., Polatin, P., Gatchel, R. J., & Indahl, A. (2000). Exploration of physicians' recommendations for activities in chronic low back pain. *Spine, 25,* 2210–2220.

Ritvo, P. G., Irvine, M. J., Lindsay, E. A., Kraetschmer, N., Blair, N., & Shnek, Z. M. (1997). A critical review of research related to family physician-assisted smoking cessation interventions. *Cancer Prevention Control, 1,* 289–303.

Robinson, J. S., Schwart, M. M., Magwene, K. S., Krengel, S. A., & Tamburello, D. (1989). The impact of fever health education on clinic utilization. *American Journal of Diseases of Children, 143,* 698–704.

Rossignol, M., Abenhaim, L., Suguin, P., Neveu, A., Collet, J. P., Ducruet, T., & Shapiro, S. (2000). Coordination of primary health care for back pain. A randomized controlled trial. *Spine, 25,* 251–259.

Schers, H., Braspenning, J., Drijver, R., Wensing, M., & Grol, R. (2000). Low back pain in general practice: Reported management and reasons for not adhering to the guidelines in the Netherlands. *British Journal of General Practice, 50,* 640–644.

Schroth, W. S. (1996). Educational and behavioral interventions for back pain in primary care. Point of view. *Spine, 21, 2858.*

Shekelle, P. G., Kravits, R. L., Beart, J., Marger, M., Wang, M., & Lee, M. (2000). Are nonspecific practice guidelines potentially harmful? A randomized comparison of the effect of nonspecific versus specific guidelines on physician decision making. *Health Services Research, 34,* 1429–1448.

SHEP Cooperative Research Group. (1991). Prevention of stroke in antihypertensive drug treatment in older persons with isolated hypertension: Final results of the Systolic Hypertension in the Elderly Program. *Journal of the American Medical Association, 265,* 3255–3264.

Smith, G. R., Rost, K., & Kashner, T. M. (1995). A trial of the effects of standardized psychiatric consultation on health outcomes and costs in somatizing patients. *Archives of General Psychiatry, 52,* 238–243.

Spitzer, W. O., Leblanc, F. E., Dupuis, M., Abenhaim, l., Belanger, A. Y., Bloch, R., Bombardier, C., Cruess, R. L., Drouin, G., Duval-Hesler, N., Laflamme, J., Lamoureux, G. Nachemson, A., Page, J. J., Rossignol, M., Salmi, L. R., Salois-Arsenault, S., Suissa, S., & Wood-Dauphinee, S. (1987). Scientific approach to the assessment and management of activity-related spinal disorders: A monogaph for clinicians. Report of the Task Force on Spinal Disorders. *Spine, 12*(Suppl.), 1–59.

Swedlow, A., Johnson, G., Smithline, N., & Milstein, A. (1992). Increased costs and rates of use in the California workers' compensation system as a result of self-referral by physicians. *New England Journal of Medicine, 327,* 1502-0516.

Turk, D. C., & Rudy, T. E. (1987). Towards a comprehensive assessment of chronic pain patients. *Behaviour Research and Therapy, 25,* 237–249.

Turner, J. A. (1996). Educational and behavioral interventions for back pain in primary care. *Spine, 21,* 2851–2859.

Turner, J. A., LeResche, L., Von Korff, M., & Ehrlich, K. (1998). Primary care back pain patient characteristics, visit content and short-term outcomes. *Spine, 23,* 463–469.

Van Tulder, M. W., Koes, B. W., & Bouter, L. M. (1997). Conservative treatment of acute and chronic nonspecific low back pain: A systematic review of randomised controlled trials of the most common interventions. *Spine, 22,* 2128–2156.

Van Tulder, M. W., Koes, B. W., Metsemakers, J. F. M., & Bouter, L. M. (1998) Chronic low back pain in primary care: A prospective study on the management and course. *Family Practice, 15,* 126–132.

Von Korff, M. (1999). Pain management in primary care: An individualized stepped-care approach. In R. J. Gatchel & D. C. Turk (Eds.), *Psychosocial factors in pain* (pp. 360–373). New York: Guilford Press.

Von Korff, M., Barlow, W., Cherkin, D., & Deyo, R. A. (1994). Effects of practice style in managing back pain. *Annals of Internal Medicine, 121,* 187–195.

Von Korff, M., Deyo, R. A., Cherkin, D., & Barlow, W. (1993). Back pain in primary care: Outcomes at one year. *Spine, 18,* 855–862.

Von Korff, M., Gruman, J., Schaefer, J., Curry, S. J., & Wagner, E. H. (1997). Collaborative management of chronic illness. *Annals of Internal Medicine, 127,* 1097–1102.

Von Korff, M., & Moore, J. (2001). Stepped care for back pain: Activating approaches for primary care. *Annals of Internal Medicine, 134*(Suppl. 9, Pt. 2), 911–917.

Von Korff, M., Moore, J. E., Lorig, K., Cherkin, D. C., Saunders, K., Gonzalez, V. M., Laurent, D., Rutter, C., & Comite, F. (1998). A randomized trial of a lay person-led self-management group intervention for back pain patients in primary care. *Spine, 23,* 2608–2615.

Von Korff, M., Ormel, J., Keefe, F. J., & Dworkin, S. F. (1992). Grading the severity of chronic pain. *Pain, 50,* 133–49.

Von Korff, M., & Saunders, K. (1996). The course of back pain in primary care. *Spine, 21,* 2833–2837.

Von Korff, M., Wagner, E. H., Dworkin, S. F., & Saunders, K. (1991). Chronic pain and use of ambulatory health care. *Psychosomatic Medicine, 35,* 61–79.

Waddell, G. (1991). Low back disability: A syndrome of Western civilization. *Neurosurgery Clinics of North America, 2,* 719–738.

Waddell, G. (1992). Biopsychosocial analysis of low back pain. *Baillieres Clinical Rheumatology, 6,* 523–557.

Waddell, G. (1996). Keynote address for primary care forum. Low back pain: A twentieth century health care enigma. *Spine, 21,* 2820–2825.

Waddell, G., Feder, G., & Lewis, M. (1997). Systematic reviews of bed rest and advice to stay active for acute low back pain. *British Journal of General Practice, 47,* 647–652.

Winkler, R., Underwood, P., Fatovich, B., James, R., & Gray, D. (1989). A clinical trial of a self-care approach to the management of chronic headache in general practice. *Social Science Medicine, 29,* 213–9.

15

A Cognitive-Behavioral Approach to the Prevention of Chronic Back Pain

Steven James Linton

Recent research suggests that applying cognitive-behavioral (C-B) techniques in health care settings could be an effective method for preventing the development of disabling chronic back pain. Although this application will certainly not eliminate all the pain, probably will not work for all, and may be difficult to implement properly, it nevertheless seems to represent a breakthrough. This is why. The new application of C-B techniques keys on isolating the right person, at the right time point, as well as providing the proper intervention to meet the patient's "risk profile." Thus, this approach addresses the classic problems of whom to offer an intervention to, when, as well as what the content of the intervention should be. Indeed, fresh results show that these methods may reduce considerably the probability of a patient developing a back-related disability.

This chapter presents an overview of a C-B approach to the prevention of chronic pain. To understand this approach, this chapter first provides a brief background that highlights the reasons that chronic problems develop. Subsequently, the chapter delves into the process of identifying patients at risk for developing long-term dis-

ability. Most important, this chapter presents psychological approaches to intervention in some detail. Insights into administering such an intervention and coordinating it in a health care team emerge. Finally, this chapter examines outcomes to underscore the potential of the approach.

Why Does Acute Pain Become Chronic?

Need for Prevention

The need for prevention is borne out by epidemiological studies that continue to show that back pain is a serious problem resulting in immeasurable suffering, work loss, and high costs (Crombie, Croft, Linton, Le Resche, & Von Korff, 1999). The literature demonstrates considerable suffering, disability, and economic loss for individual sufferers (Linton, 1998). Unfortunately, the problem is prevalent. For example, 15% of the population in the United States suffered from one or more chronic musculoskeletal disorders in 1990, and it is estimated that this number will increase to 18.4% (60 million people) by

2020 (National Research Council, 2001). Indeed, in our own study we found that 66% of 20- to 60-year-olds in the general population reported spinal pain during the past year (Linton, Hellsing, & Halldén, 1998; Linton & Ryberg, 2000). For more than a quarter of these people, the pain was a somber problem that disrupted their life considerably. Consequently, in 1999 more than 1 million Americans were on sick leave from work because of musculoskeletal pain (National Research Council, 2001). Moreover, among disabled workers in the United States between 51 and 60 years old, nearly 90% reported a musculoskeletal disorder as the reason for disability (National Research Council, 2001).

Not surprisingly, musculoskeletal pain results in a considerable number of health care visits. More than 130 million health care encounters were recorded in the United States alone during 1999 (National Research Council, 2001). In fact, the National Ambulatory Medical Care Survey of 1989 placed musculoskeletal disorders as second only to respiratory conditions as the most common reason for seeking health care (National Research Council, 2001). Yet, a relatively small number of sufferers account for a large portion of the costs. Reid, Haugh, Hazard, and Tripathi (1997) have summarized a variety of studies that report that about 5–10% of back pain patients develop a long-term pain problem. These cases, however, consume the majority of the resources (Linton et al., 1998; Reid et al., 1997; Skovron, 1992; Smedley, Inskip, Cooper, & Coggon, 1998; Williams, Feuerstein, Durbin, & Pezzullo, 1998). It is estimated that the cost in the United States was $215 billion in 1995 (National Research Council, 2001). A recent study in the Netherlands, a country of 15 million people, estimated the cost to be $150 million per hour (van Tulder, Koes, & Bouter, 1995)! The numbers are similar in Sweden, where the total cost in 1995 was estimated at 30 billion kronor (about $3 billion) (Nordlund & Waddell, 2000). It is interesting that the division between direct costs (e.g., for treatment) and indirect costs (compensation benefits) is highly skewed, with more than 90% of the expenditures being for indirect costs (Nordlund & Waddell, 2000; van Tulder et al., 1995). Consequent-

ly, there is a clear need for early, preventive interventions.

Role of Psychological Factors

Even though back pain is a multidimensional process, it appears that psychological events are instrumental in the transition from an acute injury to a chronic disability. Indeed, the way we view our pain, the communication we have with loved ones and health care professionals, and the pain relief we receive may all affect the development of the problem. Although we clearly are a long way from fully understanding the process of chronification, psychological factors have nevertheless been reported to be more potent predictors than either biomedical or biomechanical factors (Burton, Battié, & Main, 1999; Linton, 2000c; Turk, 1997). Consequently, a psychological model may help us to understand better why acute back pain sometimes develops into a persistent, disabling problem.

A key to the model is an understanding of the natural history of back pain where recurrent problems are the rule. First, an episode of back pain normally takes about 8 weeks to subside (van den Hoogen, Koes, van Eijk, Bouter, & Devillé, 1998), even though patients may expect it to go away within a few days. Second, back pain is normally recurrent (van den Hoogen, Koes, Devillé, van Eijk, & Bouter, 1997; van den Hoogen et al., 1998; Von Korff, 1994). Thus, once a person has a problem there is great likelihood for a new episode, usually within a year; the average being 8 weeks (van den Hoogen et al., 1998). In the development of a chronic problem, the interval between episodes may gradually become shorter and the length of the episodes longer. During the bouts, people will attempt a variety of ways to cope with the pain and the resultant disability. The intensity of the pain itself may change thoughts and beliefs about the pain.

The recurrent nature of back pain allows ample opportunities for learning. Keeping in mind the large number of people who deal with their back pain effectively, this learning ordinarily seems to be helpful in coping with the problem. However, for some people, coping strategies that seem to work in the short term may enhance the development of a persistent problem in the long term. The process is gradual. Rather than the "straight line" often depicted in the literature, the road to chronic pain is crooked. Some periods with little or no pain is common. With small alterations taking place during episodes of pain, a change in lifestyle may occur. However, because of the gradual nature of the change, the person may not be aware of the process until a major development is already a fact.

The problem may reach a plateau where further development of the problem is subsequently triggered by a critical event. These events seem to be individual. An example might be when a patient attempts to return to work and the supervisor states, "Your back is too weak for this work." This event might be critical in changing the patient's beliefs about his or her back and ability to work ("If my supervisor doesn't believe I can do the job, I must be really bad."). Again, rather than a smooth, linear development, the concept of critical events means that change may occur in small or large increments.

The risk factors associated with the development of persistent pain seem to be individual. Although anxiety and fear–avoidance may be important for one person, monotonous work and a poor relationship with a supervisor may be critical for another. Likewise, the pertinent risk factors may change over time. For example, anxiety and fear may be crucial in the acute stage, while depression and catastrophizing may become more important as the problem becomes unrelenting.

Taken as a whole, learning processes may support pain behaviors so that the problem evolves into a persistent one. The more frequent the problem occurs, the more time psychological factors such as learning have to operate and establish a "sick role" lifestyle. Cognitive processes are involved in a reciprocal process where attributions, pain beliefs, coping, and so on, are linked to the development of long-term disability. Even though some healing may take place, these psychological processes may influence the perception of pain, pain behaviors, and suffering.

Psychological Risk Factors

An examination of psychological risk factors casts light on the model concerning the development of chronic pain and provides an impetus for using such factors for early identification. A vast literature on the relationship between various psychological factors and back pain is available. In a recent review, more than 900 articles were identified (Linton, 2000c). Unfortunately, there have been considerable methodological difficulties in studying psychological processes. These problems include sample composition and size, severity of the pain, inadequate measures of the predictors, time of outcome, outcome criteria, design of the study, possible treatment between assessments, and the use of self-ratings as both the independent and dependent variable (Linton, 2000c; Turk, 1997). Consequently, in light of evidence-based psychology, one approach is to review the best available evidence.

I located 37 studies that employed a prospective design and thus are relevant for determining risk factors for the development of a back pain problem (Linton, 2000b). Only studies with prospective design were employed, to increase the validity of the findings (e.g., compared to cross-sectional studies). In prospective designs, the psychological factors are first measured and then subjects are followed over time and the outcome is subsequently assessed. This method increases the likelihood that the psychological factors are causally related to the outcome. The results are summarized here, but the details of the review are available in the literature (Linton, 2000b, 2000c). Interestingly, 26 studies actually examined the development of a back pain problem by using a new onset or further development of a problem after acute onset. Psychological factors were consistently found to be related to the onset and development of back pain problems. Although these factors only accounted for a certain portion of the variance, they were found to be more important in the development of pain and disability than were most biomedical or biomechanical variables.

Significant risk factors represented cognitive, emotional, and behavioral variables. For example, stress, distress, or anxiety was found to be related to back pain in all the studies investigating it. Moreover, mood and depression were consistently reported to be significant risk factors. Cognitive variables such as beliefs about the pain were related to outcome. In particular, fear–avoidance beliefs were a stable factor having a particularly significant relationship with the development of dysfunction. Behavioral aspects included coping strategies where passive strategies were related to poor outcome. Finally, high levels of pain behavior and dysfunction were a risk factor for future back pain problems. Thus, psychological factors are related to back pain from its inception to the development of a persistent problem, and they seem to be pivotal in the transition from acute to chronic pain.

Interestingly, the psychological risk factors were often relatively good predictors of future back pain problems. For example, Burton, Tillotson, Main, and Hollis (1995) studied over 250 patients seeking care for a new episode of acute back pain and followed them for 1 year. At consultation, patients received a clinical examination and an interview and they competed a battery of questionnaires said to measure pain, disability, distress, pain beliefs, fear–avoidance and coping strategies. At the follow-up, outcome was determined with regard to disability. Results of multivariate analyses indicated that the psychological variables were by far the most potent predictors, accounting for 69% of the variance. As an example, it was found that catastrophizing was seven times better as a predictor of outcome than the best clinical or historical variable. As there are several other studies indicating that psychological variables are related to outcome, I believe that these variables might be valuable for screening purposes. Although the data show that prediction is far from 100% accurate, employing such factors in a risk assessment might substantially increase precision.

Other reviews of the literature draw similar conclusions. Weiser and Cedraschi (1992) conducted a systematic review. They concluded that psychological distress, depression, anxiety, and stress are potent risk factors while coping and illness beliefs were related to recovery. In a review specifically examining the role of psychological factors in the development of persistent pain, Turk (1997) found that psychosocial factors were better predictors of chronicity than are clinical or physical factors. Important variables were pain severity, distress, anxiety, substance abuse, depression, stress, coping, and perceived health.

Psychosocial workplace factors have also been associated with the development of persistent back pain. Bongers, de Winter, Kompier, and Hildebrandt (1993) found that a lack of social support and low control were related to back pain. Hoogendoorn, van Poppel, Bongers, Koes, and Bouter (2000) found strong evidence that social support at work and job satisfaction are risk factors, whereas there was insufficient evidence for work pace, perceived demands, content, and job control. Likewise, I found that psychological workplace factors were linked to back pain (Linton, 2001); however, it was not possible to establish the relationship to the transition from acute to chronic. Indeed, the American National Research Council (2001) acknowledged in its report that several work-related psychosocial factors were associated with musculoskeletal disorders.

Conclusions

Although methodological problems restrict the conclusions that may be drawn from the literature, the findings are surprisingly consistent. The methodological problems include selection bias, inappropriate comparison groups or designs, inappropriate use of tests, intercorrelation of measures, and overinterpretation of correlational data (Linton, 2000b; Turk, 1997). Additional work is necessary to understand when, how, and why these factors operate. Nevertheless, there is surprising consistency in the results reported. Several reviews come to a similar conclusion: Psychological factors are clearly related to back pain, especially the transition from acute to chronic pain.

The development of chronic pain is a complex, multidimensional process in which psychological factors play an important role in enhancing or catalyzing the development of the problem. The evidence and theories available do not suggest that back pain is psychogenic. Rather, once an injury occurs, psychological factors may influence the course of development. Usually this is advantageous. The person copes adequately and recovers. However, sometimes the process results in further development of the problem. Thus, psychological factors interplay with other types of variables but are comparatively powerful in predicting outcome.

Consequently, psychological factors might be used in prevention in two critical ways. First, because psychological factors are predictors of future problems, they might be used for early identification of patients at risk for developing persistent pain and dysfunction. Indeed, these factors might serve to screen patients. Second, the content of early preventive interventions might be tailored after the psychological factors identified. To date, most preventive interventions have been based on biomedical or biomechanical theories. A logical approach would be to provide an intervention that addresses the psychological elements identified as important determinants of development.

Early Identification

As a large number of people seek care for back pain but only a minority develops a persistent problem, early identification would render the advantage of being able to concentrate limited resources on those most in need. Without a doubt, identifying the right person at the right point in time is a major challenge. In this section I focus on identifying patients who may risk developing long-term dysfunction because of their back pain. The aim is to identify the right person at the right time point.

Right Person

RED AND YELLOW FLAGS

Although this chapter focuses on psychological techniques, such techniques are in practice used in conjunction with those of other professionals. To aid in applying this knowledge to clinical settings, the idea of red and yellow flags has been introduced (Kendall, Linton, & Main, 1997). The concept of "red flags" denotes the relatively rare, but serious, diseases that need to be addressed in a medical examination (Kendall et al., 1997). These "red flags" include, for example, signs and symptoms related to fractures, tumors, neurological damage, and infections. "Yellow flags," on the other hand, refer to psychosocial factors that may hinder recovery. "Yellow flags" may assist clinicians in screening patients and deter-

mining the risk for developing long-term problems.

Screening refers to a first, gross evaluation. It is not a final product but, rather, the start of a clinical process. Patients determined to potentially be at risk for developing problems will need further attention to assess them properly. Consequently, screening allows clinician to focus their time on further assessing only those individuals who are at risk for developing further problems. The additional assessment may or may not show a need for early intervention. However, for those who do show a need, the next step is to address the problems isolated in the screening assessment. Consequently, screening is the first step in early preventive health care–based interventions.

Translating risk factors into an effective screening procedure is not a straightforward process. In fact, we found that primary care physicians and physical therapists did not believe that they could predict accurately which patients would develop chronic problems (Linton, Vlaeyen, & Ostelo, 2002). This may well be because doctors and physical therapists are best aquainted with the biomedical variables that unfortunately are not as salient predictors as are psychological factors. Moreover, given the time pressure in most primary care settings, clinicians may be at a loss about which factors to ask. Finally, health care providers may be concerned about how to bring up such "sensitive" issues as yellow flags.

Fortunately, there are questionnaires available to assist in assessing "yellow flags." For example, Main and colleagues (Main & Watson, 1995; Main, Wood, Hollis, Spanswick, & Waddell, 1992) developed an instrument based on a measures of depression and distress (DRAM) and showed that it helped identified patients seeking orthopedic care who were at risk of a poor outcome. In an exciting development that entails a method for use in primary care settings, Gatchel, Polatin, and Kinney (1995) employed the Minnesota Multiphasic Personality Inventory (MMPI), questionnaires, and a clinical diagnostic interview to assess patients seeking care for acute back pain. Scores on several psychological factors correctly classified 87% of the patients' work status 6 months later (see Gatchel & Dersh, Chapter 2, this volume). The Vermont

Screening Questionnaire (Hazard, Haugh, Reid, Preble, & MacDonald, 1996) consists of only 11 items but is designed as an aid for predicting future compensation among people filing an injury report. They showed that the instrument was a good predictor with 94% sensitivity and 84% specificity. However, the study only covered those filing an injury claim and suffered from a substantial dropout and refusal rate.

SCREENING PROCEDURE

Based on the evidence and experience from our clinic, a procedure for the clinical screening of patients in health care settings is presented. We developed the Örebro Musculoskeletal Pain Screening Questionnaire (OMPSQ) to aid clinicians in primary care in evaluating "yellow flags" (Linton,

1999; Linton & Halldén, 1998). Table 15.1 contains the 25 items that assess various psychosocial risk factors. These items range from the experience of the pain itself to its consequences. The questionnaire is self-administered and takes, on average, about 7 minutes to complete. Thus, it is may be completed while the patient waits to see a physician. Patients make their ratings on 0–10-point scales. Except for the first four background items that are not included in the scoring, all questions are weighted equally. With a little experience, scoring and reviewing the questionnaire takes clinicians as little as 2–3 minutes. Thus, a total score may be calculated. Likewise, the individual items may be viewed to scrutinize the patient's unique profile.

Research indicates that the questionnaire may be a helpful tool. First, it has been

TABLE 15.1. An Overview of the Items in the Örebro Musculoskeletal Pain Screening Questionnaire

Question	Variable name
1. What year were you born?	Age
2. Are you male or female?	Gender
3. Were you born in Sweden?	Nationality
4. What is your current employment status?	Employed
5. Where do you have pain?	Pain site
6. How many days of work have you missed (sick leave) because of pain during the past 12 months?	Sick leave
7. How long have you had your current pain problem?	Duration
8. Is your work heavy or monotonous?	Heavy work
9. How would you rate the pain you have had during the past week?	Current pain
10. In the past 3 months, on the average, how intense was your pain?	Average pain
11. How often would you say that you have experienced pain episodes, on the average, during the past 3 months?	Frequency
12. Based on all the things you do to cope or deal with your pain on an average day, how much are you able to decrease it?	Coping
13. How tense or anxious have you felt in the past week?	Stress
14. How much have you been bothered by feeling depressed in the past week?	Depression
15. In your view, how large is the risk that your current pain may become persistent?	Risk chronic
16. In your estimation, what are the chances that you will be able to work in 6 months?	Chance working
17. If you take into consideration your work routines, management, salary, promotion possibilities, and workmates, how satisfied are you with your job?	Job satisfaction
18. Physical activity makes my pain worse.	Belief: increase
19. An increase in pain is an indication that I should stop what I am doing until the pain decreases.	Belief: stop
20. I should not do my normal work with my present pain.	Belief: not work
21. I can do light work for an hour.	Light work
22. I can walk for an hour.	Walk
23. I can do ordinary household chores.	Household work
24. I can do the weekly shopping.	Shopping
25. I can sleep at night.	Sleep

found to have adequate test–retest reliability (Linton, 1999). Second, it has predictive validity. In a first evaluation with 137 consecutive primary care patients with acute spinal pain, we found that the items were all related to future pain, function, or sick leave (Linton & Halldén, 1997, 1998). Discriminant analyses showed, moreover, that five items were particularly related to future sick leave. These were (1) the belief that one should not work with current pain levels, (2) the perceived chance of working in 6 months, (3) functional problems when doing light work, (4) stress, and (5) the previous number of sick disability leave days. A total score analysis indicated a sensitivity (correctly identified those on sick leave at follow-up) of 87% and a specificity (correctly identified those as healthy, i.e., not on sick leave, at follow-up) of 75% for *three* classes of sick leave outcome, whereas chance would be 33%.

From the distribution of scores, we determined cutoff points for this population. We found that a score of 105 or above represented high risk, 90 to 105 medium risk, and under 90 low risk. However, this is a simple rule of thumb. The cutoff point is highly influenced by the population at hand as well as the goal of the screening. At times, for instance, it may be important to identify all patients who will develop a problem—even at the expense of a relatively large number of false positives. In other situations, one may only wish to identify those "certain" of developing the problem and false negatives would be accepted.

Some replications suggest that the OMPSQ may work in other situations. A study conducted in New Zealand (Kendall, personal communication, December 10, 2000) on a population of more than 100 acute pain patients showed that the 105 cutoff score was related to future disability. Hurley and colleagues (2000) also examined the predictive validity of the questionnaire in 118 patients presenting at physical therapy departments. The outcome employed was return to work. They found a sensitivity of .80. Although the 105 cutoff worked well, they also found that 112 was the optimal cutoff score for this population and purpose. Finally, Ekter-Andersen, Ørbaek, Ingvarsson, and Kullendoorf (2000) applied the questionnaire to people out of work for

back pain reported to the National Insurance Authority in Sweden. They found that the questionnaire predicted future disability. Not surprisingly, given that the population under study is already on sick leave, the cutoff score was higher. These studies suggest that the questionnaire has good predictive validity. The cutoff point is sensitive to the population and the goals of the screening assessment, but the original values listed previously may serve as a rule of thumb.

Although the total score provides a rough estimate of risk, the specific items provide insight into the patient's personal risk profile. This may be the most important use of the OMPSQ. Having established that there may be a risk of future problems, attention then turns to what factors are enhancing this process? The individual items may provide insight into which areas should be investigated in further assessment or treatment.

To make the evaluation, responses may be scanned with an eye for extreme answers. In addition, an overall picture of the problem should emerge when combining the information from the various questions. It also provides a lead-in to discuss sensitive issues. For example, one may ask: "I note on item 14 that you have been feeling depressed during the past week. Could you tell me more about this?" Examining combinations of items often generates questions for the patient. For example, high scores on the fear–avoidance items might be interpreted differently if the patient has acute and intense pain. Although the total score provides a prediction of future disability, the individual items help identify important areas that may be related to the problem.

Next, providing the patient with feedback presents an opportunity for learning and developing a "shared understanding" of the problem. I recommend that patients be provided with positive feedback for those behaviors that are normal or outstanding (e.g., coping well with the pain, being active despite the pain, and having an enjoyable job). Further, the results from the OMPSQ may be combined with the other examinations to provide a well-rounded result. Including the yellow flags lets the patient know that these are important and legitimate issues to be dealt with. However, it is important to provide the information in a concrete way. This is why I avoid discussing the results in terms of "risk" as patients many times do not fully understand the scientific concept and it does not relate to what the patient will need to do. Instead, the relevance of the results may be underscored, follow-up questions posed, and the bearing of the results on treatment explored. At best, the instrument provides an opportunity for an overall assessment and will guide the clinician in further assessment and treatment.

Clinicians often wonder at what time point screening should take place as well as if every patient should be included. At this point there is no scientific basis for answering the question. Some would argue that as many patients get better with few complications, the screening procedure might be saved for those seeking a second visit. Others may feel that it is important to include this information from the start as most patients have had some previous pain problems. To establish a sound routine, one option is to include the screening procedure for all spinal pain cases from the start. Thus, no patient is missed and a firm routine is established. However, the screening procedure has much less value for those already having a chronic problem as compared to those with acute or subacute pain. As chronic sufferers make up about 25% of the visits for spinal pain (van den Hoogen et al., 1998) in primary care, this number should be kept in mind.

A final question is, Who should administer the screening procedure? This is a question of professionalism. The questionnaire is fashioned for self-administration but needs to be dealt with properly to work. Skill is involved in presenting the questionnaire to the patient, scoring, and above all interpreting the scores. The subsequent interaction with the patient is crucial and involves the aforementioned skills plus communication skills. Consequently, although a variety of health care practitioners may certainly administer, score, and interpret the results, training is needed. Moreover, I suggest that the instrument be used in a team situation in which a behavioral psychologist may be consulted for training and questions. The psychologist will not need to meet every patient but should be useful in maintaining quality in the process as well as being a consultant for difficult patients. By using a

screening procedure, the "right person" may be identified who is in need of a preventive intervention.

Right Time Point

To prevent long-term disability, the intervention needs to be initiated at an early time point, but when is the best time? One line of thought has been to "wait out" the natural course of the problem. According to this idea, as most people recover from their back pain within a few weeks, early interventions should focus on those whose problem persists after 6 to 8 weeks (Frank et al., 1996). Indeed there is evidence that early, multidimensional rehabilitation produces significant improvements for this group (Frank et al., 1996; Morley, Eccleston, & Williams, 1999; Turk, 1996; van Tulder et al., 2000; Waddell, 1998). Another view has been to intervene before the problem arises for true primary prevention. These range from adjusting the workplace to teaching people how to best avoid or cope with their back. However, the research to date shows that interventions aimed at nonpatient populations (e.g., a workforce or the general population) have had little success (Linton & van Tulder, 2001). Indeed, our review found that people without a pain problem may not be motivated to participate, as compliance is often quite low. Worse, for some people, focusing on possible back problems may exacerbate the problem. Finally, providing help for all people, even those with no problem at all, would be resource intensive.

A health care visit for spinal pain appears to represent an ideal time point for initiating a program of early identification and preventive intervention. First, although most people will "recover" from their current epiosode of pain, there is no innate reason for waiting until the problem persists several weeks before beginning. This is particularly true because back pain tends to be recurrent in nature. Second, limiting the process to those who seek medical help will, in itself, greatly reduce the number of people in need of the service. Because most people will at some time have back pain, screening people at workplaces or in the general public, or offering all with back pain an intervention, would be costly and labor intensive. Therefore, restricting the program to those seeking health care services may be a good way of optimizing the program. Third, as medical care has been sought for the problem, the patient has indicated an interest for participating in an intervention. This would seem to enhance the potential for adherence.

The foregoing screening procedure also provides an opportunity for assessing the patient's interest in an early intervention oriented toward preventing future problems. Thus, rather than simply "referring" patients to an early intervention, patients may be asked about their interest in participating in such a treatment. Finally, incorporating preventive interventions into primary health care appears to be necessary in light of mounting evidence that these techniques are also effective in the treatment of acute and subacute problems. As a result, until further research is available, there are numerous advantages to employing a visit to a health care provider as an opportune time point for initiating an early identification and intervention program.

Early Interventions: "Proper Content"

Once the right person has been identified at the right time point, the next step is to provide a proper intervention, but the content of such an intervention has been a matter of debate. In this section I explore new psychological approaches that may be used as a complement to other types of care. These interventions are meant to address the psychological factors known to be operational in the transition from acute to chronic pain.

Perhaps the most important reason early, preventive interventions fail is because they do not address the factors associated with the development of a chronic problem. The evidence presented thus far in this chapter suggests that psychological factors are key ingredients in the transition from an acute to a chronic pain problem. Consequently, a significant part of the treatment might be psychological in nature. Yet, most preventive interventions are based on other theories of why the pain becomes persistent or are dictated by convenience, which is not surprising given the fact that health care facilities are biologically oriented. Moreover, relieving the pain has traditionally been the main goal of

treatment, not preventing long-term problems such as disability. Finally, psychological techniques that might be adapted for use in early intervention programs have not been available. Regardless of the reasons, there has been a dire need for attempts to directly address even the psychological aspects of preventing a chronic pain problem.

Fortunately, a number of attempts have recently been reported where psychological methods have been tested in primary care settings with the aim of preventing long-term pain and disability. One of the first reports of an application was by Fordyce, Brockway, Bergman, and Spengler (1986). As the operant model of chronic pain has isolated low activity levels, and overuse of medications as central parts of the problem (Fordyce, 1976), the early intervention focused on preventing these. Doctors learned to provide patients with specific advice about activities focusing on what patients should do and being specific about any limitations. In addition, doctors were taught to limit sick leave and restrict prescription medications to a limited number (if needed at all) taken on a time rather than pain contingency. The results of this randomized controlled study indicated that disability levels 1 year later were lower in the experimental group. Thus, the study shows that the way clinicians deal with patients can have a significant effect on outcome. In addition, it supports the idea that prevention is possible by addressing some behavioral aspects such as medications and activities.

Indeed, the communication with the patient at the first visit appears to be vital. Waddell, Feder, and Lewis (1997), for example, reviewed the literature on providing advice for back pain patients. They found that advice for bed rest was counterproductive, whereas advice to remain active despite the pain produced a significantly better long-term result with regard to pain and disability. Consequently, the content and manner in which patients are cared for may offer an opportunity for prevention.

Von Korff and colleagues (1998) presented one of the first interventions designed to help patients deal specifically with psychological aspects of the problem in the hope of preventing future problem. The intervention was based on lay-led groups for arthritic pain and focused on self-care (Von Korff,

1999). Trained lay leaders assisted participants in a well-organized four-session program including problem-solving skills, activity management, and educational videos. An evaluation was conducted on 255 patients about 8 weeks after a primary care visit for back pain and participants were randomized to the cognitive-behavioral group or a control group. At the 1-year follow-up the cognitive-behavioral group had significantly reduced worry and disability relative to the treatment-as-usual control. Participants in the lay-led group also had a significantly more positive view toward self-care, but there was no significant difference with regard to pain intensity or medication use. Similar results have been reported in two other reports using similar methods (Moore, Von Korff, Cherkin, Saunders, & Lorig, 2000; Saunders, Von Korff, Pruitt, & Moore, 1999; see Pruitt & Von Korff, Chapter 14, this volume).

In our own research we have elaborated a six-session program for participants that enables them to derive their own coping program designed to prevent future back pain-related problems. Participants met in groups of 6 to 10 people for 2 hours once a week for 6 weeks. The therapy followed a written manual, and the therapists were trained behavior therapists. Each session contained a review of homework, a short presentation of educational material, problem solving, the presentation of new skills, and final homework assignments. The end product for participants was a personalized coping program.

To test the utility of our approach, we compared it to treatment as usual in a randomized controlled trial (Linton & Andersson, 2000). Participants suffered acute or subacute pain, perceived that they had a risk of developing a chronic problem, but had not been out of work more than 3 months during the past year. Two hundred and forty-three people fulfilling the criteria were randomly assigned to one of three groups. The first group received a previously evaluated pamphlet that provided straightforward advice about the best ways to cope with back pain. It emphasized remaining active and thinking positively. The second group also received information, but more traditional in nature as well as more substantial in quantity. This information was based on a back school approach and was delivered in six packages. It also included the latest information available from the authorities on back pain. The third group received the C-B group intervention described earlier (see also Turk, Chapter 7, this volume). All three groups had usual access to health care facilities.

Results at the 1-year follow-up indicated a significant preventive effect. Although the comparison groups reported benefits, the risk for a long-term sick absence was ninefold lower for the C-B intervention group relative to the groups receiving information (see Figure 15.1). The group intervention also produced a significant decrease in perceived risk, as well as significantly fewer physician and physical therapy visits compared to the comparison groups. All three groups improved on the variables of pain, fear–avoidance, and pain-related cognitions. Thus, long-term disability and health care use was "prevented" in the C-B group.

A second test was conducted to study the effects of the group intervention on a group of nonpatients from the general population (Linton & Ryberg, 2001). Participants reported four or more episodes of relatively intense spinal pain during the past year but had not been out of work more than 30 days. Two hundred and fifty-three volunteers were randomly assigned to the C-B group intervention or a treatment as usual comparison group. The experimental group received the standardized program described previously. Both groups had usual access to health care facilities. At the 1-year follow-up, results showed that the C-B group, relative to the comparison group, had significantly better outcomes on fear–avoidance, number of pain-free days, and amount of sick leave. The risk for long-term sick leave during the follow-up was three times lower in the C-B group as contrasted with the treatment as usual comparison group. Consequently, it was concluded that despite the well-known strong natural recovery rate, the C-B intervention produced a significant preventive effect on back pain disability.

Content of Cognitive-Behavioral
Preventive Intervention

In the course of research, a manual has been produced that describes the content and

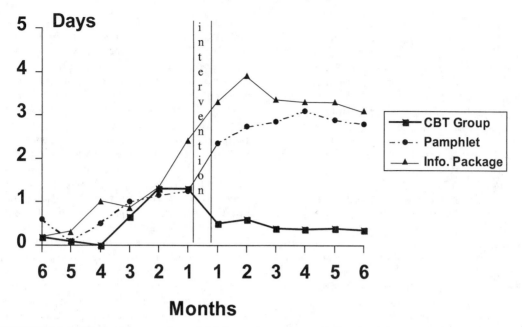

FIGURE 15.1. The average number of sick leave days per month for the three groups during the last 6 months of baseline and the follow-up. Note that the two groups receiving usual care plus information have a significantly higher level of sick leave. From Linton and Ryberg (2001). Copyright 2001 by the International Association for the Study of Pain. Reprinted by permission.

course of the C-B preventive intervention (Linton, 2000a). A summary of the main points is provided here. The goal of the course is for participants to develop their own individualized coping program.

Participants should enjoy coming to the sessions. To ensure this enjoyment, each person should have the opportunity to learn new information or skills, develop insight by discussing the application of the information, and be able to practice relevant skills under supervision. In addition, sessions should provide for emotional support, social interaction, and humor. The therapist then must ensure that all participants are active and that a friendly, productive atmosphere is achieved where people are at ease within the group. Consequently, a good deal of planning and work go into making the course valuable to every participant. The description of the outline for sessions provides more detail as to how this is achieved.

Administering these groups requires several skills, which is why our clinic has employed behavioral therapists who have good knowledge and some experience using such

techniques. For example, to form successful groups, the therapist needs to selectively reinforce positive participation. Creating a positive atmosphere to a considerable extent depends on the therapist's ability to promote constructive discussion that allows every participant to talk and develop his or her own skills. Humor is used as one method of reducing anxiety and increasing interest. In fact, our clinic has developed cartoons and short stories that may produce laughter at the same time that they illustrate an important point. However, the humor is always directed toward a neutral person (or the therapist), but never at a member of the group. We also teach and encourage members to reinforce each other's behavior. Besides developing a positive atmosphere, the therapist needs to be fluent in pain psychology and C-B techniques.

Each session shares a general format. To achieve the goals of learning new information and skills and obtaining emotional release and social support, the sessions are structured. First, the introduction provides a welcome and sets the tone for the session. Here, homework assignments are reviewed in a "no-fault" atmosphere and trouble-shooting is used to help improve application and fine-tune skills. *Every* participant summarizes his or her homework.

Second, a *short* lecture is provided to introduce the topic for the session. In addition to facts, the lecture will help people to relate the topic matter to their own situation. Although most therapists are tempted to expand on this section, it is vital that it judiciously be restricted to a maximum of 15 minutes.

Problem solving is the third part of the session. A short, written case study is given to each member. Pairs are formed to solve problems associated with the case study and these are directly related to the theme of the session. The purpose of the case study is to provide a concrete but neutral third person for discussion purposes. Problem solving is designed to enhance the skill as well as to integrate the information and skills into the participant's own life. The pairs are given approximately 15 minutes to solve the problems.

The fourth part of the session includes skills training. New skills are presented as potential elements of the coping program members are developing. The therapist describes the skill and its possible application. It is then demonstrated. Step-by-step instructions are given and group members learn how to do the skill. To create an optimal coping program, participants are asked to learn each skill and implement it in a behavioral trial during the week. However, the

final decision as to whether the skill will be included is up to the participant.

The session is rounded off with a homework assignment and an evaluation of the session. To evaluate whether a specific skill is useful, participants are asked to use the skill during the coming week. Examples of homework are provided, but the actual assignments are individualized. To maximize the enjoyment, we present homework as the "weekly adventure" whose main purpose is to get an accurate feel for which techniques may work for the individual participants. Finally, feedback is obtained in a formal summary of the day. Each person is asked to briefly state what he or she has learned and what positive and negative aspects of the session he or she has experienced.

Each session focuses on a particular problem area, and Table 15.2 provides an overview. The first session deals with the causes of back pain and how it might be prevented from becoming a chronic, disabling problem. The role of structural and soft tissue injuries in relation to activity is stressed. In particular, the difference between "hurt" and "harm" is brought out in the lecture. Further, the consequences of pain are described as well as the fact that some will develop persistent problems. A model is presented that underscores gradual lifestyle changes and mentions the role of work, family, and psychological factors. Thus it becomes clear that prevention is a worthwhile endeavor. The problem solving focuses on why the individual in the case study

TABLE 15.2. An Overview of the Content of the CBT Intervention

Session	Focus	Skills
1	Causes of pain and the prevention of chronic problems	Problem solving, applied relaxation, learning about pain
2	Managing your pain	Activities, maintaining daily routines, scheduling activities, relaxation training
3	Promoting good health, controlling stress at home and at work	Warning signals, cognitive appraisal, beliefs
4	Adapting for leisure and work	Communication skills, assertiveness, risk situations, applying relaxation
5	Controlling flare-ups	Plan for coping with flare-up, coping skills review, applied relaxation
6	Maintaining and improving results	Risk analysis, plan for adherence

Note. From Linton and Ryberg (2001). Copyright 2001 by the International Association for the Study of Pain. Reprinted by permission.

developed chronic pain and what he or she could have done to prevent it. The skills for the session are problem solving and pain control, including cognitive and applied relaxation skills.

The subsequent sessions deal with activities, self-care, work, and leisure. The sessions share basic aspects. First, participant's beliefs are challenged through the problem-solving case study and in discussion. Second, alternate ways of thinking (e.g., self-statements) and behavioral skills are taught as possible ways of coping better. Third, the new C-B skill is tested in real life through homework assignments. In this way a wide variety of common beliefs and behaviors may be dealt with in a group format.

The task of planning a coping program begins in session five. In addition, the session includes planning for eventual flare-ups. Consequently, a focus is on application of the skills over time. Participants work on developing their coping program with a special section on dealing with a flare-up. The final session is used to fine-tune the coping program and deal with long-term maintenance. We discuss adherence to the program from a self-help point of view where conscious decision is underscored.

In session six, the final coping plan is reviewed and the focus turns to maintaining the plan over time. Rather than prodding participants a self-determination approach is used. As participants have chosen the content of their coping package, they are also given charge of maintenance. Work centers on making planned changes only in the program. Thus, if an element of the program does not seem to be working, it could be eliminated. Likewise, in some situations, such as flare-ups, more coping strategies may be needed and thus could be added to the program. However, having a part of the program inadvertently disappear is not good, as it would not be a conscious choice. As a result, a key is to periodically make a progress check. To enhance this process, participants book progress checks into their calendar. This check only takes a few minutes and basically is a review of how well the program is working. It concludes with a decision as to whether the program should be changed in any way or continued as is. Again, the rule is planned changes only. To assist in identifying factors that may be beneficial or a hindrance to doing the coping program as planned, participants also complete an adherence roadmap (Keefe, Beaupré, & Gil, 1996). Participants liken their future to a car trip in which one destination is relapse and the other success. Thus, they try to identify "the road" to each of these destinations. The identified factors may then be employed in developing the maintenance plan for the coping program.

A follow-up session may be scheduled. Some groups also may chose to meet on their own periodically.

Potential Problems

Although the system described here for "the right person, at the right time point, with the correct intervention" offers many seeming advantages, there are also potential problems. Indeed, the methods reviewed here are recent, and considerable research is needed to develop and assess their effectiveness. Perhaps the most frequent problem is that the system in a sense goes against the grain of the medical model and is therefore difficult for staff to administer without training. Training should not be underestimated as it takes time and effort to understand why the methods should work as well as to hone the skills. Consequently, it is advantageous to work in teams in primary care (e.g., with a doctor, physical therapist, and psychologist). In this way, efforts may be coordinated and training may be incorporated into clinical practice.

Related to training is the problem of inadvertently reinforcing "sick behavior." By focusing on screening and early intervention, personnel might actually reinforce concern and inappropriate behaviors. If this happens, the overall results would be worse than treatment as usual. Thus, it is important to practice interactions with patients in training settings to ensure that the program is administered properly.

Another potential difficulty is the logistics of delivering the program in health care settings such as primary care. Many such units do not have psychologists and the amount of time afforded each patient is quite limited. The procedure in this chapter is designed to fit into routines for providing these patients medical care. In part the problem may involve "beliefs" concerning the psychological nature of the programs. Certainly, a new medical treatment procedure that relieved back pain would be incorporated even if some costs and time were involved in administering it. Yet, planning is necessary as proper administration does take time. It should be kept in mind, however, that most patients seeking primary health care facilities are not "at risk." Thus, only a minority of the patients will have screening profiles that dictate more consideration. And, of those with a "risk" profile, only a limited number will be candidates for an early intervention. Consequently, the time and resources needed for the program are limited.

The potential for incorrectly classifying the risk of patients may generate concern. Indeed, the screening procedure is relatively crude and both false negatives and false positives will undoubtedly be generated. Although the goal of future research is to reduce the number of these, such "errors" are present in virtually all tests, including biological ones. Fortunately, the consequences of such a mistake should not be particularly large. First, if a false negative is identified and the problem does not remit, the patient will seek additional care, which should trigger a warning flag to reassess the situation. Some time is lost, but there should still be ample opportunity to deal with prevention. Certainly, applying the program may be an improvement on the current situation in which patients may not be identified until the problem *is* chronic. Second, if a false positive is identified and early intervention is given to someone who would have recovered anyway, the prevention may still be of some value. Because back pain is recurrent, the person may in fact nevertheless have been on his or her way to developing a persistent problem even if the current episode would have resolved. Moreover, the intervention suggested in this chapter focuses on coping skills that presumably are of value even if the problem is not dire. Finally, by adjusting the cutoff level, the number of "misses" may be adjusted. Thus, although we need to improve accuracy, the consequences of mistakes do not seem to be large. One scenario is that extra costs are incurred by providing the intervention to someone not truly in need of it.

A final potential problem is the coordination of the program between different professionals. Indeed, doctors, nurses, physical therapists, psychologists, and other health care professionals may be involved. Again, this is why working in a team may have advantages. The team may initiate the program with special training that identifies roles for each member and teaches skills. Periodic meetings allow for monitoring and adjusting the program. They also provide an opportunity for continuing education in that special cases may be brought up for discussion.

Although the program described here is based on the latest scientific reports, more research is needed to determine the effects as well as to improve on them. To date, the screening procedure appears to improve considerably upon clinical guessing, but yet it is rather crude. Future work should improve on accuracy. Moreover, to date we have little scientific knowledge to help us determine the best time point for an early intervention. Few studies have directly addressed this question and thus attention needs to be turned to this issue. Finally, the C-B programs thus far have involved a "package" of techniques. More data are needed to determine efficacy in various settings. In addition, the content, length, and administration of these programs might be improved by turning the spotlight on such aspects. Taken together, then, there is a true need for continued research to shed light on procedures for the early identification and intervention to prevent chronic pain and disability.

Recapitulation

Spinal pain continues to be a prevalent problem that too often develops into persistent pain and disability. The demand for prevention, however, has not yet been adequately fulfilled. Recent developments suggest that a key to successful prevention is identifying the right person, at the right time point, and then offering an appropriate intervention. Models of the evolution of chronic pain as well as contemporary research underscore the importance of psychological factors in the transition from acute to chronic pain. Screening procedures have consequently employed these factors to help identify patients at risk for developing long-term problems early on. There are tools to assist in identifying the right person. The research is not conclusive concerning the right time point. Given the dismal results of preventive programs for nonpatients and the problem of getting people without a true pain problem to participate in prevention programs, a primary care setting would appear to be a good point at which to intervene. Patients may be motivated to participate and the health care setting offers a convenient organization from which to administer the program.

Because psychological factors enhance the evolvement of a persistent problem, it is logical that psychological methods might be an appropriate preventive intervention. C-B group interventions have shown promise in randomized, controlled studies. Basically these groups focus on assisting participants to develop their coping and self-help skills to better deal with the problem. They appear to have their biggest effect on function and may help prevent disability. More work is needed to develop and assess this system and in particular the intervention. However, the data at this point suggest that such early, preventive programs might hinder the development of persistent pain and disability for an untold number of people.

References

Bongers, P. M., de Winter, C. R., Kompier, M. A., & Hildebrandt, V. H. (1993). Psychosocial factors at work and musculoskeletal disease. *Scandinavian Journal of Work and Environmental Health, 19*, 297–312.

Burton, A. K., Battié, M. C., & Main, C. J. (1999). The relative importance of biomechanical and psychosocial factors in low back injuries. In W. Karwowski & W. Marras (Eds.), *The occupational ergonomics handbook* (pp. 1127–1138). Boca Raton, FL: CRC Press.

Burton, A. K., Tillotson, K. M., Main, C. J., & Hollis, S. (1995). Psychosocial predictors of outcome in acute and subchronic low back trouble. *Spine, 20*, 722–728.

Crombie, I. K., Croft, P. R., Linton, S. J., Le Resche, L., & Von Korff, M. (1999). *Epidemiology of pain* (Vol. I). Seattle, WA: IASP Press.

Ektor-Andersen, J., Ørbaek, P., Ingvarsson, E., & Kullendoorf, M. (2000). *Yellow flags screening for psychosocial factors related to musculoskeletal pain.* Unpublished report, Department of Social Medicine, Lund University.

Fordyce, W. E. (1976). *Behavioral methods for chronic pain and illness.* St. Louis, MO: Mosby.

Fordyce, W. E., Brockway, J. A., Bergman, J. A., & Spengler, D. (1986). Acute back pain: A control-group comparison of behavioral vs traditional managment methods. *Journal of Behavioral medicine, 9*, 127–140.

Frank, J. W., Brooker, A. S., DeMaio, S. E., Kerr, M. S., Maetzel, A., Shannon, H. S., Sullivan, T. J., Norman, R. W., & Wells, R. P. (1996). Disability resulting from occupational low back pain: Part II: What do we know about secondary prevention? A review of the scientific evidence on prevention after disability begins. *Spine, 21*, 2918–2929.

Gatchel, R. J., Polatin, P. B., & Kinney, R. K. (1995). Predicting outcome of chronic back pain using clinical predictors of psychopathology: A prospective analysis. *Health Psychology, 14*, 415–420.

Hazard, R. G., Haugh, L. D., Reid, S., Preble, J. B., & MacDonald, L. (1996). Early prediction of chronic disability after occupational low back injury. *Spine, 21*, 945–951.

Hoogendoorn, W. E., van Poppel, M. N. M., Bongers, P. M., Koes, B. W., & Bouter, L. M. (2000). Systematic review of psychosocial factors at work and in the personal situation as risk factors for back pain. *Spine, 25*, 2114–2125.

Hurley, D., Dusoir, T., McDonough, S., Moore, A., Linton, S. J., & Baxter, G. (2000). Biopsychosocial screening questionnaire for patients with low back pain: Preliminary report of utility in physiotherapy practice in Northern Ireland. *Clinical Journal of Pain, 16*, 214–228.

Keefe, F. J., Beaupré, P. M., & Gil, K. M. (1996). Group therapy for patients with chronic pain. In R. J. Gatchel & D. C. Turk (Eds.), *Psychological approaches to pain management: A practitioner's handbook* (pp. 259–282). New York: Guilford Press.

Kendall, N. A. S., Linton, S. J., & Main, C. J. (1997). *Guide to assessing psychosocial yellow flags in acute low back pain: Risk factors for long-term disability and work loss.* Wellington, New Zealand: Accident Rehabilitation & Compensation Insurance Corporation of New Zealand and the National Health Committee.

Linton, S. J. (1998). The socioeconomic impact of chronic pain. Is anyone benefitting? *Pain, 75*, 163–168.

Linton, S. J. (1999). *Manual for the Örebro Musculoskeletal Pain Screening Questionnaire: The early identification of patients at risk for chronic pain.* Örebro, Sweden: Author.

Linton, S. J. (2000a). *Cognitive-behavioral therapy in the early treatment and prevention of chronic pain: A therapist's manual for groups.* Örebro, Sweden: Author.

Linton, S. J. (2000b). Psychologic risk factors for neck and back pain. In A. Nachemsom & E. Jonsson (Eds.), *Neck and back pain: The scientific evidence of causes, diagnosis, and treatment* (pp. 57–78). Philadelphia: Lippincott Williams & Wilkins.

Linton, S. J. (2000c). A review of psychological risk factors in back and neck pain. *Spine, 25,* 1148–1156.

Linton, S. J. (2001). Occupational psychological factors increase the risk for back pain: A systematic review. *Journal of Occupational Rehabilitation, 11,* 53–66.

Linton, S. J., & Andersson, T. (2000). Can chronic disability be prevented? A randomized trial of a cognitive-behavior intervention and two forms of information for patients with spinal pain. *Spine, 25,* 2825–2831.

Linton, S. J., & Halldén, K. (1997). Risk factors and the natural course of acute and recurrent musculoskeletal pain: Developing a screening instrument. In T. S. Jensen, J. A. Turner, & Z. Wiesenfeld-Hallin (Eds.), *Proceedings of the 8th World Congress on Pain: Progress in pain research and management* (Vol. 8, pp. 527–536). Seattle, WA: IASP Press.

Linton, S. J., & Halldén, K. (1998). Can we screen for problematic back pain? A screening questionnaire for predicting outcome in acute and subacute back pain. *Clinical Journal of Pain, 14,* 209–215.

Linton, S. J., Hellsing, A. L., & Halldén, K. (1998). A population based study of spinal pain among 35 to 45 year olds: Prevalence, sick leave, and health-care utilization. *Spine, 23,* 1457–1463.

Linton, S. J., & Ryberg, M. (2000). Do epidemiological results replicate? The prevalence and health-economic consequences of back and neck pain in the general public. *European Journal of Pain, 4,* 1–8.

Linton, S. J., & Ryberg, M. (2001). A cognitive-behavioral group intervention as prevention for persistent neck and back pain in a non-patient population: A randomized controlled trial. *Pain, 90,* 83–90.

Linton, S. J., & van Tulder, M. W. (2001). Preventive interventions for back and neck pain: What is the evidence? *Spine, 26,* 778–787.

Linton, S. J., Vlaeyen, J. W. S., & Ostelo, R. (2002). *The back pain beliefs of general practitioners and physical therapists. Are professionals fear-avoidant?* Manuscript submitted for publication.

Main, C. J., & Watson, P. J. (1995). Screening for patients at risk of developing chronic incapacity. *Journal of Occupational Rehabilitation, 5,* 207–217.

Main, C. J., Wood, P. L. R., Hollis, S., Spanswick, C. C., & Waddell, G. (1992). The distress and risk assessment method: A simple patient classification to identify distress and evaluate the risk of poor outcome. *Spine, 17,* 42–52.

Moore, J. E., Von Korff, M., Cherkin, D., Saunders, K., & Lorig, K. (2000). A randomized trial of a cognitive-behavioral program for enhancing back pain self care in a primary care setting. *Pain, 88,* 145–153.

Morley, S., Eccleston, C., & Williams, A. (1999). Systematic review and meta-analysis of randomised controlled trials of cognitive behaviour therapy and behaviour therapy for chronic pain in adults, excluding headache. *Pain, 80,* 1–13.

National Research Council. (2001). *Musculoskeletal disorders and the workplace.* Washington, DC: National Academy Press.

Nordlund, A. I., & Waddell, G. (2000). Cost of back pain in some OECD countries. In A. Nachemson & E. Jonsson (Eds.), *Neck and back pain: The scientific evidence of causes, diagnosis, and treatment* (Vol. I, pp. 421–425). Philadelphia: Lippincott Williams & Wilkins.

Reid, S., Haugh, L. D., Hazard, R. G., & Tripathi, M. (1997). Occupational low back pain: Recovery curves and factors associated with disability. *Journal of Occupational Rehabiliation, 7,* 1–14.

Saunders, K. W, Von Korff, M., Pruitt, S. D., & Moore, J. E. (1999). Prediction of physician visits and prescription medicine use for back pain. *Pain, 83,* 369–377.

Skovron, M. L. (1992). Epidemiology of low back pain. *Baillière's Clinical Rheumatology, 6,* 559–573.

Smedley, J., Inskip, H., Cooper, C., & Coggon, D. (1998). Natural history of low back pain: A longitudinal study in nurses. *Spine, 23,* 2422–2426.

Turk, D. C. (1996). Efficacy of multidisciplinary pain centers in the treatment of chronic pain. In M. J. M. Cohen & J. N. Campbell (Eds.), *Pain treatment centers at a crossroads: A practical and conceptual reappraisal* (Vol. 7, pp. 257–273). Seattle, WA: IASP Press.

Turk, D. C. (1997). The role of demographic and psychosocial factors in transition from acute to chronic pain. In T. S. Jensen, J. A. Turner, & Z. Wiesenfeld-Hallin (Eds.), *Proceedings of the 8th World Congress on Pain: Progress in pain research and management* (Vol. 8, pp. 185–213). Seattle, WA: IASP Press.

van den Hoogen, H. J. M., Koes, B. W., Devillé, W., van Eijk, J. T. M., & Bouter, L. M. (1997). The prognosis of low back pain in general practice. *Spine, 22,* 1515–1521.

van den Hoogen, H. J. M., Koes, B. W., van Eijk, T. M., Bouter, L. M., & Devillé, W. (1998). On the course of low back pain in general practice: A one year follow up study. *Annals of Rheumatic Diseases, 57,* 13–19.

van Tulder, M. W., Koes, B. W., & Bouter, L. M. (1995). A cost-of-illness study of back pain in The Netherlands. *Pain, 62,* 233–240.

van Tulder, M. W., Ostelo, R., Vlaeyen, J. W. S., Linton, S. J., Morely, S. J., & Assendelft, W. J. J. (2000). Behavioral treatment for chronic low back pain: A systematic review within the framework of the Cochrane Back Review Group. *Spine, 25,* 2688–2699.

Von Korff, M. (1999). Pain management in primary care: An individualized stepped/care approach. In R. J. Gatchel & D. C. Turk (Eds.), *Psychosocial factors in pain* (pp. 360–373). New York: Guilford Press.

Von Korff, M., Moore, J. E., Lorig, K., Cherkin, D. C., Saunders, K., González, V. M., Laurent, D.,

Rutter, C., & Comite, F. (1998). A randomized trial of a lay-led self-management group intervention for back pain patients in primary care. *Spine, 23,* 2608–2615.

Von Korff, M. (1994). Perspectives on management of back pain in primary care. In G. F. Gebhar, D. L. Hammond, & T. S. Jensen (Eds.), *Proceedings of the 7th World Congress on Pain: Progress in pain research and management* (Vol. 2, pp. 97–110). Seattle, WA: IASP Press.

Waddell, G. (1998). *The back pain revolution.* Edinburgh: Churchill Livingstone.

Waddell, G., Feder, G., & Lewis, M. (1997). Systematic reviews of bed rest and advice to stay active for acute low back pain. *British Journal of General Practice, 47,* 647–652.

Weiser, S., & Cedraschi, C. (1992). Psychosocial issues in the prevention of chronic low back pain— a literature review. *Baillière's Clinical Rheumatology, 6,* 657–684.

Williams, D. A., Feuerstein, M., Durbin, D., & Pezzullo, J. (1998). Health care and indemnity costs across the natural history of disability in occupational low back pain. *Spine, 23,* 2329–2336.

16

Preparing Patients for Implantable Technologies

Daniel M. Doleys

Preparing the patient for preimplant trialing and/or implantation of a drug administration system (DAS) or spinal cord stimulator (SCS) for the treatment of chronic pain should be considered part of, or at least an extension of, the evaluation process. Ideally, the process should include an involved family member or support person as well as the patient. Recent studies in fact have documented a lower level of estimated benefit by significant others compared to the patient (Doleys, Coleton, & Tutak, 1998; Willis & Doleys, 1999). A detailed discussion of the psychological evaluation of the chronic pain patient is beyond the scope of this chapter but can be found elsewhere (Doleys, 2000; Doleys & Doherty, 2000; Doleys & Olson, 1997). However, some issues are particularly relevant, if not unique, to the psychologist's role in evaluating and preparing the patient and warrant comment.

The psychologist should clarify his or her relationship to the implanting physician with the patient. For example, the preparation process may be more prolonged and detailed if the psychologist is the "referring doctor" regarding implantation versus functioning as a consultant. If the role is that of a consultant, as it often is, the psychologist

should reveal the relationship with the referring physician (employer, interdisciplinary team member, independent practitioner, etc.). Noting the absence of any financial relationship with the referring physician or manufacturer of the implantation device encourages the patient to accept the evaluation and preparation as more objective.

Disclosure of one's experience and the goals of the evaluation and preparation should be undertaken. In some instances, the psychologist may be asked simply to evaluate the patient without regard to any proposed procedures. Other objective(s) of the referral may include (1) "clearing" the patient for implantation, (2) evaluation and education and preparation of the patient, (3) evaluation and treatment if necessary, and (4) evaluation and provision of a treatment algorithm.

A pretrial psychological evaluation is *not* required by all insurance companies. For example, it is mandated by Medicare for SCS but not DAS. Some commercial insurance companies may require it but others do not. Workers' compensation insurance companies often reimburse for a psychological evaluation but are most interested in the potential impact of SCS or DAS on return to work and future expenses. Historically, only about 20% of patients not working prior to implantation do so after. I have encountered cases in which an insurance company required the evaluation but would not provide reimbursement for it. Thus, the financial burden fell on the patient.

Once involved in the evaluation and preparation process, especially if rendering an "accept or reject" decision, the psychologist is subject to medical–legal exposure. I was involved in reviewing a case in which the patient, claiming failure and injury related to implantation of a device, sued not only all those involved in the medical procedure but the psychologist as well. The patient claimed that the psychologist should have known that he (the patient) was not a good candidate for a successful outcome and should have rejected him to begin with. This suit occured even though the patient appeared to be enthusiastically seeking the implant at the time of evaluation.

Consideration must be given to how the evaluation material will be used. That is, will it be protected as confidential with only a summary sent; will a detailed report be sent to the implanter and therefore become part of the patient's medical chart; will the results of the evaluation and any decision be revealed to the patient by the psychologist or referring physician? Limitations regarding confidentiality and informed consent issues should be reviewed early on. The psychologist must be aware of any tendency to "advocate" for the referral source, procedure, or patient. One must guard against tendencies toward theoretical, procedural, and/or disciplinary narcissism.

The psychologist must be able not only to recognize the presence of psychological factors (Doleys, Klapow, & Hammer, 1997) but to identify their functioning as mediators, modulators, or maintainers of the chronic pain (Doleys, 2000) and therefore their potential relevance to long-term outcome(s). Furthermore, there may be times, such as severe complex regional pain syndrome I (CRPS I), peripheral vascular disease, and cancer, at which the severity of the physiological symptoms will take precedence over the psychological factors (Rush, Polatin, & Gatchel, 2000).

The impact of psychological factors and therefore the role of the psychologist is not and should not be limited to the pretrial period and the outcome of testing. Figure 16.1 illustrates a variety of occasions on which psychological factors and the psychologist can play a role in the trialing, implantation, and maintenance process. Importantly, although frequently considered "reversible," the preimplantation trial, implantation, and management of SCS or DAS should not be approached with impunity by either the psychologist or the physician.

Preparing the Psychologist

Proper preparation and education of the patient and support people can only occur if the psychologist is well informed. The psychologist should have a fundamental understanding of the basic SCS and DAS technology and therapy. Recent issues of *Neuromodulation* ("Intrathecal therapy," 1999) and the *Journal of Pain and Symptom Management* ("Current status," 1997; and "Polyanalgesic consensus," 2000) have been devoted to these topics. Reviewing the manufacturer material on various types of devices, including totally implantable versus external and such topics as battery life, is basic. Ideally, the psychologist will have an opportunity to attend a workshop or training course relating to implantation technology or be present in the surgical suite to observe the procedure(s)—not that it is the psychologist's responsibility to detail the surgical procedure, but his or her credibility is enhanced by having some "firsthand" experience.

A fundamental understanding of various electrode combinations and types (Barolat, 1998; Barolat et al., 2001; Krames, 2000) as well as the more commonly accepted pharmacological preparations used in the DAS (Hassenbusch & Portenoy, 2000) will equip the psychologist to introduce these topics and encourage the concerned patient to review the details with his or her implanter. Such basis information as the importance of concordant paresthesias (Barolat, Massoro, He, Zeme, & Ketcik, 1993) and hypothesized mechanisms of action in the utilization of SCS should be in the psychologist's repertoire. Most device manufacturers provide a variety of videotapes and pamphlets that can be used to enhance the psychologist's understanding as well as to educate the patient.

PRETRIAL SELECTION

Psychological testing

MMPI, MPI, Oswestry McGill, etc.

Psychological variables (depression, anxiety, reinforcement contingencies, social support)

Role of variables in pain perception management (i.e., cooperation, compliance)

Patient/significant other education

Pretrial treatment

One to one; group

Attribution/expectations

Trial structure

Prolonged; medication adjustment (monitored)

Accept/reject/accept with reservation

Outcomes

Expectations; management issues; baseline measures

TRIAL

Variables to monitor

Pain, function, medication intake, psychological, perception, affective, somatic, cognitive, etc.

Measurements

NRS, VAS, McGill, Beck, Oswestry, MPI, etc.

Adjunctive treatment

Relaxation, individual, medication

Implant versus not

Withdraw catheter/lead; immediate implant; delayed implant

POSTIMPLANT

Adjunctive therapy

Cognitive-behavioral (individual, group); rehabilitation

Outcome measures

When, what; failure versus success

Guidelines for "adjustments"

Patient management

Flare-ups, decreased effect, "side effects," "troubleshooting" (family, behavior, person variables, contingency change)

FIGURE 16.1. This figure presents the various times during the pretrial selection, preimplant trial, and postimplant management that various behavioral psychological issues, assessments, and therapies can be used. MMPI, Minnesota Multiphasic Personality Inventory; MPI, Multidimensional Pain Inventory; NRS, Numerical Rating Scale; VAS, Visual Analog Scale.

The clinician should have at least a passing familiarity with the published literature regarding outcomes (Anderson & Burchiel, 1999; Brown, Klapow, Doleys, Lowery, & Tutak, 1999; Krames, 1999a, 199b; Paice, Penn, & Shott, 1996). Individual implanters' success rates may differ and should be acknowledged, but if a contentious situation arises it is likely to be the published results that will be referred to. "Side effects" and complications vary considerably from implanter to implanter (Maron & Loeser, 1996; Naumann, Erdine, Koulousakis, Van-Buyten, & Schuchard, 1999; Turner, Loeser, & Bell, 1995). An understanding of both the potential positive and negative factors associated with long-term SCS and DAS therapy will help in educating the patient. In the presence of such education and knowledge, the patient is most likely to be less alarmed when correctable situations arise.

Taking advantage of available opportunities to see the patient during the preimplant trial, posttrial, and after implant can provide valuable information useful in the preparation of subsequent patients. In much the same way as there is a hypothesized "learning curve" for novice implanters, so too will the psychologist's skills be enhanced by experience. Many idiosyncrasies and subtleties will be encountered that are not described in the more scientifically oriented published literature. This practical experience will help to ensure that the psychologist does not approach this process with indifference or naivete.

It is generally ill advised for the psychologist to focus solely on the psychological assessment of the patient without a basic understanding of the contribution that the pain pattern and suspected etiology play in determining whether implantation should be considered and which of the two devices may be most appropriate. In general, pain can be divided into mechanical, neuropathic, and nociceptive types. Mechanical pain is exacerbated by physical actions of the body such as increased back pain with bending or twisting in the presence of spondylolisthesis. Neuropathic pain is characterized by allodynia, hyperalgesia, and possible alterations in temperature sensitivity, to name a few. Nociceptive pain is that which arises from somatic structures, including bony and soft tissue. Some have considered visceral pain such as intersticial cystitis and pancreatitis as a separate category. In most cases, patients will have pain of mixed etiology. It is common to find a postsurgical patient with a combination of neuropathic pain from a radiculopathy, mechanical pain as a result of structural abnormalities or instability, and soft tissue pain such as myofascial pain.

Historically, though the lines are becoming more blurred, SCS therapy has been the choice in treating neuropathic pain in the extremity such as found in a radiculopathy, causalgia, or CRPS-I (formerly reflex sympathetic dystrophy, RSD). The application of DAS was favored in the setting of a more generalized or axial pain considered to be predominantly nociceptive versus neuropathic as might be identified in arthritis, degenerative disc disease, and the like. Although still considered experimental in some settings, SCS therapy has found favor in disorders such as angina, peripheral vascular disease, and pelvic pain, to name a few. The accumulated experience with various infused substances, including opioids, anesthetics, calcium channel blockers, and alpha–2 blockers (Hassenbusch & Portenoy, 2000), has presented new avenues for the application of the DAS.

A basic understanding of the foregoing would help the psychologist to communicate more effectively and thoroughly with the patient and family. Assessment of the patient's comprehension of his or her particular problem, the potential benefit to be derived from the implantation technology, and the type of technology most suitable would be enhanced. The degree to which this information is provided by the prospective implanter versus a psychologist requires clarification. Nonetheless, it is clearly better to give too much information than too little. The importance of consistent information cannot be overemphasized, thus highlighting the necessity of clear communication between the psychologist and the prospective implanter.

In summary, the psychologist must be familiar not only with psychological testing and its interpretation but how such outcomes relate to a fundamental understanding of the patient's complaints of pain, the available therapies, and the potential impact of using DAS or SCS. One of the most common complaints I have encountered has been from patients reporting, after the fact, that they were either inadequately informed or misinformed of the process and had they had more detailed information they might have chosen a different direction or had a better outcome. A significant part of patient satisfaction seems to be associated with creating expectations that, as much as possible, parallel the subsequent experience. The psychologist's unique contribution in this regard is developing an understanding of the patient's personality and psychological status and appreciating those situations in which information may need to be provided in a more detailed and perhaps repetitive fashion.

Multifactorial Nature of Pain: Patient's Role in Treatment

Patients referred for evaluation and preparation for implant technology may be medically oriented. It is crucial that they receive instructions regarding a basic understanding of pain, especially chronic pain. Brief instruction as to the biological, psychological, and sociological aspects of pain can be helpful. Helping patients to comprehend the various components of the pain experience, including sensory–discriminative, cognitive, and affective aspects, may help to "demedicalize" their approach and encourage an appreciation of the importance of a multifactorial approach to their problem. Some patients view such information as tantamount to diagnosing pain as being "all in their head." This misconception should be corrected. In some instances this defensive protestation may mask a deceptive strategy on the part of the patient to manipulate the psychologist and prospective implanter into overlooking possible "secondary gain" issues. Importantly, one should recognize that it is much easier to get a patient to accept implantation technology than to relinquish the device once it is implanted. The percentage of patients considered to have a poor or unsatisfactory long-term outcome cannot be explained by frequency of technical failure or device complication as poor patient selection, preparation and management are more probable causes (Dahm, Nitescu, Appelgren, & Curelaru, 1998; Krames, 1996; Krames & Olson, 1997; North, Kidd, Zahurak, James, & Long, 1993).

Patients and occasionally implanters, intentionally or unintentionally, view the SCS or DAS as the primary if not sole approach to pain control. Educating the patient regarding the role of psychological and behavioral factors may empower them and foster an appreciation for the impact they can have on the outcome. I have occasionally used the treatment of diabetes as an example. I point out the importance, if not necessity, of proper diet, weight control, and exercise for maximum benefit rather than having the diabetic patient rely solely on the prescribed insulin. Encouraging pain patients to take an "active" role in their therapy is needed to avoid an overreliance on the implanted device. A brief discussion of other pain control strategies such as distraction, relaxation, self-hypnosis, pacing, and cognitive-behavioral therapy is appropriate. The degree to which the patient rejects this notion may clue the psychologist and physician to the presence of a potentially demanding and dependent individual.

Psychological Evaluation

A comprehensive psychological/behavioral evaluation of the patient can be demanding, especially when one is being considered for implantation (Doleys, 2000; Doleys & Doherty, 2000; Doleys & Olson, 1997; Krames & Olson, 1997). Particularly relevant to the topic at hand is identifying those patients who will require more individualized preparation because of their tendencies toward histrionics, somatic preoccupation, compulsiveness, and worry. In much the same way as the classroom teacher must deliver educational material in a fashion most suitable to a patient's learning style, taking into account learning deficits such as dyslexia or attention deficit, so too should the psychologist be aware of personality and behavioral tendencies that necessitate a specific educational style.

It appears that many of the patients we encounter function at approximately the sixth-grade level despite their actual level of education. Oftentimes this means patients may hear only a fraction of what is actually said and understand only a fraction of what they hear in a medically oriented discussion. Patients often nod in apparent acknowledgement out of confusion and fear of asking questions. Assuming there is some basis in fact, it highlights the importance of acquiring feedback from the patient and family as to their level of comprehension of what is about to take place and appropriate expectations. For the foregoing reasons it may be prudent to use a combination of written material, audiotapes, videotapes, and follow-up visit(s).

For many implanters, especially those with extensive surgical experience, the implantation of an SCS or DAS is a relatively simple matter. Patients are frequently informed that compared to other procedures such as their laminectomy or fusion, implant surgery is a rather "minor" procedure. This type of forecasting, unfortunately, does not take into account individual patient differences in regard to their perception of any surgery. The more anxious, somatic, and "histrionic" patient is likely to find any procedure to be a "major" one. Having witnessed this in clinical practice, I have frequently encouraged patients to review the manufacturer-prepared videotape on the surgical procedure.

This use of the videotape demonstrating the implant procedure has met with mixed responses from patients and referring implanters alike. Some implanters have expressed a desire that viewing not be done, believing that it is too frightening to patients and will deter them from the procedure. Indeed, this view is partly true. Several patients after reviewing the tape requested postponement of the trial in lieu of considering alternative approaches. It takes little imagination to hypothesize what response such patients might have had if they had proceeded at that point in time to trialing and implant. It is important to be mindful that the technology continues to improve with time. There may be cases in which time is of the essence, but in many situations postponing the trial and implant until the patient is properly prepared and motivated can pay dividends.

The foregoing speaks to a specific issue, that is, whether patient selection and trialing of a device are focused primarily on avoiding "false positives," namely, the implantation of a patient who is thought to be acceptable but ultimately has a poor outcome, or "false negative," the nonimplantation of a patient who may have had a positive outcome. By virtue of the "reversibility" of these procedures and technology, the threshold for trialing and implantation is often set low. As often as not, patients may be approved for a trial not because they evidence features thought to be associated with a positive outcome (see Table 16.1) but rather because they have failed certain other procedures and the pain practitioner may have little else to offer them. In this regard it is important to note that a "positive response" to a preimplant trial while appearing necessary for a positive outcome is not in and of itself sufficient to predict a positive outcome (Nitescu, Dahm, Appelgren, & Curelaru, 1998).

Informing patients that there are no other options and that they are destined for a life of unmanageable pain if they do not consider an SCS or DAS may predispose many patients to a feeling of desperation and heighten the possibility of a profound short-term "placebo" response. This may be one possible explanation as to why a significant percentage of patients, as much as 50% in some SCS reports, no longer report adequate analgesia or continued use of their SCS within 1–2 years following implantation (Barolat, Ketcik, & He, 1998; North et al., 1993; Turner et al., 1995). Likewise, it may help to account for the rapid acceleration and frequent adjustments in opioid dosing following implantation of the DAS despite the fact of a significant analgetic response being reported during the preimplant trial period (Doleys, Coleton, & Tutak, 1998; Willis & Doleys, 1999).

Behavioral Report

The psychological report can address issues regarding the pain pattern, suspected pathology, and psychological status of the

TABLE 16.1. Hypothesized Behavioral/Psychological Indicators for Appropriateness to Undergo Implantable Technology Trial

1. Generally stable psychologically
2. Cautious
3. Effectively defensive
4. Moderate levels of self-confidence and self-efficacy
5. Realistic concern regarding "illness" and proposed therapy
6. Mild depression appropriate to the situation
7. Generally optimistic regarding outcome
8. Ability to cope with flare-ups, complications, and side effects appropriately
9. Appropriately educated regarding procedure and device
10. Supportive and educated family/support person
11. History of compliance and cooperativeness with previous treatment
12. Behavior and complaints consistent with identifiable pathology
13. Behavioral/psychological evaluation consistent with patient's complaints and reported psychosocial status
14. Comprehends instruction(s) and other information
15. Patient/significant other have appropriate expectation(s)
16. Patient able/willing to "tolerate" electrical stimulation/paresthesia with SCS and medication adjustments with DAS

patient. Potential "red flags" and psychological factors relevant to the preimplant trial, postimplant management, and long-term outcomes should be noted. In some instances, preimplant trial therapy (i.e., one or more sessions of cognitive-behavioral therapy) to assist in patient preparation may be appropriate.

Table 16.2 identifies six areas that can be reviewed in the psychological evaluation and report. Obtaining information on these points will help to direct the preparation of the patient. In some cases, for example, the patient may be identified as a potential candidate for consideration of implant technology if other psychological issues (e.g., depression) are addressed and stabilized. The patient, family member, and physician must be informed and educated as to the potential negative impact of certain psychological states on the patient's responsiveness to and acceptance of implantable technology. Patients who are determined to be extremely

TABLE 16.2. General Areas to Be Assessed during the Psychological Evaluation

- Any untreated or undertreated major affective disorder
- Axis II (personality/character) disorder: effects of such disorder on the perception of pain, compliance, cooperation, etc.
- Any untreated or undertreated alcohol or drug problems, present or past
- Expectations/attributions regarding pain and proposed therapy
- Nonphysical factors: their contribution to the patient's pain perception and behavior
- Type and degree of social support

sensitive to, and focused on, internal sensations, as might be the case in highly somatic or "hypochondriacal" patients, may, for example, have difficulty dealing with a SCS as it produces an ongoing paresthesias. Similarly, patients that may be predisposed to somatic delusions (e.g., schizoid personalities or schizophrenics) and may require additional treatment prior to considering a trial period.

There has been a tendency in the past to categorically deny certain types of patients as being appropriate candidates. In fact, Nelson, Kennington, and Novy (1996) have identified a variety of "exclusion" factors. It is important to recognize that these factors are based on theory and experience with other types of therapies and not necessarily the outgrowth of controlled experimental or clinical studies involving implantable devices. Some patients can be helped by psychological or pharmacological intervention to become better candidates. It is my belief that "successes are created not just discovered."

An example of the foregoing is a 48-year-old patient who was seen for comprehensive pain rehabilitation therapy following a crush injury to the right foot. In the process of therapy it was discovered that the patient had been "hearing voices" since the age of 15 and attributed his chronic problems with marijuana, which led to recent imprisonment, to that voice. The patient did evidence a pain pattern and pathology considered quite suitable for SCS therapy. The degree of relief that could be obtained through behavioral, psychological, and pharmacological therapy was realized but he remained symptomatic. The addition of Zyprexa (olanzapine) produced remarkable alteration in his hallucinations. He subsequently went on to an adequate SCS trial and implant. Upon first examination he would have been thought, and rightly so, to be a poor candidate by virtue of his history of drug abuse, criminal record, and auditory hallucinations. Proper preparation of the patient resulted in his becoming an acceptable candidate and proceeding to a successful postimplant outcome.

Not all such cases will have a successful outcome. It is believed, however, that it is incumbent upon the psychologists not only to identify those patients most likely to have a positive outcome but to assist those who have the potential to become candidates to achieve such an outcome. Unfortunately, efforts in this area may be thwarted by lack of insurance coverage, patient cooperation, and absence of appropriate social support. In some instances I have encouraged patients and families to advocate their cause to the insurance company, noting that the absence of an appropriate evaluation and preimplant therapy may have a negative impact on the outcome due to no fault of the implanter, the device, or patient. The easiest solution is to reject any questionable patients without concern for their future. However, this may not be the most humane, ethical, or moral approach.

Different psychological profiles and factors may suggest the need to emphasize certain aspects of implantable technology and therapy and can be incorporated into the overall report: depression, for example, if a consequence of pain may spontaneously improve with appropriate implant therapy. Patients with long-standing depression may require intervention and the use of adjunctive antidepressants for the depression prior to implantation. The highly somatic individual may be overly sensitive to physical sensations, such as the SCS paresthesia and the presence of an implanted generator or DAS. Prognosis for degree of pain relief may need to be more conservative in the case of "histrionic" or somatic patients. Those thought to possess obsessive–compulsive tendencies may be at risk to "fiddle with" the equipment. Although rare, cases of patients twirling the DAS system resulting in dislodgement of the catheter have been described anecdotally.

Patients with limited or maladaptive coping skills, as might be identified by a low K scale on Minnesota Multiphasic Personality Inventory (MMPI; Keller & Butcher, 1991) may require aggressive cognitive-behavioral therapy before and after implantation. Elevations on Scale 8 (Schizophrenia) may identify a patient predisposed to misinterpreting or overinterpreting physical sensations. Some patients with "schizophrenic" tendencies may find it difficult to tolerate persistent stimulation. For this reason, a pretrial with a transcutaneous electrical nerve stimulator (TENS) unit as well as a more lengthy preimplantation trial with a temporary lead should be considered. Patients with low Scale 9 (Hypomania) on the MMPI may lack the motivation or desire to improve activity. They may require a more structured functional restoration program and could be more at risk to identify uncontrolled activity-related pain even after implantation as a means to justify a more sedentary lifestyle.

Elevations in Scales 4 (Psychopathic Deviate) and 9 on the MMPI may reflect a difficulty in setting and responding to appropriate limits. Such patients may pose management problems and once implanted may evidence disruptive and manipulative behavior. Elevations in Scales 1, 2, and 3 (Hypochondriasis, Depression, Hysteria, respectively) are fairly common among chronic pain patients (Doleys et al., 1997). They may represent the presence of maladaptive stress or coping strategies as well as the presence of psychologically relevant issues that should be attended to preimplant trial or preimplant. This, of course, is made quite difficult by the enormous variation and in some cases absence of insurance coverage for the necessary and needed psychological therapies. Unfortunately, in such cases, patients and physicians alike feel compelled to pursue implantable technology in an effort to modulate symptoms. It is only after the device has been implanted that the "preexisting" psychological and behavioral abnormalities declared themselves. A poor outcome is then inadvertently associated with the technology rather than the absence of insurance coverage to properly prepare and

manage the patient from a psychological perspective. Patients should be encouraged to address this issue with their insurance company and perhaps local politicians. Attending physicians should consider identifying this oversight as a potential contribution to a less than desirable outcome.

These preexisting or coexisting psychological factors should be viewed as no less relevant than factors such as obesity, diabetes, and hypertension are viewed when planning surgeries for pain or other disorders. Although important, a disproportionate amount of emphasis has been placed on the "predictability" of the positive preimplant trial when in fact such a trial does not, particularly in psychologically distressed and behaviorally disordered patients, necessarily correlate with positive outcome longterm (Nitescu et al., 1998). Likewise, a "normal" MMPI preimplant trial is not always associated with the best outcome (Doleys & Brown, 2001).

Preparation of Patients to Live with Implantable Technologies

Preparation of the patient and family member depends to some degree on the problem being treated and the location of the device. Historically, SCS and DAS have been applied for the treatment of various pain disorders. Early in their history, devices were preferentially implanted with the SCS leads or the DAS catheter tip in the upper lumbar and lower thoracic area. Clinical experience and improved technology has resulted, for better or worse, in positioning of the electrodes or catheter tip further up the spine in the upper thoracic or cervical area. Implications for the patient include the possibility of positional sensitivity (Cammeron, & Alo, 1998; Olin, Kidd, & North, 1998), where turning of the head such that the SCS stimulation may vary from one arm or location in the arm to the other. From a DAS perspective, the closer the catheter to the brain, the more concern there must be for cognitive and other side effects occurring as a result of medication flow to brain structures. The flow of medicine can be influenced by the use of use of more lipophilic (i.e., fat soluble) medications such as fentanyl versus the more hydrophilic (i.e. water soluble) medications such as morphine (Royal, Wiese-meyer, & Gordin, 1998).

Not only are the SCS leads and DAS catheters being located in a broader variety of places, but implantation therapy has found applicability to a larger population. Occipital neuralgia, pelvic pain, interstitial cystitis, and urinary incontinence, though not currently FDA (Food and Drug Admin-istration)-approved indications, are being addressed with increased regularity. Recent-ly, Neuromodulation Society Meetings (March 2001) found preliminary but active discussions on the application of SCS of the vagus nerve for treating tremor, depression, and even obesity. The SCS therapy is being explored for treating intractable angina, is-chemic pain, peripheral vascular disease, and phantom limb pain. The use of the DAS with baclofen for the treatment of spasticity is FDA approved, well established, and ef-fective (Maythaler, Guin, Renfroe, Grabb, & Hadley, 1999). Although information about the technical aspects of the SCS and DAS will be similar, patients and family members may need to be educated as to condition-specific issues.

Expectations and the manner in which the efficacy of the therapy is evaluated will vary. For example, a 68-year-old female with pain of arthritis and failed back surgery will more likely be concerned about a reduction in visual analog or numeric pain ratings whereas the focus for a 38-year-old male with 14 years of formal education suf-fering from a monoradiculopathy following an on the job injury and laminectomy may be assessed regarding improvement in func-tion and return to work. Adequate time, therefore, needs to be devoted to expecta-tions, outcome measures, and what would be considered a "good to excellent" result. Patient satisfaction is more frequently associated with a correlation be-tween expected outcome and actual out-come versus the magnitude of the outcome. That is, patients expecting a 50–60% relief in pain would be satisfied with such and would consider the therapy successful whereas a patient expecting 80–100% relief would be disappointed.

The role of the psychologist in clarifying expectations and outcome measures will vary depending on the relationship with the attending physician and implanter. Within an interdisciplinary model where the team works cooperatively, the psychologist may be well aware of standard expectations and outcomes and be able to communicate and clarify these to the patient and significant others. In other instances in which the psy-chologist functions as a consultant, he or she may need to direct the patient and sig-nificant other to discuss this topic with the attending physician and help to ensure ade-quate understanding and agreement. It may be helpful, especially in the case of a less ed-ucated or elderly patients, to have the goals of therapy specified in writing.

Candidates for implantation technology, especially whose improvement in function-ing is a primary goal, should understand the concepts of "breakthrough" pain and "inci-dent" pain. From my perspective, break-through pain may represent a natural varia-tion in pain intensity that can be dictated by a variety of factors such as the underlying disease process, stress, diurnal pattern, weather changes, and so forth. Efforts should be made to address these factors through nonpharmacological mechanisms such as exercise, modality therapy, relax-ation, hypnosis, cognitive-behavioral thera-py, and the like. Encouraging the use of medications, particularly short-acting opi-oids or benzodiazepines, on a regular or daily basis can be maladaptive. It also en-courages patients to rely on the medical community to address all aspects of their problem rather than assuming some degree of responsibility.

"Incident pain" can be thought of as pain resulting from unusual activity. Incident pain might occur, for example, on holidays or special occasions when the patient is an-ticipating or has exceeded his or her usual activity tolerance and may require some ad-ditional analgesia. My recommendation is to prescribe 10–15 short-acting analgetic tablets per month to provide support to the patient but discourage overreliance on these preparations.

The barriers to increased function even in the presence of reduction in pain are many and varied. Over time, the patient may have found inactivity to be rewarding, as can sometimes be indicated by a low Scale 9 on the MMPI. Fear of reinjury and avoidance of responsibility such as work are other pos-sibilities. Depression, whether preexisting or a consequence of the pain, may have become associated with anhedonia and approach levels of severity requiring separate intervention. Some patients are so deconditioned that efforts to move may be associated with shortness of breath, muscular discomfort, and so on. Finally the absence of any functional or activity related goals may contribute as well.

Maladaptive reinforcement contingencies (e.g., attending to inappropriate pain complaints and behaviors) require discussion. Some family members may have found themselves reinforcing inactivity by providing assistance to pain patients in doing functional activities that they are capable of doing themselves (e.g., bringing food and medication). This in part may explain the tendency for subjective estimates of pain to improve more than those related to increased functioning (Doleys, Coleton, & Tutak, 1998; Willis & Doleys, 1999). Furthermore, spouses appear to view outcomes less favorably than patients because of continued inactivity on the part of the patient (Willis & Doleys, 1999).

It is important to help the patient's family members to realize what psychological issues are not likely to resolve even with improvement in pain and function. Certain types of depression, sexual problems, marital conflict, personality disorders, and addiction issues are but a few that are likely to persist. Not only will the presence of these problems require additional psychological intervention, but if unattended could compromise the short- and long-term efficacy of implantable therapy frustrating patient, physician, and family member alike.

As one can easily imagine, changes in underlying pathology, activity level, and psychological status of the patient will be ongoing and may result in the deterioration of the effect observed during the preimplant trial and immediate postimplant. Patients and family members must appreciate that in the setting of chronic pain, the use of this technology, and many other therapies, is designed to "manage" rather than cure the pain, and that maximum results require a "process" and not just a one-time intervention. This is particularly true with the DAS, where it may take several months to identify the most effective medication, combination medications, and flow rate.

The patient should be introduced to the concepts of conditioned nociception, plasticity, facilitation, and sensitization (Doubell, Mannion, & Woolf, 1999). This is particularly true in the setting of neuropathic pain. In this situation, spinal mechanisms responsible for nociceptive input can undergo continual modification, which can result in an alteration and in some cases exacerbation of the pain experience. These changes may be unrelated to any activity or psychological state of the patient. These changes can provoke a feeling of apprehension or uncertainty. Patients and family members need to be reassured that adjustments can be made in both the SCS and DAS to help to accommodate to these changes. It is equally important that those involved in the care of the patient not become so mesmerized by the implanted "machinery" that they ignore the "mechanism(s)" involved in nociceptive activity. All too often apparent exacerbations are responded to by modifying stimulation parameters or adjusting infused medications rather than a more detailed assessment of potential contributing medical and behavioral/psychological factors.

In the case of the DAS, patients need to be aware that problems relevant to utilization of oral medications, such as pharmacological dependence, tolerance, withdrawal, constipation, and the like, are also present with intraspinal opioids (Doleys, Dinoff, et al., 1998; Naumann et al., 1999; Willis & Doleys, 1999). Some patients, as well as misguided practitioners and other professionals, assume that these problems encountered through other routes of administration can be avoided by intraspinal administration. Patients are often surprised to learn that abrupt cessation of spinally administered opioids will produce withdrawal and that overinfusion can have dramatic consequences as well.

As indicated earlier, some psychological factors may be altered with suppression of pain and improvement in function and others not. Long-standing psychological maladjustment such as catastrophizing (Sullivan et al., 2001) encouraged and maintained by inappropriate reinforcement contingencies are likely to persist. Those factors such as "reactive" depression and reduced activity secondary to pain may improve with better pain control. Research has documented a weak correlation between suppression of pain and automatic improvement in activity (Jamison, Raymond, Sawlsby, Nedeljkovic, & Katz, 1998). Activity increases often have to be specifically "targeted." This may be accomplished by guiding the patient and family regarding relevant reinforcement mechanisms as well as instructions in pacing, goal setting, and so on.

Patients who have been accurately diagnosed as addicts (DuPont, 1997) present a special problem. The appropriateness of opioid therapy in this population remains controversial (Savage, 1999). As addiction is often considered a "brain disease," some would argue that the application of opioids, through whatever route of administration, will reactivate this "disease" and therefore should not be considered. Addiction, however, may exist on many levels in the same fashion as other disease entities such as diabetes and hypertension. The patient with a limited history of substance abuse, such as occasional weekend drinking and experimentation with marijuana, and who has actively participated in recovery and been abstinent and sober for an extended period, may deserve a different level of consideration than that afforded the patient who has been chronically intoxicated with one substance or another for 20 or more years and who never sought or participated actively in a recovery program. In fact, one could argue that the utilization of implantable technology, including DAS, may be a preferable approach to treating the addict with pain as it can eliminate access to oral preparations. Caution must be observed as there have been anecdotal reports of patients or spouses attempting to penetrate the DAS reservoir and catheter in an effort to withdraw the opioid for sale or other use.

Some recent attention has been paid to assessing the level of "readiness" for change. One would assume that any patient with chronic pain would be prepared to undergo changes. This, however, has not been borne out in clinical or research experience. Miller and Rollnick (1991) identified several stages of readiness, including precontemplation, contemplation, determination, action, maintenance, and relapse, which might be applicable to the pain patient. This concept of readiness-for-change has not been applied to interventional therapies, including implantable technology, but would seem intuitively relevant. The readiness-for-change model may help to explain the often observed lack of functional improvement even in the presence of significant pain relief (Jamison et al., 1998; see Jensen, Chapter 4, this volume).

In fact, this model may be applied in two different ways. Theoretically a patient could be in the determination or action phase regarding treatment of his or her pain but may be in the precontemplation or contemplation stage as to the acceptance of implantable technology. The unsuspecting physician, psychologist, and family member may be more ready for the technology than the patient and therefore may exercise undue influence resulting in the patient's submitting to the implant before he or she is prepared. This influence, of course, can have disastrous consequences on the outcome. The patient may be more likely to be attuned to even minor side effects.

Factors Specific to SCS

The patient should be informed of the importance of concordant stimulation of SCS. In general, pain relief will only be felt in the areas in which the patient experiences stimulation. For this reason patients will need to be partially alert during the implantation of the trial electrode. Patients should be encouraged to be specific about where they feel the stimulation and cognizant of the importance of it. In some cases the trial electrode will also be the "permanent" electrode with the power generator attached to it after a successful trial. In other instances the trial electrode may be removed after a successful trial in favor of implanting the more permanent one. The more somatically oriented patient may find this removal somewhat disconcerting. Such patients may have greater concern that the benefits achieved during the preimplant trial will not be replicated if the trial electrode is removed and replaced by the more "permanent" electrode. On occasion the risk of electrode migration and other anatomical and physiological factors may necessitate the implanting of a "surgical lead" that involves a laminotomy for positioning. The uninformed and unsuspecting patient may find this implantation somewhat bothersome.

The overall trialing process varies considerably. Some implanters "trial on the table" and if concordant paresthesia is achieved progress to implant, whereas others conduct a trial of several weeks in duration after which the lead is withdrawn and the patient is given several weeks to consider whether or not to implant. The degree to which activity is encouraged or restricted, in hospital versus outpatient trials and in the management of opioid medications during the preimplant trial, vary from physician to physician. These variations should be discussed and clarified.

"Positional sensitivity" can occur (Cameron & Alo, 1998; Olin et al., 1998). This sensitivity occurs when, by virtue of certain mechanical movements, the electrode position relative to the nerve pathways is altered. When closer, the patient may experience increased stimulation that although not harmful may, if unexpected, be a cause for concern. Some devices require a radio frequency coupling (RF unit). A battery-driven power source not unlike that found with a TENS unit is worn on the person. A circular-type wand is positioned over an implanted receiver and often held in place by tape or some type of elastic wrap. Other devices are totally implantable. The determination as to the most suitable device is frequently based on voltage requirements and physician and patient preference. The totally implantable SCSs are, at this point, powered by a battery. The battery life is limited and therefore the power generator will require replacement. Thus, the patient must be aware that depending on the parameters of stimulation and everyday use, the generator may require replacement every 3–5 years, though it is not necessary to change the electrodes. Electrode migration can occur. Properly implanted, minor migration can be compensated for by reprogramming. In other instances the electrode must be repositioned.

SCS, contrary to DAS, has the advantage of patient control. The patient should be advised of this and have an opportunity to be aware of where the generator will be implanted (i.e., abdomen vs. hip), and to ensure that he or she can successfully maneuver the handheld programmer over the device and manipulate the parameters. It is often helpful to encourage the patient to appreciate SCS as similar to a "pacemaker." That is, although it may activate metal-detecting devices that identify the presence of an implantable device, proper medical identification material is provided. In some instances unique electromagnetic fields may inadvertently activate the SCS, but this is rare.

Concerns have been voiced regarding the suitability of certain diagnostic procedures such as magnetic resonance imaging with implantable SCS. The issue remains unresolved, though at this time magnetic resonance imaging is not recommended. This fact may impact patient acceptance.

Some patients are quite concerned about appearance. In general, the profile of the SCS device is such that it is not detectable under normal clothing. Some manufacturers have recommended that patients not operate vehicles with the SCS on. Many patients, of course, drive without incidence. This topic requires discussion as part of the preparation process rather than after the fact.

General independence from the medical system, programmability, and patient control are unique and positive features of the SCS versus the DAS. Side effects and complications commonly associated with infusing opioids and other pharmacological agents are, of course, avoided.

Factors Specific to DAS

The author and others prefer to refer to the DAS as a drug administration system rather than a "pump." The latter term is somewhat pejorative and fails to accurately describe the device. The DAS allows for the installation of various medicines (currently morphine for pain and baclofen for spasticity are the only FDA-approved preparations) into the epidural or intrathecal space. The patient should be encouraged to be aware that it has no "curative" value but represents an efficient mechanism for administration of medicines. In general, DAS has been considered useful in the presence of an "opioid responsive" pain, where the expense of delivering opioids through other routes of administration is excessive, where the magnitude of opioid required is such that it produces untoward side effects, or wherein the underlying pathology (i.e., neuropathic pain) may be responsive to preparations that are uniquely effective when administered intraspinally and in combination with other medications such as anesthetics like bupivocaine or alpha blockers such as clonidine.

Some DAS (e.g., Medtronic Syncromed) can be programmed to deliver medicine on a variety of schedules. Other systems are considered "constant flow" and cannot be programmed. In either case the flow rate may be variable and influenced by such parameters as heat, atmospheric pressure, and amount of solution present. The patient, therefore, will have to have regular refills and is dependent on the medical system. Catheters may become kinked or dislodged, causing abrupt alteration in the infused opioid and perhaps the presence of withdrawal syndrome.

The mechanism of preimplant trialing is implanter specific and highly variable. Follett and Doleys (2002) have summarized a number of the variables to be considered. Included among these variables are the management of pretrialing oral opioids, inpatient versus outpatient, use of bolus or continuous medicines during the trial, duration of the trial, and use of epidural versus intrathecal catheter. Each combination of variables has its own proponent. In general, Follett and Doleys favor a trial that mimics the final outcome as much as possible.

These devices are generally quite robust and durable. The programmable battery-operated DAS will require replacement approximately every 5–7 years or so. The constant-flow type may withstand hundreds or thousands of refills before replacement. If opioids are infused spinally, consideration must be given to their impact on hormonal functions (Doleys, Dinoff, et al., 1998). The profile of the DAS, particularly the programmable units, can be considerably larger than the SCS and therefore more readily detectable. Patients should have the opportunity to view a sample of the device. Skillful implantation of the catheter and DAS by an experienced physician is associated with a substantially lower frequency of system-related complications such as catheter kinking and dislodgement. Some such events are inevitable and most often easily remedied.

Some of the foregoing issues are more relevant for the noncancer pain population than those who, by virtue of their cancer, have limited life expectancy. Above all, patients should be encouraged to view both the SCS and DAS as a "means to an end" rather than an end in and of itself.

Each device possesses its own unique side effects and complication profile as illustrated earlier (Schuchard, Lanning, North, Reig, & Krames, 1998). The patient and family members should be informed of these possibilities. Some suggest that by informing patients they may be predisposed to look for problems that they might otherwise ignore. Although it is possible, the danger of not attending to or reporting an obvious complication or side effect is much greater. The patient's trust and confidence may be betrayed by withholding such information.

Summary

In this chapter I have focused on patients with chronic pain predominantly in the spine and extremities. Newer applications including brain stimulation for movement disorders such as Parkinson's, vagal stimulation, sacral stimulation for pelvic pain, treatment of visceral pain, and occipital neuralgia are but a few of the developing areas. In all probability, unique patient characteristics, preparation, and management issues will emerge. The interested psychologist will be obliged to stay abreast of these developments and alter his or her approach accordingly. Unfortunately, to date, far too few studies exist that explore the potential efficacy of incorporating psychological methods into the SCS and DAS evaluation and therapy process.

In conclusion, the psychologist's role in the pretrial evaluation and preparation of the chronic pain patient being considered for implantation of an SCS or DAS can be quite significant and complex. The psychologist must be properly trained and informed. Merely interviewing the patient is often inadequate and betrays the importance of psychological influences on the experience of pain and the outcome of treatment. The growing acceptability of SCS and DAS technology can encourage a somewhat thoughtless and mechanical approach to the evaluation, preparation, preimplant trialing, and postimplant management of the chronic pain patient. It may be wise to remember that "two wrongs is only the beginning." Alternatively, "he who hesitates is probably right."

References

Anderson, V. C., & Burchiel, K. J. (1999). A perspective study of longterm intrathecal morphine in the management of chronic non-malignant pain. *Neurosurgery, 44,* 89–301.

Barolat, G. (1998). Epidural spinal cord stimulation: Anatomical and electrical properties of the intraspinal structures relevant to spinal cord stimulation and clinical correlation. *Neuromodulation, 1,* 63–72.

Barolat, G., Ketcik, B., & He, J. (1998). Long-term outcome of spinal cord stimulation for chronic pain management. *Neuromodulation, 1,* 19–29.

Barolat, G., Massaro, F., He, J., Zeme, S., & Ketcik, B. (1993). Mapping of sensory responses to epidural stimulation of the intraspinal neural structures in man. *Journal of Neurosurgery, 78,* 233–239.

Barolat, G., Oakley, J., Law, J. D., North, R. B., Ketchik, B., & Sharan, A. (2001). Epidural spinal cord stimulation with multiple electrode paddle leads is effective in treating intractable low back pain. *Neuromodulation, 4,* 59–66.

Brown, J., Klapow, J., Doleys, D. M., Lowery, D., & Tutak, U. (1999). Disease-specific and generic health outcomes: A model for the evaluation of long term intrathecal opioid therapy in non-cancer pain patients. *Clinical Journal of Pain, 15,* 122–131.

Cammeron, T., & Alo, K. M. (1998). Effects of posture on stimulation parameters in spinal cord stimulation. *Neuromodulation, 1,* 177–184.

"Current status of intrathecal therapy in non-malignant pain management: Proceedings supplement." (1997). *Journal of Pain and Symptom Management, 14*(Suppl. 1, 3), S1–S48.

Dahm, P., Nitescu, P., Appelgren, L., & Curelaru, I. (1998). Efficacy and technical complications of long term continuous intraspinal infusions of opioid and/or bupivocaine in refractory non-malignant pain: A comparison between the epidural and intrathecal approach with externalized or implanted catheters and infusion pumps. *Clinical Journal of Pain, 14,* 4–16.

Doleys, D. M. (2000). Psychological assessment for implantable therapies. *Pain Digest, 10,* 16–23.

Doleys, D. M., & Brown, J. (2001). MMPI profile as an outcome "predictor" in the treatment of non-cancer pain patients utilizing an intraspinal opioid therapy. *Neuromodulation, 4,* 93–97.

Doleys, D. M., Coleton, M., & Tutak, U. (1998). Use of intraspinal infusion therapy for non-cancer pain patients: Follow up and comparison of worker's compensation versus non-worker's compensation patients. *Neuromodulation, 1,* 149–159.

Doleys, D. M., Dinoff, B. L., Page, L, Tutak, U., Willis, K. D., & Coleton, M. (1998). Sexual dysfunction and other side effects of intraspinal opioid use in the management of chronic non-cancer pain. *American Journal of Pain Management, 8,* 5–10.

Doleys, D. M., & Doherty, D. C. (2000). Psychological and behavioral assessment. In P. P. Raj (Ed.), *Practical management of pain* (3rd ed., pp. 408–426). St. Louis, MO: Mosby.

Doleys, D. M., Klapow, J. C., & Hammer, M. (1997). Psychological evaluation and spinal cord stimulation therapy. *Pain Reviews, 4,* 189–207.

Doleys, D. M., & Olson, K. (1997). *Psychological assessment and intervention in implantable pain therapies.* Minneapolis, MN: Medtronic.

Doubell, T., Mannion, R., & Woolf, C. (1999). The dorsal horn: State dependent sensory processing, plasticity and degeneration of pain. In P. D. Wall & R. Melzack (Eds.). *Textbook of pain* (4th ed., pp. 165–181). New York: Churchill Livingstone.

DuPont, R. L. (1997). *The selfish brain: Learning from addiction.* Washington, DC: American Psychiatric Press.

Follett, K. A., & Doleys, D. M. (2002). *Seclection of candidates for intrathecal drug administration to treat chronic pain: Consideration in pre-implantatiion trials.* Unpublished manuscript, Minneapolis, MN.

Hassenbusch, S. J., & Portenoy, R. K. (2000). Special section polyanalgesic consensus conference 2000. *Journal of Pain and Symptom Management, 20,* S1–S50.

Intrathecal therapy [Special issue]. (1999). *Neuromodulation, 2*(2).

Jamison, R. N., Raymond, S. A., Sawlsby, E. A., Nedeljkovic, S. S., & Katz, N. P. (1998). Opioid therapy for chronic non-cancer low back pain. A randomized perspective study. *Spine, 23,* 2591–2600.

Keller, L. S., & Butcher, J. N. (1991). *Assessment of chronic pain patients with the MMPI-2.* Minneapolis: University of Minnesota Press.

Krames, E. S. (1996). Intraspinal opioid therapy for chronic non-malignant pain: Current practice and clinical guidelines. *Journal of Pain and Symptom Management, 11,* 332–352.

Krames, E. S. (1999a). Intrathecal Therapy [Special issue]. *Neuromodulation, 2,* 53–148.

Krames, E. S. (1999b). Interventional pain management: Appropriate when less invasive therapies fail to provide adequate analgesia. *Medical Clinics of North America, 83,* 787–823.

Krames, E. S. (2000). Overview of spinal cord stimulation: With special emphasis on the role of dual spinal cord stimulators. *Pain Digest, 4,* 6–12.

Krames, E. S., & Olson, K. (1997). Clinical realities in economic considerations: Patient selection in intrathecal therapy. *Journal of Pain and Symptom Management, 14,* S3–S13.

Maron, J., & Loeser, J. D. (1996). Spinal opioid infusion in treatment of chronic pain of non-malignant origin. *Clinical Journal of Pain, 12,* 174–179.

Maythaler, J. M., Guin-Renfroe, S., Grabb, P., & Hadley, M. N. (1999). Long-term continuously infused intrathecal baclofen for spastic-dystonic hypertonia in traumatic brain injury: One year experience. *Archives of Physical Medicine and Rehabilitation, 80,* 13–19.

Miller, W. R., & Rollnick, S. (1991). *Motivational interviewing: Preparing people to change addictive behavior.* New York: Guilford Press.

Naumann, C., Erdine, S., Koulousakis, A., VanBuyten, J. P., & Schuchard, M. (1999). Drug adverse events and system complications and intrathecal opioid delivery for pain: Origins, detection, manifestation and management. *Neuromodulation, 2,* 92–107.

Nelson, D. V., Kennington, M., & Novy, D. M. (1996). Psychological selection criteria for implantable spinal cord stimulators. *Pain Forum, 5,* 93–103.

Nitescu, P., Dahm, P., Appelgren, L., & Curelaru, I. (1998). Continuous infusion of opioid and bupivocaine by externalized intrathecal catheters in long term treatment of "refractory" non-malignant pain. *Clinical Journal of Pain, 14,* 17–28.

North, R. B., Kidd, D. H., Wimberley, R. L., & Edwin, D. (1996). Prognostic value of psychological testing in patients undergoing spinal cord stimulation: A perspective study. *Neurosurgery, 39,* 301–309.

North, R. B., Kidd, D. H., Zahurak, M., James, C. S., & Long, D. M. (1993). Spinal cord stimulation of chronic intractable pain: Experience over 2 decades. *Neurosurgery, 32,* 384–395.

Olin, J., Kidd, D. H., & North, R. B. (1998). Postural changes in spinal cord stimulation perceptual thresholds. *Neuromodulation, 1,* 171–176.

Paice, J. A., Penn, R. D., & Shott, S. (1996). In-traspinal morphine for chronic non-cancer pain: A retrospective multi center study. *Journal of Pain and Symptom Management, 11,* 71–88.

Polyanalgesic consensus conference 2000 [Special issue]. (2000). *Journal of Pain and Symptom Management, 20*(2), S1–S50.

Price, D. D. (1999). *Psychological mechanisms of pain and analgesia.* Seattle, WA: IASP Press.

Royal, M., Wiesemeyer, D. L., & Gordin, V. (1998). Intrathecal opioid conversions: The importance of lipophilicity. *Neuromodulation, 1,* 195–198.

Rush, A. J., Polatin, P., & Gatchel, R. J. (2000). Depression and low back pain: Establishing priorities in treatment. *Spine, 25,* 2566–2571.

Savage, S. R. (1999). Opioid use in the management of chronic pain. *Medical Clinics of North America, 83,* 761–787.

Schuchard, M., Lanning, R., North, R., Reig, E., & Krames, E. (1998). Neurological sequelae of intraspinal drug delivery systems: Results of the survey of American implanters of implantable drug delivery systems. *Neuromodulation, 1,* 137–148.

Sullivan, M. J., Thorn, B., Haythornthwaite, J. A., Keefe, F., Martin, M., Bradley, L. A., & Lefebvre, J. C. (2001). Theoretical perspectives on the relationship between catastrophizing and pain. *Clinical Journal of Pain, 17,* 52–64.

Turner, J. A., & Aaron, L. A. (2001). Pain-related catastrophizing: What is it? *Clinical Journal of Pain, 17,* 65–71.

Turner, J. A., Loeser, J. D., & Bell, K. G. (1995). Spinal cord stimulation for chronic low back pain: A systematic literature synthesis. *Neurosurgery, 37,* 1088–1095.

Willis, K. D., & Doleys, D. M. (1999). The effects of long term intraspinal infusion therapy with non-cancer pain patients: Evaluation of patient, significant-other, and clinic staff appraisals. *Neuromodulation, 2,* 241–253.

17

Occupational Musculoskeletal Pain and Disability

Anna R. Wright
Robert J. Gatchel

As Gatchel and Mayer (2000) have indicated, the annual cost associated with the diagnosis, treatment, lost workdays, and compensation claims associated with occupational musculoskeletal disorders in the United States alone amounts to tens of billions of dollars each year. Precise statistics on the prevalence of such work-related musculoskeletal disorders may vary from one reference source to another, primarily due to variations in the diagnostic criteria used for such disorders and variation among different jurisdictions. Such disorders can range from well-defined ones, such as disc herniation, tendonitis, and carpal tunnel syndrome, to those less well defined, such as facet syndrome, to nonspecific disorders such as cumulative trauma disorder or fibromyalgia syndrome

There can be no doubt, though, that the prevalence of musculoskeletal disorders, regardless of the vagaries of definition, is strikingly high in the United States and other developed countries. Data from the U.S. Department of Labor reveal that occupational musculoskeletal disorders are the leading cause of work disability in the United States. According to the U.S. Department of Labor, Bureau of Statistics, there were 1.7

million injuries and illnesses requiring time away from work, of which 4 of 10 were sprains and strains, typically involving the back (U.S. Department of Labor, 2000). The U.S. Department of Labor defines a musculoskeletal disorder as an injury or disorder of the muscles, tendons, ligaments, joints, cartilage, and spinal discs. In total for 1998, 593,000 musculoskeletal disorders were reported—accounting for one of three injuries and illness requiring time away from work (U.S. Department of Labor, 2000). The median amount of lost workdays was 5 per claim; however, one-fourth of the cases resulted in 21 days or more away from work (U.S. Department of Labor, 2000). Other reports for the same year found 803.2 thousand injuries cost workers time away from work stemming from sprains, strains, tears, carpal tunnel, and tendonitis (Fest, 2001). In addition, it has been estimated that the cost associated with lost workdays and compensation claims associated with such disorders range from $13 billion to $20 billion each year (AFL-CIO, 1997). A startling way of conceptualizing the costs incurred by all associated variables is to think about the distribution of wealth versus benefits paid in society. In most societies, 20% of the population usually holds 80% of the wealth; however, when assessing the distribution of benefits paid out for costs incurred by injured workers (health care benefits, short-term disability, and workers' compensation), 5% of the workers account for 80% of all benefits paid. This represents a concentration four times greater than the concentration of wealth in the society (Butler, 2000). Melhorn (2000) provides a more comprehensive review of the topic of epidemiology of musculoskeletal disorders, as does a recent publication by the National Research Council (2001).

Moreover, statistics from the U.S. Armed Forces indicate that musculoskeletal conditions are the leading cause of hospitalizations (Gardner, Amoroso, Grayson, Helmkamp, & Jones, 1999), and the leading cause of disability (Jones, Amoroso, Canham, Schmitt, & Weyandt, 1999). The military costs of musculoskeletal conditions are great in terms of both manpower losses and monetary expenditures. The Department of Defense (DOD) pays over $1.5 billion per year to disabled service members, and musculoskeletal conditions account for 40–50% of this amount. Similarly, musculoskeletal conditions are the leading cause of disability payments for the Department of Veterans Affairs (VA). The VA pays disability compensation in excess of $12 billion per year, with musculoskeletal conditions accounting for 45% of all disability cases and 34% of disability payments (Jones et al., 1999).

The critical nature of occupational musculoskeletal disorders is further highlighted by the fact that, in 1998, the National Institutes of Health (NIH) requested the National Academy of Sciences/National Research Council to convene a panel of experts (from the fields of orthopedic surgery, occupational medicine, epidemiology, human factors and ergonomics, statistics, and risk-assessment analysis) to carefully examine some major questions raised by the U.S. Congress concerning occupational musculoskeletal disorders (National Research Council, 1998). Some of the important issues raised by Congress were the following: What is the status of medical science with respect to the diagnosis, classification, and treatment of such disorders? What is the incidence of such conditions in the general population, specific industries, and specific occupational groups? Does the research literature reveal any specific guidance to prevent the development of chronic conditions?

Moreover, as further evidence of the growing worldwide concern about musculoskeletal disorders, an inaugural consensus meeting was convened in April 1998 by the World Health Organization (WHO) in Sweden (Heinegard et al., 1998). During the WHO conference, a large number of representatives from international scientific journals and societies discussed the significant problem of occupational musculoskeletal disorders and the burden on patients and society that they have created. Major concerns raised included the following: back pain is the second leading cause of sick leave; joint diseases account for 50% of all chronic conditions in patients 65 years and older; and there is an anticipation that 25% of health care expenditures in developing countries will be spent on musculoskeletal trauma-related care by the year 2010. This recognition prompted a proposal for declaring the years 2000–2010 as the "Decade of the Bone and Joint System."

Back Pain Disability as an Example of a Common Musculoskeletal Disorder

Back-related disorders represent the most prevalent source of disability in the U.S. military (Feuerstein, Berkotitz, & Peck, 1997). Indeed, in the United States, of all the occupational musculoskeletal disorders, the most research attention to date has been dedicated to low back pain disability, as this is the most expensive benign condition in industrialized countries. As Mayer and Gatchel (1988) have reviewed, it is the number-one cause of disability in persons under age 45. Over this age, it is the third leading cause of disability, becoming progressively less of a factor during later years when function and productivity become of less concern than survival. It has been estimated that, in any one year, about 3–4% of the population has a temporarily disabling low back pain episode in all industrialized countries, and that more than 1% of the working-age population is "totally and permanently disabled" by this problem. It has further been estimated that 70–85% of all people have back pain at some point in their life (Andersson, 1999). From a financial point of view, it is one of the most costly problems in the North American workplace (Krause & Ragland, 1994). Frymoyer and Durrett (1997) estimated that annual direct and indirect costs associated with spinal disability ranges from $38 billion to $50 billion. These costs become staggering when one considers that 2–7% of all adults in industrialized countries will experience chronic back pain (Andersson, 1997).

It should also be pointed out that even though most of the past clinical research has been directed at back pain disability, more recent efforts have been directed at work-related upper-extremity disorders (e.g., Mayer, Gatchel, Polatin, & Evans, 1999). This research has shown that many of the effective treatment programs developed for low back pain disability can also be applied to other musculoskeletal disorders such as upper extremity disorders. Therefore, many of the issues we discuss in this chapter concerning back pain disability are generalizable to other musculoskeletal disorders.

With the aforementioned caveats in mind, it should be noted that back pain is a brief time-limited condition almost 90% of the time, for which the treatment chosen often appears irrelevant to the outcome. From the onset of symptoms, about half the patients with acute low back pain are no longer disabled within 2 weeks; 70% have recovered in 1 month; and about 90% within 3–6 months (Andersson, 1999; Mayer & Gatchel, 1988; Mayer & Polatin, 2000). Yet, of those whose symptoms persist for more than 6 months, the majority will continue to be disabled and unable to work at the end of 1 year, and the greatest number of these will continue to be disabled even after 2 years. These chronic individuals often go on to extensive medical treatment, compensation costs, and settlement awards that make their contribution to the problem disproportionate to that of the entire group suffering acute low back pain. In fact, these 10% of the cases (i.e., the chronic cases) cost about 80% of the money in a variety of industries (see, e.g., Spitzer, LeBlanc, & Dupuis, 1987). Indeed, as Hazard (1995) has cogently noted, to significantly decrease the high cost of such chronic disability, "we need better and earlier methods for identifying patients and . . . accurate and timely identification of appropriate patients would almost certainly improve outcomes and some of the costs of unproductive care" (p. 2347).

As we discuss later in this chapter, an interdisciplinary treatment approach called *functional restoration* has been shown to be an effective modality for even the most disabled patients who are not able to recover during a normal healing period accompanied by surgery or primary or secondary nonoperative care. It is especially effective for workers' compensation patients with chronic musculoskeletal disorders. Such patients present with physical deconditioning, potential financial barriers to recovery, and psychosocial sequelae secondary to the injury, all of which need to be addressed in an integrated manner. Functional restoration is a treatment model incorporating reconditioning rehabilitation with a cognitive-behavioral orientation in a time-limited intervention. It has well-defined positive behavioral and socioeconomic outcomes, and it has well-documented success with the improvement of overall clinical and functional measures in both postoperative and nonsurgical pain patients, as well as elimination of residual disabilities. It has proven to be therapeutically efficacious, as well as cost-effective (Turk & Gatchel, 1999).

The Biopsychosocial Perspective of Pain and Disability

There are several perspectives regarding the diagnosis and treatment of occupational musculoskeletal disabilities. However, the focus of our discussion is on the biopsychosocial model, which is increasingly being shown to be the most heuristic approach to medical illnesses in general. For excellent reviews of other perspectives, the reader is referred to the work of Schultz, Crook, Fraser, and Joy (2000) and Kumar (2001).

The biopsychosocial perspective of pain and disability focuses on the complex interaction of variables—biological, psychological, medicolegal, and social variables—that patients encounter when dealing with a painful, persisting medical condition (Gatchel, 1996; Schultz et al., 2000; Turk, 1996). This model allows for an understanding of the relationship between pain and emotional factors that previous biomedical models, such as the disease model, have not adequately addressed. In the disease model of the progression of illness, the focus is on curing the disease causing the symptoms. If the disease is deemed by the physician and test findings to be cured and the symptoms persist, the patient is labeled as having a mental disorder (Turk, 1996). Unfortunately, this dualistic and archaic method of conceptualizing chronic pain patients is somewhat reinforced by the DSM-IV diagnosis of pain disorder according to the fourth edition of *Diagnostic and Statistical Manual of Mental Disorders* (DSM-IV; American Psychiatric Association, 1994; Schultz et al., 2000).

By the use of the diagnosis of pain disorder, patients are labeled as having a mental health problem. This label is applied when the following criteria are met: persisting pain that is the primary focus of concern which interferes significantly with social, occupational, or emotional functioning; the pain is judged to be exacerbated, maintained, or made more severe by psychological factors; the pain is not intentionally produced; and it is not better accounted for by another mental health disorder (American Psychiatric Association, 1994). The biopsychosocial model, unlike other models, accounts for the likelihood that patients' lives are affected greatly in a variety of ways by the persisting pain, thus requiring a comprehensive treatment approach designed to address all aspects of required care. This is in contrast to alternative, purely biological approaches designed to seek out the elusive "quick and easy" treatment plans resulting in a "medical cure." Before more thoroughly discussing the topic of treatment, we review the important issue of identification of risk factors that may contribute to the development of chronic musculoskeletal disorders in the first place.

Risk Factors

Many factors play a role in the duration of symptoms and the perception of the importance of symptoms, such as, legal, social, psychological, and work-related factors (Lawrence et al., 1998). Frymoyer and Cats-Baril (1987) were among the first to recog-

nize the importance of identifying predictive factors to determine early treatment planning. Numerous risk factors have been identified and may be best described using the following categories of factors: medical, job, compensation, social, demographic, and psychological (see Linton, Chapter 15, this volume).

Medical and Medical-Belief Risk Factors

Medical factors may be best discussed by using a further breakdown of the category. Some of the factors will relate exclusively to factual evidence found in the medical history, referred to as *medical fact*. The patient's belief or interpretation of the medical fact, referred to as *medical beliefs*, will largely influence other risk factors. For low back pain as an example, medical facts include such risk factors as severity of diagnosis and results of different clinical tests (pain during straight leg raise, positive results for the spiral range-of-motion or neurological deficit tests), as well as medical history (particularly if it includes a history of low back pain with lost work time or past surgical history) (Kumar, 2001; Lancourt & Kettelhut, 1992; Truchon & Fillion, 2000; van Poppel, 1998). Kumar (2001) also reviewed the evidence for a genetic predisposition for injury in cases of disc herniation, annular fissure with disc protrusion, age, body size, and spinal canal size. Medical beliefs include such risk factors as the following: a high subjective pain intensity persisting over a long period (Proctor, Gatchel, & Robinson, 2000; Truchon & Fillion, 2000), negative beliefs about the injury or fear of pain (Proctor et al., 2000; Truchon & Fillion, 2000), low activity level and exhibiting a significant level of pain behaviors (Proctor et al., 2000), avoidance of specific activities (Geisser, Haig, & Theisen, 2000), negative evaluation of ability to perform the job of injury (Truchon & Fillion, 2000), and patients' belief that work hampers recovery (Truchon & Fillion, 2000).

Job-Related Risk Factors

Many believe that job-related psychosocial or nonorganic factors figure more prominently than organic factors in the development and maintenance of chronic pain

(Crook & Tunks, 1996; Lancourt & Kettelhut, 1992; National Research Council, 2001). These factors include the following: high level of job stress (Lancourt & Kettelhut, 1992), job dissatisfaction (Bigos et al., 1991; Proctor et al., 2000; Truchon & Fillion, 2000; van Poppel, 1998), heavy and dangerous labor (Proctor et al., 2000; Spitzer et al., 1987), repetitive work tasks (Kumar, 2001), employment status (Proctor et al., 2000), low-wage earners (Volinn, Van Koevering, & Loeser, 1991), and poor employee/employer relations (Bigos et al., 1986).

Based on a review of the Workplace Health and Safety Agency database, Choi, Levitsky, Lloyd, and Stones (1996) found that occupational sprains and strains were found to account for the largest percentage of lost-time injuries in Ontario, Canada, during 1990. The authors found further additional risk factors unique to the workplace that had not previously been identified. Specifically, several factors were identified as targets for prevention of injury due to the high-risk association with injury: morning hours, the first 4 hours of a work shift, Mondays, and the months of January through May. Subsequently, Kuhder, Schaub, Biesi, and Krabill (1999) have also reported that sprains and strains account for the majority of work-related injuries in certain occupations (e.g., hospital workers).

Compensation Risk Factors

Compensation issues play a major role in many of the musculoskeletal disorders. Numerous studies have found that patients who are paid to remain disabled and nonproductive will behave differently from those who are uncompensated (Hadler, Carey, & Garrett, 1995; Mayer & Polatin, 2000; Proctor et al., 2000; Sanders, 2000; Sanderson, Todd, Hold, & Getty, 1995). Mayer and Polatin (2000) also note that even if patients are not receiving compensation throughout their recovery period, just the possibility of a one-time payoff based on level of impairment following treatment can affect outcomes. Indeed, Rainville, Sobel, Hartigan, and Wright (1997) analyzed outcomes for a compensated versus noncompensated consecutive cohort of patients who were referred to a spinal rehabilitation center. Treatment consisted of all patients participating in an aggressive exercise program, with a goal toward improved function. Pain, depression, and disability self-report questionnaires were administered at initial evaluation and at 3 and 12 months postdischarge. They found that patients who received compensation for disability had significantly higher rates of pain, depression, and disability than did those who had no compensation involvement; however, they had comparable treatment recommendations and compliance rates. Despite the fact that the pain, disability, and depression scores lowered for the compensation group as time went on, the scores still remained high and statistically different than those for the compensation group.

In another study, Sanderson and colleagues (1995) assessed factors influencing disability arising from low pack pain, with a specific focus on employment status and the presence or absence of a compensation claim. They found that both employment status and compensation influenced disability, but that employment status was the most important factor. Unemployed patients receiving compensation fared far worse than did employed patients claiming a compensable injury.

Social and Demographic Risk Factors

Social and demographic factors, which place an individual at greater risk for developing persisting chronic pain, include those who are experiencing personal or family difficulties at the time of injury and who have unstable family living arrangements (Lancourt & Kettelhut, 1992), older people (Proctor et al., 2000; Volinn et al., 1991), and persons who abuse substances (Proctor et al., 2000). Also, clinically we have observed that injured patients, who have a close friend or family member who is currently receiving disability or has an active workers' compensation case, are at greater risk for having persisting, unremitting pain.

Psychological Risk Factors

Psychological risk factors are often present to some degree prior to the injury but may have developed as a consequence of the injury or may be exacerbated by the injury

(Polatin, Kinney, Gatchel, Lillo, & Mayer, 1993). The presence of major psychiatric disorders, such as substance abuse, major depression, anxiety, and dysthymia, may influence treatment progress and outcomes (Crook & Tunks, 1996; Polatin et al., 1993). For this reason, it is imperative that clinicians use available information about psychological risk factors to maximize treatment outcomes, improve patient–physician collaboration, and prevent problems before they occur. Some risk factors include a patient's reliance on passive coping strategies (e.g., catastrophizing, hoping, and praying) versus active ones (trying to distract oneself) (Truchon & Fillion, 2000); the presence of psychological distress, which is a barrier for positive patient outcomes through reduced treatment compliance (Proctor et al., 2000; Riley et al., 1999); elevation of certain Minnesota Multiphasic Personality Inventory (MMPI) profiles such as the "conversion V" (Proctor et al., 2000); and depression (Proctor et al., 2000; see Linton, Chapter 15, this volume).

Finally, Gatchel, Polatin, and Mayer (1995) found evidence of a robust "psychosocial disability factor." In this study, 421 patients presenting with low back pain complaints of less than 6 months were systematically evaluated with a comprehensive psychosocial assessment battery. Contact information was verified every 3 months by telephone. Then, 1 year after the initial evaluation, all patients were contacted to participate in a structured telephone interview to document return-to-work status. Based on the responses, a logistic regression model was generated which found that the following array of variables correctly classified 90.7% of the cases in terms of work status at 1 year: self-reported pain and disability scores, scores on Scale 3 of the MMPI, workers' compensation/personal injury insurance status, and gender. A statistical algorithm was then generated to identify those acute low back pain patients who will require early intervention to prevent the development of chronic disability. Gatchel and colleagues, at UT Southwestern Medical Center at Dallas, are currently examining this algorithm. They are conducting a study in which "high risk" patients are screened for and then offered prophylactic early intervention in order to prevent the progression to chronic lumber pain and disability.

Overview of Interdisciplinary Treatment

Now that we have identified characteristics of individuals who may be at greater risk for developing persistent musculoskeletal disability, it is appropriate to discuss treatment options. The first level of care that most individuals usually encounter is at the primary care level. This is the care provided in the initial phase of injury, and it is focused on symptom control. Therapeutic modalities are generally passive, are administered by a single therapist to a large number of patients (Mayer & Polatin, 2000), may include a visit to the family doctor or an emergency room visit, and are generally accompanied by the directives to "take it easy," a prescription of pain killers or muscle relaxants, and a general statement to "avoid doing anything that causes more pain." This level of care is appropriate and adequate for 80% of the population experiencing pain following an injury. However, those who continue to experience pain graduate to the next level of care (see Pruitt & Von Korff, Chapter 14, this volume).

The secondary level of care is appropriate for a smaller number of patients than in the previous larger group of people experiencing pain. Physical and occupational therapists are the primary providers in this phase, with consultations being provided by physicians, psychologists, social workers, disability managers, and chiropractors. This level of care often occurs in a program atmosphere; however, not all the possible consultation specialists are available on site, and the patients are frequently not provided with individual attention for the length of the program (Mayer & Polatin, 2000). As in the primary level of care, approximately 80% of the smaller group who went on to the secondary level of care will return to preinjury levels of functioning. For the 5–10% of the original group who continue to experience musculoskeletal pain, it is appropriate to refer to a tertiary level of care (Mayer & Polatin, 2000; Quebec Task Force, 1987; Sternbach, 1986).

Patients who will benefit from this level of tertiary care are those for whom pain persists despite numerous treatment modalities over the course of months, or for those undergoing complex surgical procedures. The hallmark of tertiary care facilities is that they consist of physician-directed treatment teams in which all disciplines are "on site" and available to every patient (Mayer & Polatin, 2000). Interdisciplinary pain management is a prime example of a management solution for occupational musculoskeletal disorders at the tertiary level of care.

Deschner and Polatin (2000) provide a concise history of the evolution and development of the interdisciplinary approach. To summarize, single methods of treatment (i.e., medical, physical therapy, psychology, and case management) alone have not been associated with positive results in the chronic pain population. Over the past several years, providers have begun to collaborate and address the complex needs of such patients within the same physical location, thus the development of the interdisciplinary approach that is based on the biopsychosocial perspective of pain and disability discussed earlier in the chapter (see Turk & Monarch, Chapter 1, this volume).

As mentioned earlier, tertiary care is not for everyone. However, it is most effective for treating the small number of patients who do not receive pain relief after attempts at earlier interventions. By this point in time, patients have generally become a financial burden on their insurance carriers and employers in terms of lost time, disability payments, and reduced productivity. These patients also typically have complex issues involving secondary gain, medication addiction, and physical and emotional deconditioning (Deschner & Polatin, 2000). Traditionally, interdisciplinary treatment has been thought of as the treatment of choice for the most difficult patients with the most complex issues. However, it has also been found to be useful for any patient who continues to have persistent pain 3 to 6 months postinjury, regardless of presence or absence of previously identified risk factors (Crook & Tunks, 1996). The goals of interdisciplinary treatment programs are focused primarily on issues such as increased functioning in activities of daily living, a reduction in the number of medications taken, reduction in health care costs and utilization,

return to productivity/work, increase physical activity, and an increased ability to manage pain-related problems (Deschner & Polatin, 2000).

Components of Interdisciplinary Care

Part of the uniqueness of the interdisciplinary approach is in the predictability of the core components of the clinic facility and the team members. In the following section, we summarize these concepts in terms of the roles played by the treatment team members. Unlike earlier levels of care, in which the staff members are frequently part time and located off site (i.e., multidisciplinary), all core members of the interdisciplinary treatment team are full time and on site. This allows for constant formal and informal communication about patient progress and potential problems before they occur, so that solutions may be devised and implemented quickly to maximize outcomes (Deschner & Polatin, 2000). In addition, agreement among providers affords consistent advice and directives, which minimizes opportunities for patients to pit providers against one another and potentially "*subvert treatment goals*" (Deschner & Polatin, 2000, p. 631). Reinforcing this team approach are the guidelines established by the Commission on Accreditation of Rehabilitation Facilities (CARF). To receive CARF certification, treatment teams must consist of a physician, specialized nurse, physical therapist, and clinical psychologist or psychiatrist (Commission on Accreditation of Rehabilitation Facilities, 2000).

PHYSICIAN

As mentioned earlier, the physician serves as the medical director for all the patient's care. Typically, the physician has formal training varying from anesthesiology, orthopedic surgery, neurosurgery, psychiatry, occupational medicine, internal medicine, or osteopathy. The primary requirement is that the medical director has experience treating the most commonly encountered diagnoses that present among a chronic pain population (Deschner & Polatin, 2000). Patient education is also an important role for the physician, whether it be formal (leading educational classes), informal during patient contact, or seen in passing at the clinic.

NURSE

The nurse is a required team member if injections, regional anesthesia, or other medical procedures are to be offered. However, the role played by the nurse is essential to the team, because the nurse acts as a physician-extender, case manager, and provider of additional education (Deschner & Polatin, 2000). In light of the nature of the patients who present to a pain clinic, nurses typically handle numerous anxious questions about medications, side effects, refill requests, and other vague and varied requests. A nurse who has a great deal of patience and experience with this population will be most effective at reducing noncompliance, improving physician–patient communication, and maximizing treatment outcomes.

PSYCHOLOGIST

The first role of the psychologist is to complete a psychological evaluation of the patient in order to identify psychosocial barriers and current psychological functioning level. The psychologist also facilitates treatment planning by identifying the patient's primary concerns among the gamut of complex problems, only one of which may be his or her level of pain (i.e., losses secondary to financial limitations such as housing, jobs, marital problems, depression, and sexual dysfunction). This initial psychosocial assessment is necessary as psychosocial problems may originate because of persistent pain and disability but also may be activated by life disruption produced by the pain and disability (Mayer & Polatin, 2000; Wesley, Polatin, & Gatchel, 2000). From this evaluation, a treatment plan is formulated and recommendations are made, which may include individual, group, and occasionally marital or family therapy (Deschner & Polatin, 2000). Common goals identified early include helping patients cope more adaptively to psychological barriers and reducing psychosomatic correlates of stress, tension, and pain, such as depression and anxiety.

Cognitive-behavioral therapy is the most commonly used theoretical orientation when working with this population (Morley, Eccleston, & Williams, 1999; see Turk, Chapter 7, this volume). This method allows for brief, symptom-focused treatment and is generally well tolerated by the patients who are often hesitant to engage with a psychologist. This hesitance harkens back to the dualistic, anarchist thinking that plagues many. To dispel this myth that pain is "all in one's head," a great deal of education by the psychologist is necessary. Education is the key variable to dispelling this myth, and a core component of cognitive-behavioral therapy. Psychologists use examples from the patients' own life and experience to facilitate educational instruction in both the "gate control theory of pain" described by Melzack and Wall (1965) and the biopsychosocial model proposed by Turk and Rudy (1987). Both models help patients to begin to grasp the complex interactions that are likely serving to exacerbate their pain and stress.

Cognitive-behavioral therapy focuses on the learning of behaviors that occur in the chronic pain patient during the course of the pain experience. First, it is important to understand the developmental process that a chronic pain patient typically undergoes when progressing through the continuum from acute to chronic pain. Gatchel has proposed a three-stage model of the progression of pain from acute to chronic states that is well described in the literature but is summarized briefly here (Deschner & Polatin, 2000; Gatchel, 1991, 1996).

Over time, patients become acclimated to the "adoption of the sick role" based on a steadily increasing focus on pain without medical resolution and a steadily decreasing level of responsibilities socially, occupationally, and within the family. As time goes on, others take over responsibilities that previously belonged to the patients, and patients learn to accept that they are unable to do things for themselves anymore. This pattern leads to different responses within patients, depending on their preinjury emotional makeup. For some, there are significant levels of anger, for others, depression, as well as an array of other emotional and behavioral responses. For many, pain-related behavioral factors also become more apparent, such as grimacing, gait changes, more time in bed, and medication requests, all of which reinforce the assumption of the sick role (Deschner & Polatin, 2000; Tollison, Hinnant, & Kriegel, 1991).

In addition to the behavioral factors that play a role in chronic pain, many cognitive factors influence a patient's pain experience. Primarily, their perception of pain and its effect on their life circumstance will determine their response to pain and influence their ability to cope with pain (Deschner & Polatin, 2000). Motivation to recover, coexisting psychological distress, severity of injury, and perception of ability to receive adequate care will influence a patient's understanding of injury and ultimate outcome (see Jensen, Chapter 4, this volume). In addition, patients will base their interpretation of the injury on past experiences with injuries and their ability to recover, as well as on those of family members, coworkers, and friends.

Tollison and colleagues (1991; see also Turk, Chapter 7, this volume) summarized the necessary components of cognitive-behavioral therapy for the chronic pain patient, which recognizes the foregoing needs by providing (1) education about the mechanism of pain and the relationship to one's current experience; (2) instruction in self-control pain-reduction techniques such as relaxation, distraction and stress management, cognitive restructuring, and imagery; (3) reinforcement of efforts by patient to become more active in treatment; and (4) identifying and implementing prevention measures against recurrence of helpless and hopeless responses to pain. Also important in the cognitive-behavioral therapy process is instruction in coping skills training to reduce the impact of psychosocial stressors (i.e., marital distress, employment factors, financial stressors, and retraining needs). Turk (Chapter 7, this volume) also describes several essential components of cognitive-behavioral pain interventions including, education, skills acquisition, behavioral rehearsal, generalization, and maintenance.

Psychologists also serve to validate the patient's concerns about lack of relief thus far and to normalize, to a reasonable and expectable extent, the patient's experience. The role of a psychologist on an interdisciplinary team is multifaceted. The psychologist acts as a counselor, motivator, challenger, and liaison between the patient and the rest of the team. Often, the psychologist also addresses social work needs and referrals to other various agencies when deemed appropriate, (i.e., Alcoholics Anonymous, support services, housing agencies, neuropsychological resources, food banks, rehabilitation agencies, and job placement or retraining agencies). In summary, for all the patients, regardless of the method of coping or not coping and the behaviors displayed, the goal of therapy is to facilitate understanding of the relationship between emotional, behavioral, and cognitive factors that reinforce the maladaptive learned behaviors and cognitive patterns.

PHYSICAL THERAPIST

Chronic pain patients express much of their psychosocial "barriers to recovery" in the form of physical symptoms, including pain sensitivity, somatization, symptom magnification, and noncompliance with physical therapy (Deschner & Polatin, 2000). For this reason, it is imperative that physical therapists on an interdisciplinary team are familiar with the psychosocial issues and barriers most commonly encountered in chronic pain populations. This may be the first time since the injury that patients are expected to participate in active physical therapy. Active approaches to treatment likely contradict previous medical and physical therapy advice that typically promotes passive modalities. For this reason, the physical therapist should educate patients about their bodies, mechanics of movement, and how they relate to injury and job-task demands. It is during this period of education that patients begin learning to trust their bodies to act in a more active way, defying their previously learned expectations of disability. The role of the physical therapist is consequently twofold: (1) the therapist serves as a physical motivator and educator, and (2) the therapist acts as a counselor by allaying fears, anxiety, apprehension, and apathy to strides toward increased function (Turk, Okiuji, & Sherman, 2000). This level of communication and teamwork is possible because of the individual treatment approach that is a core component of interdisciplinary care (Kermond, Gatchel, & Mayer, 1991).

Complicating the many barriers to increased function are the potential reasons for secondary gain that a patient may have for not wanting to improve. A physical therapist who is aware of all of the above, and who has experience in working through these issues during the course of physical therapy, is integral to the interdisciplinary approach. To facilitate the physical therapy, the therapist uses information from collaboration with the psychologist and other team members to be aware of potential problems and also communicates with team members about the patient's progress and barriers that are still present. As with all members of the team, education plays a major role in physical therapy.

OCCUPATIONAL THERAPIST

The occupational therapist is involved in both the physical and occupational aspects of the patient's care. Unlike the physical therapist who focuses on muscle groups for "weak link" strengthening, occupational therapists help patients to work on whole-body activities that closely approximate job demands in order to facilitate the return to work. This type of therapy is twofold in its goals (1) to increase patients' confidence in their ability to return to preinjury levels of functioning and (2) to improve chances for return to work. As with all other aspects of interdisciplinary care, the occupational therapists provide a great deal of education to patients on a variety of topics, ranging from how to adjust movements for improved range of motion on the job, to interviewing skills, to improved return to work options. Occupational therapists also play a role as a case manager in terms of obtaining job descriptions to facilitate goal setting and to facilitate the actual return to work to a specific employer. These therapists are also frequently able to uncover hidden agendas on the patient's part while working with the patient on return-to-work functioning. This provides useful information for all other disciplines, so that the agenda and potential treatment barriers can be uncovered quickly (Kermond et al., 1991).

The roles of the physical therapist and occupational therapist are essential to obtaining improved levels of functioning. These therapists work with the patients on a near-daily basis and, consequently, quickly learn what activities are being avoided due to a perception of disability. The need for intervention directly aimed at resuming activities, or altering perceptions of activities to facilitate improved function, was best demonstrated by a study that found avoidance of specific activities to be a stronger predictor of disability or functional limitations than general fear of pain alone (Geisser et al., 2000).

Functional Restoration as an Example of Interdisciplinary Treatment

Functional restoration is an excellent example of an interdisciplinary management approach effectively applied to the treatment of musculoskeletal disorders. It is well described in the literature (Garcy, Mayer, & Gatchel, 1996; Jordan, Mayer, & Gatchel, 1998; Kermond et al., 1991; Mayer et al., 1998; Mayer & Gatchel, 1988; Mayer et al., 1985, 1987a, 1987b; Mayer & Polatin, 2000). To summarize, it rejects the traditional methodology for understanding chronic pain in which treatment planning is based merely on physician observation and a patient's self-report. Within a functional restoration program, there is a greater reliance on objectification of all aspects of functioning, thus allowing for treatment monitoring of otherwise difficult to observe variables (Kermond et al., 1991).

Core Concepts of Functional Restoration

Core components of functional restoration include the quantification of physical capacity; quantification of psychosocial function; reactivation for restoration of fitness; reconditioning of the injured functional unit; retraining in multiunit task performance; work simulation; multimodal disability management; vocational and societal reintegration; formalized outcome tracking; and posttreatment fitness maintenance program and monitoring (Kermond et al., 1991; Mayer, Gatchel, & Evans, 2002). Following is a brief description of concepts and terminology unique to the functional restoration approach (Mayer, Gatchel, & Polatin, 2000).

Deconditioning refers to the disuse, immobilization, and fear-related inhibition that leads to decreased function and range of motion (Gatchel, 1991). *Quantification of function* refers to the need for systematic assessment of function to determine improvement. Traditionally, improvement is determined by physician observation, results of clinical tests, and patient self-reports. By quantifying function objectively, we can better understand inconsistencies on radiographic findings (i.e., a normal MRI [magnetic resonance imaging] in the presence of continued pain complaints; (Kermond et al., 1991; Mayer et al., 2002). Quantification also allows patients to shift their focus from symptoms to repeated measures of function, thus serving as a guiding principle throughout the program (Hazard, 1998). *Disability* refers to the inability to perform usual functions of daily living and is frequently linked to prolonged episodes of severe pain. *Psychogenic pain* is a term *not* used by functional restoration as an active label but, rather, referred to as an archaic descriptor. In functional restoration, there is an active rejection of the traditional view that persistent pain is the result of a psychological cause when there is no identifiable source or medical cause for the pain. The functional restoration response answers this label by referring one back to the major tenets of the biopsychosocial model. The biopsychosocial model implies that providers will not only assess and treat the biological aspects of a pain condition but also consider the impact of the complex interactions between biological, social, psychological, and legal factors.

Quantification of psychosocial and socioeconomic factors is also essential for similar reasons as described previously. Examples include levels of depression and anxiety pretreatment and posttreatment, as well as changes in disability, occupational, marital, and living situations. There is a need for identification and treatment planning to appropriately treat possible complicating factors (i.e., emotional factors such as reactive depression, anxiety, and agitation; work-related factors such as anger and blame toward employer, job dissatisfaction, and loss of job; poor coping styles manifested in hostility and noncompliance; and organic brain dysfunction caused by factors such as age, alcohol, drugs, head injury, or limited intelligence) (Mayer et al., 2002). To track treatment outcomes, these variables must be assessed in some way. Mayer, Prescott, and Gatchel (2000) have carefully delineated a systematic way of colleting and assessing these variables. Using such a standardized assessment method provides that both the treatment team and the patient may receive feedback on the effectiveness of the treatment program based on the patient's quantifiable progress. These quantified data also allow for modifications of the program when indicated to provide more individualized effective treatment programs. Finally, quantification of physical, psychological, and socioeconomic factors also allows for intensive study of the interdisciplinary, functional restoration approach to determine treatment effectiveness.

Review of Treatment Effectiveness Studies

Mayer and colleagues note that interdisciplinary programs such as functional restoration have been found to be effective in multiple sites in the United States and other countries with varying patient populations from a range of socioeconomic variables and medical legal systems (Mayer et al., 1999). Many studies provide support for this claim (Bendix & Bendix, 1994; Burke, Harms-Constas, & Aden, 1994; Corey, Koepfler, Etlin, & Day, 1996; Hazard, 1995; Hazard et al., 1989; Hildebrandt, Pfingsten, Saur, & Jansen, 1997; Johansson, Dahl, Jannert, Melin, & Andersson, 1998). Several studies have also demonstrated the effectiveness of interdisciplinary, functional restoration for patients *following* spine surgery as compared to matched unoperated controls who had similar treatment outcomes following functional restoration (Haider, Kishino, Gray, Tomlin, & Daubert, 1998; Mayer et al., 1998). Most recently, Kishino, Polatin, Brewer, and Hoffman (2000) replicated these results using patients at a spine restoration center in California. They found that following functional restoration, the two groups (postsurgery and unoperated controls) had comparable return-to-work rates, self-reported satisfaction levels, and perceived helpfulness of the program ratings. Though the studies found similar results, the studies differed in terms of when the patients began the functional restoration program (Kishino et al., 2000; Mayer et al., 1998). Whereas one group of patients often had a long delay before beginning (approximately 1 year), the other group of patients began functional restoration almost immediately (Kishino et al., 2000; Mayer et al., 1998), suggesting that functional restoration at any time will be beneficial following surgery. All these studies provide further support for the building notion that there is hope for more conservative levels of care to treat the postspinal surgery patient, poor surgical candidates, and those who do not want surgery.

Literature reviews of the effectiveness of multidisciplinary treatment programs provide further support. After reviewing 65 studies, the treatment method was determined to be statistically superior to no treatment, waiting list, and single-discipline treatment methods (Flor, Fydrich, & Turk, 1992). The treatment benefits following participation include maintenance of gains over time, return to work, reduced pain and decreased interference caused by pain, improved mood, and decreased use of the health care system. Though the review pointed to the overwhelming effectiveness of multidisciplinary treatment, more methodologically sound studies were indicated to verify these findings (Flor et al., 1992). Subsequently, Okifuji, Turk, and Kalauokalmi (1999) conducted such an analysis and reconfirmed the substantial cost savings of multidisciplinary programs. Feuerstein and Zastowny (1996) also reviewed numerous studies and concurred that multidisciplinary treatment leads to successful outcomes following work-related injury. They attributed the treatment success to the theoretical orientation that the program is rooted in, which successfully accounts for the biological, psychological, and social factors that influence pain and disability.

In Denmark, patients with at least 6 months' disability postinjury were randomly assigned to a 3-week multidisciplinary treatment program or a no-treatment group (Bendix et al., 1996). The program was based on a functional restoration approach (Gatchel & Mayer, 1988; Hazard et al., 1989; Mayer et al., 1987a, 1987b). At 4 months' follow-up, 64% in the treatment group had returned to work, compared with only 29% in the control group. The treatment group also had significantly fewer days of sick leave, lower rates of continued health care utilization, and lower pain and disability scores. The same researchers conducted a 2-year follow-up study comparing a group of patients participating in multidisciplinary functional restoration to two, less intensive, but different training programs (Bendix, Bendix, Labriola, & Boekgaard, 1998). Overall, they found the functional restoration participants to have fared better at follow-up with respect to treatment outcomes.

Most recently, researchers at the West Coast Spinal Restoration Center in Riverside, California, compared outcomes of subacute (less than 6 months postinjury) to chronic (more than 6 months postinjury) patients following participation in a functional restoration program (Woods, Kishino, Haider, & Kay, 2000). Both groups demonstrated significant improvement on functional capacity measures from pretreatment to discharge. Subacute patients fared better than chronic patients in terms of functional gains (improved range of motion, lifting capacity, etc.). From this, they surmised that early intervention produces greater outcomes than waiting.

Though most of the foregoing studies involve patients with back injuries, particularly low back, functional restoration has also been effective in cervical spine disorders (Mayer et al., 1999; Wright, Mayer, & Gatchel, 1999) and upper extremity disorders (Evans, Mayer, & Gatchel, 2001). Many harbor the assumption that treatment of the cervical spine is much more difficult and less successful than the lumbar spine disorders. A 1-year follow-up study of cervical spinal disorder patients following functional restoration treatment demonstrated no significant differences between socioeconomic outcomes (occupational, financial, and medical variables) for cervical spinal disorder patients as compared to lumbar spinal disorder patients (Wright et al., 1999).

Summary and Conclusions

In this chapter, we have presented the strikingly high prevalence and accompanying financial costs of occupational musculoskeletal disorders in the United States today. In response to such data, there are renewed attempts to more effectively prevent and treat such disorders. A number of risk factors have been isolated that will, it is hoped, lead to better early prevention efforts. In terms of treatment, an interdisciplinary approach, such as functional restoration, has been found to be efficacious. Throughout the discussion in this chapter, the terms "multidisciplinary" and "interdisciplinary" have been used in a seemingly interchangeable manner. However, "multidisciplinary" describes a less intensive program than "interdisciplinary" care. The interdisciplinary approach involves more interactions between the staff and patient with an intensive, coordinated effort toward resumption of preinjury levels of functioning.

To achieve maximum treatment outcomes with the small number of patients who persist with musculoskeletal pain 3 to 6 months postinjury, it is recommended that an interdisciplinary approach be used. The interdisciplinary approach will serve to allay patients' fears about their situation, and it will provide a cohesive network of experts for team members and patients to consult with about problems or barriers as they arise. This intense level of communication allows for a degree of comfort and confidence by both the patient and the treatment team. Such a level of confidence is imperative when working with the complex medical, occupational, psychological, and socioeconomic issues that are prevalent in this patient population.

Acknowledgments

This work was supported in part by Grant Nos. 2R01-MH46452, 2K02-MH01107, and 2R01-DE10713 from the National Institutes of Health.

References

AFL-CIO. (1997). *Stop the pain*. Washington, DC: Author.

American Psychiatric Association. (1994). *Diagnostic and statistical manual of mental disorders* (4th ed.). Washington, DC: Author.

Andersson, G. B. J. (1997). The epidemiology of spinal disorders. In J. W. Frymoyer (Ed.), *The adult spine: Principles and practice* (2nd ed., Vol. 1, pp. 93–133). Philadelphia: Lippencott-Raven.

Andersson, G. B. J. (1999). Epidemiological features of chronic low back pain. *The Lancet, 354*, 581–585.

Bendix, A. F., Bendix, T., Labriola, M., & Boekgaard, P. (1998). Functional restoration for chronic low back pain: Two-year follow-up of two randomized clinical trials. *Spine, 23*, 717–725.

Bendix, A. E., Bendix, T., Vaegter, K., Lund, C., Frolund, L., & Holm, L. (1996). Multidisciplinary intensive treatment for chronic low back pain: A randomized, prospective study. *Cleveland Clinic Journal of Medicine, 63*, 62–69.

Bendix, T., & Bendix, A. (1994). *Different training programs for chronic low back pain—A randomized, blinded one-year follow-up study*. Paper presented at the International Society for the Study of the Lumbar Spine, Seattle.

Bigos, S. J., Battie, M. C., Spengler, D. M., Fisher, L. D., Fordyce, W. E., Hansson, T. H., Nachemson, A. L., & Wortley, M. D. (1991). A prospective study of work perceptions and psychosocial factors affecting the report of back injury. *Spine, 16*, 1–6.

Bigos, S. J., Spengler, D. M., Martin, N. A., Zeh, J., Fisher, L., Nachemson, A., & Wang, J. (1986). Back injuries in industry: A retrospective study. *Spine, 11*, 241–256.

Burke, S. A., Harms-Constas, C. K., & Aden, P. S. (1994). Return to work/work retention outcomes of a functional restoration program: A multi-center, prospective study with a comparison group. *Spine, 19*, 1880–1886.

Butler, R. J. (2000). Economic incentives in disability insurance and behavioral responses. *Journal of Occupational Rehabiliation, 10*, 7–19.

Choi, B. C. K., Levitsky, M., Lloyd, R. D., & Stones, I. M. (1996). Patterns and risk factors for sprains and strains in Ontario, Canada 1990: An analysis of the workplace health and safety agency data base. *Journal of Occupational and Environmental Medicine, 38*, 379–389.

Commission on Accreditation of Rehabilitation Facilities. (2000). *Standards manual: Medical rehabilitation June 2000–June 2001*. Phoenix, AZ: Author.

Corey, D. T., Koepfler, L. E., Etlin, D., & Day, H. I. (1996). A limited functional restoration program for injured workers: A randomized trial. *Journal of Occupational Rehabilitation, 6*, 239–249.

Crook, J. R. P., & Tunks, E. M. (1996). Musculoskeletal medicine. *Rheumatic Diseases Clinics of North America, 22*, 599–612.

Deschner, M., & Polatin, P. B. (2000). Interdisciplinary programs: Chronic pain management. In T. M. Mayer, R. J. Gatchel, & P. B. Polatin (Eds.), *Occupational musculoskeletal disorders: Function, outcomes & evidence* (pp. 629–637). Philadelphia: Lippincott Williams & Wilkins.

Evans, T. H., Mayer, T. G., & Gatchel, R. J. (2001). Recurrent chronic disabling work-related spinal disorders after prior injury claims in a chronic low back pain population. *The Spine Journal, 1*, 183–189.

Fest, G. (2001, January 15). Rules to work by. *Star Telegram*, pp. 14–16.

Feuerstein, M., Berkotitz, S. M., & Peck, C. A. (1997). Musculoskeletal related disability in U.S.

Army personnel: Prevalence, gender, and military occupational specialties. *Journal of Occupational and Environmental Medicine, 39,* 68–78.

Feuerstein, M., & Zastowny, T. R. (1996). Occupational rehabilitation: Multidisciplinary management of work related musculoskeletal pain and disability. In R. J. Gatchel & D. C. Turk (Eds.), *Psychological approaches to pain management: A practitioner's handbook* (pp. 458–485). New York: Guilford Press.

Flor, H., Fydrich, T., & Turk, D. (1992). Efficacy of multidisciplinary pain treatment centers: A meta-analytic review. *Pain, 49,* 221–230.

Frymoyer, J. W., & Cats-Baril, W. L. (1987). Predictors of low back pain disability. *Journal of Clinical Orthopedic and Related Research, 221,* 89–98.

Frymoyer, J. W., & Durett, C. L. (1997). The economics of spinal disorders. In J. W. Frymoyer (Ed.), *The adult spine* (2nd ed., Vol. 1, pp. 143–150). Philadelphia: Lippincott-Raven.

Garcy, P., Mayer, T., & Gatchel, R. J. (1996). Recurrent or new injury outcomes after return to work in chronic disabling spinal disorders. Tertiary prevention efficacy of functional restoration treatment. *Spine, 21,* 952–959.

Gardner, J. W., Amoroso, P. J., Grayson, J. K., Helmkamp, J., & Jones, B. H. (1999). Hospitalizations due to injury: Inpatient medical records data. Atlas of injuries in the U.S. armed forces. *Military Medicine, 164*(Suppl.), S1–S143.

Gatchel, R. J. (1991). Early development of physical and mental deconditioning in painful spinal disorders. In T. G. Mayer, V. Mooney, & R. J. Gatchel (Eds.), *Contemporary conservative care for painful spinal disorders* (pp. 278–289). Philadelphia: Lea & Febiger.

Gatchel, R. J. (1996). Psychological disorders and chronic pain: Cause-and-effect relationships. In R. J. Gatchel & D. C. Turk (Eds.), *Psychological approaches to pain management: A practitioner's handbook* (pp. 33–52). New York: Guilford Press.

Gatchel, R. J., & Mayer, T. G. (2000). Occupational musculoskeletal disorders: Introduction and overview of the problem. In T. G. Mayer, R. J. Gatchel, & P. B. Polatin (Eds.), *Occupational musculoskeletal disorders: Function, outcomes, and evidence* (pp. 3–8). Philadelphia: Lippincott Williams & Wilkins.

Gatchel, R. J., Polatin, P. B., & Mayer, T. G. (1995). The dominant role of psychosocial risk factors in the development of chronic low back pain disability. *Spine, 24,* 2702–2709.

Geisser, M. E., Haig, A. J., & Theisen, M. E. (2000). Activity avoidance and function in persons with chronic back pain. *Journal of Occupational Rehabilitation, 10,* 215–227.

Hadler, N., Carey, T., & Garrett, J. (1995). The influence of indemnification by workers' compensation inusrance on recovery from acute backache: North Carolina Back Pain Project. *Spine, 20,* 2710–2715.

Haider, T. T., Kishino, N. D., Gray, T. P., Tomlin, M. A., & Daubert, H. B. (1998). Functional restoration: Comparison of surgical and nonsurgical spine patients. *Journal of Occupational Rehabilitation, 8,* 247–253.

Hazard, R. G. (1995). Spine update: Functional restoration. *Spine, 20,* 2345–2348.

Hazard, R. G. (1998). Point of view. *Spine, 23,* 725.

Hazard, R. G., Fenwick, J. W., Kalisch, S. M., Redmond, J., Reeves, V., Reid, S., & Frymoyer, J. W. (1989). Functional restoration with behavioral support: A one-year prospective study of patients with chronic low-back pain. *Spine, 14,* 157–161.

Heinegard, D., Johnell, O., Lidgren, L., Nilsson, O., Rydevik, B., Wollheim, F., & Akesson, K. (1998). The bone and joint decade 2000–2010. *Acta Orthopaedica Scandinavica, 69,* 219–220.

Hildebrandt, J., Pfingsten, M., Saur, P., & Jansen, J. (1997). Prediction of success from a multidisciplinary treatment program for chronic low back pain. *Spine, 22,* 990–1001.

Johansson, C., Dahl, J., Jannert, M., Melin, L., & Andersson, G. (1998). Effects of a cognitive- behavioral pain-management program. *Behaviour Research and Therapy, 36,* 915–930.

Jones, B. H., Amoroso, P. J., Canham, M. L., Schmitt, J. B., & Weyandt, M. B. (1999). Conclusions and recommendations of the DoD injury surveillance and prevention work group. Atlas of injuries in the United States armed forces. *Military Medicine, 164*(Suppl.), 9-1–9-26.

Jordan, K. D., Mayer, T. G., & Gatchel, R. J. (1998). Should disability chronicity be an exclusion criterion for tertiary rehabilitation? Socioeconomic outcomes of early vs. late functional restoration in compensation spinal disorders. *Spine, 23,* 2110–2116.

Kermond, W., Gatchel, R. J., & Mayer, T. G. (1991). Functional restoration for chronic spinal disorders or failed back surgery. In T. G. Mayer, V. Mooney, & R. J. Gatchel (Eds.), *Contemporary conservative care for painful spinal disorders* (pp. 473–481). Philadelphia: Lea & Febiger.

Kishino, N. D., Polatin, P. B., Brewer, S., & Hoffman, K. (2000). Long-term effectiveness of combined spine surgery and functional restoration: A prospective study. *Journal of Occupational Rehabilitation, 10,* 235–240.

Krause, N., & Ragland, D. R. (1994). Occupational disability due to low back pain: A new interdisciplinary classification used in a phase model of disability. *Spine, 19,* 1011–1020.

Kuhder, S. A., Schaub, E. A., Bisesi, M. S., & Krabill, Z. T. (1999). Injuries and illnesses among hospital workers in Ohio: A study of workers' compensation claims from 1993 to 1996. *Journal of Occupational and Environmental Medicine, 41,* 53–59.

Kumar, S. (2001). Theories of musculoskeletal injury causation. *Ergonomics, 44,* 17–47.

Lancourt, J., & Kettelhut, M. (1992). Predicting return to work for lower back pain patients receiving worker's compensation. *Spine, 17,* 629–640.

Lawrence, R. C., Helmick, C. G., Arnett, F., Deyo, R. A., Felson, D. T., Giannini, E. H., Heyse, S. P.,

Hirsch, R., Hochberg, M. C., Hunder, G. G., Liang, M. H., Pillemer, S. R., Steen, V. D., & Wolfe, F. (1998). Estimates of the prevalence of arthritis and selected musculoskeletal disorders in the united states. *Arthritis and Rheumatism, 41,* 778–799.

Mayer, T., McMahon, M. J., Gatchel, R. J., Sparks, B., Wright, A., & Pegues, P. (1998). Socioeconomic outcomes of combined spine surgery and functional restoration in workers' compensation spinal disorders with matched controls. *Spine, 23,* 598–605.

Mayer, T. G., & Gatchel, R. J. (1988). *Functional restoration for spinal disorders: The sports medicine approach.* Philadelphia: Lea & Febiger.

Mayer, T. G., Gatchel, R. J., & Evans, T. H. (2002). Chronic low back pain. In R. Fitzgerald, H. Kauffer, & A. Malkani (Eds.), *Orthopaedics* (pp. 1192–1197). Chicago: Mosby.

Mayer, T. G., Gatchel, R. J., Kishino, N., Keeley, J., Capra, P., Mayer, H., Barnett, J., & Mooney, V. (1985). Objective assessment of spine function following industrial injury. A prospective study with comparison group and one-year follow-up. *Spine, 10,* 482–493.

Mayer, T. G., Gatchel, R. J., Mayer, H., Kishino, N., Keeley, J., & Mooney, V. (1987a). Prospective two-year study of functional restoration in industrial low back injury. *Journal of the American Medical Association, 259,* 1181–1182.

Mayer, T. G., Gatchel, R. J., Mayer, H., Kishino, N. D., Keeley, J., & Mooney, V. (1987b). A prospective two-year study of functional restoration in industrial low back injury. An objective assessment procedure. *Journal of the American Medical Association, 258,* 1763–1767.

Mayer, T. G., Gatchel, R. J., & Polatin, P. B. (Eds.). (2000). *Occupational musculoskeletal disorders: Function, outcomes and evidence.* Philadelphia: Lippincott Williams & Wilkins.

Mayer, T. G., Gatchel, R. J., Polatin, P. B., & Evans, T. H. (1999). Outcomes comparison of treatment for chronic disabling work-related upper extremity disorders. *Journal of Occupational and Environmental Medicine, 41,* 761–770.

Mayer, T. G., & Polatin, P. B. (2000). Tertiary nonoperative interdisciplinary programs: The functional restoration variant of the outpatient chronic pain management program. In T. G. Mayer, R. J. Gatchel, & P. B. Polatin (Eds.), *Occupational musculoskeletal disorders: Function, outcomes & evidence* (pp. 639–649). Philadelphia: Lippincott Williams & Wilkins.

Mayer, T. G., Prescott, M., & Gatchel, R. J. (2000). Objective outcomes evaluation: Methods and evidence. In T. G. Mayer, R. J. Gatchel, & P. B. Polatin (Eds.), *Occupational musculoskeletal eisorders: Function, outcomes, and evidence* (pp. 651–667). Philadelphia: Lippincott Williams & Wilkins.

Melhorn, J. (2000). Workers' compensation: Avoiding work-related disability. *Journal of Bone and Joint Surgery—American Volume, 82-A,* 1490–1493.

Melzack, R., & Wall, P. D. (1965). Pain mechanisms: A new theory. *Science, 50,* 971–979.

Morley, S., Eccleston, C., & Williams, A. (1999). Systematic review and meta-analysis of randomized controlled trials of cognitive behaviour therapy and behavior therapy for chronic pain in adults, excluding headache. *Pain, 80,* 1–13.

National Research Council. (1998). *Work-related musculoskeletal disorders: A review of evidence.* Washington, DC: National Academy Press.

National Research Council. (2001). *Musculoskeletal disorders and the workplace: Low back and upper extremities.* Washington, DC: National Academy Press.

Okifuji, A., Turk, D. C., & Kalauokalani, D. (1999). Clinical outcomes and economic evaluation of multidisciplinary pain centers. In A. R. Block, E. F. Kremer, & E. Fernandez (Eds.), *Handbook of pain syndromes* (pp. 169–191). Mahwah, NJ: Erlbaum.

Polatin, P. B., Kinney, R. K., Gatchel, R. J., Lillo, E., & Mayer, T. G. (1993). Psychiatric illness and chronic low-back pain. The mind and the spine—which goes first? *Spine, 18,* 66–71.

Proctor, T., Gatchel, R. J., & Robinson, R. C. (2000). Psychosocial factors and risk of pain and disability. In D. C. Randolph & M. I. Ranavaya (Eds.), *Occupational medicine: State of the art reviews* (Vol. 15, pp. 803–812). Philadelphia: Hanley & Belfus.

Quebec Task Force on Spinal Disorders. (1987). Scientific approach to the assessment and management of activity related spinal disorders. *Spine, 7*(Suppl.), S12–S15.

Rainville, J., Sobel, J., Hartigan, C., & Wright, A. (1997). The effect of compensation involvement of the reporting of pain and disability by patients referred for rehabilitation of chronic low back pain. *Spine, 22,* 2016–2024.

Riley, J., 3rd , Robinson, M., Wise, E., Campbell, L., Kashikar-Zuck, S., & Gremillion, H. (1999). Predicting treatment compliance following facial pain evaluation. *Cranio, 17,* 9–16.

Sanders, S. H. (2000). Risk factors for chronic disability low-back pain: An update for 2000. *American Pain Society Bulletin, 10,* 4–5.

Sanderson, P. L., Todd, B. D., Hold, G. R., & Getty, C. J. M. (1995). Compensation, work status, and disability in low back pain patients. *Spine, 20,* 554–563.

Schultz, I. Z., Crook, J., Fraser, K., & Joy, P. W. (2000). Models of diagnosis and rehabilitation in musculoskeletal pain-related occupational disability. *Journal of Occupational Rehabiliation, 10,* 271–293.

Spitzer, W. O., LeBlanc, F. E., & Dupuis, M. (1987). A scientific approach to the assessment and management of activity-related spinal disorders: A monograph for clinicians; Report of the Quebec Task Force on Spinal Disorders. *Spine, 75,* 53–559.

Sternbach, R. A. (1986). Survey of pain in the United States: The Nuprin pain report. *Clinical Journal of Pain, 2*, 49–53.

Tollison, C. D., Hinnant, D. W., & Kriegel, M. L. (1991). Psychological concepts of pain. In T. G. Mayer, V. Mooney, & R. J. Gatchel (Eds.), *Contemporary conservative care for painful spinal disorders* (pp. 133–142). Philadelphia: Lea & Febiger.

Truchon, M., & Fillion, L. (2000). Biopsychosocial determinants of chronic disability and low-back pain: A review. *Journal of Occupational Rehabiliation, 10*, 117–142.

Turk, D. C. (1996). Biopsychosocial perspective on chronic pain. In R. J. Gatchel & D. C. Turk (Eds.), *Psychological approaches to pain management: A practitioner's handbook* (pp. 3–32). New York: Guilford Press.

Turk, D. C., & Gatchel, R. J. (1999). Multidisciplinary programs for rehabilitation of chronic low back pain patients. In W. H. Kirkaldy-Willis & J. T.N. Bernard (Eds.), *Managing low back pain* (4th ed., pp. 299–311). New York: Churchill Livingstone.

Turk, D. C., Okiuji, A., & Sherman, J. J. (2000). Psychological factors in chronic pain: Implications for physical therapists. In J. W. Towney & J. T. Taylor (Eds.), *Low back pain* (pp. 351–383). Baltimore: Williams & Wilkins.

Turk, D. C., & Rudy, T. E. (1987). Towards a comprehensive assessment of chronic pain patients.

Behaviour Research and Therapy, 25, 237–249.

U.S. Department of Labor. (2000). *Lost-worktime injuries and illnesses: Characteristics and resulting time away from work, 1998* (U.S. Department of Labor Pub. No. 00-115). Washington DC: Author.

van Poppel, M. N. (1998). Risk factors for back pain incidence in industry: A prospective study. *Pain, 77*, 81–86.

Volinn, E., Van Koevering, D., & Loeser, J. (1991). Back sprain in industry: The role of socioeconomic factors in chronicity. *Spine, 16*, 542–548.

Wesley, A. L., Polatin, P. B., & Gatchel, R. J. (2000). Psychosocial, psychiatric, and socioeconomic factors in chronic occupational musculoskeletal disorders. In T. M. Mayer, R. J. Gatchel, & P. B. Polatin (Eds.), *Occupational musculoskeletal disorders: Function, outcomes & evidence* (pp. 577–608). Philadelphia: Lippincott Williams & Wilkins.

Woods, C. S., Kishino, N. D., Haider, T. T., & Kay, P. K. (2000). Effects of subacute versus chronic status of low back pain patients' response to a functional restoration program. *Journal of Occupational Rehabilitation, 10*, 229–233.

Wright, A., Mayer, T. G., & Gatchel, R. J. (1999). Outcomes of disabling cervical spine disorders in compensation injuries. A prospective comparison to tertiary rehabilitation response for chronic lumbar spinal disorders. *Spine, 24*, 178–183.

18

Cognitive-Behavioral Management of Recurrent Headache Disorders: A Minimal-Therapist-Contact Approach

Gay L. Lipchik
Kenneth A. Holroyd
Justin M. Nash

Behavioral treatments can be efficacious when used either as an alternative or as an adjunct to medication in the treatment of recurrent headache disorders. This chapter provides a brief guide to the behavioral treatment of migraine and tension-type headache. We focus on minimal-therapist-contact treatment (MTCT), or home-based treatment, because clinic-based treatment has been described elsewhere (Blanchard & Andrasik, 1985; Martin, 1993) and interest in brief cost-effective treatment that can be integrated with medical clinic appointment schedules is currently high.

First, we briefly review the epidemiology and impact of migraine and tension-type headaches and describe the clinical characteristics of these two disorders and of frequently co-occurring headaches associated with medication overuse. Next, we offer suggestions for the assessment and the selection of patients for behavioral treatment. The body of the chapter then provides a description of behavioral minimal-therapist-contact treatment, with an emphasis on clin-ical issues and predictable obstacles likely to confront therapists.

Epidemiology and Impact of Headache

In the United States alone, migraine is experienced by 18% of women and 6% of men (25 to 30 million individuals; Lipton, Stewart, Diamond, Diamond, & Reed, 2001; Stewart, Lipton, Celentano, & Reed, 1991). Tension-type headache, a more common but less disabling condition, affects 38% to 78% of people (Rasmussen, Jensen, Schroll, & Olesen, 1991; Schwartz, Stewart, Simon, & Lipton, 1998). As the frequency and severity of migraine or tension-type headaches increase, the impact of headaches on daily functioning also increases (Holroyd et al., 2000; Schwartz et al., 1998). Approximately 31% of migraine sufferers miss work, and between 58% and 76% of migraine sufferers discontinue normal household activities or cancel family or social activities (Lipton, Stewart, et al., 2001; see

Lipton, Hamelsky, & Stewart, 2001; Lipton, Stewart, & Von Korff, 1995, for additional information).

Clinical Characteristics and Diagnosis

Clinicians working with headache patients should use the diagnostic criteria of the Headache Classification Committee of the International Headache Society (IHS; Olesen, 1988). The majority of headache sufferers (probably over 95%) have benign, idiopathic headaches such as migraine and tension-type headache. These headaches may be considered episodic if they occur fewer than 15 days in the month and chronic if they occur more often. A subset of chronic headaches also is associated with overuse of acute headache medications.

Migraine

The prototypical migraine is characterized by pulsating pain of moderate to severe intensity sufficient to inhibit or prohibit daily activities. The migraine episode lasts 4 to 72 hours and is accompanied by nausea or vomiting, or both, and a heightened sensitivity to light and sound, and it is aggravated by routine physical activities (e.g., climbing stairs). The head pain is often unilateral and frequently originates behind or around the eyes and then radiates to the frontal and temporal regions and may progress to encompass the entire head. Thought, memory, and concentration may be impaired, and the sufferer may also experience lightheadedness, irritability, anorexia, diarrhea, and scalp tenderness. For the minority of headache sufferers who experience migraine with aura, the pain is preceded by temporary focal neurological symptoms that are most often visual disturbances (e.g., bright spots or stars or a scintillating scotoma) but may include sensory disturbances (e.g., parathesias), motor weakness, or syncope. Many patients with migraine headache experience tension-type headaches as well.

Tension-Type Headache

The prototypical tension-type headache is characterized by bilateral nonthrobbing (pressing–tightening, dull, band-like, or cap-like) pain of mild to moderate intensity that may inhibit, but not prohibit, daily activities. The pain is typically located in the forehead, neck, and shoulder areas. The typical tension-type headache may last 30 minutes to 7 days and is usually not aggravated by routine activities, accompanied by nausea or vomiting, or preceded by focal neurological symptoms. Tension-type headaches occurring 15 or more days a month (chronic tension-type headache) are common in clinical settings although infrequent in the population at large.

Headache Associated with Substances or Their Withdrawal

The frequent use of prescription and nonprescription analgesic medications and abortive medications (combination analgesics, opiates, nonopioid analgesics, barbiturates, ergots, and other abortive agents including triptans) can both worsen headaches and render headaches refractory to what would otherwise be efficacious drug and nondrug therapies (Diener & Tfelt-Hansen, 1993; Diener & Wilkinson, 1988; Markley, 1994; Rapoport & Sheftell, 1993). Medication overuse headache (often referred to as "rebound headache") is estimated to occur in up to 30% of people treated in headache centers (Diener & Dahlof, 2000) and should be suspected when acute medications are used 20 days monthly for at least a 3-month period. Individuals with rebound headaches are seldom pain-free and the headache characteristics overlap with those of chronic tension-type and migraine headache. Rebound headaches can only be managed effectively if the use of the offending medications is reduced or eliminated.

Assessment

Medical Evaluation

Prior to initiating behavioral treatment, a medical evaluation is needed to rule out headaches secondary to a disease state or structural abnormality. Secondary headaches often are associated with one or more of the following "red flags": (1) recent or sudden onset ("first or worst headache") of headaches; (2) recent head trauma; (3)

changing or progressive symptoms, or accompanying neurological symptoms (other than the focal neurological symptoms associated with migraine aura), (4) headache associated with fever or other signs of infection, or (5) new onset of headache in a patient over age 50 or in a patient with cancer or human immunodeficiency virus. Appearance of a "red flag" at any point during treatment is cause for referral for an additional medical evaluation. The use of medications that might aggravate headaches (oral contraceptives, antidepressants, bronchodilators, phenothaizine derivatives, sedatives) also should be assessed.

Diagnostic and Headache History

Patient assessment includes standardized tests and a clinical interview. Standardized instruments can be used to assess (1) presence of comorbid psychiatric disorders (e.g., PRIME-MD Patient Questionnaire; Spitzer et al., 1994); (2) degree of depression (Beck Depression Inventory; Beck, Ward, Mendelson, Mock, & Erbaugh, 1961), and anxiety (e.g., State–Trait Anxiety Inventory; Spielberger, Gorsuch, & Lushene, 1970, or Beck Anxiety Inventory; Beck & Steer, 1993); and (3) disability or impact of headache on work, family and social functioning (e.g., MIDAS; Stewart, Lipton, Kolodner, Liberman, & Sawyer, 1999, or the Headache Disability Inventory; Jacobson, Ramadan, Aggarwal, & Newman, 1994). The clinical interview builds on the information gathered from the questionnaires and includes a diagnostic headache evaluation, headache history, and a psychological evaluation. The diagnostic headache evaluation follows the IHS classification system criteria (Olesen, 1988). The headache history includes a review of headache precipitants, impact of headache on work, family and social functioning, and current and previous treatment (i.e., use of emergency department, medication, and alternative treatments) for headaches. The psychological evaluation includes a review of psychiatric history, mental status examination, and current psychological diagnosis (we use the PRIME-MD Diagnostic Interview; Spitzer et al., 1994). Relevant medical and social history information is also gathered.

With the increased likelihood of psychi-atric conditions in those with migraine (Breslau & Davis, 1993; Breslau, Merikangas, & Bowden, 1994) or chronic tension-type headache (Holroyd et al., 2000), screening for a psychiatric disorder is an important component of the behavioral evaluation. If a psychiatric disorder is identified, it is important to determine whether this disorder is likely to compromise the efficacy of behavioral treatment (see "Patient Selection" section).

Headache Diaries and Self-Monitoring Records

We ask patients to record medication use and headache activity four times a day (upon arising, lunchtime, dinnertime, and bedtime). These headache diaries, valuable for assessing treatment outcome, are completed for about 1 month prior to treatment (if possible), throughout treatment, for about 1 month after treatment, and at a follow-up evaluation. At other points in treatment, we ask patients to also record other relevant information such as relaxation practice, headache precipitants, or thoughts and behavior in stressful situations. At each clinic visit we review headache diaries and any self-monitoring forms to gather information useful to the treatment process, which can include information relevant to identifying patterns in headache activity, headache precipitants and early warning signs of headache onset, and difficulties in learning self-management skills.

Patient Selection

There are no firm guidelines to assist the clinician in identifying people who are well suited for behavioral treatment, especially MTCT. Nonetheless, the requirements of MTCT and the limited information from empirical data suggest that attention be paid to the following factors.

1. *Limited reading comprehension, low-intelligence, or significant cognitive impairment.* Patients with reading comprehension below the eighth-grade level; below-average intelligence; deficits in concentration, attention, or memory; or organic brain damage typically will have difficulty making effective use of the written materials and audiotapes.

2. *Misuse or overuse of medication.* Patients will need to reduce or eliminate offending medications if there is evidence of medication overuse (use of acute medications 20 days monthly). Patients who have difficulty reducing their medication use on their own may benefit from additional treatment sessions during this period. Patients overusing barbiturates or opioids may require medical supervision to eliminate these medications.

3. *Chronic daily severe headache.* Patients with near-constant headaches that are sometimes severe typically respond poorly to relaxation and biofeedback therapies, even when excessive mediation use is not an aggravating factor (Blanchard, Appelbaum, Radnitz, Jaccard, & Dentinger, 1989). Clinicians commonly assume that patients with chronic daily headache require aggressive multimodal therapy that includes prophylactic medications and multiple behavioral interventions over a longer period than that afforded in a MTCT protocol.

4. *Nonadherence.* Patient does not complete assessment questionnaires, headache diaries, or homework assignments. Some patients simply do not persist in efforts to learn or apply self-regulation skills without regular contact with a health professional. Consideration may be given to offering traditional clinic-based treatment or motivational enhancement therapy (Miller & Rollnick, 1991; see also Jensen, Chapter 4, this volume).

5. *Psychiatric comorbidity.* Patient is significantly impaired by a psychiatric disorder that requires attention (e.g., severe major depressive episode, severe anxiety disorder, posttraumatic stress disorder, somatization disorder, or psychosis) or has a personality disorder (e.g., histrionic, borderline, or dependent). The presence of psychological symptoms or a comorbid psychiatric disorder does not usually prohibit behavioral treatment. Combined psychological and pharmacological treatment should be considered (Holroyd, Lipchik, & Penzien, 1998) and additional treatment sessions may be required to address psychological problems. Cognitive-behavioral interventions for depression (Beck, Rush, Shaw, & Emery, 1979; Robinson, Berman, & Neimeyer, 1990) and anxiety (Barlow, 1993; Gould, Otto, Pollack, & Yap, 1997;

Mavissakalian & Prien, 1996) can readily be incorporated into cognitive-behavioral interventions for recurrent headache disorders.

6. *Age.* Some older patients have difficulties with attention or concentration or other problems that affect the learning of novel material. Although they typically would not benefit from MTCT, they can benefit from a clinic-based program that is modified to include weekly phone consultations, additional time to practice elementary skills before more advanced skills are introduced, and more detailed verbal and written explanations of treatment procedures (see, e.g., Arena, Hannah, Bruno, & Meador, 1991; Mosley, Grotheus, & Meeks, 1995).

Behavioral Treatment

Efficacy

Numerous qualitative and meta-analytic reviews have concluded that behavioral treatment yields a 40–60% reduction in migraine or tension-type headaches in adults, with MTCT and clinic-based treatment formats yielding similar outcomes (e.g., Blanchard, 1992; Blanchard, Andrasik, Ahles, Teders, & O'Keefe, 1980; Bogaards & ter Kuile, 1994; Haddock et al., 1997; Holroyd, in press; Holroyd & Penzien, 1986, 1990; Rowan & Andrasik, 1996). Children and adolescents may show somewhat better outcomes than adults (Hermann, Kim, & Blanchard, 1995; Holroyd, in press; Holroyd, Penzien, & Lipchik, 2001).

The U.S. Headache Consortium, a consortium of influential medical organizations,[1] drew on comprehensive evidence reports commissioned by the Agency for Health Care Research and Quality[2] (AHCRQ; Goslin, Gray, & McCrory, 2001) when they included relaxation training, thermal biofeedback combined with relaxation training, EMG biofeedback, and cognitive-behavioral therapy as empirically supported treatments in current clinical practice guidelines for the management of migraine (Campbell, Penzien, & Wall, 2000; Silberstein & Rosenberg, 2000). Similar clinical practice guidelines have yet to be developed for tension-type headache, but the initial step of evaluating the evidence base for the use of behavioral treatments has been completed (McCrory, Penzien, Hasselblad, & Gray, 2001).

Treatment Formats

Treatment can be administered individually or in a group and can be administered in a clinic-based treatment format or in an MTCT format. MTCT, or *home-based* treatment, formats were developed to reduce the cost and increase the availability of behavioral treatments

SESSION STRUCTURE

With both treatment formats, clinic sessions typically include (1) a review of self-monitoring forms and homework, (2) a discussion of any difficulties in learning and applying self-management skills up to this point, (3) the presentation of the rationale for the new headache management skill that is the focus of the present session, (4) instruction and practice in this new skill, (5) formulation of a homework assignment, and (6) summary. The goal of the skills-training portion of the session is patient demonstration of the skill during the session (e.g., role playing stress-management skills) in at least rudimentary form so that the therapist can directly observe the patient's efforts, identify problems, and provide corrective feedback.

CLINIC-BASED TREATMENT

Clinic-based treatment is likely to involve 6 to 15 or more weekly sessions, 45 to 60 minutes in length when treatment is administered individually, and 60 to 120 minutes in length when administered in a group. This treatment format offers more therapist time and attention, and allows the therapist greater opportunity to directly observe the patient than does MTCT, but requires the patient to travel more frequently to the clinic, and thus places a greater burden on the patient's schedule. Readers interested in descriptions of clinic-based treatment delivered in individual formats are referred to Blanchard and Andrasik (1985), and Martin (1993) for individual format and Scharff and Marcus (1994) for group format.

MINIMAL-THERAPIST-CONTACT TREATMENT (MTCT)

MTCT involves three to four monthly treatment sessions that are 45 to 60 minutes in length when treatment is administered individually and 60 to 120 minutes in length when administered in a group. Clinic visits are used to introduce headache management skills and to address problems encountered in acquiring or implementing these skills. The actual learning and refinement of headache management skills is guided by patient manuals and audiotapes and occurs at home. MTCT thus relies heavily on written materials and audiotapes that guide patients in learning and applying headache management skills at home.

In the protocols we describe, treatment involves four monthly clinic visits (in addition to the initial evaluation) with three brief phone consultations interspersed between clinic visits (see Table 18.1). Patient manuals and audiotapes guide patients through each of the treatment components described below.

Overview of Treatment

TENSION-TYPE HEADACHE

The primary treatment components for tension-type headache are relaxation training, cognitive-behavioral stress management (cognitive coping, problem solving), and pain management (see Table 18.1). The first month of treatment is focused on relaxation training, the second month on stress management (with an emphasis on either cognitive coping or problem solving), and the final month on the development and refinement of relaxation and stress-management skills and on the incorporation of pain management strategies into the patient's armentarium. At the final treatment session, the focus is on integrating the headache management skills that have proven effective for a given patient into a headache management plan, and on the further development and maintenance of these skills. In practice, treatment may be more individualized than this protocol suggests; although most patients are likely to follow this schedule, a few patients do well with only the relaxation and pain management components. The time devoted to each treatment

TABLE 18.1. The Structure of Minimal-Therapist-Contact Treatment

Week		Tension-type headache[a]	Migraine
1	1st clinic visit (50–60 minutes)	Orientation to self-management.	Same
		Explanation of treatment.	Same
		Introduction of progressive muscle relaxation, deep breathing, muscle stretches, imagery.	Same
2	No contact	Brief forms of relaxation.	Same
			Begin monitoring of migraine triggers/warning signs.
3	Phone consultation (15 minutes)	Address difficulties with home practice.	Same
		Preview cue-controlled relaxation, relaxation by recall, autogenic phrases.	Same
		Begin monitoring headache-related stressors.	
4	No contact	Application of quick relaxation skills to daily activities.	Same
		Begin monitoring headache-related stressors.	
5	2nd clinic visit (50–60 minutes)	Continue to refine relaxation skills if necessary.	Same
		—	Identify headache triggers and warning signs.
		Identify headache-related stressors.	Effective use of migraine medications.
		Introduce stress-management (cognitive coping or problem solving) strategies.	Develop RESCUE plan for responding to warning signs and migraines.
6	No contact	Apply and refine stress-management techniques.	Apply and refine RESCUE plan.
			Review pain management.
7	Phone consultation (15 minutes)	Address problems and refine application of stress-management techniques.	Address problems and refine RESCUE plan.
8	No contact	Continue application of stress management.	Continue with RESCUE plan incorporating pain-management skills. Preview choice of activity for 3rd treatment session.
9	3rd clinic visit (50–60 minutes)	Continue stress management, including alternate (cognitive coping or problem-solving) strategy as needed. Introduce pain management strategies.	Chosen activity is focus of this session: (1) refine skills already learned, (2) stress management, or (3) thermal biofeedback. Previous modules reviewed or new module introduced accordingly.
10	No contact	Incorporate stress-management skills into daily activities.	Practice chosen activity.

TABLE 18.1. *Continued*

Week		Tension-type headache[a]	Migraine
11	Phone consultation (15 minutes)	Address difficulties in application of stress-management skills.	Address difficulties in application of chosen skills.
12	No contact	Apply and evaluate preferred headache management skills.	Same
13	4th clinic visit (50–60 minutes)	Identify most useful headache management skills for this patient.	Same
		Develop headache management plan including coping with anticipated problems following treatment.	Same

Note. Health care professionals may request a copy of the patient manuals and audiotapes that accompany these MTCT protocols at cost from Kenneth A. Holroyd.
[a]Evaluations of this treatment (e.g., Holroyd et al., 2001) examined a version of this treatment with three, rather than four, clinic visits.

component also may vary with the patient's needs and interests.

MIGRAINE

Table 18.1 also outlines the protocol for the behavioral treatment of migraine. The first month is focused on relaxation training (as in the tension-type headache protocol). The second month is focused on the development of a RESCUE plan (*R*emain calm, *E*scape from known triggers, *S*tay away from stress or stressful situations, *C*arry your migraine medications at all times, *U*se relaxation exercises, *E*at and sleep on schedule) to respond to migraine triggers and warning signs. As part of this plan, a strategy is developed for effectively using both migraine medications and behavioral headache management strategies. The third and final month is devoted to one of three possible options: (1) continued focus on the "basic" migraine management skills that have already been covered, (2) introduction of stress-management (cognitive coping) training, or (3) introduction of thermal (hand warming) biofeedback. In addition, pain management skills (as in the tension-type headache protocol) are incorporated into the patient's armentarium.

An examination of Table 18.1 shows how migraine and tension-type headache management diverge in months 2 and 3. Although both the tension-type headache and migraine protocols include relaxation training and pain management as standard treatment components, in the migraine protocol (1) stress management is an optional component and does not include problem solving; (2) trigger identification and modification, as well as effective use of medications, receive greater attention; and (3) flexibility in the treatment components is more explicitly built into the protocol and thermal biofeedback is an optional treatment component.

Components of Behavioral Treatment

In this section, we present a description of the treatment components included in our MTCT protocols for tension-type headache and migraine. We do not present detailed descriptions of these techniques; rather, we highlight issues involved in the application of these techniques to the management of recurrent headache disorders (see Turk, Chapter 7, Arena & Blanchard, Chapter 8, and Syrjala & Abrams, Chapter 9, in this volume).

Patient Education

Recognizing and addressing countertherapeutic beliefs and instilling realistic expectancies for treatment is a necessary first step in behavioral treatment. The rigid attribution of headaches to a single, stable, uncontrollable cause (e.g., "It's just the weather," or "There's nothing I can do because it runs in my family") is likely to undermine involvement in behavioral treatment. Patients who adopt a passive stance in treatment because they assume only the therapist or only medication can help also are unlikely to put forth the effort required to learn headache management skills. Patients who expect complete or immediate relief, or who use headache management skills only when crippled by a severe headache, will likely become disillusioned and discontinue treatment.

It is critical to ensure that patients understand behavioral treatment. We use the initial part of the first treatment session to inform patients about this treatment approach, their role in the treatment, and what they can expect in terms of outcome.

1. *Structure of behavioral treatment for headache.* Orientation begins with an overview of the structure of behavioral treatment, including a brief discussion of the treatment components (e.g., relaxation, biofeedback, and stress management) and an outline of the number of sessions, timing of sessions, length of sessions, and structure of sessions.

2. *Rationale for behavioral treatment of headache.* We also provide a clear rationale for behavioral treatment of headache. We present a biopsychosocial model that conceptualizes headaches as a biological disorder in which multiple environmental, social, physical, and psychological factors play a role in the onset, course, and maintenance of headaches. The biopsychosocial model helps patients understand the relevance of psychological and behavioral interventions without conceptualizing their headaches as a psychological problem. Relaxation training is introduced as a method for reducing physical arousal and muscle tension that may be both precipitant and consequence of headaches and thermal biofeedback as a method of controlling vascular responses in migraine. Stress-management interventions (i.e., cognitive-behavioral strategies) are introduced as methods to reduce psychological reactions to stress that may trigger, aggravate, or maintain headaches. The overall rationale for behavioral treatment is introduced during the initial treatment session; at each subsequent session a specific rationale is provided for the interventions that will be introduced in that session.

3. *Treatment involves an active role from the patient and collaboration with the therapist.* Patients may enter treatment assuming they will be passive recipients of treatment, with attendance at scheduled appointments as their only responsibility. This belief will interfere with treatment adherence and is best addressed when initiating treatment. Thus, it is essential to orient patients to the collaborative process, explaining that collaboration requires active involvement of both the therapist and the patient. We explain that the role of the therapist is not to take responsibility for fixing the headaches but to provide tools for the patient to learn to better manage headaches.

4. *Homework and home-based treatment.* As part of the process of patients learning to take an active role, we stress that clinic visits are a small part of their treatment. We want patients to understand that completion of monitoring forms and practice of headache management skills at home are essential because few clinic visits are scheduled to monitor progress and learn and practice these skills. Thus, we inform patients that benefits from behavioral headache management are contingent upon regular practice.

5. *Developing realistic expectations for treatment outcome.* In helping patients to develop realistic expectations for improvement, we explain that a "cure" is not likely. We tell patients that by applying skills and making lifestyle changes, they are likely to experience moderate reductions in headache activity; a reduced need for drug therapy; improvements in affective distress, quality of life, and functioning; and a restored sense of personal control over headaches. We explain that we cannot predict who will benefit, or the exact benefit a particular patient will receive. We also warn that improvement is not likely to be observed until headache management skills are used for a number of months. Although we acknowledge that headache management skills may affect the duration and severity of headache episodes, we emphasize that behavioral treatments are to be used regularly with the

result being the *prevention* of headache episodes.

Therapist Attitude

Because patients' confidence in their ability to manage their headaches may be more important than their ability to regulate a specific physiological response (Blanchard et al., 1983; Holroyd et al., 1984), it is important for the therapist to attend to patients' perceptions of their performance as well as to their actual performance during skill training. We review the patient's performance with optimism, initially magnifying small successes and normalizing any problems as manageable phases of treatment. We encourage patients to take credit for their successes throughout treatment. We remind them, we serve primarily as teachers and coaches, while they do the more difficult work of experimenting with and refining the various headache management techniques.

Relaxation

ORIENTATION

We explain that relaxation skills may enable patients to (1) decrease their overall level of muscle tension and autonomic arousal and (2) recognize subtle signs of increased muscle tension so they can apply brief relaxation skills to prevent the buildup of additional muscle tension.

Relaxation training includes abbreviated progressive muscle relaxation (PMR) training and "quick relaxation" techniques that we encourage patients to use throughout the day. We teach a variety of "quick relaxation" skills including abdominal breathing, relaxation by recall, cue-controlled relaxation, and autogenic phrases. It is unrealistic to expect patients to become proficient in all these strategies, or to build all the strategies into their repertoire. Instead, we encourage patients to learn and try each of the strategies before deciding on those they want to build into their regular routine. Full scripts of relaxation sessions with instructions for therapists are presented elsewhere (Bernstein & Borkovec, 1973; Bernstein & Carlson, 1993; Blanchard & Andrasik, 1985; see also Syrjala & Abrams, Chapter 9, this volume). These resources also pro-

vide instructions for teaching the "quick relaxation" skills we use.

INSTRUCTION

Prior to initiating PMR training, abdominal breathing is introduced (see "Muscle Scanning and Quick Relaxation" section) and patients are instructed to practice abdominal breathing periodically during the PMR training session. Throughout the training session, we monitor behavioral signs of relaxation (see Table 18.2) and ask the patient to repeat a tension-release cycle if we notice a muscle group has not relaxed.

PMR training begins with tension-release cycles in order to relax the entire body. Muscles of the shoulders, neck, and face receive the greatest attention because they are most likely involved in headaches. At the end of PMR training, an image, selected by the patient prior to PMR practice, is used to demonstrate the use relaxation through guided imagery (see "Muscle Scanning and Quick Relaxation" section).

We suggest patients practice PMR at the least once, and preferably twice a day, in the morning and in the afternoon or evening. We require patients to keep records or logs of their home practice. The log includes the date of practice and relaxation ratings before and after practice using a rating scale from 0 (no tension, or most relaxed you can imagine) to 100 (extremely tense, or the most tense you can remember). We pay particular attention to problems that are commonly encountered during relaxation training and possible therapeutic responses, which are presented in Table 18.3.

When patients have mastered the initial muscle relaxation procedure, they are encouraged to practice briefer tension-release cycles using the audiotapes that are provided (see Table 18.2). Progress is determined by the individual needs of each patient. If an anxious patient has extreme difficulty concentrating, we may introduce only muscle stretching and abdominal breathing at the first session. Once a variety of brief relaxation techniques (see "Muscle Scanning and Quick Relaxation" section) have been mastered, the focus shifts to incorporating brief relaxation skills into daily living. Even moderate levels of muscle tension, or a situation that has been associated with tension in the

TABLE 18.2. Relaxed Behaviors Based on Poppen's Behavioral Relaxation Scale

1. *Head:* supported by chair; head not tilted; nose in midline of the body, no motion
2. *Eyes:* eyelids lightly closed with smooth appearance; no motion under eyelids
3. *Mouth:* lips parted slightly at the center of the mouth; front teeth slightly parted; no tongue movement
4. *Throat:* no motion (e.g., swallowing, other larynx action, twitches)
5. *Shoulders:* slightly rounded, transect same horizontal plane and rest against chair; no motion
6. *Body:* torso, hips, legs are symmetrical around midline and resting on chair; no movement
7. *Hands:* resting on armrest or lap with palms down and fingers slightly curled in a clawlike fashion
8. *Feet:* pointed away from each other at a 60- to 90-degree angle; feet not crossed at ankle; no movement
9. *Quiet:* no vocalizations or loud respiratory sounds (no talking, sighing, laughing, gasping, coughing)
10. *Breathing:* breath frequency less than observed at beginning of session; no breathing irregularities that interrupt the regular rhythm of breathing (e.g., coughing, sneezing, yawning).

Note. Based on Poppen (1988).

past, become a cue to use brief relaxation skills.

MUSCLE STRETCHING

Muscle-stretching exercises strengthen and lengthen sore and tight pericranial muscles. Gentle neck and shoulder stretches using sideways turns of the head and forward bends and diagonal bends of the neck and head are demonstrated (see, e.g., DeGood, 1997). The patient with a head-forward posture is instructed to monitor head and neck posture and to use chin tucks throughout the day to change this postural habit. The patient is instructed to perform brief gentle stretches intermittently throughout the day, as well as immediately prior to practicing PMR. We explain that as they progress, they will be more aware of muscles that tighten prior to, or early in, a headache episode. This awareness will allow them to stretch or relax muscles strategically, preventing muscle tension from developing into a full-blown headache. Muscle-stretching exercises need to be done gently so that already constricted shoulder and neck muscles are not extended so far as to induce pain or injury.

MUSCLE SCANNING AND QUICK RELAXATION

Quick relaxation techniques enable the patient to rapidly evoke the relaxation response that was learned during PMR train-

ing. Therefore, before attempting "quick relaxation" it is important that the patient is able to relax deeply when practicing the full version of PMR.

To provide information that patients can use to decide when to practice quick relaxation techniques, they are asked to periodically "scan" or monitor sensations of muscle tension, particularly in the shoulders, neck, and face, during the day. Scanning increases awareness of even low levels of muscle tension. Identifying low levels of tension then provides a cue for the early use of one of the quick relaxation techniques. Early use of relaxation techniques will help to *prevent* muscle tension from increasing and developing into a headache. Patients are encouraged to use specific cues such as a change-of-work task, the alarm on their wristwatch or computer, or stick-on colored dots placed in strategic locations to provide a signal to use "quick relaxation" skills. With practice, the external reminders may no longer be needed as patients will have integrated muscle scanning and their preferred quick relaxation techniques into their daily routine.

Abdominal Breathing. Abdominal or diaphragmatic breathing brings inhaled air to the base of the lungs, where oxygen is most efficiently transferred to the bloodstream. Abdominal deep breathing involves slow deep breaths (about 10 breaths per minute), with exhalation longer than inhalation. Ini-

TABLE 18.3. Relaxation Training: Problems and Solutions

Problems	Solutions
Patient's attitude	
1. Patient is self-critical or hesitant during training.	Identify self-critical thoughts and help patient to challenge them. Offer reassurance.
2. Patient is overly concerned about performance.	Suggest trying hard is counterproductive; instruct in alternative attitude of passive volition.
3. Patient is hesitant to relinquish control.	Discuss fears about loss of control; explain that novelty of sensations of relaxation may be triggering anxiety.
Learning the skill	
1. Patient's concentration is disturbed by distracting thoughts or feelings. This is most common problem; may want to discuss with patient prior to practice.	Encourage patient *not* to fight these thoughts but to let them pass through mind. Remind patient these thoughts will lessen as patient gets better at relaxation. Use imagery techniques (e.g., placing interfering thoughts in an imaginary trunk, thoughts floating by on clouds) or autogenic phrases (e.g., peaceful and calm) to focus attention. If they continue, and are severe, try thought stopping.
2. Patient falls asleep when practicing relaxation	Do not schedule relaxation practice just after meals or just before bedtime. Practice seated rather than lying down.
3. Patient has difficulty detecting difference between sensations of tension and relaxation.	Have patient place one hand on muscle while tensing vs. relaxing muscle. Introduce alternate tensing techniques. Use partial tensing of muscles (discrimination training) to help patient identify subtle cues of tension and relaxation.
4. Certain muscles are difficult to relax.	Repeat tensing–relaxing sequence with specific muscles; use muscle stretching exercises prior to relaxation practice.
Maintenance and generalization	
1. Patient reports no carryover effect after relaxation.	Introduce brief cue-controlled relaxation techniques to use periodically throughout the day. Identify thoughts or situations that evoke arousal.
2. Patient has difficulty detecting difference between sensations of tension and relaxation in daily situations.	Ask patient to discuss a recently stressful situation, note any muscle tension, such as clenched jaws or fists, furrowed brows, tightened shoulders.

tially patients are asked to practice abdominal breathing for 5 to 10 minutes twice daily. Patients are also asked to subvocalize the word "relax" with each exhalation, as they attend to the rhythm of their breathing. In time, the subvocalized "relax" can serve as a cue to trigger a quick relaxation response (see "Cue-Controlled Relaxation" section). When first learning diaphragmatic breathing, some patients may overly focus on the mechanics of the technique while trying to do it "correctly." Such a focus can be counterproductive to the elicitation of the relaxation response. Instructing these patients to simply observe their breathing can be helpful.

Guided Imagery. In guided imagery, a pleasant relaxing image is called to mind and attention focused on the sensory details (e.g., sensations of light, color, sound, temperature, texture, and physical activity) in this image (see Syrjala and Abrams, Chapter 9, this volume). Using imagery can be helpful in evoking a quick relaxation response as well as providing a brief respite from a stressful situation. We incorporate instructions for guided imagery into the PMR protocol to further deepen relaxation. It is not expected that all patients will have the ability to easily develop an image or use imagery as a quick relaxation strategy.

Relaxation by Recall/Cue-Controlled Relaxation. In relaxation by recall, the relaxation response is produced without tensing muscles, by mentally evoking sensations of relaxation in specific muscle groups. The patient first identifies sensations of tension in specific muscle groups (e.g., by muscle scanning) and then mentally evokes or recalls sensations of relaxation, maintaining sensations of relaxation for 30 to 40 seconds. Typically a cue or signal (e.g., the word "relax") that has been repeatedly paired with the relaxation response during PMR practice is used to evoke the relaxation response, hence the term "cue-controlled relaxation."

Autogenic Training. Autogenic training (AT) is a system of psychosomatic self-regulation that permits the gradual acquisition of autonomic control. In AT, phrases such as "my forehead is cool," "my arms feel heavy and warm," or "I feel relaxed and at peace" are subvocalized as the patient concentrates on his or her body sensations in a passive manner evoking the physiological sensations and mental state described in the phrase (Schultz & Luthe, 1959). We instruct patients to become aware of what appears to be their random thoughts and images, or "mental traffic." We suggest that they use autogenic phrases to counteract their racing, automatic thoughts in order to control their "mental traffic" and facilitate deep relaxation.

Identifying Early Warning Signs and Headache Precipitants

ORIENTATION

If patients are alerted to common migraine triggers and *early warning signs* or prodromal symptoms and these are recorded prospectively, most patients can learn to identify both headache triggers and early headache warning signs. This information is valuable because it allows patients to take more effective action to prevent or manage their headaches. Identification of previously unrecognized triggers opens up new options for the prevention of headaches. Prodromal symptoms can provide early warning signs or cues to employ behavioral headache management skills or, when appropriate, to use medication abortively.

INSTRUCTION

We assist patients in systematically recording possible prodromal symptoms and in evaluating their significance. Prodromal symptoms can be psychological, neurological, or general (constitutional, autonomic). Psychological symptoms include irritability, depression, moodiness, euphoria, restlessness, hyperactivity, fatigue, and drowsiness. Neurological symptoms include photophobia, phonophobia, hyperosmia, yawning, dysphasia, and difficulty concentrating. General symptoms can include stiff neck, food cravings, cold feeling, anorexia, increased thirst, fluid retention, frequent urination, diarrhea or constipation, or sluggishness. These prodromal symptoms differ between people but are fairly consistent within the same person.

Although prodromal symptoms may be difficult to link to migraine episodes initially, it is helpful for patients to learn to identify them so that they can predict an attack and prepare for it. To help identify prodromal symptoms, we ask patients to record any "odd" or "just not right" sensations they experienced prior to the onset of the migraine. Next, we ask patients to identify how often these symptoms occur without getting a migraine. Such identification enables patients to determine whether a symptom is truly a prodromal symptom.

An aura occurs prior to headache onset or early in a headache episode, lasts approximately 30 minutes, and is typically visual (i.e., blurred vision, photopsia, or fortification spectra) but may also include parathesias, olfactory hallucinations, motor weakness, ataxia, dysarthria or aphasia, and conscious trance-like states. Aura symptoms are reviewed so the minority patients with aura can use these early warning signs in the same fashion as they would prodromal symptoms.

We also assist patients in systematically recording possible headache precipitants and evaluating their significance. Many precipitants are relevant for both migraine and tension-type headache. General population studies indicate that stress, sleep difficulties, and hormonal factors (relevant specifically for migraine) are the most frequently identified triggers (Rasmussen, 1993). Table 18.4 lists the most common headache precipitants, or triggers, identified by people with headaches.

We explain that headache precipitants are not universal and do not necessarily precipitate an attack on every exposure. Headaches may occur hours after exposure to a headache trigger. Several precipitants occurring within close proximity are more likely to trigger a migraine than is a single precipitant. Patients begin by noting whether particular settings, times of the day or week, or activities are associated with headache onset. They also review the 12 hours or so prior to each headache onset for possible headache precipitants to determine whether a pattern emerges. Prospective monitoring often identifies triggers that had not been noticed or were overlooked.

STRESS

Stress is the most frequently identified headache precipitant for both migraine and tension-type headache (Rasmussen, 1993). The relaxation techniques and cognitive-behavioral (CB) interventions address headaches that occur in response to stress.

TABLE 18.4. Precipitating Factors for Headache Identified by Patients

Lifestyle factors
  Fatigue
  Inconsistent eating patterns
    Fasting
    Missing meals
    Insufficient food
  Sleep
    Excessive sleep
    Unrefreshing sleep
    Insufficient sleep
    Change in sleep schedule
    Sleep problems (i.e., delayed onset and
      restless sleep)

Stress
  During stress
  After stress (i.e., "let-down headache")
Smoking or passive smoke
Travel

Specific foods
  Aged cheese
  Alcoholic beverages
  Artificial sweeteners (i.e., aspartame)
  Beans
  Caffeine (coffee, tea, cola)
  Chocolate

Citrus fruit
Cured meats
Fish
Monosodium glutamate
Nuts
Yeast

Hormonal and physical factors
  Head or neck injury
  Hormone replacement therapy
  Medications
  Menstrual period (before, during, after)

Oral contraceptives
Physical exertion
Postmenopausal changes

Environment
  Altitude changes
  Air pollution
  Bright or flickering lights, glare
  Exposure to vapors or chemicals (i.e., gasoline,
    industrial fumes, cleaning products)
  Motion

Noise
Perfumes, colognes
Smoke
Strong odors
Weather changes (i.e., barometric changes)

Note. Information from Blau and Thavaplan (1988); Radnitz (1990); Rasmussen (1993); Robbins (1994).

SLEEP

People with either migraine or tension-type headache frequently identify sleep difficulties as a headache precipitant, with insufficient sleep, oversleeping, or an irregular sleep schedule identified as the most common sleep precipitants (Rasmussen, 1993; Sahota & Dexter, 1990). Patients with these sleep complaints are instructed in sleep hygiene and advised to maintain a regular sleep schedule. Practicing relaxation techniques prior to bedtime may facilitate sleep onset. CB interventions also can reduce sleep maintenance problems (Edinger, Wohlgemuth, Radtke, Marsh, & Quillian, 2001). Headaches also may arise as a consequence of a primary sleep disorder, such as sleep apnea. Thus, it is worthwhile to screen for the presence of a sleep disorder and to refer to a sleep specialist when a sleep disorder is suspected (Paiva, Batista, Martins, & Martins, 1995).

HORMONAL FACTORS

Reproductive hormones (menarche, menstruation, pregnancy, menopause, hormone replacement therapy) are associated with headache disorders, particularly migraine (for reviews, see Holroyd & Lipchik, 1997, 2000; Silberstein & Merriman, 1997). The behavioral treatments discussed in this chapter are effective in managing these headaches (for review, see Holroyd & Lipchik, 1997, 2000).

MEAL SCHEDULES AND DIETARY FACTORS

Close to 30% of people with headaches, primarily those with migraine, report that dietary factors, such as skipping or delaying meals or ingesting specific foods, beverages, or ingredients sometimes trigger their headaches (Robbins, 1994). Few double-blind studies of dietary triggers have been conducted and clinical opinions differ regarding the benefits from dietary alterations (Blau & Thavapalan, 1988; Medina & Diamond, 1978; Silberstein, Saper, & Frietag, 2001). Most people with headaches do not require severely restricted diets but should avoid foods or additives that they believe might trigger a headache. Generally, it is advised that people with migraine consume alcohol, particularly red wine, with caution. People with migraine may also benefit from a trial of limiting or eliminating monosodium glutamate, aspartame, and nitrites as these substances often trigger migraine episodes in susceptible individuals (Silberstein et al., 2001). Individuals with migraine should be cautioned that missing or delaying meals can also trigger headaches.

The role of caffeine as a potential precipitant may need to be explored if individuals with migraine regularly consume more than 300 milligrams of caffeine a day (approximately the amount found in two strong cups of coffee), because this amount of caffeine may precipitate migraines through the rebound effect or through caffeine sensitivity. People who ingest caffeine during the day may experience caffeine withdrawal at night and thus may be awakened by a migraine at night or first thing in the morning. This does not necessarily imply that caffeine must be completely avoided. Many migraine medications contain caffeine to facilitate absorption of the medication and counteract the drowsiness induced by some medications. Caffeine in medications thus must be included in calculations of caffeine intake. Prospective monitoring may help to determine whether caffeine intake or withdrawal are precipitants for a particular patient.

ENVIRONMENTAL FACTORS

People with headaches should be assisted in avoiding or restricting their exposure to various environmental factors they have identified as headache triggers. They also should be alerted to the possible effects of common environmental precipitants (see Table 18.4). Avoiding and restricting exposure to environmental precipitants can typically be accomplished with little lifestyle disruption.

Effective Use of Migraine Medications

ORIENTATION

We emphasize that effective use of headache medications may involve the application of complex decision rules; thus, making these rules explicit enables patients to use their medications more effectively. We help the patient develop and effectively apply optimal decision rules to guide the use of symptomatic and abortive medications, as well as relaxation, cognitive, and other psychological headache management techniques. The goal is both to prevent medication overuse and to maximize the effectiveness of headache medications. To assist patients in effectively using migraine medications, the therapist must be knowledgeable about headache medications and work closely with the prescribing physician.

HEADACHE MEDICATIONS

Following is a synopsis of four types of migraine medication. Detailed discussions of these medications can be found in Baumel (1994), Davidoff (1995), Saper, Silberstein, Gordon, and Hamel (1993), and Silberstein and colleagues (2001). Holroyd and colleagues (1998) present guidelines for the integration of medication and behavioral treatment.

Symptomatic medications include analgesics prescribed primarily to reduce pain such as nonsteroidal anti-inflammatory drugs (NSAIDs), mixed analgesics containing barbiturates (e.g., butalbital) or opioids (i.e., codeine), and opioids alone (i.e., oxycodone). Effective symptomatic therapy should reduce pain from mild to none or from moderate to mild within 1 to 2 hours. The use of opioid and mixed analgesics must be limited because overuse can cause rebound headaches and even addiction. NSAIDs are probably less likely to induce rebound headaches but nevertheless should be used in moderation.

Abortive medications include NSAIDs, ergotamine derivatives, and serotonin-receptor agonists (triptans such as sumatriptan, rizatriptan, naratriptan, zolmitrptan, and almotriptan). Effective abortive therapy should prevent migraine pain from becoming moderate or severe if taken when pain is mild or reduce severe or moderate pain to mild or no pain within 2 hours. These agents should be used no more than 2 to 3 days per week to avoid rebound headaches.

Antiemetics (e.g., prochlorperazine and metoclopramide) are used to treat the nausea and vomiting associated with migraines. The goal of antiemetic therapy is to reduce nausea within 1 to 2 hours and control vomiting most of the time. Antiemetics also improve the absorption of some oral medications, including analgesics, and may have antimigraine effects themselves. Patients who experience nausea and vomiting are instructed to take an antiemetic before or along with their analgesic.

Preventive or prophylactic medications for migraine include beta-blockers, calcium channel blockers, antidepressants (tricyclic, serotonin reuptake inhibitors, and monoamine oxidase inhibitors), anticonvulsants, and NSAIDs; antidepressants (for the most part tricyclics) are the primary preventive medications for tension-type headache (Holroyd et al., 1998; Silberstein et al., 2001). The goal of preventive therapy is to reduce the frequency of headaches by 50% or more.

INSTRUCTION

The symptomatic and abortive use of medication receives the greatest attention because effective use of these medications may require complex decisions that take into account the limits on the use of the medication, patients' headache symptoms (e.g., Do these symptoms predict a moderate to severe migraine?), and previous empirical observations of patients' responses to specific medications. For example, for one headache sufferer, analgesics, NSAIDs, or a single triptan dose may effectively abort a migraine when taken early in the migraine episode, but the same medication will be much less effective, even in multiple doses, when taken later in a migraine episode. In this case, overall medication use per episode can be reduced and the efficacy of the medication improved by implementing a judicious plan to initiate treatment early. Another person may be unable to confidently predict whether a mild headache will develop into a severe migraine; attempting to initiate treatment early in an episode, the person may not only fail to reduce medication consumption but may be tempted to overuse medications. Thus, effective use of medications in the acute treatment of migraine requires a systematic plan that takes multiple factors into account in each decision to treat. Decision rules also must be refined as the patient collects data by experimenting with different possible treatment options. We assist the patient in formulating decision rules for medication use that are consistent with medical advice and help the patient conduct and evaluate data from "experiments" to test different treatment options.

Responding to Early Warning Signs and Triggers

ORIENTATION

The information that has been collected about early headache warning signs and headache triggers is now used to develop an action plan that is directed at preventing and managing headaches. The prodromal symptoms and aura symptoms the patient has identified serve as signals to take actions to abort or reduce the severity of the anticipated migraines. Headache triggers provide information that can help the patient take actions to prevent or manage headaches. The goal is to replace the sense of dread, anxiety, and helplessness many people feel when anticipating a headache with a sense of self-efficacy and a plan of action.

INSTRUCTION

Decisions about effective medication use and about the use of relaxation skills are integrated in an action plan that incorporates this new knowledge about early headache warning signs and headache triggers. For example, specific early warning signs that reliably signal the onset of a migraine may now serve as a cue for a patient to use a triptan medication, apply quick relaxation skills, and limit exposure to possible triggers. This tentative action plan is then further refined on the basis of subsequent experience. As noted, we use the RESCUE acronym to remind patients of general principles underlying the RESCUE plan but develop a specific plan for each person.

- *Remain calm.* Worrying about how to work around a migraine or denying that it might occur usually makes it more long lasting and severe.
- *Escape from known triggers.* Your body may be more susceptible to triggers during the preheadache (or prodrome) phase. Avoid or minimize triggers wherever possible.

- *Stay away from stress or stressful situations.* Avoid taking on extra work. Let some things go that do not have to be completed right now. Be extra kind to yourself.
- *Carry your migraine medications with you at all times.* Make sure you have quick and easy access to your medications wherever you go. Always be prepared.
- *Use relaxation exercises.* Concentrate on the ones you find most useful. Remember that relaxation may help control some of the physical changes associated with migraine.
- *Eat and sleep on schedule.* This is not the time to skip meals or go without sleep. Do not try to finish everything you think you have to do before the migraine begins.

Cognitive-Behavioral Stress Management

Experience with clinic-based cognitive-behavioral therapy (CBT) for headache is helpful before attempting to administer CBT in a home-based format. Basic descriptions of CBT can be found in A. Beck and colleagues (1979), Beck and Emery (1985), J. Beck (1995), Greenberger and Padesky (1995), Persons (1989), and Turk, Chapter 7, this volume.

ORIENTATION

We suggest that stress management is an important headache management skill because stress is the most frequently reported headache trigger. For patients who view stress as unrelated to their headaches, we note that the occurrence of a headache itself is stressful. We also may focus on related targets (e.g., anxiety), or with migraine we may skip stress management (see Table 18.1). In brief treatment the goal is for patients to acquire a set of basic stress-management skills and sufficient confidence (self-efficacy) in their ability to apply and further develop their rudimentary skills in increasingly difficult situations following treatment.

Stress management begins with a description of the stress reaction (i.e., physical, emotional, and cognitive components), the role of stress in triggering and aggravating headache episodes, and the role of cognition in shaping the stress reaction. The therapist explains that stress reactions have three components: physical (e.g., neck tension and rapid heart rate), emotional (e.g., frustration and anxiety), and cognitive (e.g., worry). Thoughts and beliefs or the cognitive component is central in that it can render the person vulnerable to stress. We explain that stress-generating thoughts have three characteristics. They (1) are automatic (i.e., occur habitually without any conscious effort or awareness), (2) distort the situation or the patient's coping options to some extent, and (3) have a negative emotional and physical impact. We further suggest that stress reactions can be managed with strategies that counteract, challenge, or reappraise stress-generating thoughts.

To illustrate how thoughts mediate the stress reaction, we use generic examples of the way thoughts associated with common stressors (e.g., work demands, social situations, refusing demands, criticism, or headaches themselves) can trigger or magnify a stress reaction. We attempt to use examples that are relevant to the particular patient and to phrase the examples in the patient's own words. Examples begin with identification of a specific stressful situation, preferably one that is associated with headaches for the patient; identification of the emotional, physical, and cognitive components of the stress reaction; and an analysis of how thoughts shaped the stress reaction. This analysis is most effective when a detailed account of the patient's reactions to stress is obtained from daily diaries rather than from a general retrospective reconstruction of the patient's stress reaction (Holroyd & Andrasik, 1982).

To assist patients in observing headache-related stress reactions, patients are asked to complete thought monitoring forms similar to those used in CBT (Beck et al., 1979; Greenberger & Padesky, 1995). These stress analysis worksheets require patients to identify stressful situations and their thoughts and feelings during the stressful situation. Completion of these worksheets helps patients observe relationships between cognitions, emotions, and physical reactions. The worksheets also provide the therapist with valuable information about the patient's current coping skills (or lack thereof).

INSTRUCTION

We use two general approaches to *cognitive restructuring.* Self-talk strategies (Meichenbaum, 1977) may help patients control situation specific stress-generating thoughts (e.g., "I'll never meet my sales goal by the end of the month."). Strategies for identifying and challenging the beliefs or assumptions that underlie stress-generating thoughts ("If I don't meet my sales goal I'm a failure.") help patients control a class of stress-generating thoughts that appear in different guises across similar stressful situations. The first step in applying either of these cognitive restructuring approaches is to identify a stressor and a cognitive target.

Identifying a Stressor and Cognitive Target. Reviewing information from the patient's stress analysis worksheets, we generate a list of stressful situations, emphasizing stressors that are associated with headaches. Patients typically identify several stressful situations. We choose a stressor that we believe can be addressed in brief treatment.

Once an appropriate stressful situation has been identified we proceed to the collaborative identification of a cognitive target; that is, we choose the stress-related cognitions that will be the focus of the session. The targeted cognitions may be stress-generating *thoughts* associated with a specific situation or an underlying *belief* or assumption that distills the common meaning or theme from many stress-generating thoughts. For example, a patient who reported experiencing frequent headaches in response to new sales goals that she feared she was unable to meet recorded the thought "I have let the company down (by not meeting this month's sales goal)." This thought appeared (on the basis of other evidence) to be related to the belief that "if I fail to meet this goal or make a mistake, I am a failure."

Stress-generating beliefs commonly reflect perfectionism, excessive need for approval, and excessive need for control. To identify beliefs, look for a theme that explains a pattern of stress reactions exhibited by the patient; that is, the situations the patient finds stressful and the patient's thoughts, emotions, and behavior in these stressful situations.

Stress-generating thoughts and behaviors occurring in the treatment session itself provide special therapeutic insight and leverage because the patient's behavior can be observed directly rather than inferred from patient report and diary recordings. For example, when a patient describes stressful situations that appear to be associated with nonassertive behavior, we might ask ourselves: "Does this patient's timidity and self-critical posture with me provide information about the stressful situation she describes at work? Might her boss continue to add to her responsibilities because she never protests or gives a clear indication she is distressed by this? Has she reported thoughts that might further explain her inability to refuse new demands? Has she refused a homework assignment, disagreed with me, or shown other sparks of independence in therapy?" If the answer to this final question is no, we might ask ourselves "Is this a good point to obtain the patient's input before I proceed with this hypothesis?" If the answer is yes, we might think "What enabled her to show this independence here (but not at work) that we might capitalize on in managing stress at work?" Once a cognitive target is identified, it is important to make an explicit agreement with the patient that this cognitive target will be the focus of the session.

Challenging Stress-Generating Thoughts. When the identified cognitive target involves stress-generating thoughts, adaptive coping statements can be generated to interrupt the flow of these thoughts. Methods of challenging stress-generating thoughts might include evaluation of evidence for the stress-generating thought: "Lets see what evidence we can find for (the statement implicit or explicit in the stress-generating thought)." We then assist the patient in finding both confirming and disconfirming evidence for this thought and in weighing the evidence. It is important that the therapist adopt an inquiring stance and remain open to any outcome, including the confirmation of the stress-generating thought. Verbal challenges may proceed to the generation of alternative adaptive coping statements. For example, to manage the thought "I'll never meet my sales goal by the end of the month," adaptive coping statements might include statements such as "At this time, there is no way to tell how far I'll get this month. Instead I'll focus on the task at hand and I'll see how far I get" and "I'll focus on what I can do; if I need to, I'll find a way to work toward meeting my goal next month." Coping self-statements are best developed collaboratively so the patient is not a passive recipient of a prepackaged coping statement. The act of collaboratively formulating coping statements that feel "right" or "potent" may be more therapeutic than the exact coping statement that results from this exercise. A useful coping statement is typically stated in the patient's own words and framed within the patient's belief system so that it undermines problematic beliefs "from within." Adaptive coping statements can be particularly helpful in short-circuiting stress-generating thoughts that occur in reaction to specific, circumscribed, and time-limited stressors.

Challenging Stress-Generating Beliefs. When the identified cognitive target involves a stress-generating belief, the patient may be pushed to examine it. Stress-generating beliefs can be challenged in much the same way as stress-generating thoughts. Other techniques for working with stress-generating beliefs include decatastrophizing or the "what if" technique, and cost-benefit analysis (see Beck & Emery, 1985). For example, perfectionistic beliefs such as "I must never make a mistake or I am a failure" are often defended on the grounds that they are necessary for high achievement. However, when the costs as well as the benefits of this belief are listed, the list can highlight costs such as time devoted to unimportant tasks (they need to be done perfectly), anxiety ("I might fail"), and frustration (" I have to do better") in achievement situations and avoidance of opportunities (exploring new opportunities requires a tolerance for initial failure).

Alternative views techniques that encourage the patient to generate alternative explanations for events that confirm a stress-generating belief can be particularly helpful. The patient might be asked "What might Ann [a respected friend, relative or coworker] think if you refused this new responsibility?" or "What would you say to Ann if she was asked to do this and declined with the explanation that her workload was full?" It can be helpful in working with alternative views to reverse roles with the patient, where the therapist plays the patient, adopting and defending the patient's belief system, while the patient plays the therapist, attempting to challenge the targeted dysfunctional belief. For example, the woman described earlier who failed to meet the sales goal for 1 month might be asked, "What would you say to a colleague who failed to meet the sales goal?" or "What would you think about a colleague if he or she didn't meet this goal?"

All CBT sessions culminate in a homework assignment that is designed to continue or extend the work done in the session. Homework assignments that are developed collaboratively and incorporate input from the patient are most likely to be carried out. Typical homework tasks include engaging in a specific behavior that is avoided because of a stress-generating belief; asking a significant other what he or she would think of this behavior; or collection of additional diary data on thoughts, feelings, and behaviors in stressful situations. For example, a patient who believes "I must be perfect, never make a mistake, or I am a failure" might be asked to intentionally make a small mistake and carefully record the consequences. Alternatively, the patient might inquire of coworkers (or family members, if more appropriate) how they would feel and think about the patient if the patient made a specific feared mistake.

PROBLEM SOLVING

Problem solving focuses directly on actions that can be taken to alter the stressful situation. Problem solving guides patients through the steps of identifying the problem, generating possible coping strategies, choosing a preferred coping strategy, and implementing and evaluating the chosen coping strategy (D'Zurilla, 1989, 1990). As was noted previously, the problem or stressful situation should be one that is likely to be manageable in brief treatment. In describing the problem we limit the description to a well-defined circumscribed situation and include only the facts and not one's own appraisal of the problem (e.g.,

"Forty-five minutes before my work day ended I was handed five new tasks," instead of "At the last possible moment I was handed an impossible number of tasks that I'm expected to get all done before I leave."). In generating possible solutions, the focus is on brainstorming to generate as many possible coping strategies as possible. The goal is to move patients beyond the mode of considering a single problematic coping strategy. Choosing a coping strategy often involves cognitive restructuring, as beliefs that restrict the choice of options the patient considers (e.g., "The only choice I have is to stay here until all the tasks are completed") need to be challenged. In selecting a coping strategy, we focus on a solution that is viable, can be implemented before the next treatment contact (phone contact or clinic visit), and is likely to have an impact on the stressful situation (e.g., "I can talk to my supervisor about how I can prioritize the tasks I have in the time I have remaining" vs. "I have to quit and start looking for a new job"). Frequently the chosen coping strategy requires that the patient engage in a previously avoided behavior. Once a coping strategy is chosen we may discuss problems likely to be encountered in executing the coping strategy and role-play its execution.

Table 18.5 presents problems commonly encountered during CB stress management and possible therapeutic responses.

Thermal Biofeedback

ORIENTATION

Thermal biofeedback was initially identified as a treatment for migraine 30 years ago at the Menninger Foundation (Sargent, Green, & Walters, 1972). Although the exact mechanism of thermal biofeedback is not well understood, the voluntary hand-warming response appears to induce changes in vascular activity that can prevent or abort migraines. Like relaxation training, thermal biofeedback is a preventive strategy, not an acute intervention. To maximize its preventive effects, daily practice is important. Additional information about the use of thermal biofeedback in the treatment of migraine can be found in Holroyd and colleagues (1998), Blanchard and Andrasik

TABLE 18.5. Cognitive-Behavioral Stress Management Therapy: Problems and Solutions*

Problems	Solutions
Treatment rationale	
1. Patient does not see her/his behavior as influencing stress responses or headaches.	Use personal examples to illustrate how cognitions influence stress responses. Review rationale using concrete examples.
Monitoring stress and identifying a target problem	
1. Patient presents a large number of stressful situations.	Be alert to common themes that cut across multiple problems. List problems from largest to smallest. Choose manageable problem as an initial focus. Structure session to maintain focus on a selected problem.
2. Headaches are not clearly stress related, or patient unable to identify stress-related thoughts.	Review headache records and analyze situations associated with headache. First, use physical cues, stressful events associated with headaches to recognize onset of episode, then identify concrete thoughts present prior to onset. Use events that occur in therapy as opportunity to identify automatic thoughts occurring in the "here and now."
3. Headache always present.	Identify factors associated with exacerbation rather than onset of headache. Consider focusing on potential aggravating factors (e.g., chronic stress, depression, anxiety or worry, and lack of sleep).
4. Patient's and therapist's preferred target problem differ.	Openly discuss difference of opinion; defer to patient if patient's preference strongly held.
Coping skills training and application	
1. Patient does not attempt, or attempts but "fails" homework assignment.	Examine patient's thoughts about homework assignment for clues to maladaptive thoughts/beliefs. Frame assignments as opportunity to learn. Break assignment into easier tasks. Change homework assignment (focus) if necessary.
2. Patient believes external pressures prevent change (e.g., inflexibility in job situation).	Be alert to thoughts or beliefs that prevent patient from seeing alternatives. Experiment with small change (e.g., muscle stretching during bathroom break). Discuss persons who the patient identifies as effective copers for models of feasible change. Brainstorm without requiring that alternatives generated be perceived as feasible.
3. Maladaptive thoughts seem self-evidently true to patient.	Offer variety of alternative explanations of same "facts." Evaluate the evidence for and against maladaptive appraisals. Reverse roles with patient.
4. Friction or difficulties in therapeutic alliance.	Openly discuss conflict. Be alert to possibility that difficulty provides information about patients coping. Admit errors.

Note. Based on Holroyd, Lipchik, and Penzien (1998).

(1985), and Arena and Blanchard (Chapter 8, this volume).

INSTRUCTION

The goal is to teach patients to warm their hands through volitional peripheral vasodilation with the assistance of sensory feed- back. Thermal biofeedback involves the use of a temperature-sensitive probe (a thermis- tor) and an electronic device that converts the temperature signal to a feedback dis- play, which is typically visual but may be auditory. We usually place the thermistor on the ventral pad of the last digit of the index finger. We use medical tape to hold the thermistor in close contact with skin but avoid encircling the finger completely as it is important to avoid creation of a tourniquet. We keep the room relatively warm (around 75°F) because it is difficult to warm one's hands in a cool room. For MTCT biofeedback, we give patients a small digital biofeedback device sensitive to 0.1°F with a screen that updates every 2 seconds (Bio-Medical Instruments, Inc; www.bio-medical.com, available for less than $20). More sensitive and quickly responding instruments can be obtained at a somewhat higher cost, and crude alcohol-in-glass thermometers can be obtained for 50 cents.

It is important for patients to develop a sense of internal control over the hand-warming response. We encourage patients to experiment with a variety of hand-warming techniques. For example, we suggest they experiment with imagery (e.g., warming hands before a fire), sensory (e.g., focus on physical sensations that accompany handwarming), and verbal (e.g., autogenic phrases) techniques. We ask patients to practice between 10 to 20 minutes twice daily.

Pain Management

ORIENTATION

The same relaxation and stress-management skills that are used to prevent headaches can also be used during headache episodes to manage the pain associated with the headache. We review the use of quick relaxation skills during a headache episode and instruct patients in additional pain management techniques including attention control or attention-diversion strategies, additional guided imagery, pain transformation, and the application of CBT to catastrophizing thoughts triggered by the anticipation of a headache episode. Readers unfamiliar with attention control, guided imagery, and pain transformation are referred to Martin (1993), Philips and Rachman (1996), and Syrjala and Abrams (Chapter 9, this volume).

INSTRUCTION

A brief description of pain management techniques is provided herein.

Attention Control or Attention Diversion. Concentrating on an undemanding mental task for a brief period may help to shift attention away from pain. The task should be neutral, repetitive, or pleasant. Some examples include singing or reciting words to a favorite song, making a mental list of plans for an upcoming holiday or event, or mental arithmetic.

Pain Transformation. Pain transformation involves mentally modifying the characteristics of the pain sensation so that these sensations become less aversive. It is important that the image fit the pain. For example, if head pain is experienced "as if my head is in a vise," patients may imagine the vise loosening, or the vise disintegrating. Patients who report prominent muscle tightness or muscle pain with their headaches may imagine tight muscles as a rope tied in knots, then imagine the knotted rope unwind and go limp, with tension leaving the muscles as they unwind.

Application of CBT to Headache Episodes. Cognitive-behavioral stress-management skills can be especially helpful for patients who experience anxiety when anticipating their headaches, or for patients who experience high levels of affective distress in response to their headaches. CBT can help patients identify and modify thoughts that occur as a headache begins or in anticipation of a headache. For example, common stress-generating thoughts include the following: "These headaches are never going to go away," or "This headache will make it impossible to do anything today." Coping statements that reflect a more balanced appraisal, including thoughts such as "I am learning many things that I can do to cope with this headache" or "I can still get something done even when I have a headache," can be of help to some patients.

Maintenance of Self-Management

ORIENTATION

The goal of treatment is long-term headache management. We explain to patients that further improvement or even the maintenance of current improvements probably will require continued effort. Patients are encouraged to continue to incorporate headache management skills into their daily routine as well as to be on the lookout for the lapses in behavior that can lead to problems in headache control. We reassure patients that the continued practice of headache management skills will require less time and effort than was required when they were learning the skills.

INSTRUCTION

MTCT provides only an introduction to headache management skills; therefore, we plan what the patient will work on when clinic contacts end and identify events likely to cause a reoccurrence or worsening of headaches. We help patients identify obstacles to effective self-management and develop plans for coping with these obstacles. We assist patients in identifying behaviors (such as increased use of medications, sleep difficulties, ineffective coping with stress) in addition to an increase in headache activity that might suggest they are off track with their headache management program and discuss how to handle such temporary setbacks. Finally, we remind patients that life is full of challenges, and they might need an occasional "checkup" or booster session.

Discussion

We presented a brief clinical guide for the MTCT of migraine and tension-type headache addressing, when possible, clinical issues that are likely to confront therapists. MTCT formats can reduce the cost and increase the availability of behavioral treatment and reduce barriers to the integration of behavioral treatments into the medical setting. MTCT formats and other recent innovations in the delivery of behavioral treatments for headache (Holroyd, in press) have the potential to improve the dissemination of behavioral treatments into the health care system. The last two decades have seen the emergence of empirically supported psychological treatments for a number of pain disorders, but these treatments are rarely available in the medical settings in which most patients are seen. Ideally, in the next decade we will see not only continued progress in the development and evaluation of behavioral treatments but also the effective dissemination of these treatments into the health care system where they can benefit greater numbers of patients.

Acknowledgments

Support for this chapter was provided, in part, by a grant from the National Institute of Neurological Disorders and Stroke of the National Institutes of Health (NS32374).

Notes

1. American Academy of Family Physicians, American Academy of Neurology, American Headache Society, American College of Emergency Physicians, American College of Physicians, American Osteopathic Association, and National Headache Foundation.
2. Previously the Agency for Health Care Policy and Research.

References

Arena, J. G., Hannah, S. L., Bruno, G. M., & Meador, K. J. (1991). Electromyographic biofeedback training for tension headache in the elderly: A prospective study. *Biofeedback and Self-Regulation, 35,* 187–195.

Baumel, B. (1994). Migraine: A pharmacological review with newer options and delivery modalities. *Neurology, 44*(Suppl. 3), S13–S17.

Beck, A. T., & Emery, G. (1985). *Anxiety disorders and phobias: A cognitive perspective.* New York: Basic Books.

Beck, A. T., Rush, A. J., Shaw, B. F., & Emery, G. (1979). *Cognitive therapy of depression.* New York: Guilford Press.

Beck, A. T., & Steer, R. A. (1993). *Beck Anxiety Inventory.* San Antonio, TX: Psychological Corporation.

Beck, A. T., Ward, C. H., Mendelson, M., Mock, J., & Erbaugh, J. (1961). An inventory for measuring depression. *Archives of General Psychiatry, 4,* 561–571.

Beck, J. S. (1995). *Cognitive therapy: Basics and beyond.* New York: Guilford Press.

Bernstein, D. A., & Borkovec, T. D. (1973). *Progressive relaxation training: A manual for the helping professions.* Champaign, IL: Research Press.

Bernstein, D. A., & Carlson, C. R. (1993). Progressive relaxation: Abbreviated methods. In P. Lehrer & R. L. Woolfolk (Eds.), *Principles and practice of stress management* (pp. 53–85). New York: Guilford Press.

Blanchard, E. B. (1992). Psychological treatment of benign headache disorders. *Journal of Consulting and Clinical Psychology, 60,* 537–551.

Blanchard, E. B., & Andrasik, F. (1985). *Management of chronic headaches: A psychological approach.* Elmsford, NY: Pergamon Press.

Blanchard, E. B., Andrasik, F., Ahles, T. A., Teders, S. J., & O'Keefe, D. M. (1980). Migraine and tension headache: A meta-analytic review. *Behavior Therapy, 11,* 613–631.

Blanchard, E. B., Andrasik, F., Arena, J. G., Neff, D. F., Saunders, N. L., Jurish, S. E., Teders, S. J., & Rodichok, L. D. (1983). Psychophysiological responses as predictors of response to behavioral treatment of chronic headache. *Behavior Therapy, 14,* 357–374.

Blanchard, E. B., Appelbaum, K. A., Radnitz, C. L., Jaccard, J., & Dentinger, M. P. (1989). The refractory headache patient: I. Chronic, daily, high-intensity headache. *Behaviour Research and Therapy, 27,* 403–410.

Blau, J. N., & Thavapalan, M. (1988). Preventing migraine: A study of precipitating factors. *Headache, 28,* 481–483.

Bogaards, M. C., & ter Kuile, M. M. (1994). Treatment of recurrent tension headache: A meta-analytic review. *Clinical Journal of Pain, 10,* 174–190.

Breslau, N., & Davis, G. C. (1993). Migraine, physical health and psychiatric disorder: A prospective epidemiologic study in young adults. *Journal of Psychiatric Research, 27,* 211–221.

Breslau, N., Merikangas, K., & Bowden, C. L. (1994). Comorbidity of migraine and major affective disorders. *Neurology, 44*(Suppl. 7), S17–S22.

Campbell, J. K., Penzien, D. B., & Wall, E. M. (2000, May 15). *Evidence-based guidelines for migraine headache: Behavioral and physical treatments.* US Headache Consortium [On-line]. Available: http://www.aan.com/public/practiceguidelines/headache_gl.htm

Davidoff, R. A. (1995). *Migraine: Manifestations, pathogenesis, and management.* Philadelphia: Davis.

DeGood, D. E. (1997). *The headache and neck pain workbook: An integrated mind and body program.* Oakland, CA: New Harbinger.

Diener, H. C., & Dahlof, G. H. (2000). Headache associated with chronic use of substances. In J. Olesen, P. Tfelt-Hansen, & K. M. A. Welch (Eds.), *The headaches* (pp. 871–877). Philadelphia: Lippincott Williams & Wilkins.

Diener, H. C., & Tfelt-Hansen, P. (1993). Headache associated with chronic use of substances. In J. Olesen, P. Tfelt-Hansen, & K. M. A. Welch (Eds.), *The headaches* (pp. 721–728). New York: Raven Press.

Diener, H. C., & Wilkinson, M. E. (1988). *Drug-induced headache.* New York: Springer-Verlag.

D'Zurilla, T. J. (1989). Clinical stress management. In A. M. Nezu & C. M. Nezu (Eds.), *Clinical decision making in behavior therapy: A problem-solving perspective* (pp. 371–400). Champaign, IL: Research Press.

Edinger, J. D., Wohlgemuth, W. K., Radtke, R. A., Marsh, G. R., & Quillian, R. E. (2001). Cognitive behavior therapy for treatment of chronic primary insomnia. *Journal of the American Medical Association, 285,* 1856–1864.

Goslin, R., Gray, R., & McCrory, D. (2001, May 15). *Behavioral and physical treatments for migraine headache. Technical review 2.2* [On-line]. Available: http://www.clinpol.mc.duke.edu

Gould, R. A., Otto, M. W., Pollack, M. H., & Yap, L. (1997). Cognitive behavioral and pharmacological treatment of generalized anxiety disorder: A preliminary meta-analysis. *Behavior Therapy, 28,* 285–305.

Greenberger, D., & Padesky, C. A. (1995). *Mind over mood: A cognitive therapy manual for clients.* New York: Guilford Press.

Haddock, C. K., Rowan, A. B., Andrasik, F., Wilson, P. G., Talcott, G. W., & Stein, R. J. (1997). Home-based behavioral treatments for chronic benign headache: A meta-analysis of controlled trials. *Cephalalgia, 17,* 113–118.

Hermann, C., Kim, M., & Blanchard, E. B. (1995). Behavioral and pharmacological intervention studies of pediatric migraine: An exploratory meta-analysis. *Pain, 60,* 239–256.

Holroyd, K. A. (in press). Assessment and psychological treatment of recurrent headache disorders. *Journal of Consulting and Clinical Psychology.*

Holroyd, K. A., & Andrasik, F. (1982). A cognitive-behavioral approach to recurrent tension and migraine headache. In P. E. Kendall (Ed.), *Advances in cognitive-behavioral research and therapy* (Vol. 1, pp. 276–320). New York: Academic Press.

Holroyd, K. A., & Lipchik, G. L. (1997). Recurrent headache disorders. In S. J. Gallant, G. P. Keita, & R. Royak-Schaler (Eds.), *Psychosocial and behavioral factors in women's health care: A handbook for medical educators, practitioners, and psychologists* (pp. 365–384). Washington, DC: American Psychological Association.

Holroyd, K. A., & Lipchik, G. L. (2000). Sex differences in recurrent headache disorders. In R. B. Fillingim (Ed.), *Sex, gender and pain: From the benchtop to the clinic* (pp. 251–279). Seattle, WA: IASP Press.

Holroyd, K. A., Lipchik, G. L., & Penzien, D. B. (1998). Psychological management of recurrent headache disorders: Empirical basis for clinical practice. In K. S. Dobson & K. D. Craig (Eds.), *Best practice: Developing and promoting empirically supported interventions* (pp. 193–212). Newbury Park, CA: Sage.

Holroyd, K. A., O'Donnell, F. J., Stensland, M., Lipchik, G. L., Cordingley, G. E., & Carlson, B. (2001). Management of chronic tension-type headache with tricyclic antidepressant medication, stress-management therapy, and their combination: A randomized controlled trial. *Journal of the American Medical Association, 285,* 2208–2215.

Holroyd, K. A., & Penzien, D. B. (1986). Client

variables in the behavioral treatment of recurrent tension headache: A meta-analytic review. *Journal of Behavioral Medicine, 9*, 515–536.

Holroyd, K. A., & Penzien, D. B. (1990). Pharmacological vs. nonpharmacological prophylaxis of recurrent migraine headache: A meta-analytic review of clinical trails. *Pain, 42*, 1–13.

Holroyd, K. A., Penzien, D. B., Hursey, K. G., Tobin, D. L., Rogers, L., Holm, J. E., Marcille, P. J., Hall, J. R., & Chila, A. G. (1984). Change mechanisms in EMG biofeedback training: Cognitive changes underlying improvements in tension headache. *Journal of Consulting and Clinical Psychology, 52*, 1039–1053.

Holroyd, K. A., Penzien, D. B., & Lipchik, G. L. (2001). Behavioral management of headache. In S. D. Silberstein, R. B. Lipton, & D. J. Dalessio (Eds.), *Wolff's headache and other headache pain* (7th ed., pp. 562–598). New York: Oxford University Press.

Holroyd, K., Stensland, M., Lipchik, G., Hill, K., O'Donnell, F., & Cordingley, G. (2000). Psychosocial correlates and impact of chronic tension-type headaches. *Headache, 40*, 3–16.

Jacobson, G. P., Ramadan, N. M., Aggarwal, S. K., & Newman, C. W. (1994). The Henry Ford Hospital Headache Disability Inventory (HDI). *Neurology, 44*, 837–842.

Lipton, R. B., Hamelsky, S. W., & Stewart, W. F. (2001). Epidemiology and impact of headache. In S. D. Silberstein, R. B. Lipton, & D. J. Dalessio (Eds.), *Wolff's headache and other head pain* (7th ed., pp. 85–107). New York: Oxford University Press.

Lipton, R. B., Stewart, W. F., Diamond, S., Diamond, M. L., & Reed, M. (2001). Prevalence and burden of migraine in the United States: Data from the American Migraine Study II. *Headache, 41*, 646–657.

Lipton, R. B., Stewart, W. F., & Von Korff, M. (1995). Migraine impact and functional disability. *Cephalalgia, 15*, 4–9.

Markley, H. G. (1994). Chronic headache: Appropriate use of opiate analgesics. *Neurology, 44* (Suppl. 3), S18–S24.

Martin, P. R. (1993). *Psychological management of chronic headaches: A functional perspective.* New York: Guilford Press.

Mavissakalian, M. & Prien, R. (Eds.). *Long-term treatment of anxiety disorders.* Washington, DC: American Psychiatric Association.

McCrory, D., Penzien, D., Hasselblad, V., & Gray, R. (2001). *Behavioral and physical treatments for tension-type and cervicogenic headache.* Des Moines, IA: Foundation for Chiropractic Education and Research.

Medina, J. L., & Diamond, S. (1978). The role of diet in migraine. *Headache, 5*, 1020–1026.

Meichenbaum, D. A. (1977). *Cognitive-behavior modification: An integrative approach.* New York: Plenum Press.

Miller, W. R., & Rollnick, S. (1991). *Motivational interviewing: Preparing people to change addictive behavior.* New York: Guilford Press.

Mosley, T. H., Grotheus, C. A., & Meeks, W. M. (1995). Treatment of tension headache in the elderly: A controlled evaluation of relaxation training and relaxation combined with cognitive-behavior therapy. *Journal of Clinical Geropsychology, 1*, 175–188.

Olesen, J. C. (1988). Classification and diagnostic criteria for headache disorders, cranial neuralgias, and facial pain: Headache Classification Committee of the International Headache Society. *Cephalalgia, 8*(Suppl. 7), 1–96.

Paiva, T., Batista, A., Martins, P., & Martins, A. (1995). The relationship between headaches and sleep disturbances. *Headache, 35*, 590–596.

Persons, J. B. (1989). *Cognitive therapy in practice: A case formulation approach.* New York: Norton.

Philips, H. C., & Rachman, S. (1996). *The psychological management of chronic pain: A treatment manual* (2nd ed.). New York: Springer.

Poppen, R. (1988). *Behavioral relaxation training and assessment.* Elmsford, NY: Pergamon Press.

Radnitz, C. L. (1990). Food-triggered migraine: A critical review. *Annals of Behavioral Medicine, 12*, 51–65.

Rapoport, A. M., & Sheftell, F. D. (1993). Headache associated with medication and substance withdrawal. In C. D. Tollison & R. S. Kunkel (Eds.), *Headache: Diagnosis and treatment* (pp. 227–231). Baltimore: Williams & Wilkins.

Rasmussen, B. K. (1993). Migraine and tension-type headache in a general population: Precipitating factors, female hormones, sleep pattern and relation to lifestyle. *Pain, 53*, 65–72.

Rasmussen, B. K., Jensen, R., Schroll, M., & Olesen, J. (1991). Epidemiology of headache in a general population—a prevalence study. *Journal of Clinical Epidemiology, 44*, 1147–1157.

Robbins, L. (1994). Precipitating factors in migraine: A retrospective review of 494 patients. *Headache, 34*, 214–216.

Robinson, L. A., Berman, J. S., & Neimeyer, R. A. (1990). Psychotherapy for the treatment of depression: A comprehensive review of controlled outcome research. *Pyschological Bulletin, 108*, 30–49.

Rowan, A. B., & Andrasik, F. (1996). Efficacy and cost-effectiveness of minimal therapist contact treatments of chronic headache: A review. *Behavior Therapy, 27*, 207–234.

Sahota, P. K., & Dexter, J. D. (1990). Sleep and headache syndromes: A clinical review. *Headache, 35*, 80–84.

Saper, J. R., Silberstein, S., Gordon, C. D., & Hamel, R. L. (1993). *Handbook of headache management: A practical guide to diagnosis and treatment of head, neck, and facial pain.* Baltimore: Williams & Wilkins.

Sargent, J. D., Green, E. E., & Walters, E. D. (1972). The use of autogenic feedback training in a pilot study of migraine and tension headaches. *Headache, 12*, 12–124.

Scharff, L., & Marcus, D. A. (1994). Interdisciplinary outpatient group treatment of intractable headache. *Headache, 34*, 73–78.

Schultz, J., & Luthe, W. (1959). *Autogenic training: A psychophysiologic approach in psychotherapy* (Vol. 1). New York: Grune & Stratton.

Schwartz, B. S., Stewart, W. F., Simon, M. S., & Lipton, R. B. (1998). Epidemiology of tension-type headache. *Journal of the American Medical Association, 279*, 381–383.

Silberstein, S. D., & Merriman, G. (1997). Sex hormones and headache. In P. Goadsby & S. D. Silberstein (Eds.), *Blue books of practical neurology: Headache* (pp. 143–176). Boston: Butterworth Heinemann.

Silberstein, S. D., & Rosenberg, J. (2000). Multi-specialty consensus on diagnosis and treatment of headache. *Neurology, 54*, 1553–1554.

Silberstein, S. D., Saper, J. R., & Frietag, F. G. (2001). Migraine: Diagnosis and treatment. In S. D. Silberstein, R. B. Lipton, & D. J. Dalessio (Eds.), *Wolff's headache and other head pain* (7th ed., pp. 121–237). New York: Oxford University Press.

Spielberger, C. D., Gorsuch, R. L., & Lushene, R. E. (1970). *STAI manual for the State–Trait Anxiety Inventory ("Self-Evaluation Questionnaire")*. Palo Alto, CA: Consulting Psychologists Press.

Spitzer, R. L., Williams, J. B. W., Kroenke, K., Linzer, M., deGruy, F. V., Hahn, S. R., Brody, D., & Johnson, J. G. (1994). Utility of a new procedure for diagnosing mental disorders in primary care: The PRIME MD 1000 study. *Journal of the American Medical Association, 272*, 1749–1756.

Stewart, W. F., Lipton, R. B., Celentano, D. D., & Reed, M. L. (1991). The epidemiology of severe migraine headache from a national survey: Implications of projections to the US population. *Cephalalgia, 11*(Suppl. 11), 87–88.

Stewart, W. F., Lipton, R. B., Kolodner, K., Liberman, J., & Sawyer, J. (1999). Reliability of the migraine disability assessment score in a population-based sample of headache sufferers. *Cephalalgia, 19*, 107–114.

19

Treatment of Patients with Fibromyalgia Syndrome

Dennis C. Turk
Jeffrey J. Sherman

Fibromyalgia syndrome (FMS) consists of a pervasive set of unexplained physical symptoms with generalized pain and hypersensitivity to palpation at specific body locations ("tender points," or TPs; Wolfe et al., 1990; see Figure 19.1) as the cardinal features. In addition, patients with FMS typically report a range of functional limitations and psychological dysfunction, including persistent fatigue, sleep disturbance, feelings of stiffness, headaches, irritable bowel disorders, depression, anxiety, cognitive impairment, and general malaise, sometimes referred to as "fibro fog" (Baumstark & Buckelew, 1992). FMS may have an insidious onset without any identifiable cause, may develop following a flu-like illness, or may rapidly develop following an identified trauma such as a motor vehicle accident or emotional distress (Clauw & Chrousos, 1997; Turk, Okifuji, Starz, & Sinclair, 1996).

This chapter provides a brief overview of models that have been postulated to explain FMS, describes a perspective on FMS that draws heavily on the biopsychosocial model (see Turk & Monarch, Chapter 1, this volume), provides an overview of treatment issues, and makes some general recommendations regarding the treatment of patients with FMS based on a cognitive-behavioral perspective (see Turk, Chapter 7, and Keefe, Beaupre, Gil, Rumble, & Aspnes, Chapter 11, this volume). We emphasize features unique to FMS and how these must be addressed in the treatment of this population.

Extent of the Problem, Course, and Severity

FMS is one of the most common disorders evaluated in outpatient rheumatological clinics accounting for up to 20% of all patients seen (White, Speechley, Harth, & Østbye, 1995). The population prevalence of FMS is estimated to range from .66% to 10.50% (Schochat, Croft, & Raspe, 1994). The variability may result from differences in classification criteria as not all these studies used the 1990 American College of Rheumatology (ACR) criteria (Wolfe et al., 1990). Although there are some reports of FMS in children as young as 10 years old (Breau, McGrath, & Ju, 1999), FMS occurs predominantly between the second and sixth decade of life.

FMS is more commonly observed in women, with a female to male ratio of 7 to

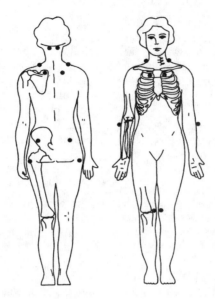

Tender points located in nine bilateral sites, namely:

Occiput: at the suboccipital muscle insertions.
Low cervical: at the anterior aspects of the intertransverse spaces at C5–C7.
Trapezius: at the midpoint of the upper border.
Supraspinatus: at origins, above the scapula spine near the medial border.
Second rib: at the second costochondral junctions, just lateral to the junctions on upper surfaces.
Lateral epicondyle: at 2 cm distal to the epicondyles.
Gulteal: in upper outer quadrants of buttocks in anterior fold of muscle.
Greater trochanter: posterior to the trochanteric prominence.
Knee: at the medial fat proximal to the joint line.

FIGURE 19.1. Location of tender points

1 in those seeking treatment. In community samples, however, the ratio is closer to 3 to 1, females to males. Although FMS seems relatively common in the general population, the severity of the symptoms in the "population-based" FMS tends to be less severe and disabling compared to those FMS patients who seek treatment (Prescott et al., 1993).

The Torment of FMS

Beyond the pain and related symptoms, FMS sufferers are confronted with a poorly understood disorder that is not well accepted by health care providers, employers, or the legal system. People with FMS often look well despite the symptoms, and many people question the severity and seriousness of their condition. The lack of objective medical findings to confirm the diagnosis can result in confusion and frustration. Patients often wonder, "How can I be in so much pain and yet look normal on all the tests." Moreover, not only is the sufferer affected but significant others are often confused and frustrated. Relationships can suffer as the costs of pain extend well beyond the physical and begin to affect the emotional, occupational, social, and recreational life of those afflicted.

To work effectively with FMS patients, it is important to appreciate their suffering and the difficulties associated with having a chronic condition for which no apparent physical cause can be identified. This appreciation is important in establishing rapport with patients and in understanding aspects of their behavior that might, at times, seem surprising. The extent of this suffering and of the puzzling responses sometimes heard from FMS patients is apparent in the following interaction that occurred during our first session. Although some would feel relief when hearing that their symptoms reflect a "benign" and nonprogressive condition, one of our patients appraised this information negatively:

PATIENT: It won't kill me, but sometimes I think I would be better off if this was cancer.

THERAPIST: How do you mean, "better off"?

PATIENT: People understand cancer, they give support for cancer, cancers can be cured, tumors removed. When I tell people that I have fibromyalgia they don't know what I mean or they think I'm making this up or that it's all in my head.

THERAPIST: So you mean you'd be "better off" in the sense that you'd be better understood and supported rather than better off physically?

PATIENT: Yes.

THERAPIST: Would it be helpful then if in treatment we discussed ways to make yourself better understood by others and that would help you to receive support by asking for what you need from others?

PATIENT: Yes.

This interaction provided an important therapeutic inroad. In a later session during our group intervention we discuss assertiveness and work with patients to improve their communication skills in order to better explain their condition to others. We also role-play interactions that the patient may have with others who are naïve to FMS or who provide support for the patient with FMS.

Patients with FMS often present to psychologists on the recommendation of their physician. Because FMS sufferers are sensitive to suggestions that their symptoms are largely psychological, it is important for the psychologist to address this concern at the onset. We do so by reviewing some of the possible causal mechanisms and suggesting to the patient that we work collaboratively to set realistic therapeutic goals and pursue them in short-term therapy.

Causal Mechanisms

Typically, as was the case in the chronic pain literatures, etiological factors of un-remitting pain have been viewed in a dichotomous fashion—either physical or psychological. Because this model appears to be inadequate, several attempts have been made to integrate information into more comprehensive models that incorporate both physical and psychological contributors. We briefly describe some of the most prominent models of FMS.

Physiological Models

The pathophysiological mechanisms underlying FMS are poorly understood. Radiographic and laboratory findings tend to be negative. The earliest attempts to uncover the etiology of FMS were dominated by the biomedical model, which assumes that reported pain was caused by demonstrable or occult physical abnormality particularly related to the muscle anatomy (Bengtsson, Henriksson, & Larsson, 1986) and physiological processes including oxygen availability and depletion (Bengtsson & Hendriksson, 1989; Drewes, Andreasen, Schroder, Hogsaa, & Jennum, 1993), tension myalgia resulting from spasms, overuse, or poor posture (Zidar, Backman, Bengtsson, & Henriksson, 1990).

A number of neurochemical and physiological factors have also been studied in FMS patients, including (1) dysregulation of hypothalamic–pituitary–adrenal [HPA] axis (Crofford, Engleberg, & Demitrack, 1996; van Denderen, Boersma, Zeinstra, Hollander, & van Neerbos 1992); (2) serotonin imbalance (Wolfe, Russell, Vipraio, Ross, & Anderson, 1997); (3) insulin-like growth factor-I dysregulation (i.e., somatomedin C) (Bennett, Clark, Campbell, & Burckhardt, 1992); (4) sleep deficiency (Drewes, Svendsen, Nielsen, Taagholt, & Bjerregåd, 1994); and (5) physical deconditioning (Nørrengaard, Bülow, Mehlsen, & Danneskiold-Samsose, 1994). However, to date, no definitive physical basis for FMS has been identified. What is most notable in the studies examining various neuroendocrine substances in FMS seems to be the large intragroup variability observed in any of the substances tested. Thus, although FMS patients may statistically be different from people without FMS, the large individual differences within FMS patients may make it difficult to interpret the results.

Psychological Models

Failure to identify a direct association between physical pathology and the high degree of psychiatric comorbidity in FMS has led some to suggest that FMS should be viewed as predominantly a psychogenic disorder. Concurrent depression is diagnosed in 14–71% of FMS patients and far exceeds the prevalence of depression in community populations (see, e.g., Ahles, Khan, Yunus, Spiegel, & Masi, 1991; Walker et al., 1997). The high prevalence rate of depression in FMS, has led some to hypothesize that the affective disorder is the primary mechanism underlying FMS (Alfici, Sigal, & Landau, 1989; Hudson, Hudson, Pliner, Goldenberg, & Pope, 1985). Some clinical investigators who have observed the similarity and overlap of symptoms in FMS, chronic fatigue syndrome (CFS), irritable bowel syndrome (IBS), and temporomandibular disorders (TMDs) have proposed that FMS is one of several overlapping "functional somatic syndromes" (Barsky & Borus, 1999; Morriss et al., 1999). At the present time, arguments and empirical evidence do not support the psychogenic models.

Once the patient has been cleared as medically stable, we do not, in practice, distinguish between biomedical or psychological explanations for the pain problem because the distinction itself implies a mind–body dualism. Instead, we introduce some of the following psychosocial concepts to the patient as likely contributors to pain and to their quality of life.

STRESS

Many FMS patients report that their symptoms began following physical or emotional stress (see, e.g., Clauw & Chrousos, 1997; Turk, Okifuji, Starz, & Sinclair, 1996). There is little doubt that living with FMS and related symptoms serves as an ongoing stressor. For example, as part of a treatment study currently in progress, we asked FMS patients to specify what factors were associated with improvement and exacerbation of their symptoms. The majority (65%) indicated that stress was an aggravating factor. On the other hand, stress-reducing strategies, such as taking warm baths and relaxation, were noted as ameliorating factors by over 50% of the sample. Several possible explanations might account for these differences, including such predisposing factors as genetics, learning history, anxiety sensitivity, and the normal distribution of sensory sensitivity.

HYPERVIGILANCE

The diffused and generalized nature of FMS has led some investigators to consider impairment or dysfunction in information processing as a critical factor in FMS. The hypervigilance model for chronic pain suggests that some patients may be more sensitive to pain signals as a result of increased attention to somatosensory stimuli. Research investigating sensory processing of FMS patients has consistently demonstrated that FMS subjects exhibit lower pain threshold than do age-matched and sex-matched healthy people (e.g., Kosek, Ekholm, & Hansson, 1996; McDermid, Rollman, & McCain, 1996). Based on these results, Rollman and Lautenbacher (1993) proposed a "hypervigilance model" in which heightened sensory vigilance is a predisposing factor in FMS. Furthermore, vigilance to sensory information in FMS may not be limited to pain. Some data indicate that FMS patients are more sensitive to cold, noise, and environmental irritants (McDermid et al., 1996; Nørrengaard et al., 1994).

COGNITIVE BELIEFS AND APPRAISALS

Research has often demonstrated that cognitive factors (e.g., beliefs and appraisals) play an important part in determining adaptation to symptoms in chronic pain patients (e.g., Turk & Rudy, 1986). As has been observed in many chronic pain syndromes, maladaptive thoughts and information processing seem to be closely associated with functional limitations and affective distress observed in FMS. Cognitive factors are not generally considered to be etiological. However, research examining the effects of maladaptive cognition on maintenance and aggravation of chronic pain suggests that physical pathology, which may have initiated the symptoms, plays a diminished role over time. On the other hand, perception and interpretation of the symptoms contribute to an internal representation of FMS. The dysfunctional representation is likely to facilitate an environment that supports "sick behaviors" and reduction of activities; in turn, patients experience decreased levels of social reinforcement and sense of accomplishment, along with progressive physical deconditioning, all of which will facilitate further disability, distress, and pain. Other maladaptive cognitions such as catastrophizing contribute to the depression (Hassett, Cone, & Sigal 2000) and the physical disability (M. Y. Martin et al., 1996) associated with FMS.

Lower self-efficacy beliefs, in particular, have been shown to be related to greater pain, disability, and depressive mood in FMS (Buckelew, Murray, Hewett, Johnson, & Huyser, 1995; Turk & Okifuji, 1997). FMS patients with lower self-efficacy who underwent a 6-week training intervention involving physical training and exercise had lower posttreatment physical activity when compared to those with higher self-efficacy. Furthermore, improvements in self-efficacy during treatment were associated with lower tender point scores and pain intensity (Buckelew et al., 1996).

Multidimensional Model

At this point, the most appropriate way to conceptualize FMS is much like the conceptualization of other chronic illnesses, as having both physical and psychological components. Perhaps the earliest multidimensional model of pain was the gate control model proposed by Melzack and his colleagues (Melzack & Casey, 1968; Melzack & Wall, 1965). The gate control model focused on the sensory–discriminative, motivational–affective, and cognitive–evaluative components of pain. It postulated a hypothetical gating system within the spinal cord that could be activated or inhibited by noxious sensory input as well as interpretive process and a person's current mood state. Thus, it proposed that the resulting pain was an amalgam on afferent input and downregulation by psychological processes.

Although physical, psychological, and multidimensional models help to inform research and the clinician, too much of a focus on etiology can be viewed as excessively detailed for the patient. There is, however, a need to demonstrate understanding to the patient and to convey information about the processes that contribute to chronic pain in order to plan and guide treatment decisions. In our treatment program, we present to the patient a simplified version of the gate control theory of pain (Wall & Melzack, 1965; see also Keefe et al., Chapter 11, for a discussion of the applicability of the gate control model for use with chronic pain patients) and use it as a heuristic means for helping patients understand the role of both physical and psychological factors in the experience of pain. The accuracy and details of the model are less important than it conceptual simplicity. Because one goal of treatment is providing the patient with an understanding of how physical and psychological factors interact to maintain chronic pain, educating the patient on a model that is easy to grasp and to communicate to others is integral to treatment. We present this model to the patient in Figure 19.2 and describe a situation familiar to most everyone:

THERAPIST: Has anyone in the group ever stubbed their toe on the side of a coffee table?

GROUP: (*Knowing nods.*)

THERAPIST: Good. If I asked you at that moment and for the next several minutes after stubbing your toe, to make it hurt more, what would you do?

PATIENT 1: Look at it. Worry that I broke it.

THERAPIST: Exactly! What if I asked you to make it better, to decrease the pain from stubbing your toe?

PATIENT 2: Not pay any attention to it. Ignore it.

PATIENT 3: Rub it, or put ice on it.

THERAPIST: Each of these will work but let's look at each and how they work. Rubbing and icing are physical ways to close the gate. By providing a counterstimulus, different nerve fibers work and block the pain message, that is, they prevent the message from getting to that area of the spine where the gate can open or close. Two of the other ways to close the gate were mentioned, ignoring the pain and continuing on with your activity help to block the gate because the brain is otherwise occupied.

PATIENT 4: Is that why little kids are more likely to cry when they fall down if you make a fuss over it?

THERAPIST: Yes! If a child falls and the parent just encourages him to continue playing, then

FACTORS THAT OPEN THE GATE

- ○ Physical factors
    - ⇑ Extent of injury
    - ⇑ Inappropriate activity level
- ○ Emotional stress
    - ⇑ Depression
    - ⇑ Anxiety
    - ⇑ Worry
    - ⇑ Tension
    - ⇑ Anger
- ○ Psychological factors
    - ⇑ Focusing on the pain
    - ⇑ Boredom due to minimal involvement in life activities
    - ⇑ Nonadaptive attitudes

FACTORS THAT CLOSE THE GATE

- ○ Physical factors
    - ⇓ Medication
    - ⇓ Counterstimulation (heat, rubbing)
    - ⇓ Appropriate activity level
- ○ Relative emotional stability
    - ⇓ Relaxation
    - ⇓ Positive emotions (happiness, optimism)
    - ⇓ Rest
- ○ Psychological factors
    - ⇓ Life involvement, increased interest in life activities
    - ⇓ Intense concentration/distraction
    - ⇓ Adaptive attitudes/ positive thoughts and feelings

FIGURE 19.2. Factors that open and close the "pain gate."

the child continues to be active. The result is that there is less painful input getting through to his brain from that scraped knee. It's still the same scraped knee but his sense of it, or if you will, his perception and appraisal of it, is different. It's now something to be ignored rather than a threat to his integrity and safety. On the other hand, the child is more likely to cry if the parent runs to the child, acts worried, and calls attention to the scrape on his knee.

The latter part of this interaction led to a discussion on maladaptive thinking. In session, we began to discuss the role of worrying and catastrophizing in pain perception. This role was discussed in the context of "opening the gate," but in later sessions we revisited the topic as it applies not only to pain but also to the depression and sense of hopelessness that often accompany pain (see Figure 19.2).

In general, biopsychosocial models of pain have been proposed to integrate physical, psychosocial, and behavioral contributions to pain perception and adaptation (see Turk & Monarch, Chapter 1, this volume). These models attempted to extend the gate control model to consider pain as a dynamic, developmental process. As chronic pain extends affecting more and more of a pain sufferers' life, psychosocial and behavioral come to play an expanding role not only in the perception of pain but in the resulting emotional and functional adaptation. Flor, Birbaumer, and Turk (1990) proposed a biobehavioral model that not only focused on pain onset and evolution but integrated predispositional factors such as prior learning history, genetic makeup, and personality.

More recently, Okifuji and Turk (1999) proposed a dynamic-process model designed to incorporate the current understanding of FMS. In this model, FMS is characterized as a disorder of information processing due to the dysregulated stress-response system. It is a diathesis (predisposition)–stress model that integrates premorbid factors, precipitating factors, and stress responses in the development and maintenance of the symptoms associated with FMS.

Patient Heterogeneity

A number of investigators have suggested that FMS patients may not be a homogeneous group. Rather, there may be subgroups of FMS sufferers. Studies have focused on differences depending on symptom onset, for example, idiopathic versus traumatic (Greenfield, Fitzcharles, & Esdaile, 1992; Turk, Okifuji, Sinclair, & Starz, 1996; Waylonis & Perkins, 1994). Turk and Flor (1989) suggested that FMS may be a heterogeneous disorder consisting of several patient subgroups with different constellations of physical and psychological features. They argued that delineation of the relevant subgroups would facilitate the identification of the mechanisms underlying the symptoms of FMS and the development of treatments customized to address specific needs of different patient groups.

As noted, investigators have begun to conceptualize FMS as a multifactorial, biopsychosocial disorder (e.g., Bennett et al., 1991; Masi & Yunus, 1990). Interestingly, however, biomedical and psychosocial factors contributing to the clinical picture may have only modest relationships with each other. Turk and Rudy (1988) suggested that

there are a range of psychosocial and behavioral factors that are important in understanding chronic pain patients and that may differentiate subgroups. They developed an empirically derived taxonomy of chronic pain patients based on patients' responses to the West Haven–Multidimensional Pain Inventory (MPI; Kerns, Turk, & Rudy, 1985)—Dysfunctional (DYS), interpersonally distressed (ID), and adaptive copers (AC). Table 19.1 describes the characteristics of these three subgroups.

The results of the study by Turk, Okifuji, Starz, and Sinclair (1996) indicate that the majority of the FMS patients (87%) can be classified into one of the three primary groups: DYS, ID, and AC that had been previously identified for diverse chronic pain populations (e.g., Jamison, Rudy, Penzien,

TABLE 19.1. Subgroups of Chronic Pain Patients Based on the Multidimensional Pain Inventory (Kerns et al., 1995)

Relative to other chronic pain patients . . .

DYSFUNCTIONAL patients report:
- Higher levels of pain
- Higher levels of perceived interference of pain with their lives
- Higher levels of emotional distress
- Lower levels of perceived control over their lives
- Lower levels of activity

INTERPERSONALLY DISTRESSED patients report:
- Lower levels of perceived support
- Higher levels of negative (punishing) responses from significant others
- Lower levels of solicitous responses from significant others
- Lower levels of distracting responses from significant others

ADAPTIVE COPER patients report:
- Lower levels of pain (although still seeking treatment)
- Lower levels of perceived interference of pain with their lives
- Lower levels of emotional distress
- Higher levels of perceived control over their lives
- Higher levels of activity

Mosley, 1994; Turk & Rudy, 1988; 1990; Turk, Sist, et al., 1998). The three FMS groups differed significantly in opioid use, depression, pain severity, perceived disability, and level of marital satisfaction. Such differences were observed even though the groups exhibited comparable degrees of physical pathology and levels of physical functioning. The results revealed that the patients in the DYS group reported higher level of pain severity and opioid use than those in the ID and AC groups. The ID and DYS groups also differed significantly from the AC group in depression. The extent of marital satisfaction differentiated the two groups, with the ID patients reporting a significantly lower level of satisfaction with their marriage than the DYS patients.

The distinct characteristics associated with each patient subgroup suggest that prescription of a uniformed intervention for all patients might result in less than optimal outcomes because the specific needs of some patients will not be directly addressed. It may be more appropriate to customize treatment to meet their specific clinical needs (Turk, 1990). For example, although the patients in both DYS and ID groups were depressed, depression in the latter group may be closely related to marital and interpersonal problems. Meaningful improvement, therefore, may not be achieved without addressing interpersonal or marital issues for ID FMS patients. Being able to prescribe specific treatments based on patient characteristics, rather than the more typical one-size-fits-all approach, is likely to benefit a greater number of patients and ultimately be more cost-effective. The value of customizing treatment to the three subgroups identified has recently been demonstrated in several studies (Bergstrom, Jensen, Bodin, Linton, & Nygren, 2001; Carmody, 2001; Dahlstrom, Widmark, & Carlsson, 1997; Strategier, Chwalisz, Altmaier, Russell, & Lehmann, 1997; Talo, Forssell, Heikkonen, & Puukka, 2001; Turk, Rudy, Kubinski, Zaki, & Greco, 1996).

Turk and colleagues (1996) noted a general lack of the association between perceived disability and objective functional ability in FMS. It appears that there are FMS patients who, despite negligible physi-

cal dysfunction, believe that they are significantly disabled. This perception may actually facilitate reduction of activity and consequently greater disability, thereby contributing to a self-fulfilling prophecy.

Importantly, the nature of relationships between observed level of physical functioning and perceived disability seems to vary across patient groups. Patients in the AC group demonstrated a statistically significant association between those two variables, whereas the patients in the other two groups did not. The differential associations among disability and physical functioning across subgroups further support the notion that meaningful grouping of FMS patients can be performed on a basis of patients' psychosocial and behavioral responses to their chronic pain conditions.

Psychosocial differences in FMS patients also relate to outcome in treatment. Turk, Okifuji, Sinclair, and Starz (1998) evaluated the effectiveness of a rehabilitation approach for FMS patients that consisted of six, 4-hour sessions spaced over a period of 1 month. Three sessions were conducted during the first week and then one session each of the next three weeks. Each session included information about FMS presented by a physician. In addition, a physical therapist focused on aerobic exercises, an occupational therapist on pacing and body mechanics, and a psychologist who focused on the role of stress and pain management techniques (e.g., relaxation, attention diversion, and problem solving). In general, the results of the treatment were effective in reducing pain, depression, and disability at the end of treatment and at a 6-month follow-up for the total sample of patients. Careful examination of the results, however, revealed that the DYS patients responded quite well to the treatment and the AC patients somewhat less so. The ID patients, however, appeared to achieve no benefit from the treatment. These results demonstrate the differential response to treatment for the different subgroups and support the need to reconsider the components of treatment provided. For example, the ID patients are characterized by their perceptions of low levels of support from significant others. Nothing in the treatment directly addressed interpersonal problems or attempted to improve communication patterns. The failure to address directly these concerns may have impeded benefit from the more general information, exercise, and pain coping strategies included in the comprehensive treatment.

The importance of differences of FMS patient in response to treatment was also reported by Vlaeyan and colleagues (1997). These investigators developed a treatment based on reducing fear believed to be an important factor in FMS patients' avoidance of activities. The treatment included information about psychosocial factors that influence pain and ergonomic principles as applied to daily activities (i.e., education). One group received coping skills training and applied relaxation skills training in addition to the educational component. The authors found that patients who had lower levels of fear responded somewhat better to the treatment that included the cognitive component, whereas the high fear patients showed somewhat better outcomes in response to the education and discussion alone without including the coping skills training.

To summarize, it is important to acknowledge that FMS patients are not a homogeneous group (Turk, Okifuji, Sinclair, & Starz, 1996). It is reasonable to assume that large individual differences existed prior to the development of FMS and that these differences persist or are magnified in response to the stress associated with a chronic condition. Thus, although the evolving processes may be present in all FMS patients, the degrees to which the processes become dysregulated may vary across people due to differences in the predispositional factors (Okifuji & Turk, 1999). Subgroups may respond to an identical intervention in different manners. Consequently, the "one-size-fits-all" approach of treating FMS patients is not likely to be effective. Identification of patients' characteristics and matching them to specific treatment may be needed to maximize clinical efficacy.

Assessment

A comprehensive interview with the patient and, whenever possible, his or her significant other is essential (see Turk, Monarch, & Williams, in press). This interview not only provides important assessment information but also can begin to help the patient and significant other understand the role of pain in emotional and physical functioning; conversely, the role of thoughts, feelings, and behavior in physical functioning; and the effect of environmental consequences (Turk et al., in press).

We have already mentioned the MPI (Kerns et al., 1985). In addition, we use the Center for Epidemiological Studies Depression Scale (Radloff, 1977), the Oswestry Disability Index (Fairbank, Couper, Davies, & O'Brien, 1980), and the Locke–Wallace Marital Adjustment Scale (Locke & Wallace, 1959) for married patients. Depending on the results of this screening, additional measures may be selected to assist in providing in depth information about areas of concern (Turk et al., in press).

The most important thing to keep in mind about assessment is that the information obtained should be used to assist in treatment planning and decision making. Gathering copious information that will not be used is time-consuming and inappropriate. Because most FMS patients are already concerned about being referred to a psychologist and fear that their symptoms will be attributed solely to emotional problems, it is incumbent upon the psychological evaluator that he or she takes time to explain to the patient the purpose of the assessment

ASSESSOR: As you are well aware, living with disabling and distressing symptoms such as pain create a great deal of stress on you. They affect all areas of your life, physical, emotional, and social. Many people with fibromyalgia become anxious, depressed, frustrated, and angry—angry at doctors, significant others, their bodies, and themselves. These are normal reactions to the presence of symptoms with an unknown cause and no cure. I'm, not sure if you have had such feelings but let me tell you what I have told others with fibromyalgia.

There is no question that your pain is real, nor is there any question that living with pain causes a lot of problems. I want to try to learn more about you and your situation so that I can work with other health care providers to develop a treatment plan that address all of these important contributors to your life and your pain.

Have you noticed that you are irritable and

feeling like your body is letting your down? That no one understands how you feel?

PATIENT: It's really hard when no one understands. It just is so hard to get going and to deal with so many problems when you don't have energy. My family try to help but they don't know how bad I feel.

ASSESSOR: I can understand, that's what I want to do, to learn more about how fibromyalgia has affected your mood and your life so that we can work on these areas as well as on your pain, feelings of fatigue, and weakness.

Treatments Commonly Used for FMS Patients

FMS patients report a host of somatic and psychological symptoms. Although no organic pathology has been identified, patients' quality of life is substantially compromised. In the past few decades, a number of approaches have been tested for the treatment of FMS. We outline the most prominent here. Despite the extensive research efforts, however, no treatment has proven to be universally effective. In the following section, we describe our own short-term cognitive-behavioral treatment (CBT) approach for FMS.

Unidimensional Treatments

A wide variety of pharmacological (e.g., corticosteroids: Clark, Tindall, & Bennett, 1985; nonsteroidal anti-inflammatory agents: Russell, Fletcher, Mchalek, McBroom, & Hester, 1991; benzodiazepines: Russell et al., 1991; tricyclic antidepressants: Carette, Bell, & Reynolds, 1994; selective serotonin reuptake inhibitors [SSRIs]: Goldenberg, Felson, & Dinerman, 1986), aerobic exercise (e.g., L. Martin et al., 1996; Wigers, Stiles, & Vogel, 1996), and psychological (relaxation: e.g., Günther, Mur, Kinigadner, & Miller, 1994; Nicassio et al., 1997; biofeedback: Ferraccioli et al., 1987) interventions have been used in an attempt to treat FMS patients. The rationales for these different modalities seem reasonable in some but not all instances, and yet the results are rather modest.

The results of the unimodal treatment outcome studies have led some to pessimism and resignation about the ability to treat FMS patients successfully. Solomon and Liang (1997) have questioned the appropriateness of rheumatologists continuing to treat FMS patients given limited results. Although we are sympathetic to the concerns raised, as we will note later, we believe that one of the major problems is that FMS patients are being treated as a homogeneous set. It is more likely that there are subgroups of FMS patients and that treatment will be more effective when it is matched to the unique characteristics of each group. Thus, at this point it may be premature to rule out the potential value of these unimodal therapies described. Moreover, we note that some of these individual therapies may be incorporated within comprehensive programs.

Multidisciplinary Treatments

In the past few decades, a growing number of investigators have emphasized the importance of addressing multiple factors associated with FMS (e.g., Bennett, 1996). Various types of multidisciplinary treatment programs have been developed for FMS, although programs tend to include some common components including physical exercise, education, and some type of cognitive treatments to improve coping (e.g., Burckhardt, Mannerkorpi, Hendenberg, & Bjelle, 1994, Mengshoel, Forseth, Haugen, Walle-Hansen, & Førre, 1995). Patients may need to learn proper exercise techniques, to use relaxation as pain and stress management and to internalize new and adaptive cognitive and behavioral coping strategies during sessions. Nielson, Walker, and McCain (1992) developed a comprehensive inpatient program consisting of exercise, relaxation training, coping training, family education, and pacing and demonstrated that their program was effective in reducing pain, emotional distress, pain behaviors, and a maladaptive cognitive set. A subsequent study (White & Nielson, 1995) demonstrated the maintenance of treatment benefit at 30-month follow-up in emotional distress and pain behaviors. Unfortunately, they did not assess typical FMS symptoms such as fatigue and sleep problems.

Other investigators (Bennett et al., 1996) developed comprehensive outpatient programs consisting of CBT, exercise, medication management, and pacing. Bennett and colleagues (1996) provided weekly 90-minute sessions over 6 months. As noted earlier, Turk, Okifuji, Sinclair, and Starz (1998) provided six half-day sessions over 4 weeks. In both programs, patients reported significant improvements in various FMS-related areas including reducing pain, fatigue, distressed mood, and perceived functioning. The demonstrated efficacy of the multidisciplinary treatment programs suggests that the combination of medical, physical, and CBT components should be the treatment of choice for all FMS patients. Certainly, the treatment effects on average were statistically significant. However, the large individual variation in treatment response was also present. We attribute that variation in treatment response to existing, often overlooked, psychosocial differences suggesting that matching treatment to clinical needs of subgroups of FMS patients may be critical in optimizing treatment efficacy.

General Treatment Recommendations

After careful assessment of salient issues faced by the patient, some or all of the following therapeutic foci might apply to treatment of FMS patient. Our strategy has been to direct treatment toward MPI profile characteristics. For example, ACs may need only support, reading recommendations to help them self-manage their symptoms, and recommendations for appropriate stretches and exercise increased in a gradual and reasonably paced manner. FMS patients with DYS profiles may need considerably more support, supervision, and a reactivation program that includes physical therapy and psychotherapy. In this subgroup, CBT will likely focus on acquisition of behavioral skills such as relaxation and alteration of maladaptive thoughts contributing to depression, hopelessness, isolation, and deconditioning. FMS patients with an ID profile may need CBT for depression and in addition may need training in assertive and effective communication styles. Such patients may also be candidates for couple counseling. We treat all FMS patients in groups based on their psychosocial and behavioral characteristics and the subgroups classification based on their response to the MPI (for a discussion of group treat-

ment, see Keefe et al., Chapter 11, this volume). What follows is an overview of general treatment recommendations that we believe are appropriate for all FMS patients regardless of their unique psychosocial and behavioral characteristics. We follow this overview with a review of some of the components in our treatment matching intervention based on the MPI subgroups.

Education

As noted previously, information and reassurance are essential for treating FMS. The lack of a definitive explanation for the symptoms often produces fear—fear that something serious but as yet unidentified is causing the symptoms, that the symptoms will become progressively worse, of being told that there is nothing that can be done, of being told that the problems are all caused by psychological factors (imaginary), and that they will be simply told to learn to live with symptoms without being told how. Consequently, we begin our intervention with information about the nature of FMS, the possible causes (described previously), and the treatment that we feel is most effective and safe for FMS, that is, reactivation through exercise and CBT to alter some of the automatic thoughts that increase the likelihood for depression, anxiety, fear, and relapse from a self-management treatment.

Education includes a discussion of the distinction between acute pain and chronic pain. Acute pain is rightly seen as a signal of "harm" or potential damage or danger to the body. In the case of chronic pain and FMS, however, the pain is no longer a signal of damage to the body. Thus, we make the distinction between "hurt" and "harm." Indeed, we admit to patients that we will be asking them to engage in the very activities they might fear. We ask them to increase physical activity and exercise. From our first session, we admit that a reconditioning program will likely "hurt" as muscles become sore after months or years of disuse, but we reassure them that we will not ask them to perform any exercises that will harm them.

Acceptance

The idea of acceptance, rather than cure, is often a wise course to follow with FMS patients. However, some patients view acceptance as synonymous with failure, that is, an admission that "I'll never be better." We view acceptance as necessary before adopting significant lifestyle and behavior changes and convey that message to our patients. Rather than viewing acceptance as "living with the FMS," we view it as "living despite FMS." A patient offers her account of coming to acceptance:

"Somewhere along the line, I began to come out of the fog and take control of my life. I have done a great deal of soul searching and assessment of myself. I discovered how my need to control and lack of acceptance of my reality was hindering my ability to enjoy life. I realized I could not allow the pain and discomfort to be my sole focus. I realized that how I responded to this situation was going to make the difference. I could either continue to fight it, or I could accept what was, grieve what I lost, and move on. Until that point, no one else had really understood how much I had lost, and that I had a right to, and needed to, grieve. After that breakthrough, I could, and I chose to move on. My faith has helped and I began to view this as an opportunity and a blessing, as well as a chance to work on being the person I always wanted to be. Rather than spend my energy waiting on finding either answers or a cure, I decided to do something in the meantime. That is why I am back in school."

Focus on Functional Gains Rather Than on "the Disease"

Treatment of an FMS patient can often be obstructed by a patient with a rigid conviction that something is medically wrong and needs to be corrected or cured. This belief can obstruct progress in a therapy that focuses on a rehabilitative model and striving to make functional gains. It is best to discuss such a belief with the patient and mutually consider whether or not it is sufficiently strong to make the case incompatible with a treatment strategy that focuses on self-management. If patient and therapist agree to embark on treatment, therapy should always focus on functional gains rather than etiology or cure. One effective comparison is treatment of a condition such as diabetes. Once the pancreas is found to

be impaired, treatment does not focus on curing the pancreas, but, rather, treatment focuses on keeping glucose levels within a healthy range by dietary change, exercise, checking blood levels regularly, and, if indicated, medication management.

Goal Setting

We focus on goal setting as a means to use therapy time efficiently and direct behavior into achievable, reinforcing units. A focus on goal setting achieves multiple purposes. First, people with FMS need to have realistic goals and their goal setting can inform treatment decisions. If a patient enters treatment with the goal of "being completely pain free," perhaps treatment should focus first on education about FMS, a discussion about how treatment for FMS, as with treatment of all chronic illness (it is often helpful to make the analogy of other chronic conditions such as heart disease and diabetes), involves making significant lifestyle changes and maintaining these changes during symptom flare-ups and remissions.

A second function of goal setting is to provide an evaluation of the concordance between the patient's expectations and those of his or her health care provider. Clinicians must be careful to ensure that treatment goals are mutually understood and agreed on. For example, people may be willing to tolerate some degree of pain if they are able to have increased energy for work or other activities. Health care providers must also take into account which areas of functioning are most important for their patients' quality of life (see, e.g., Gorbatenko-Roth, Levin, Altmaier, & Doebbeling, 2001).

Goal setting is the first assignment in our intervention and we ask patients to write down several goals. We request that they make their goals short term (e.g., achievable during the 6-week intervention, operational (e.g., measurable), and within their control. This step can be difficult for some FMS patients who may have low self-efficacy and few coping skills. One patient returned in the second session and remarked that she was unable to think of any appropriate short-term goals despite genuine consideration of the assignment. She stated that she became increasingly uncomfortable and frustrated while doing the assignment. Further discussion revealed that the only goals that she could produce were vague goals that were primarily under the control of others. For example, she wanted to "be happy, to have better behaved children and a more attentive, understanding husband, and less deadline pressure at work." Therapy helped this patient rephrase her wishes into operational, controllable units. We focused on identifying the activities that would make her happier. Other group members helped by sharing their behavioral goals such as being able to walk a mile at the end of the program, dance without interruption for one song, or lose a certain amount of weight. This patient then considered ways that she could change how she communicates her needs in order to help her husband be more attentive. She also considered time-management strategies as a goal to reduce deadline pressures at work.

The nature of patient goals may be somewhat different for different subgroups of FMS patients. For example, DYS patients might focus on behavioral change to improve mood, ID patients may need to establish goals related to communication with significant others, whereas AC patients may have goals related to pacing of activities.

Self-Management of Physical Symptoms Using Relaxation

Relaxation is an integral part of the self-management behavioral program for patients with FMS. There are many different methods to help patients learn to relax (e.g., controlled breathing, progressive muscle relaxation, and autogenic training), no one of which is better than any other. Moreover, different people will find different methods more conducive to their styles. Thus, when we present information about relaxation we note the following:

THERAPIST: Relaxation is important because it can help control your muscles and also can help distract you from unpleasant thoughts and feelings. There are a lot of different ways to relax. Have you tried any on your own?

PATIENT 1: Yes, I take hot baths.

THERAPIST: Good, that is one way to try to relax your body. Do you find this helps you?

PATIENT 1: Yes, sometimes it does and I play soft music in the background, it sets a nice mood for me.

THERAPIST: So you try to relax by physical means of the warm water and to calm you thoughts by the music. Anyone else try other ways to relax?

PATIENT 2: I find that talking to my daughter about my granddaughter is relaxing.

THERAPIST: Yes, this is another way to relax our minds by distracting ourselves by doing other things and take our minds off of how we are feeling. So there are both physical and mental ways to relax. I will teach you some others that may be helpful for you. There are many different methods and different people find different ones useful at some times but often find that they can use different methods at different times. I don't know which ones will be most helpful for you. But as I teach you to use different ones, I want you to try them out at home. Give each one a chance and this way you will learn several and can switch around if you need to from one technique to another.

For a detailed discussion of relaxation, see Syrjala and Abrams (Chapter 9, this volume).

Imagery

One of the most commonly used means of diverting attention from an unpleasant stimulus is focusing attention on events external to bodily sensations. Emergency room doctors have learned the useful technique of attention diversion. Talking with adults about something that interests them or asking children to pretend they are watching a favorite television program and then to describe what is happening are two such strategies used routinely in performing painful emergency procedures when it is not possible to use an anesthetic. We discuss imagery as a strategy that patients may use when they are feeling overwhelmed by their pain and other symptoms or when they are having difficulty sleeping at night and are focusing on their bodies and distressing aspects of their lives.

"Perhaps you sometimes have daydreamed about an incident so vividly or have become so involved in reading a book or watching a movie that you completely forgot what you were doing. The more involving the image is, the less attention you can give to other events, and therefore the less pain you will experience. Although you may not frequently experience such an event, it is possible for everyone to do so, with some practice. Peoples' imagination can be so powerful that their muscles actually respond to their imagination. For example, muscles can tense during anxious images and relax during pleasant ones. Try involving yourself in the following image right now and see just how vivid you can make it."

We inform the patient that this strategy will become easier with practice, like any other skill. We also emphasize that the inclusion of the various senses enhances the vividness of the image and facilitates the imagery process.

There are an infinite number of images people can use. We try to help patients identify ones that will be engaging for them and have them practice these at home for a week. Some patients have difficulty doing this on their own, so we may make an audiotape to help guide them along. Other patients have tried to focus on a picture or poster to help them with their image. We try to make this a "no lose" situation by emphasizing that there are many types of images and we can work with them to find one might be helpful, but if they are reluctant we can give greater attention to relaxation methods. The idea is to help patients develop a repertoire of coping strategies that they can use on their own. For more about imagery, see Syrjala and Abrams (Chapter 9, this volume).

Pacing and Increasing Activities

In addition to the fears noted previously, FMS sufferers often develop an association between physical activity and pain and subsequently a fear that by engaging in activities they will make themselves worse (Vlaeyan et al., 1997). Understandably, this fear leads to avoidance of activity to prevent more pain, fatigue, and injury. In a sense they have learned that if something causes distress or pain, it should be avoided. Thus, treatment focuses on breaking the association between activity and pain by encouraging patients to gradually increase the pace

of their activity and endurance and lessen fatigue.

We introduce exercise into our treatment program under the guidance of a physical therapist. In the group session we discuss some of the barriers to exercise. For some patients with FMS, the idea of increasing activity is anathema. Often, individuals with FMS associate activity with pain, that is, increases in activity result in increased pain and an escape from pain results from reducing activity. Thus, pacing is a way to break the association between activity and pain. This concept is introduced by the following typical discussion:

THERAPIST: Does this pattern sound familiar to anyone? You wake up one morning and feel OK, not pain free but the pain is more tolerable than it has been in a long time.

GROUP: (*Nods yes.*)

THERAPIST: Good, that is a pattern in FMS, the symptoms, wax and wane. Some days are better than others.[1] Does anyone try to take advantage of those better days? Perhaps you do this by catching up on work deadlines, grocery shopping, laundry, errands. So that during the time that you feel better, your activity increases dramatically, like a "yo-yo."

GROUP: Nods yes.

THERAPIST: (*while graphing an activity line rising on the board*), "What is happening to pain while your engaging in all of these activities?" [See Figure 19.3.]

PATIENT 1: The pain is rising slowly.

PATIENT 2: Sometimes the pain just flares out of nowhere.

THERAPIST: (*while graphing the pain line that corresponds to the activity line*) So, I know that this is an over generalization and of course there are individual differences but in general, the pain seems to follow the activity?

GROUP: Yes.

THERAPIST: Then what happens to activity when the pain gets really bad? (*Draws a dramatically downward sloping activity line.*) What is learned here, is that pain follows activity and pain remits with inactivity. We want you to learn another way of behaving and increasing activity called pacing of activity. [See Figure 19.4.]

The remainder of the session is spent teaching patients the principles of pacing. A pac-

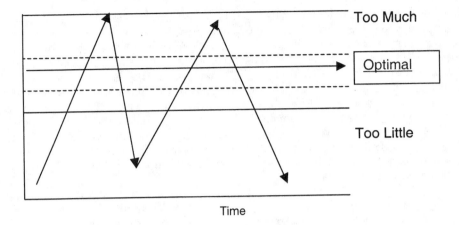

FIGURE 19.3. The yo-yo pattern.

ing exercise calls for them to set up a daily time quota for a particular activity and to spend only the preset amount of time on the activity (see Figure 19.5). The quota is based on a portion of the person's known capacity for that activity. Patients are asked to perform the activity for several days, up to the point where they are beginning to feel pain or fatigue or other signs that they have reached their limit (see Figure 19.5). Using this as a baseline, they then set up a manageable activity plan, with gradually increasing activity levels that they are likely to be able to maintain. Activity schedules should be established in advance and should not be based on their pain, fatigue, or other symptoms. This assignment often requires a significant conceptual adjustment. Patients have typically adjusted their activity based on their pain and fatigue levels, trying to maximize their activity on good days. More conscientious or high-achieving patients also have difficulty with the notion of starting a project or task and not necessarily completing it. Thus, it is important to stress that proper pacing involves not only performing to the quota on days with more pain but also preventing oneself from doing too much on days with less pain.

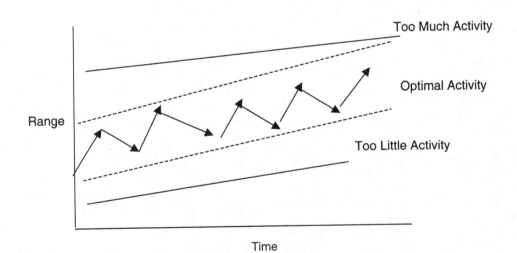

FIGURE 19.4. Balanced growth.

Pacing Graph

Activity: *Walking (example)*

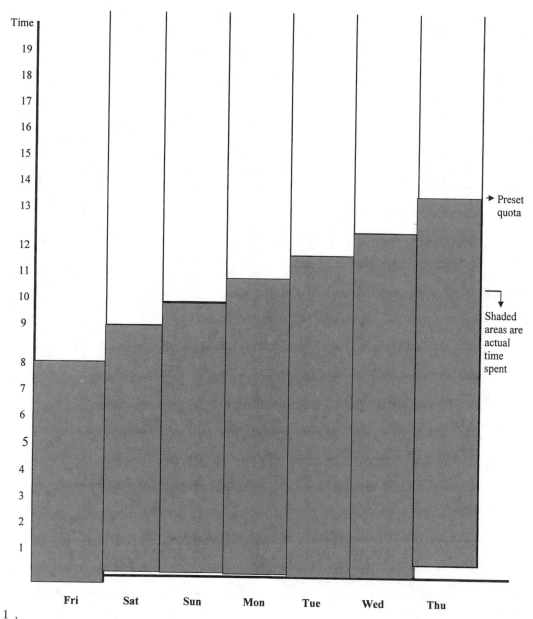

1 . Pick an activity.
2. Set baselines.
   Take a couple of days to do an activity (or part of an activity) until pain, fatigue, or weakness make you stop.
3. Average the work that you do to set the first quota.
   The first quota should be about 80% of your average from the previous couple of days.
4. Set subsequent quotas.
   These can be time or amount of work. Use these quotas as the ceiling and floor for subsequent activity.
5. Keep records and graphs.
6. Reward yourself.

FIGURE 19.5. Steps to pacing.

Sleep

A common symptom of FMS is poor sleep. We encourage patients to follow a "sleep hygiene" plan. This includes establishing a standard wakeup time, getting out of bed during extended wakenings, avoiding sleep-incompatible behaviors in bed, eliminating daytime napping, and avoiding activities near bed time that might interfere with sleep (see Table 19.2).

Cognitive Dysfunction

Along with sleeping problems, many patients with FMS report significant cognitive impairment (Glass & Park, 2001). They report difficulty concentrating, attending to new material, and less frequently difficulty with short-term and long-term memory. The term "fibro fog" is commonly used to describe the clinical presentation. The data are still unclear as to the existence or extent of cognitive impairment in FMS patients. Attention and concentration deficits may be more related to sleep deficits, medication, physical deconditioning, and depression than to FMS uniquely (Landro, Stiles, & Sletvold, 1997). Perceived memory deficits of FMS patients are often disproportionately greater than their objective deficits (Grace, Nielson, Hopkins, & Berg, 1999). It is helpful to discuss and demonstrate the same memory and attention strategies with FMS patients as one would discuss with any population reporting cognitive impairment—that is, use of day planners, selective attention, repetition strategies, laundry lists, and "to-do" lists.

Maladaptive Thoughts

Many people with FMS subcribe to a number of negative and maladaptive thoughts about themselves and their plight. We directly address the relationship between thoughts, feelings, behavior, and physiology.

"It is easy to indulge in negative thinking when you have FMS. Your pain drags on, and a part of your reaction to that situation comes in the form of thoughts and feelings of fear and frustration. These negative thoughts can be so automatic that you may not be aware of how frequently they occur and how debilitating they are. You need to take the time now to examine your negative thinking and understand its effect on your ability to manage your pain.

"Right now try to recall some of your typical negative thoughts. See if they sound like any of these:

- "I have no control over my pain."
- "I'll never get better."
- "This is going to get worse and worse until I go crazy."
- "This should never have happened to me."
- "No one else can ever really understand this pain."

TABLE 19.2. Do's and Don'ts for a Good Night's Sleep

Do's	Don'ts
1. Have a comfortable bedroom, clean linens, pillows, and a mattress that doesn't squeak.	1. Don't use radios, TVs, stereos in the bedroom
2. Have a comfortable level of lighting.	2. Don't drink or eat caffeinated beverages or foods (coffee, tea, chocolate) after about 2:00 P.M.
3. Have a quiet, cool room.	3. Don't drink alcohol after about 7:00 P.M.
4. Have a set time to wake and go to sleep.	4. Don't nap during the day.
5. Reserve the bedroom for sleep and sexual activity.	5. Try not to let yourself get too sleepy during the day (try exercise for an energy boost or consider other midday energy boosters).
6. Daily exercise.	6. Don't exercise close to bedtime.
7. Allow yourself a transition period before bedtime.	7. Don't concentrate on important things immediately prior to going to bed.
8. Develop a "going to bed ritual."	8. Don't change your sleep habits from day to day.
9. Establish daytime routines.	9. Don't go back to bed until you feel sleepy.
10. Get out of bed if you haven't fallen asleep after 20 minutes. Go to another room and do something that is not interesting, stimulating, or exciting.	

- "It's all my [job's, boss's, doctor's, family's, spouse's] fault that I'm in this mess."

"Do any of these statements sound familiar to you? These are only a few of many pain-related messages. You may have others of your own that are unique to your situation.

"What you think becomes what you feel. Once you get started, the momentum of your negative thoughts continues to carry you down and down, unless you do something to break out of the pattern. By changing the way you think you can learn to change the negative things you say to yourself that fuel your fears, depression, and anger and inevitably makes your pain worse.

"Take a few days to jot down all thoughts that occur to you concerning your pain. Note when and where these thoughts occur. Take an observer's stance while writing down your thoughts. In other words, try not to censor or debate your thoughts; simply write down all that come to you, whether they're about yourself or others. Remember that it takes practice to become familiar with your brand of negative thinking. Automatic thinking is lightning fast; if you can identify only one thought in a week, that's fine. In time, more thoughts will come to you. After the week, look back on your list of statements. Compare them to the following characteristics of typical negative thinking [hands out Table 19.3]. Think which of the ones on the list you do most often."

We ask patients to complete a dysfunctional thought diary over a week and to record when their symptoms are worse, what they were doing at the time, what they were thinking, how they felt, and how their thoughts and feelings might affect what they did.

Stress

Many patients with FMS fail to see the relationship between stress and their physical health or feel that the stress in their life is unavoidable or unmanageable. We introduce the concept of stress by comparing the stress associated with having a chronic illness to other common stressors.

"Chronic pain drains your energy much like the stress of a demanding job or a nagging family problem. When you have chronic pain, life stressors seem like insurmountable obstacles in your path. Your family is affected and your ability to do your job or chores around the house can be severely curtailed, perhaps leading to financial worries.

"As one person with FMS said, 'I feel like I use all my energy doing battle with the pain—I have no stamina or joy left over for important things in my life, like my family and job.'"

"When you're in pain, you need to learn and practice stress management for two simple reasons. First, chronic pain and fatigue are themselves stressors. It reduces your ability to function, to cope, and to feel good. If you can't function, you feel useless. If you can't cope, then other stressors begin piling up. Second, you tense your muscles in response to pain and its by-products.

"Begin by realizing that there is a stress component to your pain. Physical tension, mental anxiety and fatigue can make coping more difficult. You can minimize the domino effect of stress and pain by learning to manage the tension component in your life. Learn to identify stress in your body and its interplay with your symptoms.

"Self-knowledge is the first step to gaining control. You need to learn about the stresses in your life. You can help yourself by learning to identify your typical unhelpful stress patterns and by beginning to eliminate them from your daily routine. This can be done with regular and consistent daily practice of one or more of the techniques discussed in the program. These techniques have different names and use different processes, but they are all designed to do the same thing . . . to relax your body so that you can cope better with your pain and stress.

"To help you learn about stress in your life, I would like you to complete this stress diary over the next week [see Figure 19.6]. Bring it with you next week and we can see what you learned about yourself."

In session we advocate several stress-management techniques. We begin by having patients identify stressors and distinguish between stressors they can or cannot control. We focus on modifying the stressors they can control and practicing other skills such as relaxation, time management, and effective communication for those stressors that they cannot control.

TABLE 19.3. Eight Styles of Negative Thinking

1. *Blaming.* You make someone or something else responsible for your pain. "My lousy boss is to blame for my job accident." "My family demands so much from me, I can't afford the time or money to take care of this pain." Some people go too far in the other direction and focus all the blame entirely on themselves. "It's all my fault that this happened to me." If you continually put yourself down in this way, the insidious nature of self-blame can lead to lethargy and depression. This self-defeating stance can also serve as an excuse for inactivity.

2. *"Should" statements.* The words *should, must,* or *ought* appear regularly in chronic pain negative thinking and are examples of irrational thoughts. Shoulds are usually a put-down, implying that you were stupid, foolish, or weak for not living up to some standard. "I *should* have thought of good body mechanics before I lifted that box." "I *shouldn't* have been in such a hurry when I slipped on the ice." "I *must* keep up with all my responsibilities, pain or no pain." "I *shouldn't* react to pain like this."

3. *Polarized thinking.* Everything is "black or white," "good or bad." There is no gray area in the middle for improvement. Polarized thinking assumes things must go perfectly or else. If you have a pain relapse, then you're likely to think that the program you're using is no good or it's a sure sign of your ineptness. This thinking leads to damaging overgeneralizations. You have one relaxation session where you are unable to decrease your pain, and you assume that you'll *never* be able to decrease your pain. Overgeneralizations are often couched in terms of absolute statements-cue words are *all, every, none, never, always, everybody,* and *nobody.*

4. *Catastrophizing.* People who engage in this kind of thinking react to life situations by imagining the worst possible outcome and then reacting to their fear-provoking scenario as if it will surely come true. "I *know* that the only option left open to me is to have surgery. I'm sure I'll be laid up for months. What if the operation is a failure?" "What if" statements characterize this thinking, and greatly add to anxiety levels. "What if my pain *never* gets better, and I have to live like an invalid for the rest of my life? What if my spouse leaves me? What if I am unable to work?"

5. *Control fallacies.* Some chronic pain sufferers see themselves as "externally controlled" by others, such as those in the medical profession. By assigning a doctor or a clinic total power over their fate, they make themselves helpless victims of their pain and of the system. In effect, they absolve themselves of any responsibility Others may see themselves as powerless to change a dysfunctional family situation. On the other hand, people who see themselves as "internally controlled" believe that they have complete responsibility for everything and everyone. "Everyone depends on me. The family will fall apart if I don't recover quickly from this mess."

6. *Emotional reasoning.* This line of thinking assumes that what you feel *must* be true. If you feel guilty about needing time to heal, then taking the time must be wrong and needing the time must be your fault. If you're frightened that the pain will never stop, then you *believe* it will never stop. If you feel grief at the thought that you'll never run again, then you must be right-you won't run again. You let your feelings rule your reasoning ability. The strength of the feeling creates conviction, but later things may seem different as the emotional storm dies down.

7. *Filtering.* Some people have a tendency to see their pain through tunnel vision, filtering out any potentially positive aspects. These people make things worse than they are by focusing only on the pain and nothing else. The process of filtering can also be very selective. You may choose to remember only those things that support your angry feelings, thus pulling your negative memories out of context and isolating you from positive experiences.

8. *Entitlement fallacy.* People often feel that they are "entitled" to a pain-free existence. They believe they shouldn't have to suffer pain or loss. They feel cheated, that life is being unfair. People who harbor the entitlement fallacy feel that the luxury of ignoring or taking their bodies for granted is their right. And if they lose some capacity due to chronic pain, they feel that their life has been diminished.

These eight styles of thinking are related to each other. In fact, if you have a tendency toward one line of thinking, you will probably catch yourself doing several of the others. While the categories are a helpful way of showing how negative thinking works, don't be surprised if you have trouble labeling your own thoughts, since the boundaries between styles can blur. It's also quite possible to bombard yourself with a number of negative thoughts all at once in a lightening-fast mental shorthand. You rapidly heap negative thought upon negative thought until you feel overwhelmed and ready to give up. Be patient with yourself and allow yourself to gradually become familiar with your unique way of negative thinking.

	A	B
Date and time	Activating event (pain or other distressing situation)	Rating (1–100)
9/14 8:35 A.M.	1) Back pain while driving	50
9/15 9:15 A.M.	2) Boss yelled at me	30
	3)	
	4)	
	5)	

1. Record in Column A a situation in which you have increased pain and/or are feeling emotionally upset about your pain. Provide relevant details such as where you were, who you were with, and what you were doing.
2. Write down in the "Rating" column (B) the intensity of the feeling on a scale from 0–100 (with 100 being extremely intense).

FIGURE 19.6. Diary of Stressful Events.

Relapse

We discuss relapse in the same context of acceptance. FMS is a chronic condition and most often, symptoms of FMS wax and wane. Periods of symptom reduction are often followed with periods of flare-up. During our intervention, we describe a relapse prevention model. We view the behavioral change involved in treatment for FMS as a dynamic process involving a series of stages. First, patients often believe that a physician must do something for them in order for pain relief to occur and that they will be passive recipients of a medical cure. Later, when confronted with the realization that management rather than cure is the most likely treatment, patients begin to consider behavioral change as a viable treatment option. Ideally, soon after considering change, FMS patients seek treatment for their depression, manage or reduce the stress in their lives, actively seek to improve relationships, engage in relaxation to reduce muscle tension, and perform whatever other activities they choose to manage their conditions.

At some point thereafter, the behaviors become habits and patients engage in exercise as part of a normal daily routine, practice relaxation on a daily basis, and use pacing consistently to moderate their activity levels. Almost invariably, patients experience some relapse. That is, they have a pain flare-up or fail to engage in the behaviors that have helped to keep them manageable. We present this as a process where people can find themselves relapsing and need to reinstitute their self-management plan. We acknowledge that there will be good and bad days as everyone experiences "ups and downs." We suggest that the key to consistent recovery is not the absence of symptoms but the willingness to reenter the process of recovery with independent action even after a flare-up.

The challenge for patients is twofold: (1) to recognize when they are relapsing and (2) to return to the use of their self-management skills. We assist this process by assigning a relapse prevention worksheet. Patients are asked to list the behaviors, thoughts and feelings that act as cues or predictors that a relapse is likely to occur. They are then asked to list the behaviors that have helped in the past and to develop a written plan for engaging in those behaviors.

Some Treatment Modules That Can be Matched to Patient Characteristics

Depression

Over 60% of patients treated in our program reveal clinically significant levels of depressive mood. Our research suggests that the DYS and ID patients are significantly more depressed than the AC. Here we can see the advantage of subgrouping patients. It makes little sense to focus on depression, as is commonly done with general pain rehabilitation programs, for patients such as the ACs, as they are not in need of attention to affective distress.

CBT focuses on the person's thoughts, feelings, and behaviors. It also addresses the role of environmental factors in maintaining and exacerbating symptoms while facilitating disability (see Turk, Chapter 7, this volume). Although CBT is not a cure, it can help people gain control of their symptoms and regain control of their lives. One patient describes how lack of control over symptoms and significant functional impairment led to depression:

"Initially, my life was turned upside down due to pain. . . . I was confident that the pain I had been experiencing would eventually decrease, and I would be able to return to normal. I worked hard to make that happen and drove my family and supervisor crazy pushing myself so hard. When 6 months later I was still unable to function at a level acceptable to me, I became more frustrated and depressed. I was sent to more doctors and each time I would get my hopes up that there would be an explanation, and each time I was told there was nothing wrong. With no concrete explanations as to why this was occurring, I began to feel helpless. By this time, I had to take another leave of absence from work. I couldn't understand why I could not seem to handle what was occurring, or control it. I began to feel crazy and isolated. I had to quit my job of 10 years. A job I really enjoyed and did well. I lost my belief in myself to handle adversity

and I lost my sense of identity that was at that time, tied to my job. . . . I began to isolate myself. I do not like to make commitment I cannot keep and since I could no longer predict how I would feel on any given day, I made no commitments. I stopped talking about how I felt and I stopped doing anything that made the pain worse, which was just about everything. I simply stopped trying to get better. I hated the way I looked, I felt fat, unattractive and pitiful. I lost me, or at least who I believed myself to be. I lost all sense of who I was and for me, which was worse than the pain. My relationships with family and friends changed drastically because I was terribly uncomfortable with not being able to be the person I once was. I also felt worthless because I could no longer be the strong one and do for others. I felt I had no value."

For the clinician, this vignette is rife with material for a CBT approach. Examination of dysfunctional thoughts can influence attitudinal components of coping responses. Attention should be given to raising patients' awareness of their negative thought patterns, such as catastrophic thoughts, black–white thinking, or unrealistically global or negative thinking; filtering, or biased awareness of negative information; and unrealistic appraisals of control and self-efficacy. Efforts should be made to enable patients to develop more adaptive cognitions that permit more hope, or a belief that there may be something they can do that can make things better.

The foregoing vignette also offers several behavioral targets for therapy. Review of the patient's statements reveal several past behaviors that contributed to this patient's depression and pain dysfunction. She reports isolating herself from friends and family, changing relationships to accommodate her perceived inability to commit and to be the person she was before, and upset over her physical appearance. Identification of the behaviors elicited that contributed to her depression and dysfunction facilitated taking action and trying new behaviors. In addition to exercise goals, her behavioral goals included making a phone call each day, face-to-face contact with a friend once a week, rejoining her study group, and contact with her family once a week. Each behavior helped to alter her self-concept in the direction of a person who is addressing her situation and away from a more passive, patient sufferer. Such behavior can facilitate a patient's taking action or trying new behaviors, which in turn encourages the patient to make further efforts, all of which can alter the patient's self-concept in the direction of a person who is addressing his or her situation and away from a more passive, patient sufferer.

We use an ABCD model to help the patient identify and alter maladaptive thoughts and behaviors:

The ABCD Model

"The ABCD model is a useful tool in structuring your approach to understanding negative thinking about pain.

"*A* is the '*activating event*' or *stressor*. In this case, let's make it a muscle spasm in your back that keeps you from fulfilling a commitment.

"*B* is your '*belief system,*' or your thoughts and attitudes about the stressful event. For example, you may think, 'Now I can't do what I said I would—they'll think I'm weak. I can't do anything anymore.'

"*C* stands for the '*consequences*' of the activating event, or basically, your feelings. When you think poorly of yourself, as in *B,* you *feel* guilty, frustrated, depressed.

"*D* is a way to change the above sequence of events. *D* means '*disputing*' the negative thinking you discover in *B,* which can affect how badly you feel in *C.*

"It takes a little getting used to breaking your thoughts and feelings down into this structured format. Once you do, however, you'll be more familiar with your own typical pattern and will be able to more automatically and rapidly dispute the negative thinking that gets in your way.

"Work this *A-B-C* process several times until you feel comfortable with it. Note your stress levels as you work it. Also note that A doesn't actually cause your negative feelings. B causes the feelings. B is your *perception of the event,* and determines your reaction to it. Beliefs can aggravate the consequences of an event or ameliorate them. Negative thoughts and feelings also create a pain-making feedback loop. The more negative thoughts, *B,* the more negative feelings, *C.* Then as you feel more anxious, depressed, and so on, you start thinking how horribly anxious or depressed you are, and this only serves to intensify your negative feelings."

Interpersonal Problems

It has been our experience that a high percentage of patients with FMS best fit an ID profile on the MPI (Turk, Okifuji, Sinclair, & Starz, 1996). People with such profiles show high levels of pain and depression and report low social support or high levels of negative or punishing responses from significant others. For these people we guide treatment toward effective communication skills and role-playing assertive interactions with others. The FMS patient with ID may need to learn new communication skills to facilitate cooperation from others, including family, friends, and coworkers. As people become less preoccupied or burdened by their illness experience, they may need to practice teaching others how much, or how little, they wish to discuss or focus on their symptoms and help others to see them in their new, more active, light. One role-play in particular begins with the therapist acting the role of friend or family member. After the patient briefly winces in pain, the therapist asks about FMS. This interaction often begins in an emotionally loaded fashion:

THERAPIST: (*after patient winces*) What's wrong?

PATIENT: It's just my fibro.

THERAPIST: You still have fibromyalgia? When are they going to figure it out? Are you going to be like this forever?

The subsequent role-plays involve patients finding an effective way to convey information about the chronicity and nature of FMS, how symptoms are managed rather than cured, and how they are learning new skills to help them to effectively manage the symptoms.

Assertiveness

Assertiveness training is particularly important for assisting people in making their different attitudes and behaviors actually work in their interpersonal contexts. For example, as one shifts from an attitude of feeling responsible for everything to a perspective that allows for acknowledgement of limits and asking for help, he or she may need to learn new communication skills to facilitate cooperation from others, including family, friends, and coworkers. We first teach patients the distinction between different communication styles (i.e., passive, aggressive, and assertive) and then role-play typical interactions.

We use the mnemonic of *DEAR MAN* to help patients learn a strategy for getting what they want or need in interpersonal situations. The mnemonic corresponds to the following steps:

- *Describe* the current situation;
- *Express* your feelings and opinions about the situation;
- *Assert* yourself by asking for what you want;
- *Reinforce* the other person by explaining the positive effects of getting what you want; be
- *Mindful* and stay focused on your objectives;
- *Appear* effective, competent, and non-apologetic; and be willing to
- *Negotiate*.

Using this technique, significant others (e.g., spouses, other family members, and partners) can be taught how they can be most helpful to the affected person, whether through instrumental, direct problem-solving support or through emotional support and validation of the person's experience and efforts. Attention to family interactions is also crucial in addressing problems of FMS and other chronic illnesses (e.g., Schmaling & Sher, 2000; see Kerns, Otis, & Wise, Chapter 12, this volume).

Psychosocial interventions provided in groups allow for sharing of concerns and advice and for validation of individual experiences. Less disabled participants can gain a greater awareness of their progress and can provide advice and hope to more disabled patients, often more plausibly than can a nonpatient health care provider. More disabled participants can learn from others who have managed to make progress and enjoy good outcomes in spite of their symptoms.

Medications

Medication that targets key symptoms (i.e., fatigue, sleep, and depression) should also be considered adjuncts to exercise and CBT (Goldenberg et al., 1986; O'Malley et al., 2000). Providing some symptomatic relief may enable patients to sleep better and to engage in paced physical activities. In particular, antidepressant medication may work because it addresses actual depression symptoms, but it may also be helpful in improving sleep quality or in somehow reducing pain severity, even at doses that are typically lower than those used for depression. It is interesting to note that low dose tricyclic antidepressants have been shown to be effective with FMS but newer selective serotoning reuptake inhibitors (SSRIs) have not had as positive an outcome. To our knowledge, there have been no blinded, randomized controlled-trials with long-term follow-ups evaluating the effectiveness of such combined treatments.

Concluding Comments

Preliminary studies using a CBT approach have been generally positive in reducing symptoms and related distress but not in eliminating all symptoms of FMS (e.g., Nielson et al., 1992; Turk, Okifuji, Sinclair, & Starz, 1998; Turk, Okifuji, Starz, & Sinclair, 1998). Larger-scale studies with appropriate control groups and adequate follow-up periods are required to confirm the effectiveness of the CBT approach. To date, only one study (Turk, Okifuji, Starz, & Sinclair, 1998) has addressed the question of the characteristics of FMS treatment responders. Research is need to determine what set of FMS patients, with what characteristics, can benefit from generic CBT combined with activity therapy. The failure of many patients to achieve and maintain positive outcomes indicates, most assuredly, that one size does not fit all (Turk, 1990).

Acknowledgments

Preparation of this chapter was supported in part by grants from the National Institute of Arthritis and Musculoskeletal and Skin Diseases

(AR/AI44724, AR47298) and the National Institute of Child Health and Human Development/National Center for Medical Rehabilitation Research (HD33989).

Note

1. Early in treating FMS patients, we made the mistake of saying "good" day and once said "you wake in the morning and feel 'no' pain." The group made very clear that they rarely have "good" days, and that the never wake with "no" pain. Stating "better" days is far more likely to result in agreement.

References

Ahles, T. A., Khan, S. A., Yunus, M. B., Spiegel, D. A., & Masi, A. T. (1991). Psychiatric status of patients with primary fibromyalgia, patients with rheumatoid arthritis and subjects without pain: A blind comparison of DMS III diagnoses. *American Journal of Psychiatry, 148,* 1721–1726.

Alfici, S., Sigal, M., & Landau, M. (1989). Primary fibromyalgia syndrome—a variant of depressive disorder. *Psychotherapy and Psychosomatics, 51,* 156–161.

Barsky, A. J., & Borus, J. F. (1999). Functional somatic syndromes. *Annals of Internal Medicine, 130,* 910–921.

Baumstark, K. E., & Buckelew, S. P. (1992). Fibromyalgia: Clinical signs, research findings, treatment implications, and future directions. *Annals of Behavioral Medicine, 14,* 282–91.

Bengtsson, A., & Henriksson, K. G. (1989). The muscle in fibromyalgia—a review of Swedish studies. *Journal of Rheumatology, 19,* 144–149.

Bengtsson, A., Henriksson, K. G., & Larsson, J. (1986). Muscle biopsy in primary fibromyalgia. Light-microscopical and histochemical findings. *Scandinavian Journal of Rheumatology, 15,* 1–6.

Bennett, R. M. (1996). Multidisciplinary group programs to treat fibromyalgia patients. *Rheumatic Diseases Clinics of North America, 22,* 351–367.

Bennett, R. M., Burckhardt, C. S., Clark, S. R., O'Reilly, C. A., Wiens, A. N., & Campbell, S. M. (1996). Group treatment of fibromyalgia: A 6 month outpatient program. *Journal of Rheumatology, 23,* 521–528.

Bennett, R. M., Campbell, S., Burckhardt, C., Clark, S., O'Reilly, C., & Wiens, A. (1991). A multidisciplinary approach to fibromyalgia management. *Journal of Musculoskeletal Medicine, 8,* 21–32.

Bennett, R. M., Clark, S. R., Campbell, S. M., & Burckhardt, C. S. (1992). Low levels of somatomedin C in patients with the fibromyalgia syndrome. A possible link between sleep and muscle pain. *Arthritis and Rheumatism, 35,* 1113–1116.

Bergstrom, G., Jensen, I. B., Bodin, L., Linton, S. J., & Nygren, A. L. (2001). The impact of psychologically different patient groups on outcome after a vocational rehabilitation program for long-term spinal pain patients. *Pain, 93,* 229–237.

Breau, L. M., McGrath, P. J., & Ju, L. H. (1999). Review of juvenile primary fibromyalgia and chronic fatigue syndrome. *Developmental and Behavioral Pediatrics, 20,* 278–288.

Buckelew, S. P., Huyser, B., Hewett, J. E., Parker, J. C., Johnson, J. C., Conway, R., & Kay, D. R. (1996). Self-efficacy predicting outcome among fibromyalgia subjects. *Arthritis Care Research, 9,* 97–104.

Buckelew, S. P., Murray, S. E., Hewett, J. E., Johnson, J., & Huyser, B. (1995). Self-efficacy, pain, and physical activity among fibromyalgia subjects. *Arthritis Care and Research, 8,* 43–50.

Burckhardt, C. S., Clark, S. R., & Bennett, R. M. (1993). Fibromyalgia and quality of life: A comparative analysis. *Journal of Rheumatology, 20,* 475–479.

Burckhardt, C. S., Mannerkorpi, K., Hedenberg, L., & Bjelle, A. (1994). A randomized, controlled trial of education and physical training for women with fibromyalgia. *Journal of Rheumatology, 21,* 714–720.

Carmody, T. P. (2001). Psychosocial subgroups, coping, and chronic low-back pain. *Journal of Clinical Psychology in Medical Settings, 8,* 137–148.

Carrette, S., Bell, M. V., & Reynolds, W. J. (1994). Comparison of amitriptyline, cyclobenzaprine, and placebo in the treatment of fibromyalgia: A randomized, double-blind clinical trial. *Arthritis and Rheumatism, 37,* 32–40.

Clark, S., Tindall, E., & Bennett, R. M. (1985). A double blind crossover trial of prednisone versus placebo in the treatment of fibrositis. *Journal of Rheumatology, 12,* 980–983.

Clauw, D. J., & Chrousos, G. P. (1997). Chronic pain and fatigue syndromes: Overlapping clinical and neuroendocrine features and potential pathogenic mechanisms. *Neuroimmunomodulation, 4,* 134–153.

Crofford, L. J., Engleberg, N. C., & Demitrack, M. A. (1996). Neurohormonal perturbations in fibromyalgia. *Bailliere's Clinical Rheumatology, 10,* 365–378.

Dahlstrom, L. Widmark, G., & Carlsson, S. G. (1997). Cognitive-behavioral profiles among different categories of orofacial pain patients: Diagnosis and treatment implications. *European Journal of Oral Sciences, 105,* 377–383.

Drewes, A. M., Andreasen, A., Schroder, H. D., Hogsaa, B., & Jennum, P. (1993). Pathology of skeletal muscle in fibromyalgia: A histo-immunochemical and ultrastructural study. *British Journal of Rheumatology, 32,* 479–483.

Drewes, A. M., Svsenden, L., Nielsen, K. D., Taagholt, S. J., & Bjerregåd, K. (1994). Quantification of alpha-EEG activity during sleep in fibromyalgia: A study based on ambulatory sleep monitoring. *Journal of Musculoskeletal Pain, 2,* 33–53.

Fairbank, J. C. T., Couper, J., Davies, J. B., & O'Brien, J. P. (1980). The Oswestry Low Back Pain Disability Questionnaire. *Physiotherapy, 166,* 271–273.

Ferraccioli, G., Ghirelli, L., Scita, F., Nolli, M., Mozzani, M., Fontana, S., Scorsonelli, M., Trident, A., & Derisio, C. (1987). EMG-biofeedback training in fibromyalgia syndrome. *Journal of Rheumatology, 14,* 820–825.

Flor, H., Birbaumer, N., & Turk, D. C. (1990). The psychobiology of chronic pain. *Advances in Behavior Research and Therapy, 12,* 47–84.

Glass, J. M., & Park, D. C. (2001). Cognitive dysfunction in fibromyalgia. *Current Rheumatology Reports, 3,* 123–127.

Goldenberg, D. L., Felson, D. T., & Dinerman, H. (1986). A randomized, controlled trial of amitriptyline and naproxen in the treatment of patients with fibromyalgia. *Arthritis and Rheumatism, 29,* 1371–1377.

Gorbatenko-Roth, K. G., Levin, I. P., Altmaier, E. M., & Doebbeling, B. N. (2001). Accuracy of health-related quality of life assessment: What is the benefit of incorporating patients' preferences for domain functioning? *Health Psychology, 20,* 136–140.

Grace, G. M., Nielson, W. R., Hopkins, M., & Berg, M. A. (1999). Concentration and memory deficits in patient with fibromyalgia syndrome. *Journal of Clinical and Experimental Neuropsychology, 21,* 477–487.

Greenfield, S., Fitzcharles, M. A., & Esdaile, J. M. (1992). Reactive fibromyalgia syndrome. *Arthritis and Rheumatism, 35,* 678–681.

Günther, V., Mur, E., Kinigadner, U., & Miller, C. (1994). Fibromyalgia—the effect of relaxation and hydrogalvanic bath therapy on the subjective pain experience. *Clinical Rheumatology, 13,* 573–578.

Hassett, A. L., Cone, J. D., & Sigal, L. H. (2000). The role of catastrophizing in the pain and depression of women with fibromyalgia syndrome. *Arthritis and Rheumatism, 43,* 2493–2500.

Hudson, J. I., Hudson, M. S., Pliner, L. F., Goldenberg, D. L., & Pope, H. G. (1985). Fibromyalgia and major affective disorder: A controlled phenomenology and family history study. *American Journal of Psychiatry, 142,* 441–466.

Jamison, R. N., Rudy, T. E., Penzien, D. B., & Mosley, T. H. (1994). Cognitive-behavioral classifications of chronic pain: Replication and extension of empirically-derived patient profiles. *Pain, 57,* 277–292.

Kerns, R. D., Turk, D. C., & Rudy, T. E. (1985). The West Haven–Yale Multidimensional Pain Inventory (WHYMPI). *Pain, 23,* 345–356.

Kosek, E., Ekholm, J., & Hansson, P. (1996). Sensory dysfunction in fibromyalgia patients with implications for pathogenic mechanisms. *Pain, 68,* 375–383.

Landro, N. I., Stiles, T. C., & Sletvold, H. (1997). Memory functioning in patients with primary fibromyalgia and major depression and healthy controls. *Journal of Psychosomatic Research, 42,* 297–306.

Locke, H. J., & Wallace, K. M. (1959). Short-term marital adjustment and prediction tests: Their reliability and validity. *Family Living, 21,* 251–255.

Martin, L., Nutting, A., Macintosh, B. R., Edworthy, S. M., Butterwick, D., & Cook, J. (1996). An exercise program in the treatment of fibromyalgia. *Journal of Rheumatology, 23,* 1050–1053.

Martin, M. Y., Bradley, L. A., Alexander, R. W., Alarcon, G. S., Triana-Alexander, M., Aaron, L. A., & Alberts, K. R. (1996). Coping strategies predict disability in patients with primary fibromyalgia. *Pain, 68,* 45–53.

Masi, A. T., & Yunus, M. B. (1990). Fibromyalgia—What is the best treatment? A personalized, comprehensive, ambulatory, patient-involved management program. *Balliere's Clinical Rheumatology, 4,* 333–370.

McDermid, A. J., Rollman, G. B., & McCain, G. A. (1996). Generalized hypervigilance in fibromyalgia: Evidence of perceptual amplification. *Pain, 66,* 133–144.

Melzack, R., & Casey, K. L. (1968). Sensory, motivational and central control determinants of pain: A new conceptual model. In D. Kenshalo (Ed.), *The skin senses* (pp. 423–443). Springfield, IL: Thomas.

Melzack, R., & Wall, P. D. (1965). Pain mechanisms: A new theory. *Science, 50,* 971–979.

Mengshoel, A. M., Forseth, K. O., Haugen, M., Walle-Hansen, R., & Førre, O. (1995). Multidisciplinary approach to fibromyalgia. A pilot study. *Clinical Rheumatology, 14,* 165–170.

Morriss, R. K., Ahmed, M., Wearden, A. J., Mullis, R., Strickland, P., Appleby, L., Campbell, I. T., & Pearson, D. (1999). The role of depression in pain, psychophysiological syndromes and medically unexplained symptoms associated with chronic fatigue syndrome. *Journal of Affective Disorders. 55,* 143–148.

Nicassio, P. M., Radojevic, V., Weisman, M. H., Schuman, C., Kim, J., Schoenfeld-Smith, K., & Krall, T. (1997). A comparison of behavioral and educational interventions for fibromyalgia. *Journal of Rheumatology, 24,* 2000–2007.

Nielson, W. R., Walker, C., & McCain, G. A. (1992). Cognitive behavioral treatment of fibromyalgia syndrome: Preliminary findings. *Journal of Rheumatology, 19,* 98–103.

Nørregaard, J., Bülow, P. M., Mehlsen, J., & Danneskiold-Samsose, B. (1994). Biochemical changes in relation to a maximal exercise test in patients with fibromyalgia. *Clinical Physiology, 14,* 159–167.

Okifuji, A., & Turk, D. C. (1999). Fibromyalgia: Search for mechanisms and effective treatments. In R. J. Gatchel & D. C. Turk (Eds.), *Psychosocial factors in pain: Critical perspectives* (pp. 227–246). New York: Guilford Press.

O'Malley, P. G., Balden, E., Tomkins, G., Santoro, J., Kroenke, K., & Jackson, J. L. (2000). Treatment of fibromyalgia with antidepressants: A meta-analysis. *Journal of General Internal Medicine, 15,* 659–666.

Peters, M. L., Vlaeyen, J. W. S., & van Drunen, C. (2000). Do fibromyalgia patients display hypervigilance for innocuous somatosensory stimuli? Application of a body scanning reaction time paradigm. *Pain, 86,* 283–292.

Prescott, E., Jacobsen, S., Kjoller, M., Bulow, P. M., Danneskiold-Samsoe, B., & Kamper-Jorgesen, J. (1993). Fibromyalgia in the adult Danish population: I. Prevalent study. *Scandinavian Journal of Rheumatology, 22,* 238–242.

Radloff, L. S. (1977). The CES-D: A self-report depression scale for research in the general population. *Applied Psychological Measurement, 1,* 385–401.

Rollman, G. B., & Lautenbacher, S. (1993). Hypervigilance effects in fibromyalgia: Pain experience and pain perception. In H. Værøy & H. Merskey (Eds.), *Progress in fibromyalgia and myofascial pain* (pp. 71–81). Amsterdam: Elsevier.

Russell, I. J., Fletcher, E. M., Michalek, J. E., McBroom, P. C., & Hester, G. G. (1991). Treatment of primary fibrositis/fibromyalgia syndrome with ibuprofen and alprazolam. A double-blind, placebo-controlled study. *Arthritis and Rheumatism, 34,* 552–560.

Schochat, T., Croft, P., & Raspe, H. (1994). The epidemiology of fibromyalgia. *British Journal of Rheumatology, 33,* 783–786.

Schmaling, K. B., & Sher, T. G. (Eds.). (2000). *The psychology of couples and illness: Theory, research, and practice.* Washington, DC: American Psychological Association Press.

Solomon, D. H., & Liang, M. H. (1997). Fibromyalgia: Scourge of humankind or bane of a rheumatologist's existence? *Arthritis and Rheumatism, 40,* 1553–1555.

Strategier, L. D., Chwalisz, K., Altmaier, E. M., Russell, D. W., & Lehmann, T. H. (1997). Multidimensional assessment of chronic low back pain: Predicting treatment outcomes. *Journal of Clinical Psyhology in Medical Settings, 4,* 91–110.

Talo, S., Forssell, H., Heikkonen, S., & Puukka, P. (2001). Integrative group therapy outcome related to psychosocial characteristics in patients with chronic pain. *International Journal of Rehabilitation Research, 24,* 25–33.

Turk, D. C. (1990). Customizing treatment for chronic pain patients: Who, what, and why. *Clinical Journal of Pain, 6,* 255–270.

Turk, D. C., & Flor, H. (1989). Primary fibromyalgia is more than tender points: Toward a multiaxial taxonomy. *Journal of Rheumatology, 16,* 80–86.

Turk, D. C., Monarch, E. S., & Williams, A. D. (in press). Psychological evaluation of patients diagnosed with fibromyalgia syndrome: Comprehensive approach. *Rheumatic Disease Clinics of North America.*

Turk, D. C., & Okifuji, A. (1997). Evaluating the role of physical, operant, cognitive, and affective factors in the pain behaviors of chronic pain patients. *Behavior Modification, 21,* 259–280.

Turk, D. C., Okifuji, A., Sinclair, J. D., & Starz, T. W. (1996). Pain, disability, and physical functioning in subgroups of patients with fibromyalgia. *Journal of Rheumatology, 23,* 1255–1262.

Turk, D. C., Okifuji, A., Sinclair, J. D., & Starz, T. W. (1998). Interdisciplinary treatment for fibromyalgia syndrome: Clinical and statistical significance. *Arthritis Care and Research, 11,* 186–195.

Turk, D. C., Okifuji, A., Starz, T. W., & Sinclair, J. D. (1996). Effects of type of symptom onset on psychological distress and disability in fibromyalgia syndrome patients. *Pain, 68,* 423–430.

Turk, D. C., Okifuji, A., Starz, T. W., & Sinclair, J. D. (1998). Differential responses by psychosocial subgroups of fibromyalgia syndrome patients to an interdisciplinary treatment. *Arthritis Care and Research, 11,* 397–404.

Turk, D. C., & Rudy, T. E. (1986). Assessment of cognitive factors in chronic pain: A worthwhile enterprise? *Journal of Consulting and Clinical Psychology, 54,* 760–768.

Turk, D. C., & Rudy, T. E. (1988). Toward an empirically derived taxonomy of chronic pain states: An integration of psychological assessment data. *Journal of Consulting and Clinical Psychology, 56,* 233–238.

Turk, D. C., & Rudy, T. E. (1990). The robustness of an empirically derived taxonomy of chronic pain patients. *Pain, 42,* 27–35.

Turk, D. C., Rudy, T. E., Kubinski, J. A., Zaki, H. S., & Greco, C. M. (1996). Dysfunctional TMD patients: Evaluating the efficacy of a tailored treatment protocol. *Journal of Consulting and Clinical Psychology, 64,* 139–146.

Turk, D. C., Sist, T. C., Okifuji, A., Miner, M. F., Florio, G., Harrison, P., Massey, J., Lema, M. L., & Zevon, M. A. (1998). Adaptation to metastatic cancer pain, regional/local cancer pain and non-cancer pain: Role of psychological and behavioral factors. *Pain, 74,* 247–256.

van Denderen, J. C., Boersma, J. W., Zeinstra, P., Hollander, A. P., & van Neerbos, B. R. (1992). Physiological effects of exhaustive physical exercise in primary fibromyalgia syndrome (PFS): Is PFS a disorder of neuroendocrine reactivity? *Scandinavian Journal of Rheumatology, 21,* 35–37.

Vlaeyen, J. W. S., Nooyen-Haazen, I. W. C. J., Boossens, M. E. J. B., van Breukelen, G., Heuts, P. H. T. G., & The, H. G. (1997). The role of fear in the cognitive-educational treatment of fibromyalgia. In T. S. Jensen, J. A. Turner, & Z. Wiesenfeld-Hallin (Eds.), *Proceedings of the 8th World Congress on Pain: Progress in pain research and management* (Vol 8, pp. 693–704). Seattle, WA: IASP Press.

Walker, E. A., Keegan, D., Gardner, G., Sullivan, M., Katon, W. J., & Bernstein, D. (1997). Psychosocial factors in fibromyalgia compared with rheumatoid arthritis: I. Psychiatric diagnoses and functional disability. *Psychosomatic Medicine, 59,* 565–571.

Waylonis, G. W., & Perkins, R. H. (1994). Post-traumatic fibromyalgia. A long-term follow-up. *American Journal of Physical Medicine and Rehabilitation, 73,* 403–412.

White, K. P., & Nielson, W. R. (1995). Cognitive behavioral treatment of fibromyalgia syndrome: A follow up assessment. *Journal of Rheumatology, 22,* 717–721.

White, K. P., Speechley, M., Harth, M., & Østbye, T. (1995). Fibromyalgia in rheumatology practice: A survey of Canadian rheumatologists. *Journal of Rheumatology, 22,* 722–726.

Wigers, S. H., Stiles, T. C., & Vogel, P. A. (1996). Effects of aerobic exercise versus stress management treatment in fibromyalgia: A 4.5 year prospective study. *Scandinavian Journal of Rheumatology, 25,* 77–86.

Wolfe, F., Russell, I. J., Vipraio, G., Ross, K., & Anderson, J. (1997). Serotonin levels, pain threshold, and fibromyalgia symptoms in the general population. *Journal of Rheumatology, 24,* 555–559.

Wolfe, F., Smythe, H. A., Yunus, M. B., Bennett, R. M., Bombardier, C., Goldenberg, D. J., Tugwell, P., Campbell, S. M., Abeles, M., Clark, P., Fam, A. G., Farber, S. J., Fiechtner, J. J., Franklin, C. M., Gatter, R. A., Hamaty, D., Lessard, J., Lichtbroun, A. S., Masi, A. T., McCain, G. A., Reynolds, W. J., Romano, T. J., Russell, I. J., & Sheon, R. P. (1990). The American College of Rheumatology 1990 criteria for the classification of fibromyalgia: Report of the multicenter criteria committee. *Arthritis and Rheumatism, 36,* 160–172.

Zidar, J., Backman, B., Bengtsson, A., & Henriksson, K. G. (1990). Quantitative EMG and muscle tension in painful muscle in fibromyalgia. *Pain, 40,* 249–254.

20

Treatment of
Whiplash-Associated Disorders

Lex Vendrig
Kevin McWhorter
Pieter van Akkerveeken

The term "whiplash" coined by Crowe (1958) during a meeting of the Western Orthopaedic Association in San Francisco has become a controversial issue. People talk about "having whiplash," meaning that they have persisting symptoms after an automobile accident. The costs in Western countries of chronic symptoms after whiplash injury in personal disability, work loss, and disability claims appears to be substantial and can even be termed "epidemic" (Cassidy, 1995).

What is whiplash exactly? It is usually used to refer to the rapid and sudden extension and flexion of the neck following a motor vehicle or other accident. The Quebec Task Force on whiplash-associated disorders (Spitzer et al., 1995) restricts the term "whiplash" to the mechanism of the injury: During rear-end car collisions people are subjected to an extension–acceleration force that may result in a ligamentous, nervous, muscular, and/or bony injury of the neck. The combination of symptoms and signs caused by the injury is currently labeled whiplash-associated disorders (WADs). The term "whiplash" itself does not indicate a diagnosis. The diagnosis, or in other words the anatomic lesion, is usually classified following the grading system proposed by the

Quebec Task Force (Spitzer et al., 1995). It should be emphasized that the Quebec classification is not a comprehensive classification. It only differentiates with regard to the quality of the lesion in relation to neck pain. The authors of the Quebec Task Force described four classes of WADs based on severity of signs and symptoms (see Table 20.1) The Quebec classification has some prognostic value. Hartling, Brison, and Arderen (2001) showed that risk for symptoms at 6, 12, 18, and 24 months increased with increasing grade.

Neck pain is the most prominent complaint in patients after whiplash injury. Other symptoms frequently reported by these patients include headache, dizziness, concentration and memory problems, irritability, fatigue, and sleep disturbances (Barnsley, Lord, & Bogduk, 1994).

After a grade 1 and 2 (the least severe), the majority of people report neck pain. The pain often radiates from the occiput, at one or both sides, into the shoulder along the trapezius muscle. Many of those suffer also from occipital headache. Some may have a frontal headache. Patients with a grade 1 lesion may complain of neck pain and stiffness that usually occurs a couple of hours after the accident. This is the only symptom

TABLE 20.1. The Quebec Task Force-Suggested Clinical Classification of Whiplash-Associated Disorders

Grade	Clinical presentation[a]
0	No complaint about the neck No physical sign(s)
I	Neck complaint of pain, stiffness or tenderness only No physical sign(s)
II	Neck complaint AND musculoskeletal sign(s)[b]
III	Neck complaints AND neurologic sign(s)[c]
IV	Neck complaints AND fracture or dislocation

Note. From Spitzer et al. (1995). Copyright 1995 by Lippincott Williams & Wilkins. Reprinted by permission.

[a]Symptoms and disorders that can be manifest in all grades include deafness, dizziness, tinnitus, headache, memory loss, dysphagia, and temporomandibular joint pain.

[b]Musculoskeletal signs include decreased range of motion and point tenderness.

[c]Neurological signs include decreased or absent deep tendon reflexes, weakness, and sensory deficits.

and at examination no tenderness or a reduced range of motion of the neck is observed. Patients with a grade 2 lesion have neck pain and stiffness within half an hour or so. At examination positive signs of tenderness and muscle spasm of the trapezius muscle are present. These findings differentiate a grade 2 lesion from a grade 1. Patients with a grade 2 lesion may also report other symptoms, such as dizziness, jaw pain, and even back pain. In patients with a grade 3 lesion, objective findings indicating neurological pathology such as a cord lesion, a nerve root, or cervical plexus lesion are observed. A grade 4 lesion is characterized by a fracture, a fracture dislocation, or a rupture of a cervical disc.

There has been a controversy as to whether a grade 1 and 2 injury results in a physical lesion as indicated by physical and/or radiological examination. Gundry and Fritts (1997) showed that magnetic resonance imaging (MRI) is capable of detecting even small injuries of ligaments, muscle, and bone. Minor muscle or ligament injury may be missed. MRI studies have failed to demonstrate physical pathology, not only in the chronic phase but also within 2 to 4

days after the accident. Borchgrevink, Smevik, and Nordby (1995) examined 52 patients by MRI within 2 to 4 days after a whiplash accident. They found no evidence of lesions of the cord or brain or evidence of significant injuries of ligaments, muscles, or bones. They concluded that only minor lesions that can be overlooked by MRI may be present. Ronnen, De Korte, and Brink (1996) examined 100 patients with MRI within the first 3 weeks after the whiplash accident. They also did not find any evidence of significant tears of ligaments or muscles. Consistent with Borchgreink and colleagues (1995), they concluded that if any lesions are present they would likely be microscopic and minor or have already healed at the time of the MRI examination. It is apparent that the vast majority of patients after grade 1 and 2 whiplash injuries have no significant physical lesion. At most, such patients have experienced only minor tears of muscles and/or ligaments that heal within a short period.

Patients with a grade 3 or 4 lesions, on the other hand, have conversely demonstrable pathology of ligaments, muscles, bones, and/or nervous tissue. Despite the lack of objective evidence of significant pathology in WADs, grade 1 and 2, about 10–15% of patients develop chronic symptoms (e.g., Pennie & Agambar, 1991). How can we explain this contrast? Which mechanisms lead to chronicity of the symptoms? In answering this question, we propose three hypotheses: (1) the "physical injury hypothesis," (2) the "disuse hypothesis," and (3) the "muscle spasm hypothesis."

The Physical Injury Hypothesis

According to the physical injury hypothesis, chronic symptoms are caused by a persisting physical lesion that has yet to be discovered. Some people suggest a lesion of the brain; others suggest a lesion in the cervical spine or a combination of those two (Pearce, 1994). There is little scientific evidence to support physical injury hypothesis. A number of neurophysiological studies have failed to demonstrate electroencephalograph abnormalities indicating a brain lesion following a whiplash injury.

Otte, Mueller-Brand, Nitzscke, Wachter,

and Ettlin (1997), in a number of excellent studies using ECD, PET scans, and SPECT-technology, proved the absence of brain lesions. They demonstrated that the mere presence of neck pain produces the abnormalities observed by brain imaging. Bicik, Radanov, and Schafer (1998) also used PET scans in patients with chronic symptoms after whiplash injury. They concluded that the abnormal findings on the scan correlated best with depression. These findings reinforce the results of MRI studies published by Borchgrevink and colleagues (1995) and Ronnen and colleagues (1996).

Theoretically, chronic patients may have other persisting lesions in the neck such as soft tissue injuries and/or lesions of the facet joints and discs. MRI, as discussed earlier, does not demonstrate any sign of a persisting soft tissue lesion. Although a number of studies have confirmed that the facet joint is a potential source of chronic neck pain, the preponderance of evidence does not support a whiplash trauma as the cause of that source of pain (Ferrari, 1999).

The Disuse Hypothesis

According to the disuse hypothesis, following a motor vehicle accident people may be so distressed that they develop avoidance behavior. That is, they are afraid to move their head and neck freely and therefore they avoid motion because of fear for pain or potential disaster, such as paraplegia. Subsequently the neck musculature, in particular of the trapezius muscle, is reduced, resulting in muscle atrophy. Indeed, it has been observed that decreased regional bloodflow in atrophic muscles is associated with neck pain (Larsson, Alund, Cai, & Ake Oberg, 1994). The consequence of the disuse is the development of a "negative spiral" from which the patient can hardly escape. However, some patients with chronic symptoms after whiplash do reveal hyperactivity or spasm of the trapezius muscle that is generally not compatible with muscle atrophy (Nederhand, IJzerman, Hermens, Baten, & Zilvold, 2000).

The core idea of the disuse hypothesis is that symptoms such as pain may become chronic while the physical lesion, which originally caused the symptoms, has healed.

This proces of "chronification" has been addressed from several perspectives: "negative reinforcement," "illness behavior," "fear–avoidance beliefs," or "somatization." There is a vast amount of research data in the area of behavioral medicine to support the involvement of behavioral factors in this chronification process (see Vlaeyen et al., Chapter 10, this volume). With regard to clinical management of patients after whiplash injury in rehabilitation programs, the disuse hypothesis underlies many different sorts of interventions. In fact, many activities applied by physiotherapists, manual therapist, or chiropractics, to name a few, have the effect that patients expose themselves to movements, which they avoided until then. The mechanism is interruption of the negative spiral. Despite being plausible, there is, to our knowledge, no direct evidence supporting or rejecting the disuse hypothesis following whiplash injury.

The Muscle Spasm Hypothesis

Many patients with chronic symptoms have a hyperactive trapezius muscle, also called a muscle spasm. This muscle spasm may result in a restricted range of motion of the neck and often in a fixed position of the head in light flexion and rotation. Other chronic patients suffer episodically from this hyperactivity even though they can move their head freely in other periods. The stiffness of the neck in those patients may occur suddenly or come along gradually and may last several hours or several days. This muscle hyperactivity occurs for the first time shortly after the trauma in a grade 2 lesion or a couple of hours after a grade 1 lesion as a result of a protective reflex. Generally, this reflex disappears within days or weeks. Indeed, in the majority of people with a grade 1 or grade 2 lesion the stiffness of the neck is resolved within a couple of weeks. However, in 10–20% this hyperactivity persists or reoccurs frequently. We postulate that the persistent hyperactivity might be due to classical conditioning. The injury is the unconditioned stimulus (US) and the muscle spasm the unconditioned response (UCR), that is, the protective reflex. What may happen is that otherwise harmless stimuli (CSs) may become triggers that provoke the unconditioned reponse. Thus, the muscle spasm becomes a conditioned response (CR). CSs may be different for each person with chronic symptoms (e.g., driving a car, a frightening thought, and neck movements). The pain itself is not a UCR or CR but the mere result of the muscle spasm. Moreover, other symptoms such as fatigue and dizziness (overstimulation of the proprioceptive system) can be related to hyperactivity of the trapezius muscle. The pain itself may become a trigger (CS) that provokes muscle spasms (CR); hence a vicious circle is set in motion.

Over time patients may become more disabled, see their lives becoming less fascinating, and employ less activities. In terms of classical conditioning, this increase may be due to "stimulus generalization." That is, the number of CSs increases. Whether or not the explanation in terms of the conditioning paradigm is correct, the "phenomenon" of stimulus generalization is seen in many chronic patients. That is, the pain and other symptoms are provoked in more and more situations. For example, the patient first avoided some specific activities and started to avoid related activities in general.

There is no direct evidence currently available to support or reject the validity of the muscle spasm hypothesis, although there are a growing number of studies demonstrating a hyperactivity of the trapzezius muscle in patients with chronic neck pain complaints. Nederhand and colleagues (2000) demonstrated the hyperactivity of the trapezius in WAD grades 1 and 2.

The "disuse" and "muscle spasm" hypotheses seem to complement each other. To date, the effect of stimulus generalization may be that the CSs are avoided, resulting in muscle disuse. And, in return, such disuse may lower the threshold for the muscle spasms. The implication of the disuse and the muscle spasm hypotheses for the management of patients with chronic symptoms after a whiplash injury is that any intervention that stimulates patients to expose themselves to activities or calm down their hyperactive muscles will be helpful in increasing muscle strength and decrease muscle spasm.

With regard to scientific evidence, we are confronted with the difficult situation that we have strong evidence in disfavor of the "injury hypothesis" but with a lack of research data to support or reject the disuse and muscle spasm hypotheses. The psychological approach to whiplash, to which this chapter is devoted, has therefore a small empirical basis. However, as shown before, we have some indirect evidence to demonstrate that the approach followed "makes sense."

The remainder of this chapter is divided into two sections: assessment and treatment. It has not been our intention to provide a definitive manual for the assessment and treatment of patients following whiplash injury. We conclude this chapter with a brief discussion of some considerations regarding whiplash that go beyond clinical or scientific arguments (i.e., the effect of the attitude in society regarding whiplash).

Assessment

To carry out an effective treatment, it is important that the preparatory phase focuses on collecting information from various angles regarding the patient's situation. These angles include the beliefs and behavior of the patient, the social context in which this behavior manifests itself, and the patient's motivation to change his or her behavior. Assessment and treatment are not independent. The experience of going through an assessment means that some patients already start to change their beliefs regarding whiplash. Moreover, during the assessment a trusting relationship is established with the patient, something that is essential for an effective treatment.

We will discuss two stages of assessment: (1) the first-stage screening, designed to identify patients who are at risk of developing chronic symptoms; and (2) the second stage, where more extensive analysis takes place before multidisciplinary treatment is initiated.

Recovery after Whiplash: A Model

As previously mentioned, the majority of people involved in rear-end collisions do not develop pain. For the small group who do develop pain, two subgroups can be identified: people who experience a normal recovery as opposed to those who continue to be affected by pain or other symptoms beyond what is considered a normal healing time.

According to the Quebec Task Force (Spitzer et al., 1995), the average (median) time for recovery is 30 days (recovery—defined as the resumption of normal daily activities, including work). Investigators have shown that the effects of the injury (pain resulting from damage to muscles, tendons, and ligaments) usually are completely resolved after a few weeks to months (Spitzer et al., 1995). Thus, the main question, which should be a focal point of the assessment, is: Why do people continue to be limited in their activities of daily living beyond the healing time? Specifically, we are referring to patients who show little sign of improvement in their daily functioning after a period of approximately 4 weeks.

We hypothesize that behavioral factors (i.e., the "disuse hypothesis" and "muscle spasm hypothesis") may be a primary reason why the symptoms persist beyond the expected healing. We mentioned some of the arguments supporting these two hypotheses previously.

Figure 20.1 illustrates the reasons why symptoms following a whiplash injury may persist beyond a normal healing time. This model distinguishes between "direct" and "indirect" effects related to the accident. The direct-injury effects primarily concern bodily injury (e.g., Quebec grade 2—injury to ligaments and musculotendenous areas). The indirect-injury effects are related to patients' reactions to what has happened to them as a result of the accident, both mentally and physically. These reactions (such as catastrophizing, the muscle tension cycle, depression, and posttraumatic stress disorder) can further intensify the pain sensations initially related to the direct-injury effects. We hypothesize that in the acute phase, the direct effects dominate, whereas in the chronic phase the indirect effects play a greater role. However, in the patient's experience the symptoms are still the same, whether it concerns the acute or chronic phase. It is difficult for the person to understand that "under" the same symptoms, different processes are operating with the passage of time. This is perhaps one of the reasons why some whiplash patients are reluctant to admit behavioral factors.

First-Stage Assessment

PROGNOSTIC FACTORS

Research regarding chronic symptoms after a whiplash accident recognizes the influence of psychosocial factors when pain does not subside within a normal recovery period (Ferrari & Russell, 1999). In support of this research, volunteers who have undergone a rear-end collision did not develop chronic pain symptoms (Castro et al., 1997). One possible explanation could be the volunteers' belief that they could experience no more than a temporary period of neck pain. In a later study, Castro and colleagues (2001) found some volunteers (20%), after being exposed to a placebo rear-end collision (i.e., a simulated impact without biomechanical stress), developed acute symptoms. Such symptoms can be explained only by psychological factors. Further evidence supporting the role of psychosocial factors during recovery is seen in the great variation between countries (e.g., Lithuania vs. Cana-

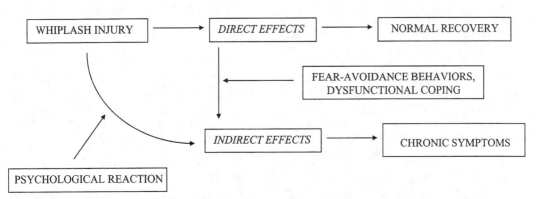

FIGURE 20.1. Model of recovery after whiplash injury.

da) concerning the prevalence of chronic pain after rear-end collisions.

Investigators have identified a number of specific whiplash-related prognostic factors including decreased mobility of the neck directly after the accident (e.g., Gargan, Bannister, Main, & Hollis, 1997); previous head trauma (e.g., Radanov, Begré, Sturzenegger, & Augustiny, 1996); female sex (e.g., Harder, Veilleux, & Suissa, 1998); older age (e.g., Harder et al., 1998); and severity of initial reaction to the accident, such as intense neck pain and headache and changes in psychological functioning (Radanov et al., 1996). Some recent studies report negative predictors measured shortly after the accident including: a strong posttraumatic stress response (Drottning, Staff, & Malt, 2001); perceived lack of control (interference) of the symptoms (Bunketorp, Olsson, Carlsson, & Styf, 2001); decreased neck mobility (Jensen & Kasch, 2000; Kasch, Bach, & Jenssen, 2001); and disturbed well-being and avoidance of activities (Gaitsch et al., 2001).

RISK ASSESSMENT

It is important to screen patients to identify those who may be at risk to develop chronic symptoms after a whiplash injury. The "triage" technique might be helpful. Once we have identified at-risk patients, we can use more comprehensive instruments to tailor the treatment (second-stage assessment).

Because most patients recover within a few weeks after the whiplash injury, the "right time" to conduct the risk assessment is about 6 weeks after the injury (i.e., in the subacute phase). The most important question is, Which variables should be included in this risk assessment? One way to decide is to assess risk factors derived from epidemiological research. A major disadvantage of relying solely on epidemiological research, however, is that we do not know whether such variables are "causal" or "secondary." For example, is decreased mobility of the neck a risk factor as such or secondary to a more "central" variable such as fear–avoidance beliefs? What we need is some *model* of how symptoms become chronic.

We propose a risk assessment model that includes two components: distress and illness behavior. A questionnaire that has our preference regarding the assessment of distress is the Distress Risk Assessment Method (DRAM; Main, Wood, Hollis, Spanswick, & Waddell, 1992), which is a combination of the Modified Zung and the Modified Somatic Perception Questionnaire. The DRAM has been specifically developed for chronic pain patients. The Short Form Health Survey (SF–36; Ware & Sherbourne, 1992) can also be used for this purpose. The SF–36 has been recommended for outcome prediction research because of its brevity, good psychometric properties, and growing clinical use with patients who have a variety of chronic medical conditions (Gatchel, Mayer, Dersh, Robinson, & Polatin, 1999). With regard to the assessment of illness behavior, one can think of questionnaires such as the Illness Behavior Questionnaire (IBQ; Pilowsky & Spence, 1975) or the Fear–Avoidance Beliefs Questionnaire (FABQ; Waddell, Newton, Henderson, Somerville, & Main, 1993). However, the disadvantage of these questionnaires is that they have not been developed for patients after whiplash injury and miss some typical features of this group of patients. Therefore, we developed our own questionnaire to assess illness behavior in subacte whiplash patients. This questionnaire, the Whiplash Recovery Inventory (WRI), is shown in Figure 20.2. We must emphasize that it concerns an experimental version. The WRI is designed to assess four variables: (1) "expectations regarding recovery"; (2) "beliefs regarding symptoms and physical activity"; (3) "work resumption expectations"; and (4) "negative experiences with health care." We are currently investigating the psychometric properties of the WRI and SF–36, including the predictive validity, in a large population of patients with subacute symptoms after a whiplash injury.

Second-Stage Assessment

Further psychological assessment of patients after whiplash injury may take place as part of a multidisciplinary treatment approach. We discuss several essential aspects of the psychological interview.

WHIPLASH BELIEFS

Research indicates that cognitive processes are major determinates in the development

With this questionnaire, we would like to find out what your experiences are after the whiplash injury, and how you feel about your symptoms and your recovery.

We would like you to circle a number to indicate how much you agree or disagree with each statement.

It is essential that your answers are based on your own personal feelings; what others think is not relevant.

Please answer all of the statements.

For each statement, please circle a number from 1 to 4 indicating how much you agree or disagree with the statement. The numbers have the following meaning:

1 = completely disagree
2 = moderately disagree
3 = moderately agree
4 = completely agree

Recovery:

1. I expect to make a full recovery within a few months	1	2	3	4
2. As a result of the accident, my neck will always be vulnerable	1	2	3	4
3. My recovery is taking longer than I expected	1	2	3	4
4. My injury has not yet healed	1	2	3	4
5. The symptoms have significantly decreased since the accident	1	2	3	4

Activity and pain:

6. The pain I am experiencing is a result of bodily injury	1	2	3	4
7. If I were to ignore my pain, it would become worse	1	2	3	4
8. In my present situation, it would be unwise to be physically active	1	2	3	4
9. It is important not to surpass my pain threshold	1	2	3	4
10. I should try to avoid unexpected movements as much as possible	1	2	3	4

Work:

11. People at work are inconsiderate toward my disabilities	1	2	3	4
12. With my present complaints I cannot do my normal work	1	2	3	4
13. Within a few months, I will be able to do my normal work	1	2	3	4
14. My symptoms get worse as a result of my work	1	2	3	4
15. My supervisor understands my present situation	1	2	3	4

Medical care:

16. My general practitioner takes my symptoms seriously	1	2	3	4
17. Regarding my symptoms I receive conflicting medical advice	1	2	3	4
18. In my opinion, not enough is done to treat my symptoms	1	2	3	4
19. As a whiplash patient, I feel I am not taken seriously	1	2	3	4
20. The treatments that I received so far have had little effect	1	2	3	4

Note. Scoring: The scores of items 1, 5, 13, 15, and 16 must be reversed.

FIGURE 20.2. Whiplash Recovery Inventory (WRI).

of symptoms (Pennebaker, 1982). Pain does not directly represent a nocioceptive stimulus but an end product, which includes individual beliefs and cultural factors. This appears also to be the case in people who have experienced a whiplash injury. In Western countries, there is, even on a preconscious level, widespread knowledge concerning the expected symptoms after a whiplash injury (Ferrari & Russell, 1999). In the course of their journey after the whiplash injury, these people are frequently bombarded with advice from medical, insurance, and legal professionals, which is often quite subjective and in some cases biased. Remarks by doctors and therapists such as "whiplash can lead to many symptoms" and "not all brain lesions can be shown on MRI" only intensify these people's fear and create beliefs concerning the illness, hence "whiplash beliefs."

Whiplash beliefs frequently concern the attribution of symptoms. That is, the whiplash patient may be attributing nonaccident symptoms to the accident. Frequently, this association is unjustly made. We have had some cases in which patients who were symptom-free for 6 months after the accident request service concerning their whiplash symptoms 2 years after the accident occurred. It is their belief that the symptoms are a result of the accident, which in a later phase become too irritable to ignore. The more recent symptoms as well as past symptoms, which were considered insignificant at the time, are linked to the focal point of the accident, itself. Some typical whiplash beliefs can be found in the WRI, shown in Figure 20.2.

PAIN BEHAVIOR

At the present time, research has not yet focused on the prevention of fear–avoidance beliefs and behaviors in patients after whiplash injury. However, there is no doubt that these aspects play a significant role in the process of chronicity. Immediately after the accident, the patient can be fearful. Patients' fears may start when paramedics remove them from the automobile on a special stretcher, apply a hard collar, and warn them not to move (Ferrari & Russell, 1999). In a later stage of the recovery process, patients may receive well-meaning but contradictory advice from therapists and physicians, which may lead to confusion and apprehension. Often, the advice is, "Stay active, but stop immediately if you feel pain." Also, the advice of friends, family, and neighbors can further enhance fear–avoidance beliefs.

A reduction in activities of daily living, in quality and quantity, as well as the avoidance of spontaneous movement, can indicate the presence of inadequate pain behavior. Some patients fixate their heads, rotating their entire body to look beside or behind them. The use of a neck collar strongly suggests the presence of pain behavior. Some patients use their collars selectively; for example, only during long periods of driving or in the course of a long, eventful day. Therefore, questioning patients concerning the detailed use of their collars gives further insight into their whiplash-related beliefs and pain behaviors. Not only do patients exhibit fear–avoidance behavior in relation to pain in the neck but in many cases patients complain of chronic fatigue and a reduced ability to concentrate, combined with or without neck pain symptoms. Patients can actually provoke a feeling of fatigue by reducing their activities, including work, and resting too much. To illustrate, one of our patients planned 2 hours extra sleep on Tuesday because she wanted to visit the cinema Thursday evening. We provide some typical beliefs regarding symptoms and activity in the WRI (Figure 20.2).

POSTTRAUMATIC STRESS DISORDER

As a result of the accident, some patients can have a prolonged emotional response. In our facility, we quite frequently see patients who have recurring, fear-provoking dreams related to the accident, which last for several weeks to months. According to the fourth edition of the *Diagnostic and Statistical Manual of Mental Disorders* (DSM-IV; American Psychiatric Association, 1994), we speak of posttraumatic stress disorder (PTSD) if there are symptoms of intrusion (intrusion of unpleasant memories concerning the accident), avoidance (e.g., avoidance of driving or driving on highways), and increased irritability (extreme jumpiness and/or concentration difficulties). We have seldom treated a whiplash patient who met all PTSD criteria according to DSM-IV. However, many patients exhibit temporary PTSD symptoms, shortly after the accident, which can lead to an increased risk of chronicity. In more specific terms, the increased arousal associated with a PTSD leads to abnormal muscle activity and increased pain. Drottning and colleagues (2001) showed a strong posttraumatic stress response to be associated with poor outcome 1 year after the accident.

It should be realized that avoidance behaviors are subtle and can be masked by other symptoms. We have frequently treated patients who avoided driving because of "physical hindrance." These patients often reveal that fear is the real reason they avoid driving.

Sometimes feelings related to a posttraumatic reaction can be expressed as inadequate anger and resentment, in excessive proportions. In these cases, patients take on the role of the victim with feelings of anger. As part of the assessment, it is important to realize that behind every aggressive opinion lies a greater degree of frustration and vulnerability. The psychologist is faced with the challenge of bringing the patient gradually in contact with these underlying feelings as well as assisting the patient in developing adequate coping strategies to interrupt this vicious cycle.

EMOTIONAL DISTRESS

In addition to neck pain and headache, whiplash patients frequently report sleep disturbances, depressive symptoms, anxiety, and fatigue (Stovner, 1996). Several mechanisms may act on the etiology and the maintenance of such emotional distress.

First, certain beliefs and maladaptive coping strategies lead to catastrophizing and depressive reactions. Catastrophizing has been linked consistently to depression and disability (see, e.g., Gil, Williams, Keefe, & Beckman, 1990). A fear-inducing concept of whiplash in society may aggravate this process. A "negative spiral" may develop in which self-sustaining mechanisms operate. As a result of the constant pain, the disrupted sleep, and the associated feelings of fatigue, the patient becomes fatigued, and in some cases, patients adapt a more passive existence. Again, they react with feelings of fear and depression.

It is important to identify exactly what adaptations patients have made since the accident, as well as the reasoning behind these actions. These adaptations can eventually lead to the emotional distress. In many cases, these adaptations are passed on from patient to patient as result of fear-inducing illness models specific to the culture. In addition, individual, patient-specific characteristics associated with catastrophizing may lower the threshold for this process. A large number of studies have shown that

symptoms can be maintained quite easily through operant conditioning.

There are, however, also cases in which the maladaptive coping style is more clearly related to the person than to the situation itself. In these cases the whiplash injury can be seen as a "breaking point." Sometimes, a fragile balance can be maintained for years through "overcompensation" before the accident. That is, the individual could get going through extra effort. This is sometimes seen in young adults where a fast-paced career path can lead to the discovery of areas of personal doubt or shortcomings. In everyday life, there appear to be no problems; actually, everything seems to be going the individual's way. This is probably why many whiplash patients indicate that psychological reasons play no role in their situation. Before the accident, they had few problems in their lives and they blame everything on the accident. From another perspective, the whiplash injury can deprive patients of overcompensation, which was heavily relied on in their everyday lives. For example, a person could have difficulty coping with the death of a close friend. To cope with this loss, the person throws himself into his work as a distraction. A traffic accident can trigger a loss of balance in his life and eventually lead to an emotional crisis.

NEUROPSYCHOLOGICAL ASSESSMENT

Memory and concentration problems are frequently reported among whiplash patients. Epidemiological research reveals that directly after the injury between 20 and 60% of victims report concentration problems and 6 months later between 5–21% (Stover, 1996). Many whiplash patients seeking multidisciplinary treatment report cognitive problems. Minor brain injury could be an explanation for these cognitive difficulties based on the fact that most whiplash patients underperform compared to what is expected on cognitive tests. The use of neuropsychological assessment cannot identify the presence of brain damage. This type of assessment can only identify patients who score below healthy controls.

We hypothesize that brain injury is not caused by accidents resulting in a grade 1 or 2 injury based on the following arguments:

1. The first study on this topic (Yarnell & Rossie, 1988) revealed major debilitation after minor whiplash head injury after the examination of a small group of chronic whiplash patients. This study, however, lacked of a control group. Recent, prospective studies using larger samples and adequate control groups reveal that severe cognitive deficits are not common among whiplash patients. These studies do show that whiplash patients score lower on complex speed tasks such as the Paced Auditory Serial Addition Task (PASAT) (e.g., Kessels, Aleman, Verhagen, & van Luijtelaar, 2000; Radanov, Dvorak, & Vallach, 1996).

2. The performances of whiplash patients are worse than those of healthy subjects, but the scores are comparable to the scores of chronic pain patients without a history of head injury (Olsnes, 1989; Taylor, Cox, & Mailis, 1996).

3. Underperformance appears to be a substantial problem among whiplash patients: In the context of litigation, 61% of whiplash patients appear to underperform compared to 29% of whiplash patients not involved with litigation who underperform (Schmand et al., 1998).

4. Whiplash patients show a substantial improvement of cognitive functioning within 6 months after the accident (Radanov, Di Stefano, Schindrig, Sturzenegger, & Augustiny, 1993). Brain-injured patients do not demonstrate such an improvement (van Zomeren & Deelman, 1978).

In summary, there is strong scientific evidence that the speed of information processing of whiplash patients is somewhat delayed. However, this observation may not be regarded as the evidence for minor brain injury among whiplash patients. As discussed earlier, there is instead evidence for the absence of brain injury in patients with chronic symptoms after whiplash injury. Brain injury is just one of many possible factors affecting cognitive functioning. Optimal cognitive functioning, as natural as it may seem, is in fact a fragile process; it immediately starts to show deficits when a shortage of sleep, fatigue, fever, pain, or drugs are present. Van Zomeren and Saan (1997) identified seven factors in the literature that may disturb the cognitive functioning of whiplash patients. The empirical support varied from "strong and direct" to "weak and indirect": pain (e.g., Radanov et al., 1992), sleep disturbances, depression (e.g., King & Caine, 1996), drugs (e.g., Radanov et al., 1993), abnormal illness behavior (Schmand et al., 1998), fear–avoidance of cognitive effort (self-protection), secondary gain factors.

When Should a Neuropsychological Assessment be Applied? In clinical practice, at least in The Netherlands, neuropsychological assessment is frequently used as part of the assessment of patients after whiplash injury. From a scientific point of view, this is rather surprising because of the previously mentioned information regarding the lack of evidence supporting the presence of minor brain injury. Furthermore, cognitive problems are also common in disorders such as depression and chronic pain, while in these areas, neuropsychological assessment is not carried out as routinely as for whiplash patients.

In general, we advise a reserved policy regarding neuropsychological assessment of whiplash patients. The danger lies in the chance that the symptoms, which already have a great degree of emotional influence on the patient, could also be given a medical label. In other words, the neuropsychological assessment could strengthen the "whiplash beliefs." Neuropsychological testing should certainly not take place when there are no cognitive symptoms.

Despite the recommendations against testing, in some cases neuropsychological testing could be of value. We want to stress the importance of having a clear-cut goal when using a test battery. In our opinion, the primary goal lies in the determination of cognitive performance and not brain injury. The selection of which neuropsychological instruments to use lies beyond the scope of this chapter (cf. Lezak, 1995, for further reading on this topic).

We feel the neuropsychological assessment is appropriate in the following situations:

- If the patient subjectively experiences memory or concentration problems.
- To reinforce the feeling that one's complaints are taken seriously.
- For reassurance to demonstrate that the

cognitive performances of the patient are "normal."

- As an aid to help patients to understand their cognitive difficulties.

We feel that neuropsychological testing can be especially useful in achieving the last goal on the previous list. Neuropsychological assessment provides tangible evidence that supports the verbal advice of the therapist. Improving the situation entails creating insight (through such testing) into these symptoms and mechanisms that have led to the present situation. Initially, many patients report that they have a memory disorder. Neuropsychological testing can provide evidence to the contrary. However, in many cases, an attention problem is identified; the ability to recall is lacking, not because of forgetfulness but because of a lack of attention. This problem can lead to a discussion as to the possible reason why attention has become less optimal.

In conclusion, our clinical experience indicates that the fear–avoidance mechanism frequently plays a role by cognitive symptomatology of patients with chronic symptoms. Some patients react so heavily to their cognitive symptoms that it becomes a phobia. This is especially the case when patients exhibit traits related to perfectionism. Their preoccupation with their perceived memory problem results in a reduced overall functioning and a worsening of the whole situation. Some patients develop rather unique strategies to avoid difficult situations. This may include organizing their lives through a system of Post-it Notes or using their partner as an "external memory bank." Frequently, the fear of making a mistake intensifies the emotions related to the aforementioned situation. For example, a nurse is apprehensive about returning to her work because of the possibility of making a mistake while making her medication rounds. This had happened on one occasion since her accident. The first step toward coping with these beliefs involved relabeling the idea that she had a "memory disorder" as "performance anxiety."

SOCIAL ENVIRONMENT

According to Fordyce (1976), the patient's social environment represents an important influence on pain behavior. Therefore, we strive to meet with the patient's partner at least once. Most of the time, the meeting takes place when the assessment results are discussed. It is important to remember that the social environment of the patient should not be limited to the partner. The influence of friends, other family members, and colleagues should not be underrated. According to Turk, Kerns, and Rosenberg (1992), two different responses from the social environment can further reinforce pain behavior. These are overprotective, illness-confirming responses and, second, responses that give the patient the impression that he is not being taken seriously. For example, if the patient says that the quality of his relationship has improved since the accident, the possibility of illness confirmation exists. If the quality of the relationship has decreased since the accident, the possibility of interpersonal distress exists.

MEDICOLEGAL ISSUES

Vast amounts of epidemiological research data indicate that the process of litigation and battling with insurance companies contributes to the behavior of reporting chronic symptoms (Ferrari & Russell, 1999). The following examples illustrate the impact of litigation.

In Lithuania, no preconceived notion of chronic pain arising from rear-end collisions exists and thus no fear of long-term disability. There is little involvement with the therapeutic community and insurance companies and no litigation. Symptoms after whiplash injury tend to be brief and do not involve to the so-called late whiplash syndrome (Obelieniene, Schrader, Bovim, Miseviciene, & Sand, 1999).

The change from a "tort-compensation" system (all damage, including inconvenience as well as pain and suffering are included in the settlement) into a "no-fault" system (only medical costs and lost income are compensated) resulted in a 28% decrease of whiplash claims. Even more surprising was a greater than 50% decrease in the duration of the symptoms, from 433 days to 203 days (Cassidy et al., 2000).

For the assessment, it is important to find out what a claim or possible claim means to the patient. A few possibilities are compensation for pain and suffering, revenge directed at the person who caused the accident, and compensation for damage to a career. Or, is the claim considered to be a legal formality? We advise discussing the advantages and disadvantages of a claim. For example, one advantage might be that a settlement may provide some degree of financial security; on the other hand, a disadvantage might be that legal battles and ongoing attention to symptoms do not contribute to a quick recovery. Some patients think that short-term financial gain ensures, in the long run, a higher quality of life. If the claim is one of the central issues, then progress toward healthy coping behavior could threaten the end result of the claim. We prefer that a settlement be reached before the start of a multidisciplinary treatment; however, this is often not the case. In the limited number of cases in which settlement is reached before treatment, we believe that the patient achieves a sense of "closure of the whiplash chapter" in his or her life. In terms of operant conditioning (Fordyce, 1976), medicolegal issues can be regarded as strong reinforcers of the patient's symptoms.

THE INTERVIEW

If there is one factor that determines the quality of the interview, it must be the communication skills of the therapist. Whiplash patients are, in our experience, one the most difficult groups of chronic pain patients with whom to work. The reasoning for this can be found in the culture, more specifically Western society. Whiplash patients are really victims twice. First, as a result of the accident and, second, from the tug of war between groups in society, whose interests, often financial ones, are biased by the recognition or nonrecognition of the patient's dilemma (e.g., insurance companies vs. attorneys). The struggle at a societal level can definitely influence the interaction between the whiplash patient and the clinician. Therefore, high expectations are placed on the clinician concerning his or her ability to deal with these issues and ultimately to assist patients in improving the chances of getting on with their lives.

We suggest beginning the interview without any type of explanation and using an open manner in questioning, such as the following: "What are your greatest concerns or difficulties at this moment?" The patient's direct answer to this question often is the central problem in a nutshell. One patient tells about his pain symptoms, the other tells of her frustrations around not working, and the next tells about the contradictory advice from her physicians and therapists. The clinician should write down the patient's response to the opening question verbatim. In some cases, it is helpful to use testing, other than neuropsycholoigcal testing, to collect extra information regarding the situation. These test results can be used as a baseline before treatment. The use of additional psychological testing in the treatment of chronic pain can be found in the literature and is not further discussed here.

As mentioned earlier, the main goal of the psychological interview is to answer the question why the patient continues to experience reduced functioning beyond the healing time for the whiplash injury. It is important to avoid discussion about whether the symptoms are "psychological" in origin. It might help in avoiding such discussion to use the model shown in Figure 20.1. The clinician should talk with the patient in terms of recovery, what has helped the patient to recover until so far, and what has not? How does the patient experiences his or her present situation? The clinician should not make the mistake of taking the commonplace, such as "I feel upset through the pain," for granted. He or she should ask instead, "What exactly makes you feel upset with the pain?" It may also be helpful to investigate together with patients the aspects in which they are their "own worst enemy" regarding the recovery. For example, patients with perfectionistic traits have difficulty accepting that things are not going perfectly. They cannot meet their high standard in their work. This "underperformance" can cause them a lot of stress, which works against their recovery. Talking in terms of "your own enemy" may help patients to distance from their physical discomfort. They learn that "parts" inside them influence their well-being. It is useful to help patients recognize that that there are factors within themselves working against recovery. The clinician can ask the patients what coping abilities they should learn so that their recovery will go more easily?

The interview should contain an inventory of emotional disturbances such as depression, anxiety disorders, PTSD, examination of the patient's preinjury functioning (be alert to signal overcompensation), use of medication and supportive devices, examination of the social context, including medicolegal issues, and, most important, evaluation of the patient's motivation to change.

We advocate giving the patient feedback. In this way, the multifactorial nature of the whiplash problem is stressed.

The topics included are part of the second stage assessment are summarized in the list contained in Table 20.2. The greater the number of checked items, the greater degree of complexity. This checklist can be used as a guide for a tailored treatment for the patient.

Treatment

The scientific research that has been carried out in the past years concerning whiplash has focused primarily on epidemiological and diagnostic questions. A surprising contrast in the area of treatment outcome studies can be observed. On the one hand, research increasingly supports the hypothesis that psychosocial factors influence the process of chronicity after a whiplash injury. However, on the other hand, there is almost no mention of the use of multidisciplinary treatment approaches for whiplash patients. As far as we know, no randomized clinical trials on this topic have been published. In a recent uncontrolled study (Vendrig, van Akkerveeken, & McWhorter, 2000), we presented the results of a multimodal treatment approach for whiplash patients (the details of this approach are outlined next). The results indicated that at 6-month follow-up, pain was reduced in 46%; disability reduced to normal in 38%; cognitive and behavioral complaints eliminated in 90%; return to normal work in 65%; ceased drug use in 58%; and ceased pursuing medical care in 81%.

The following guidelines are based primarily on clinical experience. First, a short summary of the guidelines for the treatment of acute and subacute whiplash symptoms is provided. Second, we expand on our multidisciplinary treatment approach for patients with chronic symptoms.

Management of Whiplash in the Acute Phase (0–6 Weeks)

The best treatment of choice in this phase, is no treatment at all. In a randomized clinical trial, Borchgrevink and colleagues (1998) identified better outcome for patients who were encouraged to continue engaging in their normal, preinjury activities than for patients who took sick leave from work and were immobilized during the first 14 days after the injury. The importance of an active approach has also been identified in other studies (Peeters, Verhagen, Bie, & Oostendorp, 2001). The following recommendations are based on Spitzer and colleagues (1995); Peeters, Verhagen, Bie, and Oostendorp (2001); Scholten-Peeters et al., 2002; and Cole, Cassidy, Carroll, Frank, and Bombardier (2001).

TABLE 20.2. Checklist for Psychological Assessment in Whiplash Patients

	Present	Absent
1. Incorrect "whiplash beliefs"	0	0
2. Fear–avoidance beliefs/behavior	0	0
3. Frequent use of analgesia or alcohol abuse	0	0
4. PTSD symptoms	0	0
5. Emotional distress	0	0
6. Preinjury vulnerabilities or "overcompensation"	0	0
7. Subjectively experienced cognitive deficits	0	0
8. Overprotective partner or interpersonal distress	0	0
9. No intention to come to a settlement of the claim	0	0
10. Work-related disabilities or work-resumption undermining factors	0	0

Of great importance is the fact that patients need to be reassured. For some patients, the symptoms can be alarming, resulting in fear–avoidance reactions and an increased neck muscular activity. These reactions can persist beyond the healing time and need to be prevented. A thorough discussion, where time is taken to explain the symptoms and the prognosis, is necessary to calm and reassure the patient. In this process, a medical examination may be necessary.

Accident-related stress often makes it difficult to concentrate. Therefore, it is recommended that patients be given written advice, to which they can refer. Included in the advice is the message that the movement of the neck and head gradually needs to increase over the following days. Rosenfeld, Gunnarsson, and Borenstein (2000) found that active exercises performed at home and supported by a physiotherapist seemed to have some beneficial effect on the outcome of acute whiplash patients. The attention of a physiotherapist is encouraged if the patient is fearful about doing this alone. The exercises need to be based on time and quantity contingent goals. If needed, pain medication can be temporarily used; for example, 24 to 48 hours, using the maximum safe dosage and also on a time-contingent basis. After this short period, pain medication needs to be decreased and stopped.

As noted, intervention in the acute phase needs to be kept to a minimum. An exception to this guideline could be the presence of an increased arousal level, sleep disturbance, emotionally lability, anxiety, and PTSD. It is essential that these symptoms be reduced as soon as possible to avoid the danger of chronicity. The family physician is, in most cases, the most appropriate person to advise the patient. Various treatment approaches are listed below: reassurance, medication, giving the partner of the patient instructions, relaxation exercises, and encouraging the patient not to fall into the trap of fear-avoidance behavior by not driving.

Management of Whiplash in the Subacute Phase (6–12 Weeks)

The subacute phase is generally considered between 6 and 12 weeks after the accident. If there is evidence of a normal recovery, in other words, the symptoms gradually decrease and daily functioning increases, no action is recommended, allowing patients to continue on their recovery path. If, after 6 weeks, pain symptoms are still present and the possibility of a slowed recovery exists, multidisciplinary consultation is indicated. In some cases, a sudden increase in symptoms is seen in patients who initially ignored their symptoms. As time passed, they failed in this effort.

If the patient does not show any improvement after 6 weeks, we advise performance of a risk assessment (e.g., using the WRI). When is a multidisciplinary intervention indicated? This type of intervention, in our opinion, is indicated when the patient shows signs of emotional distress (DRAM) and scores positive in at least three of the four areas of the WRI.

- The patient has incorrect "whiplash beliefs."
- Fear-avoidance beliefs are observed.
- The patient experiences work-related disabilities.
- The patient is unsatisfied with the received health care.

According to a chronological time scale, the patient is in the subacute phase, but as far as his or her behavior is concerned, the patient presents as a chronic pain patient. Waiting until the patient is "chronic" according to the criterion of "3 months" makes no sense. Multidisciplinary intervention is indicated.

When the patient scores positive in one or two of the four areas, a partial solution could be recommended. For example, the patient has appropriate beliefs regarding whiplash injury but exhibits emotional disturbances. In this case, referral to a qualified psychologist is sufficient. If evidence of inappropriate whiplash beliefs and fear–avoidance exists while the patient is in the subacute phase, an active graded-activity program under the supervision of a physiotherapist probably would be sufficient.

It should be emphasized that a careful medical examination by a medical specialist is recommended if the patient continues to experience symptoms. It is often difficult to make a correct medical differential diagnosis. For example, a Quebec grade 3 diagnosis has been missed. It is outside the scope of this chapter, however, to discuss this topic in more detail.

Management of Whiplash in the Chronic Phase (> 12 Weeks)

In the chronic phase, a multidisciplinary approach is indicated. The multidisciplinary approach we describe here has its roots in the functional restoration approach (Mayer & Gatchel, 1988; see also Wright & Gatchel, Chapter 17, this volume). The primary aim of this approach is returning participants to an active life and their original jobs and other functional activities. The goal is achieved by means of goal-directed, functional improvement. The most ideal setting for whiplash patients with chronic symptoms is a multidisciplinary setting.

In our program, patients with a variety of chronic pain problems participate. Thus, the program is not specific to whiplash patients, though there is customizing to individual situations within the program. There are three phases along the path: the preparatory (preprogram) phase, the intensive phase (the program), and the return-to-work (postprogram) phase.

THE PREPARATORY PHASE

This phase starts with a multidisciplinary assessment. The goal of this assessment is threefold: to build a trusting relationship with the patient, test the exclusion criteria for participating in the program, and collect baseline data. The following areas are always examined as part of a multidisciplinary assessment: full physical examination by the medical specialist, structured interview concerning the work situation performed by a occupational therapist, assessment of the pattern of movement and pain behaviors by the physiotherapist, and an assessment by the psychologist. Additional testing is sometimes required to create a complete overview of the patient's situation. This may include further diagnostic studies (CT scan and MRI), neuropsychological screening, and administration of additional psychological testing, if needed. The multidisciplinary assessment takes approximately 6 hours. One week after the multidisciplinary assessment, we discuss the results with patients and their partners. The presence and participation of the partner during the feedback of the results has a number of advantages. First, the chance that the patient forgets what has been said is reduced. Second, the feedback can lead to an open discussion with the assessment team and the two most important players in the situation. The psychologist has the chance to analyze how both people interact with each other in relation to the patient's situation.

The following exclusion criteria for multidisciplinary treatment are used:

- Structural, symptomatic pathology of the spine (Quebec grade 3 and 4; medical treatment required)
- Severe psychopathology (e.g., suicide attempts and antisocial behavior)
- No wish to return to work
- Language difficulties

Assuming that the exclusion criteria are considered to be negative, a 2- to 3-week period begins during which a number of practical actions take place. These actions include discussing the assessment results with the referral source, finalizing the financial aspects of future intervention, discussing the planning of the intervention with the employer, and discussing the intervention strategy with the patient's attorney if needed.

The rounding off of the preparatory phase includes a program introduction day, during the week before the intensive part of the training begins. In the course of this day, the patients meet and get to know the other members of the group and team. The basic principles, logistics, and rules of the program are discussed. The group members start to formulate specific goals, which upon achievement will allow them to function normally at home and on the job. The treatment team stimulates the group to formulate goals, which are positive, realistic, and measurable. Finally, the use and the role of pain medication and assistive devices such as corsets and neck collars are discussed. Sometimes these items block the patient's path to normal functioning. If this is the case and it is appropriate to do so, a goal-directed phasing-out plan is developed and agreed on with the patient.

THE INTENSIVE PHASE

Our program is of 2 full weeks' duration and 4 part-time weeks. In the third week of the program, the first step is made toward work resumption. Each day of the program is structured in the same way; four blocks of 1½ hours, where two blocks are devoted to a graded activity program for the reversal of the deconditioning process and two blocks are for the group sessions. The graded activity program is led by a physiotherapist. Each discipline is responsible for a number of group sessions containing various subjects depending on the discipline. There are also a number of additional sessions that are available depending on the logistics of the program and the response of the group to the program.

Each week begins with the so-called, goal session where the participants formulate their weekly subgoals. At the close of each week, an evaluation session takes place where the participants have the chance to discuss what they learned during the week, which subgoals were achieved, and what the next step is for the following week.

TEAM MEMBERS' RESPONSIBILITIES

In our setting, the medical specialist is usually an orthopedic surgeon or neurologist. The question that he or she is required to answer as part of the multidisciplinary team assessment is whether or not the patient's situation is resulting solely from pathophysiological abnormality. This is seldom the case. During the training program, the role of the medical specialist is basically to reassure the participants and other significant people in their life that they do not need any further traditional medical care and to give the "green light" to moving on with their lives. The education sessions of the medical specialist focus on beliefs and understanding of the origin of their symptoms.

The role of the physiotherapist in assessment and intervention is basically to determine the patient's general capacity to deal with the demands of his or her environment. More specifically, the physiotherapist determines the general level of physical deconditioning as described by Mayer and Gatchel (1988) that has taken place since the accident occurred. During the first 2 weeks of intervention, a reversal of the deconditioning process starts to take place by using the graded activity principles. The physiotherapist uses exercise equipment to stimulate the conditioning process and to decrease the patient's possible fear of movement, resulting in a reduced cervical range of motion. In this fashion, patients set realistic goals, based on measurable units and not based on how they feel that day, good or bad. This process assists patients to separate their pain symptoms, which can vary daily from what they have planned to accomplish that day. This process of grading activities can also be used in combination with the principles of graded exposure to address activities that are part of normal life, such as driving a car and diving into a swimming pool, both of which can be daunting to some patients.

The clinical psychologist, together with other members of the team, stimulates the behavioral change process. The first sessions are educational and focus on the relationships between symptoms, behaviors, and beliefs. The following group sessions deal with further assessing and changing the reinforcers of the patient's current situation.

Once these reinforcers are identified by the psychologist and acknowledged by the patient, steps can be made to empower the patient to develop adequate coping strategies in order to deal with these reinforcers in the future. The development of adequate coping strategies helps prevent potential relapse. Techniques used to assist in this process are: cognitive-behavioral therapy (see Turk, Chapter 7, this volume), assertiveness training, role-playing, and analysis of group dynamics.

During the intervention process, the occupational therapist works as a liaison between the patient and his or her current employer. Once the patient is making progress in the other team members' areas of responsibility, the occupational therapist expands on these experiences the patient has had using the graded activity principles in the exercise area and applies them to the development of a return-to-work plan. The tempo of the work resumption plan is tailor-made. It is essential that patients develop their own return-to-work plan, within certain guidelines. These guidelines are:

- Create a realistic goal-oriented graded plan.
- Be clear but not complex.
- Build up over the course of approximately 10 weeks.
- Communicate and gain support for the plan from all parties involved.
- Strive for a balance between work, family and leisure.

THE RETURN-TO-WORK PHASE

The follow-up visits are intended to monitor the patients' progress regarding their private life and returning to work. The follow-up meetings are planned at 6 weeks, 4 months, and 12 months after the close of the intensive part of the training program. Extra counseling can be carried out by the various team members depending on what is needed to support the patient in returning back to a more active lifestyle.

AIMS AND PHASES DURING THE TREATMENT

The danger of using a multidisciplinary approach with patients experiencing chronic symptoms is that partially related problems within the situation as a whole are simultaneously addressed without a well-thought-out strategy. In these cases, the treatment should be introduced in phases, which are based on the hierarchy of reinforcers identified in the assessment. Two considerations should be kept in mind when arranging this hierarchy of reinforcers (1) how close does this associated issue, that is, in terms of behavioral analysis, lie to the "central problem," and (2) how to match the treatment goal to the expectations of the patient. At times, these considerations can conflict with each other. For example, the clinician identifies that a PTSD is a central issue in the patient's situation, yet the patient expects to be treated for his pain. In such situations, a compromise should be developed where both points of view receive adequate attention.

The following information illustrates the phasing of treatment goals that can be used with whiplash patients. It goes without saying that these phases are intended to overlap. For example, correction of whiplash beliefs (Phase 1) will be further stimulated if patients gain some positive experiences with

the reconditioning training (Phase 2): They learn that they are more able than they had suspected; they correct the idea that moving is harmful.

- Phase 1: Correction of "whiplash beliefs"
- Phase 2: Treatment of fear–avoidance, pain behaviors, reconditioning
- Phase 3: Treatment of PTSD
- Phase 4: Management of emotional distress and coping strategies
- Phase 5: Neuropsychological training

Phase 1 and especially Phase 2 are of primary importance and correspond with the expectations of the average whiplash patient. It is essential that whiplash beliefs and myths be addressed in an early phase of intervention. The correct beliefs concerning the patient's situation will have a strong effect on the remaining phases in the treatment plan. For example, if patients continue to believe that they are limited in their abilities as a direct result of the accident, the chance that they will show progression in their graded activity exercise program is reduced.

In Phase 2, patients experience the disabling influence these beliefs have on them. Many patients realize that a general improvement in movement gives them a "boost" in their self-confidence, which in turn helps them better deal with related emotional issues. Issues specific to whiplash, such as wearing neck collars, chronic fatigue, and concentration problems, should be addressed in Phase 2.

The treatment goals in Phases 3 and 4 can play a central role in the situation but do not, at least initially, correspond with the patient's expectations. This is exactly the reason why these issues are addressed after certain, more relevant issues, as seen though the eyes of the patient, are addressed previously in Phase 2. The phases are meant to blend into each other for the best results.

The treatment of PTSD in a group setting is difficult; therefore, in these cases, individual counseling sessions are recommended. Phased exposure through the use of imagination or EMDR are the treatments of choice for PTSD.

In Phase 4, the focus is directed toward assisting the patient to develop more adequate coping strategies. We mean both coping strategies with the complaints and coping with personal stressors. The patients gradually gain insight in why previous coping strategies were inadequate and are stimulated to alter these strategies to deal with such situations in the future in a way that costs less time and energy, thereby reducing the influence these associated problems have on general functioning. A great variety of techniques from the cognitive-behavioral therapy can be used during this phase (see Turk, Chapter 7, this volume). One hopes that during this phase the patient becomes more sensitive to his or her own experiences and goes some steps further. Thus, new "personal stressors" come alive. Some patients also learn to see similarities between how they cope with the complaints and how they cope with other stressors. It is important to recognize that every patient has his or her process regarding such changes. Patient dropout can in many cases be prevented if the patient's "own way to change" is respected.

The treatment goals in Phase 5 are not often in need of attention because most neuropsychological deficits significantly decrease when working through the first four phases. If this is not the case, and neuropsychological deficits continue to strongly influence the general functioning of the patient, the individual attention of the psychologist is required. The goal of this counseling should be to increase the self-confidence of patient with regard to cognitive abilities. If patients experience some control over their cognitive functions, the negative spiral of emotional distress and neuropsychological deficits may be interrupted. The counseling should begin with a quick assessment of depression as memory and concentration problems are often symptoms of depression. If depression is excluded, some education regarding the origin and mechanisms of neuropsychological deficits following a whiplash injury should be given. The clinician should explain that the pain, emotional distress, and other symptoms distract the patient's concentration, and thus memory fails and the emotional distress is reinforced. The next step is that patients learn some techniques to make their cognitive functioning more simple and efficient. Some examples are selective attention, doing one thing after each other, and

internal repetition of important things that must be remembered. The concept of "graded exposure" can be applied here. The training should start with simple tasks. The cognitive tasks should be made simple so that the patient succeeds. Once some "success experiences" have occurred, tasks can be made more complex or intense. This principle can be applied to any activity: car driving, going shopping, reading the newspaper. We feel that this approach is more in correspondence with the nature of the neuropsychological deficits in whiplash patients than the application of some standard memory training.

Conclusion

The thoughts presented in this chapter are the result of more than 8 years of clinical experience with the treatment of whiplash patients. This chapter would have been totally different if it had been written when we first started. The most important change we have seen during this period is the notion of persistent symptoms after whiplash more in terms of a chronic pain problem and less as a "distinct" disease or syndrome. Research has shown that whiplash in itself is not a "disease" with well-defined and specific characteristics. Instead, whiplash is a description of the accident mechanism, nothing more, nothing less.

It has been our intention in this chapter to demonstrate good reasons for our belief that many features of musculoskeletal chronic pain in general are also applicable to whiplash. There is no reason to believe that concepts such as, for example, fear–avoidance beliefs, pain-coping strategies, or the muscle tension cycle, do not to play a role in patients with persistent symptoms after a whiplash injury. It has not been the intention of this chapter, however, to provide an in-depth discussion of all conceivable psychological aspects related to the treatment of chronic pain. Instead, we have selected those topics that, in our opinion, are most crucial in the treatment of chronic symptoms after whiplash. Therefore, this chapter should not be regarded as a treatment manual for whiplash patients.

One thing that definitely distinguishes

whiplash from many other types of chronic pain is the attention paid in the media to this subject. It is hard to take a "neutral" standpoint regarding whiplash. Some patients even ask doctors to which "side" they belong: the one that "believes" in whiplash or the one that does not. The fact that "believing" clearly plays a role indicates a lack of scientific evidence. There is clearly a lack of randomized clinical trials of treatment protocols for whiplash patients with chronic symptoms. Ideally, such research brings whiplash back to its "normal" proportions—a difficult to treat chronic pain problem but not without hope for many patients.

Perhaps more important, if we really want to reduce the "whiplash epidemic," something must change in our society. In fact, this chapter has in several places indicated that "incorrect whiplash beliefs" are in many patients the most important hindrance for improvement. Only when the whiplash beliefs are adequate will recovery take place. The origin of the whiplash beliefs can be traced back to the attitude toward whiplash in society. This attitude should change. Thus, the information about whiplash that we can download from the Internet and read in the whiplash folder by the general practitioner, the physiotherapist, and many others should be based more on scientific evidence and less on folklore. If this were the case, many chronic cases after a whiplash injury could probably be prevented. We should treat such cases well in an earlier phase and not leave chronic patients to their own devices or even make them ill with well-intended but incorrect advices and legal assistance.

Finally, this chapter focuses on the psychological aspects of whiplash. However, we do not deny the medical aspects associated with whiplash. Instead, we want to emphasize that careful medical examination and, if necessary, medical treatment is in some cases needed. In fact, those people involved who have experienced an accident may have a lesion. However, examination and treatment of medical factors related to whiplash is not more than one component of this complex problem. Certainly if the symptoms become chronic, many of the factors we have described in this chapter are contributing to major disability.

References

American Psychiatric Association. (1994). *Diagnostic and statistical manual of mental disorders* (4th ed.). Washington, DC: Author.

Barnsley, L., Lord, S., & Bogduk, N. (1994). Whiplash injury. *Pain, 58,* 283–307.

Borchgrevink, G. E., Kaasa, A., McDonagh, D., Stiles, T. C., Haraldseth, O., & Lereim, I. (1998). Acute treatment of whiplash neck sprain injuries: A randomized trial of treatment during the first 14 days after a car accident. *Spine, 23,* 25–31.

Borchgrevik, G. E., Smevik, O., & Nordby, A. (1995). MR imaging and radiography of patients with cervical hyperextension-flexion injuries after car accidents. *Acta Radiologica, 36,* 425–428.

Bicik, I., Radanov, B. P., & Schafer, N. (1998). PET with (18) fluozodeoxyglucose and hexamethylpropylene amine oxine SPECT in late whiplash syndrome. *Neurology, 51,* 345–350.

Bunketorp, O., Olsson, I., Carlsson, S. G., & Styf, J. (2001, March 8–10). *Outcome of WAD predicted by MPI.* Berne, Germany: International Congress on Whiplash Associated Disorders.

Cassidy, J. D. (1995). Scientific monograph of the Quebec Task Force on whiplash associated disorders: Redefining whiplash and its management. *Spine, 20*(Suppl.), 9–73.

Cassidy, J. D., Carroll, L. J., Cote, P., Lemstra, M., Berglund, A., & Nygren, A. (2000). Effect of eliminating compensation for pain and suffering on the outcome of insurance claims for whiplash injury. *New England Journal of Medicine, 342,* 1179–1186.

Castro, W., Meyer, S. J., Becke, M. E., Nentwig, C. G., Hein, M. F., Ercan, B. I., Thomann, S., Wessels, U., & Du Chesne, A. E. (2001). No stress—no whiplash? Prevalence of "whiplash" symptoms following exposure to a placebo rear-end collision. *International Journal of Legal Medicine, 114,* 316–322.

Castro, W., Schilgen, M., Meyer, S., Weber, M., Peuker, C., & Wötler, R. (1997). Do "whiplash injuries" occur in low-speed rear impacts? *European Spine Journal, 6,* 366–375.

Cole, P., Cassidy, D., Carroll, L., Frank, J. W., & Bombardier, C. (2001). A systematic review of the prognosis of acute whiplash and a new conceptual framework to synthesize the literature. *Spine, 26,* E445–E458.

Crowe, H. E. (1958). Whiplash injuries of the cervical spine. In *Proceedings of American Bar Association, Section of insurance, negligence and compensation law* (pp. 176–271). Chicago: American Bar Association.

Drottning, M., Staff, P. H., & Malt, U. F. (2001, March 8–10). *The one-year prevalence of posttraumatic stress response after common whiplash.* Berne, Germany: International Congress on Whiplash Associated Disorders.

Ferrari, R. (1999). *The whiplash encyclopedia. The*

facts and myths of whiplash. Gaithersburg, MD: Aspen.

Ferrari, R., & Russell, A. S. (1999). Epidemiology of whiplash: An international dilemma. *Annals of the Rheumatic Diseases, 58,* 1–5.

Fordyce, W. E. (1976). *Behavioral methods for chronic pain and illness*. St. Louis, MO: Mosby.

Gaitsch, G., Stude, P., Baume, B., Hasenbring, M., Diener, H. C., & Keidel, M. (2001, March 8–10). *Predictors of delayed recovery from post-traumatic neck pain in whiplash injury*. Berne, Germany: International Congress on Whiplash Associated Disorders.

Gargan, M., Bannister, G., & Main, C. (1997). The behavioral response to whiplash injury. *Journal of Bone and Joint Surgery, 97-B,* 523–526.

Gatchel, R. J., Mayer, T., Dersh, J., Robinson, R., & Polatin, P. (1999). The association of the SF–36 health status survey with 1-year socioeconomic outcomes in a chronically disabled spinal disorder population. *Spine, 24,* 2162–2170.

Gil, K. M., Williams, D. A., Keefe, F. J., & Beckham, J. C. (1990). The relationship of negative thougths to pain and psychological distress. *Behavior Therapy, 21,* 349–352.

Gundry, C. R., & Fritts, H. M. (1997). Magnetic resonance imaging of the musculoskeletal system. Part 8, The spine, section 2. *Clinical Orthopedics and Related Research, 343,* 260–271.

Harder, S., Veilleux, M., & Suissa, S. (1998). The effect of socio-demographic and crash-related factors on the prognosis of whiplash. *Journal of Clinical Epidemiology, 51,* 377–84.

Hartling, L., Brison, R. J., Ardern, C., & Pickett, W. (2001). Prognostic value of the Quebec Classification of Whiplash-Associated Disorders. *Spine, 26,* 36–41.

Jensen, T. S., & Kasch, H. (2000). *A prospective study of whiplash injury with ankle-injured controls*. Nice, France: Third Congress of the European Federation of IASP Chapters.

Kasch, H., Bach, F. W., & Jensen, T. S. (2001, March 8–10). *Risk for the assessment after acute whiplash injury: A one-year prospective study*. Berne, Germany: International Congress on Whiplash Associated Disorders.

Kessels, R. Aleman, A., Verhagen, W., & van Luijtelaar, E. (2000). Cognitive functioning after whiplash injury: A meta-analysis. *Journal of International Neuropsychological Society, 6,* 271–278.

King, D. A., & Caine, E. D. (1996). Cognitive impairment and major depression: Beyond the pseudodementia syndrome. In I. Grant & K. M. Adams (Eds.), *Neuropsychological assessment of neuropsychiatric disorders* (pp. 200–217). New York: Oxford University Press.

Larsson, S. E., Alund, M., Cai, H., & Ake Oberg, P. (1994). Chronic pain after soft-tissue injury of the cervical spine: Trapezius muscle blood flow and electromyography at static loads and fatigue. *Pain, 57,* 173–80.

Lezak, M. (1995). *Neuropsychological assessment*. New York: Oxford University Press.

Main, C. J., Wood, P. L., Hollis, S., Spanswick, C. C., & Waddell, G. (1992). The Distress Risk Assessment Method (DRAM): A simple patient classification to identify distress and evaluate the risk of poor outcome. *Spine, 17,* 42–52.

Mayer, T. G., & Gatchel, R. J. (1988). *Functional restoration for spinal disorders. The sports medicine approach*. Philadelphia: Lea & Febiger.

Nederhand, M. J., IJzerman, M. J., Hermens, H. J., Baten, C. T., & Zilvold, G. (2000). Cervical muscle dysfunction in the chronic whiplash associated disorder grade II (WAD-II). *Spine, 25,* 1938–1943.

Obelieniene, D., Schrader, H., Bovim, G., Miseviciene, I., & Sand, T. (1999). Pain after whiplash: A controlled prospective inception cohort study. *Journal of Neurology, Neurosurgery and Psychiatry, 66,* 279–283.

Olsnes, B. T. (1989). Neurobehavioral findings in whiplash patients with long lasting symptoms. *Acta Neurologica Scandinavica, 80,* 584–588.

Otte, A., Mueller-Brand, J., Nitzscke, E. U., Wachter, K., & Ettlin, T. M. (1997). Funtional brain imaging in 200 patients after whiplash injury. *Journal of Nuclear Medicine, 38,* 1102–1120.

Pearce, J. M. (1994). Polemics of chronic whiplash injury. *Neurology, 44,* 1993–1997.

Peeters, G., Verhagen, A., Bie, R. de, & Oostendorp, R. (2001). The efficacy of conservative treatment in whiplash patients: A systematic review of clinical trials. *Spine, 26,* E64–E73.

Pennebaker, J. W. (1982). *The psychology of physical symptoms*. New York: Springer-Verlag.

Pennie, B., & Agambar, I. (1991). Patterns of injury and recovery in whiplash. *Injury, 22,* 57–59.

Pilowsky, I., & Spence, N. D. (1975). Patterns of illness behavior in patients with intractable pain. *Journal of Psychosomatic Research, 19,* 279–287.

Radanov, B. P., Begré, S., Sturzenegger, M., & Augustiny, F. (1996). Course of psychological variables in whiplash injury—a 2-year follow-up with age, gender and education pain-matched patients. *Pain, 64,* 429–434.

Radanov, B. P., Di Stefano, G., Schnidrig, A., Sturzenegger, M., & Augustiny, F. (1993). Cognitive functioning after common whiplash. *Archives of Neurology, 50,* 87–91.

Radanov, B. P., Dvorak, J., & Valach, L. (1992). Cognitive deficits in patients after soft tissue injury of the cervical spine. *Spine, 17,* 127–131.

Ronnen, H. R., De Korte, P. J., & Brink, P. R. G. (1996). Hidden cervical spine injuries in traffic accident victims with skull fractures. *Journal of Spinal Disorders, 4,* 251–263.

Rosenfeld, M., Gunnarsson, R., & Borenstein, P. (2000). Early intervention in whiplash-associated disorders. *Spine, 25,* 1782–1787.

Schmand, B., Lindeboom, J., Schagen, R., Heijt, R., Koene, T., & Hamburger, H. L. (1998). Cognitive complaints in patients after whiplash injury: The impact of malingering. *Journal of Neurology, Neurosurgery and Psychiatry, 64,* 339–343.

Scholten-Peeters, G., Bekkering, G., Verhagen, A. P., Van der Windt, D., Lanser, K., Hendriks, E., & Oostendorp, R. (2002). Clinical practice guidelines for the physiotherapy of patients with whiplash-associated disorders. *Spine, 27,* 412–422.

Spitzer, W. O., Skovron, M. L., Salmi, L. R., Cassidy, J. D., Duranceau, J., Suissa, S., & Zeiss, E. (1995). Scientific monograph of the Quebec Task Force on whiplash-associated disorders: Redefining whiplash and its management. *Spine, 20,* 10S–73S.

Stovner, L. J. (1996). The nosologic status of the whiplash syndrome: A critical review based on a methodological approach. *Spine, 21,* 2735–2746.

Taylor, A. E., Cox, C. A., & Mailis, A. (1996). Persistent neuropsychological deficits following whiplash: Evidence for chronic mild traumatic brain injury? *Archives of Physical Medicine and Rehabilitation, 77,* 529–235.

Turk, D. C., Kerns, R. D., & Rosenberg, R. (1992). Effects of marital interaction on chronic pain and disability: Examining the down-side of social support. *Rehabilitation Psychology, 37,* 259–274.

van Akkerveeken, P. F., & Vendrig, A. A. (1998). Chronic symptoms after whiplash: A cognitive behavioral approach. In R. Gunzburg & M. Szpalski (Eds.), *Whiplash injuries: Current concepts in prevention, diagnosis, and treatment of the cervical whiplash syndrome* (pp. 183–191). Philadelphia: Lippincott-Raven.

van Zomeren, A. H., & Deelman, B. G. (1978). Long-term recovery of visual reaction time after closed head injury. *Journal of Neurology, Neurosurgery and Psychiatry, 41,* 452–457.

van Zomeren, A. H., & Saan, R. (1997). Whiplash. In B. Deelman, P. Eling, E. de Haan, A. Jennekens-Schinkel, & E. van Zomeren (Eds.), *Clinical neuropsychology* [Klinische neuropsychologie] (pp. 290–298). Amsterdam: Boom.

Vendrig, A. A., van Akkerveeken, P. F., & McWhorter, K. R. (2000). Results of a multimodal treatment program for patients with chronic symptoms after a whiplash injury of the neck. *Spine, 25,* 238–243.

Yarnell, P. R., & Rossie, G. V. (1988). Minor whiplash head injury with major debilitation. *Brain Injury, 2,* 255–258.

Waddell, G., Newton, M., Henderson, I., Somerville, D., & Main, C. J. (1993). A Fear–Avoidance Beliefs Questionnaire (FABQ) and the role of fear–avoidance beliefs in chronic low back pain and disability. *Pain, 52,* 157–168.

Ware, J. E., & Sherbourne, C. D. (1992). The MOS 36-Item Short-Form Health Survey: I. Conceptual framework and item selection. *Medical Care, 30,* 473–483.

21

Treatment of Patients with Temporomandibular Disorders

Robert J. Gatchel

Temporomandibular disorders (TMDs) are a heterogeneous collection of disorders characterized by orofacial pain, masticatory dysfunction, or both. The majority of cases of TMD involve either disc displacements, muscle disorders, internal derangements or degenerative changes of the temporo-mandibular joint (TMJ), or combined mus-cle–joint disorders. Fricton and Schiffman (1995) have estimated that the annual cost of treating chronic pain approximates $80 billion, with 40% of the cost attributed to craniomandibular pain, including that of TMD. This high cost is directly related to the unresponsiveness of this TMD popula-tion to traditional medical treatment ap-proaches. It is well established that as the duration of pain increases, patients become more refractory to intervention. Therefore, it is of utmost importance to identify pa-tients at the acute stage in order to prevent the development of chronicity and treatment difficulties.

TMD has received increasing attention from behavioral scientists during the last two decades because of the importance of psy-chosocial factors (e.g., stress, anxiety, and depression) in these disorders. Conservative estimates indicate that anywhere between 5 and 12% of all American adults experience some form of craniofacial pain at some time in their lives (Duckro, Tait, Margolis, & Deshields, 1990; Von Korff, Dworkin, LeResche, & Kruger, 1988). However, one traditional major roadblock in the scientific investigation and potential development of effective treatment for this problem had been the often poor agreement among researchers as to which symptoms to include in defining patient samples (Rugh, 1983). Other than the agreement that the two major clinical features of most TMD patients are pain and dysfunction, patients present unique combi-nations of symptoms that make it difficult to classify them as a homogeneous group. Real-izing that a major obstacle standing in the way of a further understanding of TMD was the lack of a standardized diagnostic criteria for differentiating clinical subtypes of TMD, a project was funded by the National Insti-tute of Dental and Craniofacial Research to create standardized diagnostic criteria. This project yielded "Research Diagnostic Crite-ria for Temporomandibular Disorders"

(RDC/TMD) (Dworkin & LeResche, 1992). The RDC/TMD allows standardization and replication of studies of TMD because there is now some reliable and valid diagnostic criteria that will be reproducible among clinical researchers.

The RDC/TMD

The RDC/TMD allows one to assess the patient on two axes according to specified and standardized procedures. The first axis assesses and diagnoses clinical subtypes of TMD conditions. Axis I disorders are broken down into three groups: Group I—muscle disorders; Group II—disk displacements; and Group III—arthralgia/arthritis/arthrosis. The rules for assessing diagnoses are as follows: A patient can be assigned, at most, one Group I (muscle) diagnosis. In addition, each *joint* may be assigned, at most, one diagnosis from Group II and one diagnosis from Group III. That is, diagnoses within any given group are mutually exclusive. This means that, in principle, a patient can be assigned from 0 diagnoses (no diagnosable muscle joint conditions) to five diagnoses (one muscle diagnosis plus one diagnosis from Group II and one from Group III for each joint). The second axis—Axis II—assesses pain-related disability and psychological status. Specifically, it assesses pain intensity, pain-related disability, depression, and nonspecific physical symptoms (somatization). Patients are graded as low, medium, or high for each of four categories. The development of this RDC/TMD was a major breakthrough in the assessment and diagnosis of TMD, especially given that it incorporates standardized procedures for making Axis I diagnoses and evaluating Axis II conditions. Throughout this chapter, I note when the RDC/TMD was used when reviewing a treatment-outcome study.

Traditional Treatment Of TMD: An Overview

The time course of TMD often leads to a great deal of perceptual distortion among dental observers. About 90% of the time, TMD is a brief time-limited condition for which the treatment chosen often appears irrelevant to the outcome (Greene, 1992). This, though, is also true for other forms of pain, such as low back pain (Mayer & Gatchel, 1988).

Physical Treatments

A large number of physical treatments have been used to treat TMD patients, including temporomandibular joint surgery, muscular exercises, tranquilizing drugs, corticosteroids, muscle relaxants, placebo drugs, and occlusal adjustment (Rugh & Solberg, 1976). Moreover, other nonsurgical treatment of TMD, such as patient education, occlusal splints, nonnarcotic analgesics, heat, and a soft diet is frequently recommended (Greene, 1990; Hodges, 1990; Moss & Garrett, 1984). In fact, Hodges (1990) found that 75% of 448 TMD patients in his study were successfully managed (i.e., relieved of pain, had longer pain-free periods, or were more comfortable with their TMD problems) by such treatment within 4 weeks after initiation of treatment. The treatment Hodges used consisted of patient education (a TMJ disease pamphlet from the American Dental Association and a brief demonstration of the anatomy of the TMJ using a skull), heat, massage, nonnarcotic analgesics (ibuprofen or acetaminophen), and occlusal splints. It is generally agreed that such an approach is best for initially treating TMD, although some have even advocated not using occlusional splints in the initial conservative treatment of TMD (e.g., Greene, 1992).

Glaros and Glass (1993), as well as Goldstein (1999), have provided more comprehensive reviews of traditional dental or physical treatments of TMD (see Table 21.1). Both of these reviews conclude that a purely traditional biomedical model approach is often insufficient in providing long-term improvement and management of TMD. Rather, there is growing evidence of a biopsychosocial nature of most cases of TMD, thus supporting the use of noninvasive and multidisciplinary treatment modalities. The *biopsychosocial model* of pain (Figure 21.1) emphasizes the complex and dynamic interaction among physiological, psychological, and social factors that often results in or maintains chronic pain condi-

TABLE 21.1. Traditional Dental/Physical Treatment of TMD

Irreversible techniques

- Surgery (arthroscopy; open joint surgery; replacement of articular discs)
- Occlusional equilibration
- Orthodontic treatment

Interocclusional appliances (splints)

- There is much variation in the type of splint used, varying in the degree to which the mandible is allowed to move freely or is forced into a particular position.
- There is much controversy concerning the mechanism by which splints may produce beneficial results.

Medications

- Tranquilizing drugs
- Opioid analgesics
- Nonopioid analgesics
- Local anesthetics
- Corticosteroids
- Nonsteroid anti-inflammatory drugs (NSAIDs)
- Muscle relaxants

Patient education and palliative home care

- Instructions about the biomechanics of the temporomandibular joint (TMJ)
- Avoid behaviors that can exacerbate problems (e.g., chewing gum; avoid problem foods, especially hard and chewy foods; avoid deliberately cracking or popping jaws)
- Application of heat or cold packs can often provide temporary pain relief
- Over-the-counter analgesics can be helpful
- Stretching exercises can help increase range of motion and decrease pain levels

tions such as TMD (see, e.g., Epker & Gatchel, 2000; see also Turk & Monarch, Chapter 1, this volume).

Early Psychological Treatment Approaches

Early investigators noted a high prevalence of emotional factors in TMD patients (e.g., Moulton, 1955, 1966). After interviewing 35 TMD patients, Moulton identified two personality profiles: (1) an exceedingly dependent and ingratiating type, with this syndrome leading to frustration, hostility, and reactive anger (which was expressed muscu-

larly in an attempt to suppress such unwanted emotions); and (2) a domineering, perfectionistic, and obsessive type (which was expressed by prolonged bruxism or clenching, likely leading to muscle spasm and increased pain). However, subsequent studies evaluating such emotional and personality factors associated with TMD patients have been quite diverse and mixed (e.g., Suvinen & Reade, 1995).

Although it has long been suggested that TMD patients may suffer from a variety of psychological problems, surprisingly few studies have looked at the effectiveness of psychotherapy in treating TMD patients. In an early study, Lupton (1969) found that TMD patients who received client-centered counseling alone reported as much physical symptom relief as patients who received dental treatment alone. Similarly, Pomp (1974) found that 15 of 23 patients (65%) who received brief psychotherapy had a remission of their symptoms at the conclusion of therapy. The brief psychotherapy program consisted of 12 sessions of individual therapy that focused on dealing with the stressful events that arose in the patients' lives.

Of the few studies that have examined the effectiveness of psychotherapy for TMD patients, none to date has used a cognitive-behavioral approach in treating psy-

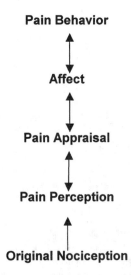

FIGURE 21.1. The biopsychosocial model of pain.

chopathology. This omission is quite interesting given that many TMD patients experience depression (see, e.g., Kinney, Gatchel, Ellis, & Holt, 1992; Speculand, Goss, Hughes, Spence, & Pilowsky, 1983), and that cognitive-behavioral approaches have been shown to be effective in alleviating the symptoms of depression (see, e.g., K. Dobson, 1989; Jarrett, 1990). It should be noted that cognitive-behavioral (cognitive-behavior) treatment represents a broad class of therapies, of which cognitive therapy is one specific type (J. Dobson & Block, 1988). Indeed, as Lewinsohn, Antonuccio, Steinmetz, and Teri (1984) have noted, even though contemporary therapeutic approaches have been divided into those that primarily emphasize "behavior" and those that emphasize "cognitions" in the etiology of depression, they are quite similar. Moreover, there is empirical support for the treatment efficacy of both approaches. For example, a review of the literature on cognitive therapy for depression revealed that most studies relied on the treatment approach outlined by Beck, Rush, Shaw, and Emery (1979), which uses both cognitive and behavioral techniques. Furthermore, K. Dobson's (1989) meta-analysis of the efficacy of cognitive therapy for depression found that cognitive therapy resulted in a greater relief of depressive symptoms than did a waiting list of no-treatment control, pharmacotherapy, and other psychotherapies. Similarly, treatments derived from "behavioral" approaches and aimed at enhancing social skills, improving pleasant activity level, and increasing general problem-solving skills have been shown to be effective (cf. Lewinsohn et al., 1984).

According to Lewinsohn and colleagues (1984), the problem confronting the practitioner is selecting from among a range of these promising cognitive and behavioral approaches. These investigators have developed a structured treatment approach that was designed to incorporate the various specific behavioral and cognitive strategies shown to be effective. However, again, in keeping with the biopsychosocial model of pain, practitioners need to be aware of the importance of evaluating and managing physical factors, as well as cognitive and behavioral issues. This is the philosophy of many recent biobehavioral treatment approaches, to be discussed next.

Biobehavioral Treatment of TMD

With the realization that psychosocial and physical factors may interact in the etiology and/or maintenance of TMD, a number of biobehavioral treatment modalities have been used with these patients. One such approach has been that of EMG biofeedback and progressive muscle relaxation training. Many researchers originally published case studies that suggested the effectiveness of biofeedback in the treatment of TMD. For example, Carlsson and Gale (1977) published a case report demonstrating that biofeedback allowed a person to regain muscle control and eliminate pain. Klonoff and Janata (1986) also conducted a case study and found that the patient reported a substantial decrease in pain after learning to maintain equal levels of electromyograph (EMG) activity in the right and left masseter muscles, and learning relaxation through EMG biofeedback treatment. Although case studies support biofeedback as an effective treatment, their generalizability is limited when compared to studies that include larger sample sizes and control groups.

In another novel biobehavioral treatment approach, Dworkin and colleagues (1994) compared the effects of usual TMD treatment (i.e., the use of splints and anti-inflammatory medication, heat and cold packs, and modification of parafunctional and dietary habits) and the effects of group-administered cognitive-behavioral treatment provided to patients before the usual dental treatment was initiated. Results of this randomized clinical trial demonstrated that although the benefits of the cognitive-behavioral intervention were not seen at a 3-month follow-up, this cognitive-behavioral treatment was associated with greater long-term (6 months) decreases in self-reported pain levels and pain interference in daily activities, relative to patients who merely received only the usual dental treatment.

Relaxation and Biofeedback

The assumption underlying these biobehavioral treatment approaches is that stress-induced muscle hyperactivity often is one important cause of the pain and dysfunction (Moss & Garrett, 1984). The research on the efficacy of using biofeedback or relaxation training to treat TMD has been generally positive. For example, Carlson and Gale (1977) found that masseter EMG biofeedback eliminated or significantly reduced temporomandibular joint pain in 8 of 11 patients. Similarly, Scott and Gregg (1980) reviewed many articles on treating TMD with biofeedback and/or muscle relaxation and concluded that biofeedback and muscle relaxation were helpful clinical interventions, especially for TMD patients who were not depressed and who had not had the pain for more than a few years. Hijzen, Slanger, and Van Houweligen (1986) found that EMG biofeedback training to increase control over masseter activity produced significantly more improvement in clinical dysfunction and subjective symptoms related to pain and mandibular movement than either a splint-treatment group or a no-treatment control group.

In a study by Burdette and Gale (1988), a treatment procedure that emphasized cognitive awareness of dysfunctional orofacial behavior and EMG biofeedback training of the masseteric area to teach masticatory muscle relaxation was administered to 37 myofascial pain-dysfunction patients. These patients displayed greater resting EMG activity in the masseter area at initial assessment relative to a control group of 23 patients. The most interesting finding, though, was that the overall results did not necessarily support a direct association between a change in the level of tonic EMG activity, or muscle tension, and relief of muscle pain. This was because only 29 of the 37 patients demonstrated significant symptom improvement; the other eight, however, did not, even though their EMG levels similarly decreased. The investigators indicated that other factors are therefore responsible for the differences between these treatment-success and treatment-failure subgroups. Such individual differences in response to treatment would be expected on the basis of the biopsychosocial model. It may be that the eight treatment-failure patients required a cognitive-behavioral therapy regimen to more directly deal with problems related to psychopathology rather than merely reducing muscle tension.

Several studies have also been conducted that have compared the efficacy of EMG biofeedback versus relaxation training. Moss, Wedding, and Sanders (1983) found that progressive relaxation training was just as effective as masseter EMG biofeedback in three of five TMD patients, and that the other two patients were not helped by either biofeedback or progressive relaxation. Funch and Gale (1984) also compared relaxation therapy with masseter EMG biofeedback and found that both treatments work equally well with TMD patients. However, they found that characteristics of the patients with successful outcomes were not similar for the two treatments. Successful patients in the relaxation therapy group tended to be younger, had their TMD a shorter period of time, and had reported other psychophysiological problems, relative to those who were successfully treated with EMG biofeedback. Similarly, Stenn, Mothersill, and Brooke (1979) compared the efficacy of masseter EMG biofeedback with relaxation training and found that subjects in both groups experienced significant reductions in scores on self-report measures of pain. Furthermore, all subjects in the Stenn and colleagues (1979) study demonstrated significant decreases in masseter muscle tension. Interestingly, patients who received biofeedback did not demonstrate more masseter muscle relaxation than those who received relaxation training. In terms of this issue of muscle relaxation versus biofeedback, the clinical research literature on the treatment of anxiety and stress actually suggests that a combined relaxation–biofeedback approach produces the greatest overall improvement across the greatest number of patients and is the preferred method (Gatchel, 1979, 1982, 1988).

Scott and Gregg (1980) have presented several criticisms of the early studies on biofeedback and relaxation treatments for TMD. They point out that there has been a lack of evidence to suggest that reduced pain ratings of patients were accompanied by lowered EMG levels. In addition, dependent measures have been generally restricted to the use of self-reported measures of pain and have often excluded other symptoms of TMD. They also indicate that few studies have employed placebo control groups and there has been a lack of follow-up data allowing for further analysis of treatment effectiveness. Moreover, Moss and Garrett (1984) concluded that no firm conclusions can be drawn regarding relaxation training and EMG biofeedback other than that these procedures appear to be effective with some

TMD patients. Thus, many of the early studies were not methodologically sound investigations (see also Mealiea & McGlynn, 1987). One of the major problems with these past studies has been the absence of diagnostic criteria, such as the recent RDC/TMD, to help delineate which TMD patients respond best to this treatment modality. This shortcoming, however, has recently been remedied by two studies (Gardea, Gatchel, & Mishra, 2001; Mishra, Gatchel, & Gardea, 2000). These studies evaluated the relative efficacy of four methods for treating chronic TMD patients: continuation of nonsurgical treatment alone and three different biobehavioral treatment approaches—relaxation–biofeedback treatment, cognitive-behavioral skills treatment (CBST), and combined relaxation–biofeedback/CBST. Separate studies addressed this issue, one looking at immediate posttreatment outcomes (Mishra et al., 2000) and the other evaluating 1-year follow-up results (Gardea et al., 2001). Both studies used the RDC/TMD for diagnosing TMD.

Finally, Crider and Glaros (1999) reported the results of meta-analyses of treatments incorporating EMG biofeedback for TMD. Through a literature search, they were able to identify 13 studies of EMG biofeedback treatment for TMD. These included six controlled studies, four comparative studies, and three uncontrolled studies. Three different outcome measures were assessed: patient pain reports, clinical examination findings, and ratings of global improvement. Results revealed that five of the six controlled studies demonstrated EMG biofeedback to be superior to no treatment or psychological placebo controls for at least one of the three outcome measures. Crider and Glaros also used the data from 12 of the studies to conduct a meta-analysis. This analysis revealed substantially greater outcomes for biofeedback treatments relative to control conditions. Follow-up outcomes also revealed no deterioration of these positive outcomes over time. Based on these analyses, the authors conclude that the existing data support the clinical efficacy of EMG biofeedback treatments of TMD.

Comparisons among Biobehavioral Treatments

In the Mishra and colleagues (2000) study, results clearly demonstrated that a chronic pain index (CPI) score (from Axis II of the RDC/TMD) significantly decreased, from pretreatment to posttreatment, for the three biobehavioral treatment groups, indicating a decrease in self-reported pain. Overall, these three treatment groups demonstrated significantly greater change than did the comparison group (continuation of nonsurgical treatment alone), with additional analysis of the CPI variable revealing no significant differences among the three biobehavioral treatment conditions. Moreover, a significant pretreatment to posttreatment group effect was found, with the relaxation–biofeedback group displaying significantly greater reductions relative to the comparison group. Also, significant differences in pre- to posttreatment CPI scores were found for the three treatment conditions but not for the comparison group condition, clearly demonstrating that all three biobehavioral treatments were effective in reducing the pain that TMD patients experience. Although the relaxation–biofeedback treatment was the most effective at reducing pain in TMD patients, the CBST and the combined treatment approaches were also more therapeutically effective than the comparison condition. Finally, all three treatment groups displayed a significant improvement in positive mood states. Again, these findings are congruent with the biobehavioral perspective of an interactive and reciprocal nature of pain and psychosocial functioning in TMD patients.

The etiology of TMD may be directly related to the hyperactivity of muscles of mastication (see, e.g., Dahlstrom, Carlsson, & Carlsson, 1982; Kight, Gatchel, & Wesley, 1999). It is not surprising, then, that relaxation–biofeedback was the most effective treatment at initially reducing pain, as it directly focuses on reducing EMG activity levels. These results also concur with those reported by Flor and Birbaumer (1993), who found that patients administered biofeedback showed more improvement at posttreatment compared to patients who received cognitive-behavioral therapy or conservative medical treatment. Relatedly, at first glance, it may seem puzzling that the combined treatment group did not have greater effects than the relaxation–biofeedback group had on reducing pain, because this group also received biofeedback in their treatment. A possible explanation is that because they were receiving CBST and biofeedback in each session, the patients' perception of the problem may have been affected. Most TMD patients view their pain as a physically based, rather than a psychologically based, problem. Thus, it is understandable that initially they might be more motivated to fully engage in biofeedback treatment, which focuses on physiology, versus a combined treatment, which includes a psychological component.

The same reasoning can be used to explain why those in the CBST group did not do as well as those in the relaxation–biofeedback treatment group. CBST is primarily a psychological treatment that focuses on psychological difficulties not necessarily related to TMD. Thus, although the skills learned by those in the CBST group helped reduce their TMD pain, it seems logical that a treatment focused on physiology would initially be more effective, especially if TMD is indeed caused by the hyperactivity of muscles.

The results of this study suggest that relaxation–biofeedback is the most effective of the three treatment conditions for *short-term* pain reduction, and there are definite advantages to this method. Besides biofeedback being more physiologically based, and thus more "engaging" for patients, it is the easiest of the three biobehavioral treatments to administer to patients. In addition, it is more time efficient than either CBST or a combined treatment.

We hypothesized that participants in all three treatment conditions would show significant improvements in emotional distress, namely, anger/hostility, confusion/bewilderment, depression/dejection, fatigue/inertia, and tension/anxiety scores from pre- to posttreatment assessment. Vigor/activity scores significantly increased among those in all three biobehavioral treatment conditions. In addition, there was a significant decrease in the total mood disturbance score, which takes into account the other six factors measured. There were no significant differences among the three treatment conditions on any of these factors. Thus, consistent with the biopsychosocial perspective, improved mood and reduction of pain seem to be interactive. These factors likely influence one another, with improved mood contributing to decreased pain, and decreased pain contributing to improved mood. Pain severity and level of mood disturbance were clearly not the only factors influencing one another, as demonstrated by the lack of significant differences in affective state scores between those in the relaxation–biofeedback group and those receiving other biobehavioral treatments.

In a follow-up study, Gardea and colleagues (2001) evaluated the 1-year posttreatment outcomes of the aforementioned four groups. A comparison of changes from initial to 1 year for the CPI and Graded Chronic Pain Scale (GCPS) scores (both measures from Axis II of the RDC/TMD) in this study found significant differences between all three biobehavioral treatment conditions combined versus the comparison group. A contrast evaluation among the biofeedback, CBST, and combined biofeedback/CBST treatment groups revealed that the most robust CPI change occurred for the combined biofeedback/CBST treatment group, relative to the comparison group. Further analyses also found that all three biobehavioral treatment groups were comparable in terms of improved GCPS response. The decrease in subjective pain (CPI) and pain-related disability (GCPS) from initial to 1 year, therefore, clearly demonstrated the efficacy of all three biobehavioral interventions in treating TMD, with the most improvement displayed by the combined treatment group. Thus, an intervention aimed at comprehensively addressing the biobehavioral needs of TMD patients greatly enhances long-term treatment outcomes. Clinicians treating TMD patients must therefore be sensitive to the psychosocial aspects contributing to the disorder, as well as the physiological underpinnings. Indeed, this is another clear illustration of the heuristic value of adopting a biopsychosocial perspective to the assessment and treatment of chronic medical/dental disorders such as TMD (Turk, 1996).

Several other investigators have added EMG biofeedback to other TMD treatments to determine whether the use of biofeedback increases treatment efficacy. An interesting study by Erlandson and Popper (1989) found that masseter EMG biofeedback alone did not result in increased mandibular range of motion or decreases in self-reported pain. However, when patients were given a prosthesis, similar to an occlusal splint, which placed their jaw in the "rest" position and were given biofeedback, they reported significant reductions in self-report of pain, had significant reductions in masseter activity, and had significant increases in mandibular range of motion. Moreover, Olson (1977) found that patients who were unresponsive to drug and splint therapy had much better treatment outcomes when they received a combination of masseter biofeedback and brief psychotherapy than when they received biofeedback alone. Finally, Gessel (1975) found that depressed patients had greater symptom relief if they received EMG biofeedback coupled with tricyclic antidepressants than if they received biofeedback alone. Gessel concluded that biofeedback alone may help patients who do not have a psychological overlay to their problem. However, when psychological factors coexist with TMD, they need to be treated along with the physical symptoms.

Finally, Turk, Zaki, and Rudy (1993) evaluated the differential efficacy of two commonly used TMD treatments—intraoral appliances (IA) and biofeedback—both separately and in combination with one another. Two separate studies were conducted. In the first, the comparative efficacy of IA treatment, a combined biofeedback and stress management (B-SM) treatment, and waiting-list control group was evaluated. Results revealed that immediately after treatment, the IA treatment was more effective that the B-SM treatment in reducing pain. However, at a 6-month follow-up, the IA group significantly relapsed, especially in depression, whereas the B-SM group maintained its improvements in both pain and depression and continued to improve. In the second study, the combination of IA and B-SM was assessed in a sample of TMD patients. Results clearly showed that the combined treatment was more effective than either of the single treatments alone (especially in pain reduction) at a 6-month follow-up. Overall, these results strengthen the argument that both physical and psychological treatments are most effective in successfully treating TMD

patients in order to ensure that therapeutic gains are to be maintained.

Summary and Conclusions

From the literature reviewed, it is quite clear that biobehavioral treatment, which is based on a biopsychosocial approach to pain, is therapeutically effective with TMD patients. Indeed, as reviewed in Table 21.2, there are now numerous studies supporting its effectiveness. According to the literature, routine nonsurgical care should, at least initially, be the standard treatment for TMD. Biobehavioral treatment fulfills this need.

Finally, now that biobehavioral treatments have been shown to be effective in the management of many chronic pain syndromes, clinical researchers are beginning to evaluate variables that predict what patients respond best to such programs (e.g., Gatchel & Epker, 1999). As Turk and Okifuji (1998) have noted, one must avoid the assumption of "pain-patient homogeneity" in terms of response to treatment. There are many individual differences or heterogeneity in such responses. As a result, there have been attempts to identify subgroups of pain patients. One such subgroup classification system used with chronic pain patients is the Multidimensional Pain Inventory (MPI), originally developed by Kerns, Turk, and Rudy (1985). The MPI is a self-report measure developed to evaluate chronic pain patients' experience of pain from a cognitive-behavioral perspective. A strength of the MPI is that its factor structure and psychometric properties have been replicated in the United States, Germany, Sweden, and the Netherlands. Subsequent to establishing the reliability and validity of the MPI, Turk and Rudy (1988) used cluster analysis to generate profile classifications that divide patients into subgroups on the basis of significant differences in their responses to the 12 scales comprising the MPI.

There are three primary MPI subgroups, or profile types, that have been found to predict response to treatment: "adaptive coper," "dysfunctional," and "interpersonally distressed." The adaptive coper profile patients typically report less pain severity, lower levels of affective distress, higher ac-

TABLE 21.2. Summary of Biobehavioral Treatment of TMD Studies (in Chronological Order)

Type of treatment	Investigators	Methodology	Findings
EMG biofeedback of masseter muscle activity	Budzynski & Stoyva (1973)	One session comparing normal volunteers receiving auditory or visual EMG activity to those instructed to relax without biofeedback.	EMG biofeedback subjects reduced activity of the masseter significantly, relatively to relaxation subjects. Results suggested the usefulness of EMG biofeedback in treating patients with myofascial pain.
EMG biofeedback, antidepressant medication	Gessel (1975)	23 MPD patients were evaluated and treated.	EMG biofeedback was found to significantly relieve symptoms in 15 of the 23 patients. Antidepressant medication effectively treated half of the remaining 8 patients.
EMG biofeedback of masseter muscle activity	Carlsson & Gale (1977)	Treated 11 patients, who had at least a 3-year history of TMD pain, with masseter muscle biofeedback. These patients had not responded to routine dental treatment.	8 patients were found to be significantly better or totally symptom free after at least a 1-year period.
Combined conservative treatment and a mild tranquilizer, combined conservative treatment and an occlusional splint, combined conservative treatment, and physiotherapy, relaxation/coping skills training, biofeedback	Brooke, Stenn, & Mothersill (1977)	Treated 194 MPD patients with either of the three combined treatments. Patients were reassessed 16–44 months after their initial visit.	75% of patients had complete or almost complete recovery from their symptoms. 11 of the patients still experiencing symptoms then participated in relaxation/coping skills training, with half also receiving biofeedback. This training consisted of 8 weekly sessions. 10 of these patients subsequently showed marked improvement on objective and subjective symptoms after completion of the additional relaxation/coping skills training.
EMG biofeedback of masseter muscle activity	Dohrmann & Laskin (1978)	15 patients diagnosed with MPD received 9 biofeedback sessions.	All 15 patients reduced their mean masseter EMG levels. Of those patients reporting pain, 11 had complete remission and 2 reported a decrease in the frequency and severity of their pain. At a 1-year follow-up, only three patients had MPD episodes that they could not relieve with biofeedback.
EMG biofeedback	Gale (1979)	Patients with a history of more than 2 years of TMD pain, who had been previously treated unsuccessfully, were administered EMG biofeedback.	91% of patients who received at least five sessions reported some improvement at 1-year follow-up. Of this 91%, 58% showed no symptoms, and only 9% showed no improvement. Moreover, there was an 80% improvement rate for patients who received one or more biofeedback sessions.

TABLE 21.2. *Continued*

Type of treatment	Investigators	Methodology	Findings
Combined relaxation training, sensory awareness training, and coping skills training (6 of the 13 MPD patients also received EMG biofeedback	Stenn, Mothersill, & Brooke (1979)	MPD patients received 7 training sessions, following a 1-week baseline period when they monitored their pain.	Significant reductions in masseter EMG levels were found across sessions and at a 3-month follow-up. No differences were found in masseter EMG levels or pain behavior between those patients who received the additional biofeedback training and those who did not.
EMG biofeedback and occlusional splint therapy	Dahlstrom, Carlsson, & Carlsson (1982)	30 patients with mandibular dysfunction were treated, half of whom used full coverage splints nightly for 6 weeks and the other half received six, 30-minute EMG biofeedback sessions.	At a 1-month follow-up, both groups displayed significant reductions in symptoms clinically and subjectively. There were no significant differences between groups.
Masseter EMG biofeedback, relaxation training	Moss, Wedding, & Sanders (1983)	A series of single-case studies comparing the relative efficacy of masseter EMG biofeedback versus relaxation training. Study 1: multiple baseline design with a chronic TMJ patient. Study 2: four single-case studies.	Study 1: Relaxation training was the treatment responsible for improvement in self-reported jaw pain and tension; masseter EMG biofeedback provided little additional benefit. Study 2: Relaxation produced clear improvements in pain and tension ratings in two patients; combined biofeedback and relaxation provided slight improvement in one patient; neither treatment was effective for one patient.
Occlusional splint therapy, relaxation therapy	Okeson, Moody, Kemper, & Haley (1983)	24 patients were randomly assigned to receive either occlusional splint therapy or a simplified relaxation therapy technique.	Occlusional splint therapy was more effective than simplified relaxation on the following outcome measures: total mean observable pain scores; mean maximum comfortable opening; mean maximum opening.
EMG biofeedback and occlusional splint therapy	Dahlstrom & Carlsson (1984)	Extended the earlier Dahlstrom, Carlsson, & Carlsson (1982) study in order to compare the long-term (1-year) outcomes.	No significant differences found between the two treatment groups; both groups maintained significant reductions in clinical and subjective symptoms.
Relaxation therapy and biofeedback	Funch & Gale (1984)	Treatments were administered for 12 weeks on a weekly basis.	No significant differences between the two treatment groups immediately following treatment, as well as 2 years following treatment.

(continued)

TABLE 21.2. *Continued*

Type of treatment	Investigators	Methodology	Findings
Combined hypnosis and cognitive coping skills, combined relaxation and cognitive coping skills	Stam, McGrath, & Brooke (1984)	61 TMD patients were assigned to either one of the combined treatment groups or a no-treatment control group. Treatment group patients received four weekly sessions.	Both treatment groups reported decreases in pain, mouth opening limitations, joint sounds, as well as an increase in maximal mouth opening after treatment; there were no significant differences between the two groups. Both groups demonstrated greater decreases in pain and limitations relative to the no-treatment control group.
EMG biofeedback of masseter muscle activity	Dahlstrom, Carlsson, Gale, & Jansson (1985)	Obtained masseter EMG recordings before and after six biofeedback treatment sessions in 20 patients with mandibular dysfunction and 20 healthy controls. The posttreatment assessment involved obtaining EMG levels during no activity and stressful activity.	The patient group had significantly greater EMG activity before biofeedback, relative to controls; however, no differences were seen after treatment, with patients showing a significant decrease in their responsiveness.
EMG biofeedback and splint therapy	Hijzen, Slanger, & Von Houweligen (1986)	48 patients were divided into 3 groups: splint treatment, EMG biofeedback, or no-treatment control. Biofeedback consisted of 10 sessions. Splint treatment and control group patients participated in the first and last biofeedback sessions in order to obtain EMG activity levels from the masseter and anterior temporalis muscles.	Only the biofeedback group evidenced significant improvement in dysfunction and a significant improvement in amount of pain experienced and degree of mouth opening.
EMG biofeedback of frontales and masseter muscle activity	Dalen, Ellertsten, Espelid, & Granningsaeter (1986)	MPD patients were assigned to either a biofeedback group (eight sessions) or a no-biofeedback control group.	At 3- and 6-month follow-ups, biofeedback group patients displayed significantly reduced frontales EMG levels, while the control group did not. Both groups improved in terms of self-reported pain intensity and duration, but the degree of improvement was significantly more pronounced relative to the control group.
EMG biofeedback	Dalen, Ellertsen, Espelid, & Granningsaeter (1986)	TMD patients were assigned to either a biofeedback treatment group or a waiting-list control.	Results demonstrated the treatment success of biofeedback, with somewhat sustained improvement at a 6-month follow-up.

TABLE 21.2. *Continued*

Type of treatment	Investigators	Methodology	Findings
Bite splint and physiotherapy, EMG biofeedback and relaxation training, transcutaneous nerve stimulation	Crockett, Foreman, Alden, & Blasberg (1986)	21 TMD patients were assigned to one of the three treatment groups.	All three treatment groups displayed some success, with no one treatment consistently superior to the others.
Cognitive awareness of dysfunctional orofacial behavior and EMG biofeedback training for masticatory muscle relaxation	Burdette & Gale (1988)	41 MPD patients were tested and treated. 23 asymptomatic subjects were also tested as controls.	Pretreatment EMG levels of both the masseteric and anterior temporal areas were significantly higher in the pain-patient group relative to the control group. Masseter EMG activity decreased significantly in the pain-treatment group. Interocclusal distance significantly increased in the pain-treatment group.
EMG biofeedback of masseter muscle activity, combined EMG biofeedback of masseter muscle activity and occlusal splint therapy	Erlandson & Popper (1989)	TMD patients were administered either biofeedback treatment alone or a combined biofeedback–occlusal splint therapy.	Masseter EMG biofeedback alone did not result in increased mandibular range of motion or decrease in self-reported pain. However, when patients were provided an occlusal splint and given biofeedback, there were significant decreases in self-report of pain, reductions in masseter activity, and increases in mandibular range of motion.
Stretch-based relaxation of masseter muscle activity	Carlsson, Okeson, Falace, Nitz, & Anderson (1991)	34 orofacial pain patients with elevated masseter activity were randomly assigned to one of two groups: postural relaxation/rest group or a stretch-based relaxation group. During and following administration of a psychosocial stressor and then the relaxation procedure, masseter-muscle EMG activity was recorded.	Patients in the stretch-based relaxation group displayed greater reductions in the left and right masseter regions relative to the postural relaxation group.
EMG biofeedback, CBT and conservative medical treatment	Flor & Birbaumer (1993)	Biofeedback and CBT consisted of eight sessions.	At posttreatment, all three groups showed improvement, with the biofeedback group displaying the greatest change. Only the biofeedback group maintained significant decreases in pain severity, interference caused by pain, affective distress, and the number of pain-related doctor visits at a 6- and 24-month follow-up.

(continued)

TABLE 21.2. *Continued*

Type of treatment	Investigators	Methodology	Findings
Biofeedback and stress management (B-SM); intraoral appliance (IA); combined B-SM and IA	Turk, Zaki, & Rudy (1993)	Study 1: 70 TMD patients assigned to IA, B-SM, or waiting-list control. Study 2: 30 TMD patients assigned to combined IA and B-SM treatment or single treatments alone.	Study 1: Immediately after treatment, IA was more effective than B-SM in reducing pain. However, at 6 months, IA significantly relapsed, whereas the B-SM group maintained its improvements in both pain and depression. Study 2: Combined treatment was more effective than either the single treatments alone at a 6-month follow-up.
Combined CBT and conservative dental treatment; conservative dental treatment alone	Dworkin et al. (1994)	CBT given in a group format of two to seven patients, and consisted of two sessions that were 2 hours each.	No difference found between the two groups at a 3-month follow-up, although the combined group displayed continued improvement in pain and interference during the 3–12-month follow-up interval while the usual conservative care group did not.
Meta-analysis of treatments incorporating EMG biofeedback for TMD	Crider & Glaros (1999)	Literature search identified 13 studies of EMG biofeedback treatments for TMD.	Analyses revealed substantially greater outcomes of biofeedback treatments relative to control conditions. Follow-up evaluations also revealed no deterioration of these positive outcomes over time.
Frontales EMG/ temperature biofeedback, CBST, combined biofeedback and CBST	Mishra, Gatchel, & Gardea (2000)	94 TMD patients (diagnosed according to the RDC/TMD) were randomly assigned to one of the three treatment groups or a no-treatment control group. Each treatment consisted of 12 separate sessions.	All three treatment groups displayed significantly decreased pain scores from pretreatment to posttreatment, while the no-treatment control group did not. Biofeedback group patients were the most significantly improved compared to the no-treatment control group. Moreover, patients in the three treatment groups displayed significant improvement in most states.
Frontales EMG/ temperature biofeedback, CBST, combined biofeedback and CBST	Gardea, Gatchel, & Mishra (2001)	A 1-year follow-up of the Mishra, Gatchel, & Gardea (2000) study.	All three treatment groups displayed significant improvement in subjective pain and pain-related disability relative to the no-treatment control group. Moreover, the combined biofeedback and CBST groups displayed the most subjective pain improvement relative to the no-treatment control group.

TABLE 21.2. *Continued*

Type of treatment	Investigators	Methodology	Findings
Combined education and medication (flurbiprofen), combined education and physical therapy exercises, combined education and masseter muscle biofeedback training	Greco, Rudy, Henteleff, Herlich, & Pullano (in press)	171 TMD patients (diagnosed according to the RDC/TMD) were randomly assigned to four sessions of one of the three combined treatment groups. Change over the 4 weeks of treatment was analyzed.	All three treatment groups demonstrated significant reductions in weekly ratings of pain severity, muscle palpation pain, pain-related interference with activities, affective distress, and perceived jaw function. However, the combined education–medication group displayed the most rapid improvement in muscle palpation pain relative to the other groups. Moreover, this group also showed more rapid changes in self-reports of pain severity and jaw function relative to the biofeedback group.

Note. CBST, cognitive-behavioral skills training; CBT, cognitive-behavioral therapy; EMG, electromyogram; IA, intraoral appliance; MPD, myofacial pain disorder; RDC/TMD, research diagnostic criteria for temporomandibular disorders; SM, stress management; TMD, temporomandibular disorders; TMJ, temporomandibular joint.

tivity levels, and less pain-related interference in their lives, relative to the other two subgroups. Interpersonally distressed profile patients typically report that their significant others are not supportive of them. Finally, dysfunctional profile patients characteristically display greater severity of pain, higher levels of affective distress, lower activity levels, and greater pain-related interference in their lives. This particular subgroup is hypothesized not to respond as well to intervention as would patients in the other two subgroups. Such individual differences are in keeping with the conclusion made by Turk and Okifuji (1998) that one must avoid the assumption of pain-patient homogeneity in terms of response to treatment. There are many individual differences or heterogeneity in such responses.

A study by Asmundson, Norton, and Alterdings (1997) reported that patients with chronic low back pain who were classified as dysfunctional on the MPI reported more pain-specific fear and avoidance than did patients in the other subgroups. Such characteristics were, in turn, related to poorer coping ability in these dysfunctional chronic pain patients. Turk and Okifuji (1998) reviewed research demonstrating the utility of the MPI in predicting treatment response with other specific chronic pain conditions.

Similar individual differences were found with TMD patients (Epker & Gatchel, 2000). Finally, Turk, and colleagues (1993) also reported differential MPI profile treatment response differences in TMD patients. In this study, a treatment program specifically tailored to the needs of dysfunctional group patients was employed. These patients were compared to a group of dysfunctional patients who did not receive such tailored treatment. It was found that the former group improved significantly more than the latter group.

These aforementioned findings indicate that it is worthwhile to take into account such individual differences in order to develop the most time- and cost-effective methods for successfully treating TMD patients. Indeed, with the advent of the biobehavioral treatment methods incorporating the biopsychosocial perspective of pain, we now have the ability to tailor our treatments in order to comprehensively deal with both physical and psychosocial concomitants of chronic pain conditions such as TMD.

Acknowledgments

The writing of this chapter was supported in part by grants from the National Institutes of Health:

2K02-MH01107, 2R01-DE010713, and 2R01-MH46452.

References

Asmundson, G. J. G., Norton, G. R., & Alterdings, M. D. (1997). Fear and avoidance in dysfunctional chronic back pain patients. *Pain, 69,* 231–236.

Beck, A. T., Rush, A. J., Shaw, B. F., & Emery, G. (1979). *Cognitive therapy of depression.* New York: Guilford Press.

Brooke, R. T., Stenn, P. G., & Mothersill, K. J. (1977). The diagnosis and conservative treatment of myofascial pain dysfunction syndrome. *Oral Surgery, 44,* 844–852.

Budzynski, T., & Stoyva, J. (1973). Eletromyographic feedback technique for teaching voluntary relaxation on the masseter muscle. *Journal of Dental Research, 52,* 116–119.

Burdette, B. H., & Gale, E. N. (1988). The effects of treatment of masticatory muscle activity and mandibular posture in myofascial pain-dysfunction patients. *Journal of Dental Research, 67,* 1126–1130.

Carlsson, S. G., & Gale, E. N. (1977). Biofeedback in the treatment of long-term temporomandibular joint pain. *Biofeedback and Self-Regulation, 2,* 161–171.

Carlsson, D. J., Okeson, J. P., Falace, D. A., Nitz, A. J., & Anderson, D. (1991). Stretch-based relaxation and the reduction of EMG activity among masticatory muscle pain patients. *Journal of Craniomandibular Disorders: Facial and Oral Pain, 5,* 205–212.

Crider, A. B., & Glaros, A. G. (1999). A meta-analysis of EMG biofeedback treatment of temporomandibular disorders. *Journal of Orofacial Pain, 13,* 29–37.

Crockett, D. J., Foreman, M. E., Alden, L., & Blasberg, B. (1986). A comparison of treatment modes in the management of mysofascial pain dysfunction syndrome. *Biofeedback and Self-Regulation, 112,* 279–291.

Dahlstrom, L., & Carlsson, S. G. (1984). Treatment of mandibular dysfunction: The clinical usefulness of biofeedback in relation to splint therapy. *Journal of Oral Rehabilitation, 11,* 277–284.

Dahlstrom, L., Carlsson, G. E., & Carlsson, S. G. (1982). Comparison of effects of electromyographic biofeedback and occlusal splint therapy on mandibular dysfunction. *Scandinavian Journal of Dental Research, 90,* 151–156.

Dahlstrom, L., Carlsson, S. G., Gale, E. N., & Jansson, T. G. (1985). Stress-induced muscular activity in mandibular dysfunction: Effects of biofeedback training. *Journal of Behavioral Medicine, 8,* 191–200.

Dalen, K., Ellerstein, B., Espelid, I., & Granningsaeter, A. G. (1986). EMG feedback in treatment of myofascial pain dysfunction syndrome. *Acta Odentologia Scandinavia, 44,* 279–284.

Dobson, J. D., & Block, L. (1988). Historical philosophical bases of the cognitive-behavior therapies. In K. S. Dobson (Ed.), *Handbook of cognitive-behavior therapies* (pp. 3–38). New York: Guilford Press.

Dobson, K. S. (1989). A meta-analysis of the efficacy of cognitive therapy for depression. *Journal of Consulting and Clinical Psychology, 57,* 414–419.

Dohrmann, R. J., & Laskin, D. M. (1978). An evaluation of electromyographic biofeedback in the treatment of myofascial pain dysfunction syndrome. *Journal of the American Dental Association, 96,* 656–662.

Duckro, P. N., Tait, R. C., Margolis, R. B., & Deshields, T. L. (1990). Prevalence of temporomandibular symptoms in a large United States metropolitan area. *Journal of Craniomandibular Practice, 8,* 131–138.

Dworkin, S. F., & LeResche, L. (1992). Research diagnostic criteria for temporomandibular disorders. *Journal of Craniomandibular Disorders: Facial and Oral Pain, 6,* 301–355.

Dworkin, S. F., Turner, J. A., Wilson, L., Massoth, D., Whitney, C., Huggins, K. H., Burgess, J., Sommers, E., & Truelove, E. (1994). Brief group cognitive-behavioral treatment intervention for temporomandibular disorders. *Pain, 59,* 175–187.

Epker, J., & Gatchel, R. J. (2000). Coping profile differences in the biopsychosocial functioning of TMD patients. *Psychosomatic Medicine, 62,* 69–75.

Erlandson, P. J., & Popper, R. (1989). Electromyographic biofeedback and rest position training of masticatory muscles in myofascial pain-dysfunction patients. *Journal of Prosthetic Dentistry, 62,* 335–338.

Flor, H., & Birbaumer, N. (1993). Comparison of the efficacy of electromyographic biofeedback, cognitive-behavioral therapy, and conservative medical interventions in the treatment of chronic musculoskeletal pain. *Journal of Consulting and Clinical Psychology, 61,* 653–658.

Fricton, J. R., & Schiffman, E. L. (1995). Epidemiology of temporomandibular disorders. In J. R. Fricton & R. Dubner (Eds.), *Orofacial pain and temporomandibular disorders* (pp. 102–131). New York: Raven Press.

Funch, D. P., & Gale, E. N. (1984). Biofeedback and relaxation therapy for chronic temporomandibular joint pain: Predicting successful outcomes. *Journal of Consulting and Clinical Psychology, 52,* 928–935.

Gale, E. N. (1979). Biofeedback treatment for TMJ pain. In B. D. Ingersoll & W. R. McCutchean (Eds.), *Clinical research in behavioral dentistry* (pp. 83–94). Morgantown: West Virginia University Foundation.

Gardea, M. A., Gatchel, R. J., & Mishra, K. D. (2001). Long-term efficacy of biobehavioral treatment of temporomandibular disorders. *Journal of Behavioral Medicine, 24,* 341–360.

Gatchel, R. J. (1979). Biofeedback and the modification of fear and anxiety. In R. J. Gatchel & K.

P. Price (Eds.), *Clinical applications of biofeedback: Appraisal and status* (pp. 148–172). Elmsford, NY: Pergamon Press.

Gatchel, R. J. (1982). EMG biofeedback in anxiety reduction. In L. White & B. Tursky (Eds.), *Clinical biofeedback: Efficacy and mechanisms* (pp. 372–396). New York: Guilford Press.

Gatchel, R. J. (1988). Clinical effectiveness of biofeedback in reducing anxiety. In H. L. Wagner (Ed.), *Social psychophysiology and emotion* (pp. 197–210). Chicester, UK: Wiley.

Gatchel, R. J., & Epker, J. T. (1999). Psychosocial predictors of chronic pain and response to treatment. In R. J. Gatchel & D. C. Turk (Eds.), *Psychosocial factors in pain: Critical perspectives* (pp. 412–434). New York: Guilford Press.

Gessel, A. H. (1975). Electromyographic biofeedback and tricyclic antidepressants in myofascial pain-dysfunction: Psychological predictors of outcome. *Journal of the American Dental Association, 91,* 1048–1052.

Glaros, A. G., & Glass, E. G. (1993). Temporomandibular disorders. In R. J. Gatchel & E. B. Blanchard (Eds.), *Psychophysiological disorders* (pp. 299–356). Washington, DC: American Psychological Association.

Goldstein, B. H. (1999). Temporomandibular disorders: A review of current understanding. *Oral Surgery, Oral Medicine, Oral Pathology, 88,* 379–385.

Greco, C. M., Rudy, T. E., Henteleff, H. B., Herlich, A., & Pullano, J. (in press). Rapidity of effects during cooperative TMD treatments: A comparison of flurbiprofen, physical therapy exercises, and biofeedback. *Clinical Journal of Pain.*

Greene, C. S. (1990). Temporomandibular joint disorders. In J. F. Harding (Ed.), *Clark's clinical dentistry* (Vol. 2, pp. 151–176). Philadelphia: Lippincott.

Greene, C. S. (1992). Managing TMD patients: Initial therapy is the key. *Journal of the American Dental Association, 123,* 43–45.

Hijzen, T. H., Slangen, J. L., & Van Houweligen, H. C. (1986). Subjective, clinical and EMG effects of biofeedback and splint treatment. *Journal of Oral Rehabilitation, 13,* 529–539.

Hodges, J. M. (1990). Managing temporomandibular joint syndrome. *Laryngoscope, 100,* 60–66.

Jarrett, R. B. (1990). Psychosocial aspects of depression and the role of psychotherapy. *Journal of Clinical Psychiatry, 51,* 26–35.

Kerns, R., Turk, D., & Rudy, T. (1985). The West Haven–Yale Multidimensional Pain Inventory (WHYMPI). *Pain, 23,* 345–356.

Kight, M., Gatchel, R. J., & Wesley, L. (1999). Temporomandibular disorders: An example of the interface between psychological and physical diagnoses. *Health Psychology, 18,* 177–182.

Kinney, R. K., Gatchel, R. J., Ellis, E., & Holt, C. (1992). Major psychological disorders in chronic TMD patients: Management implications. *Journal of the American Dental Association, 123,* 49–54.

Klonoff, E. A., & Janata, J. W. (1986). The use of bilateral EMG equalization training in the treatment of temporomandibular joint dysfunction: A case report. *Journal of Oral Rehabilitation, 13,* 273–277.

Lewinsohn, P. M., Antonuccio, D. O., Steinmetz, J. L., & Teri, L. (1984). *The coping with depression course.* Eugene, OR: Castalia.

Lupton, D. E. (1969). Psychological aspects of temporomandibular joint dysfunction. *Journal of the American Dental Association, 79,* 131–136.

Mayer, T. G., & Gatchel, R. J. (1988). *Functional restoration for spinal disorders: The sports medicine approach.* Philadelphia: Lea & Febiger.

Mealiea, W. L., & McGlynn, F. D. (1987). Treatment status of biofeedback of TMD. In J. P. Hatch, J. Fischer, & J. D. Rugh (Eds.), *Biofeedback: Studies in clinical efficacy* (pp. 201–230). New York: Plenum Press.

Mishra, K. D., Gatchel, R. J., & Gardea, M. A. (2000). The relative efficacy of three cognitive-behavioral treatment approaches to temporomandibular disorders. *Journal of Behavioral Medicine, 23,* 293–309.

Moss, R. A., & Garrett, J. C. (1984). Temporomandibular joint dysfunction syndrome and myofascial pain dysfunction syndrome: A critical review. *Journal of Oral Rehabilitation, 11,* 3–28.

Moss, R. A., Wedding, D., & Sanders, S. H. (1983). The comparative efficacy of relaxation training and masseter EMG feedback in the treatment of TMJ dysfunction. *Journal of Oral Rehabilitation, 10,* 9–17.

Moulton, R. E. (1955). Psychiatric considerations in maxillofacial pain. *Journal of the American Dental Association, 51,* 408–416.

Moulton, R. E. (1966). Emotional factors in nonorganic temporomandibular joint pain. *Dental Clinics of North America, 10,* 609–617.

Okeson, J. P., Moody, P. M., Kemper, J. T., & Haley, J. V. (1983). Evaluation of occlusional splint therapy and relaxation procedures in patients with temporomandibular disorders. *Journal of the American Dental Association, 107,* 420–424.

Olson, R. E. (1977). Biofeedback for MPD patients non-responsive to drug and biteplate therapy. *Journal of Dental Research, 56*(B), 61.

Pomp, A. M. (1974). Psychotherapy for the myofascial pain-dysfunction syndrome: A study of factors coinciding with symptom remission. *Journal of the American Dental Association, 89,* 629–632.

Rugh, J. D. (1983). Psychological factors in the etiology of masticatory pain and dysfunction. In D. Laskin, W. Greenfield, E. Gale, J. Rugh, P. Neff, C. Alling, & W. Ayer (Eds.), *The President's Conference on the Examination, Diagnosis, and Management of Temporomandibular Disorders* (pp. 85–94). Chicago: American Dental Association.

Rugh, J. D., & Solberg, W. K. (1976). Psychological implications in temporomandibular pain and dysfunction. *Oral Sciences Review, 7,* 3–29.

Scott, D. S., & Gregg, J. M. (1980). Myofascial pain of the temporomandibular joint: A review of the behavioral-relaxation therapies. *Pain, 9,* 231–241.

Speculand, B., Goss, A. N., Hughes, A., Spence, N. D., & Pilowsky, I. (1983). Temporomandibular joint dysfunction: Pain and illness behavior. *Pain, 17,* 139–150.

Stam, H. J., McGrath, P. A., & Brooke, R. I. (1984). The effects of a cognitive-behavioral treatment program on temporomandibular pain and dysfunction syndrome. *Psychosomatic Medicine, 46,* 534–545.

Stenn, P. G., Mothersill, K. J., & Brooke, R. I. (1979). Biofeedback and a cognitive behavioral approach to treatment of myofascial pain dysfunction syndrome. *Behavior Therapy, 10,* 29–36.

Suvinen, T. I., & Reade, P. C. (1995). Temporomandibular disorders: A critical review of the nature of pain and its assessment. *Journal of Orofacial Pain, 9,* 317–339.

Turk, D. C. (1996). Biopsychosocial perspective on chronic pain. In R. J. Gatchel & D. C. Turk (Eds). *Psychological approaches to pain management: A practitioner's handbook* (pp. 3–32). New York: Guilford Press, 1996.

Turk, D. C., & Okifuji, A. (1998). Directions in prescriptive chronic pain management based on diagnostic characteristics of the patient. *APS Bulletin, 8,* 5–11.

Turk, D. C., & Rudy, T. (1988). Toward an empirically derived taxonomy of chronic pain patients: Integration of psychological assessment data. *Journal of Consulting and Clinical Psychology, 56,* 233–238.

Turk, D. C., Zaki, H. S., & Rudy, T. E. (1993). Effects of intraoral appliances and biofeedback/stress management alone and in combination in treating pain and depression in patients with temporomandibular disorders. *Journal of Prosthetic Dentistry, 70,* 158–164.

Von Korff, M., Dworkin, S. F., LeResche, L., & Kruger, A. (1988). An epidemiologic comparison of pain complaints. *Pain, 32,* 173–183.

22

Treating the Patient with Pelvic Pain

Mark L. Elliott

Chronic pelvic pain (CPP) is a common and debilitating problem for women. In the general population, 14.7% of women report CPP (Mathias, Kupperman, Liberman, Lipschutz, & Steege, 1996), whereas 39% in both gynecological and family practice clinic setting suffer with CPP (Jamieson & Steege, 1996). The typical woman with CPP is married, in her early 30s, and experiences a pain intensity ranging from 5.0 to 7.0 on a scale from 0–10 (Elliott, 1996a; Mathias, et al., 1996). Reiter, Shakerin, Gambone, and Milburn (1991) estimated that at least 10% of gynecological visits involve a report of pelvic pain (and note that CPP is a frequent cause for hysterectomies).

Women with CPP are often found to have a constellation of psychological problems that cross many diagnostic categories including depression, anxiety, fear, and hostility (see, e.g., Fry, Crisp, Beard, & McGuigan, 1993; Harrop-Griffiths et al., 1988; Slocumb, Kellner, Rosenfeld, & Pathak, 1989), personality disorders (e.g., Gross, Doerr, Caldirola, Guzinski, & Ripley, 1980–1981; Walker, Katon, Neraas, Jemelka, & Massoth, 1992), somatization disorders (e.g., Ehlert, Heim, & Hellhammer, 1999), posttraumatic stress disorder

(e.g., Heim, Ehlert, Hanker, & Hellhammer, 1999), and drug abuse (Walker et al., 1995).

Sexual abuse (e.g., Elliott, 1996a; Rapkins, Kames, Darke, Stampler, & Naliboff, 1990) and physical abuse (e.g., Schei, 1991; Toomey, Hernandez, Gittelman, & Hulka, 1993) are common and consequential factors in the histories of women with CPP. CPP patients frequently experience associated psychosexual dysfunctions (Elliott, 1996a; Harrop-Grifiths et al., 1988; VanLankveld, Weijenborg, & Kuile, 1996).

There is insufficient space to illuminate the significant and mutually exacerbating interaction of CPP with psychological sequelae, neurochemical changes, muscles and nerves, and the experience of pain (for greater detail and discussion of these topics, see Grace, 1998; McDonald & Elliott, 2001; and Wesselman, 2001).

Patients with CPP also present with a spectrum of pelvic pain symptoms and pathology (McDonald & Elliott, 2001) that include some of the following:

- Endometriosis
- Dysmenorrhea
- Dyspareunia (e.g., vaginismus)

- Pelvic neuropathies (pudendal, ilio-inguinal, ilio-hypogastric, genital femoral, etc.)
- Myofascial pain and trigger points (e.g., abdominal)
- Hymeneal syndrome, vulvar vestibulitis, and vulvitis
- Parasympathetically and sympathetically maintained pelvic pain
- Interstitial cystitis
- Pelvic pain without observable pathology or of unknown etiology.

It is interesting to note that CPP patients in the general population do not typically seek medical or psychological intervention. A study of U.K. women with CPP for at least 3 months found that only 25% sought medical care (Zondervan & Barlow, 2000). Mathias and colleagues (1996) found that in the United States, 19% women suffering with CPP sought help from a gynecologist and only 1% sought help from a mental health professional.

In this chapter, I focus primarily on the evaluation and treatment issues unique to working with CPP patients. I elucidate how problems common to CPP can be addressed with various psychological evaluation and intervention techniques. More extensive information regarding treating chronic pain patients in general and with specific disorders can be found in other chapters in this volume. I describe an interdisciplinary approach for the efficacious management of CPP, thereby reducing suffering and increasing quality of life for women experiencing this devastating problem.

Overview

The diagnosis and treatment of CPP in women is complicated by a plethora of etiological considerations confounded by numerous diagnostic enigmas that cross medical and psychological specialties. Professionals with broad specialty training in the treatment of CPP are scarce. Therefore, the average CPP patient is transferred between and within medical specialties. For women with CPP, multiple health care visits, multiple diagnostic tests, multiple drug trials, and multiple treatment regimens (including multiple surgeries) are common and

cause escalating stress and psychosocial symptoms that can have a devastating effect on her occupational, social, and personal pursuits.

Assessment

The Psychologist's Role

The psychologist is an integral member of an interdisciplinary team evaluating and treating CPP (see, e.g., Rapkin & Kames, 1987; Wood, Wiesner, & Reiter, 1990). Rosenthal, Ling, Rosenthal, and Stovall (1991) state that "in treating CPP patients the emphasis has to be on rehabilitation, both physical and emotional, rather than solely searching for 'the cause' or 'the cure'" (p. 38).

Sometimes the role of the psychologist is primarily as a consultant who augments treatment planning for medical and pharmacological interventions. For instance, a psychologist can be helpful when the medical team is considering a more invasive medical procedure (e.g., spinal cord stimulation). The consult might include illumination of potential psychological contraindications as well as suggestions regarding options to increase long-term medical efficacy (see Doleys, Chapter 16, this volume). A more substantial role includes evaluation and then treatment for some of the following problems:

- Decreased medical efficacy due to (1) traumatic history, (2) poor coping skills, and (3) depression
- Treatment compliance and limit setting
- Excessive pain behavior and/or secondary gains
- Over- or undercompensation regarding activity

A psychologist who is considering whether to work with CPP patients must understand the differences between this population and other chronic pain populations (e.g., chronic back pain and daily headaches). Psychologists working with CPP patients must develop a good background in abdominal/pelvic anatomy and physiology in addition to an understanding of sexual problems and their treatment (see McDonald & Elliott, 2001).

Review of Clinical Information

The psychological evaluation of patients with CPP begins with a review of medical and psychological records. The medical history is important to understanding the presenting psychophysiological status of CPP patients. Many have experienced multiple office visits, diagnostic tests, and procedures that result in significant emotional distress that can directly affect their presenting pelvic pain symptomatology.

Initial clinic questionnaires are also important for the collection of psychological information and for helping the patient feel that they are not alone with their problem. The breadth and depth of questions can normalize some of their psychosocial concerns. In our clinic, patients with CPP complete two questionnaires. The first is a general pain clinic questionnaire that examines the etiology, characteristics, intervention attempts, and psychosocial impact of their pain. The second questionnaire investigates sexual history (including abuse) and the impact of CPP on current sexual function. A copy can be found in McDonald and Elliott (2001).

Initial Consultation

The psychological consult is implemented after reviewing available records and internal questionnaires. The CPP patient's fear that she is seeing the "shrink" because her pain is "all in her head" must be addressed and reassured immediately. Most CPP patients are relieved to hear that I think their pain is *real* and to hear an explanation how psychophysiology affects their pain condition. This association is presented as a reason for the psychological evaluation and possible interventions.

I then review the development and characteristics of their pelvic pain. It is important to understand what activities or situations make the pelvic pain worse and under what conditions the pain is better. I also review previous intervention attempts (e.g., surgical, pharmacological, and psychological) and the patient's psychological experience with these attempts.

During the consult, I explore the following areas: pelvic pain characteristics, personality and psychosocial factors; relationship and sexual problems; and stressors.

Current coping skills and resources are also assessed. Normalization of the psychosocial sequelae associated with CPP is important during this first meeting. Special awareness is directed to verbal or physical evidence of somatic preoccupation in addition to a history of physical or sexual abuse. CPP patients may need time to develop a therapeutic alliance before she can give more extensive details about her abuse.

CPP patients are acutely aware if the clinician exhibits any discomfort or hesitance regarding abuse or sexuality questions. They have a propensity to interpret the discomfort in negative, unsupportive, if not punishing, ways. It is important for clinicians to remember that if they psychologically *open a patient up* by having her talk about the abuse, it is obligatory that they have future meetings to manage the patient's emotional reactions and vulnerability. A one-shot evaluation is not the time to discuss childhood abuse in detail.

Couple Consultation

I usually exclude the partner from the initial consult. However, if the partner is adamant about attending the consult, he or she is allowed to participate for the first few minutes to address concerns and questions. An overprotective, unsupportive, or dominating partner has this behavior pointed out in a sympathetic but firm way. I attempt to address the partner's questions and reassure their often legitimate fears. They are offered an opportunity to come back with their partner at a later date.

The subsequent couple consult is often a mixture of data collection and education. Many partners do not understand the characteristics or the interventions associated with CPP. Sexual issues are usually of paramount concern. These questions provide an opportunity to illuminate the effect of persistent sexual pressure on the psychophysiology of CPP. With some hope regarding possible successful interventions, many partners become more supportive and less petulant.

Psychological Evaluation

The psychological evaluation of a patient with CPP is critical for the development of an effective medical and psychological treatment plan. Each clinical setting has different needs, resources, and psychological expertise in working with CPP patients. Clinicians new to the treatment of CPP may consider a comprehensive evaluation process until more familiarity is achieved.

The increase in health maintenance organizations and capitated health care has tragically decreased reimbursement and directly effected payment for psychological evaluation and treatment. Therefore, the cost of testing is an important consideration. Only a few insurance companies (workers' compensation insurance in some states) pay for psychological testing. Forcing an extensive evaluation may create an unfair (and additional) financial burden for the CPP patient.

It is also important to consider the amount of time it takes to administer and interpret each of the different tests or combinations of tests. Some CPP patients have difficulty sitting for hours to complete a battery of tests. When working with a physician (as a solo practitioner or as a part of team) it is most helpful when the request for a psychological evaluation is implemented from the onset of treatment, if not the diagnostic process, and not when all other options are depleted.

CPP patients often need a psychological evaluation with psychometric testing when any of the following are observed:

- Using opioids for *nonmalignant* pain
- Long-term use of opioids
- History of pharmacological noncompliance or abuse
- History of medical noncompliance
- Considering an invasive procedure
- History of physical or sexual abuse or trauma
- Pain disability greatly disproportionate to pathology
- Strong affect during medical or psychological workup
- Apparent poor coping skills
- Prior psychiatric hospitalization or suicide attempt

Psychometric Instruments

The list of possible psychometric tests is vast and is not presented here. (For a good general resource for the assessment of chronic pain, see Turk & Melzack, 2001; more specifically for CPP, see Elliott, 1996b; Steege, Stout, & Somkuti, 1993; Wesselman, 2001).

Over the years, I have administered a Minnesota Multiphasic Personality Inventory (MMPI) to almost every CPP patient in our clinic but use other psychological testing sparingly. The MMPI is the most common tool used in the evaluation of pain patients (Keller & Butcher, 1991; Piotrowski, 1997) and more recently has been described for CPP patients (Wood et al., 1990). I have found the MMPI to be an excellent tool for illuminating the psychological symptoms (not diagnostic categories) that are critical to medical and psychological treatment planning for CPP patients.

Caution is warranted when interpreting the profiles of CPP patients. CPP patients often have significant elevations on scales 1 (Hypochondriasis) and 3 (Hysteria) and less elevation on scale 2 (Depression) (see, e.g., Keller & Butcher, 1991). This configuration has been described as the "conversion 'V'" and sometimes overinterpreted in reports as evidence of a "conversion reaction." I recommend against using this specific interpretation or diagnosis without substantial collaborating medical evidence. In my experience with many CPP patients, this configuration is rarely (if ever) consistent with a conversion pain disorder but instead represents a hypersensitivity to somatic/pain sensations compounded by a disconnection from adaptive expression of affect. I have found the fairy tale *The Princess and the Pea* a useful way to describe this MMPI configuration. Many of our patients agree that they would "feel the pea" under all the mattresses. This helps them put into perspective their somatic preoccupation.

Patient Diaries and Logs

Patient diaries and logs are integral to the evaluation and treatment process. I use three different types that include (1) hourly activity log, (2) daily sleep log, and (3) daily feeling/stress and pain graph.

The hourly activity log has the CPP patient monitor her activities on a frequent and regular basis. These would include work and domestic activities, recreational activities, and even rest. A sleep log provides nightly information about approximate-falling-asleep times, number of nightly sleep disruptions, and time of awakening in the morning. The log also gives information about the causes of sleep disturbance (e.g., rumination and too much coffee). I also implement the use of a feeling/stress and pain graph. I ask patients to record the level of their pain and 2–3 different emotions on a 0–5 scale once or twice per day. The consult and psychometric testing (when available) provide the emotions to be recorded. They might include anxiety, fear, rumination, anger, depression, loneliness, or irritability.

Triage and Referral

The psychologist must proceed with caution when giving feedback to physicians regarding the psychological evaluation. A *psychogenic* diagnosis (or misinterpretation) can damage the patient's access to consistent, helpful, or efficacious medical intervention (McGowan, Pitts, & Clark, 1999). I have also found that some physicians are quite reluctant to treat (or continue to treat) a woman with a psychogenic pelvic pain diagnosis. In fact, a psychogenic diagnosis is a convenient excuse to discontinue treatment when dealing with the enigmatic (often frustrating) characteristics of working with CPP patients.

The psychologist may need to educate referring physicians on the import of a supportive, educative referral process. The physician must be sensitive to the patient's likely perception of being dumped or seen as having pain caused (only) by psychopathology. I often provide referring physicians (internal or external) with the didactic on the psychophysiology of emotions and the effect on pain, which often helps them more efficaciously bridge to psychological evaluation and treatment.

Treatment Approaches

The most effective treatment modality for CPP involves an integrated interdisciplinary or multidisciplinary approach. As early as 1977, Beard, Belsey, Lieberman, and Wilkinson recognized the importance of an interdisciplinary approach for successful treatment of CPP. They found that many

(11/18) CPP patients with a negative laparoscopy showed marked improvement or were pain free with a combination of reassurance or therapy. Later, Beard, Reginald, and Pearce (1988) reported that women receiving *stress analysis* or *pain analysis* therapies were significantly improved at the end of treatment compared to a minimal intervention control group.

Kames, Rapkin, Naliboff, Afifi, and Ferrer-Brechner (1990) found that a comprehensive 6–8-week program for CPP patients resulted in 67% reporting pain improvement at the end of treatment and 65% at 6-month follow-up. Social and sexual activity were reported improved by 44% and 27%, respectively, at the end of treatment and 65% and 79%, respectively, at the 6-month follow-up. At the 6-month follow-up, 92% reported that they were improved and that they were satisfied or highly satisfied with the treatment program.

Peters and colleagues (1991) used an integrated treatment group (including medical, psychological, dietary, environmental, and physiotherapy interventions) that resulted in significant improvement in pain experience, daily activity, and associated symptoms compared to a *standard* approach. A similar treatment approach not only helped to reduce pain symptoms in 75% of 200 CPP subjects but also decreased the percentage of hysterectomies from 15–20% to 6% (Gambone & Reiter, 1990).

One interesting study examined the psychological factors associated with patients who refuse participation in a multidisciplinary program (Wexler, 1995). No significant psychological differences were found between the participating patients and the controls. However, the patients who refused participation were found to have consistently higher levels of overall psychological pathology, including higher levels of hypochondriasis, hysteria, and dissociation.

Wood and colleagues (1990) advocate the use of a 10-session method for the treatment of CPP. Their program involves a systematic use of cognitive-behavioral therapy, sex therapy, and relaxation training and self-hypnosis techniques. I have found that an "integrated hierarchical psychological approach" (Elliot, 1996b) is most effective for my CPP patients. Based on the issues illuminated in the consult, I start with the most basic interventions (i.e., Level 1) and move to "higher" levels only when the ongoing techniques are insufficient to reduce pain, reduce psychological distress, and increase function. For example, CPP patients who have a history of sexual abuse may do well with the first two levels but may ultimately need psychodynamic therapy to reduce preconscious defenses that preclude treatment efficacy.

- *Level 1:* Didactics and behavioral homework
- *Level 2:* Psychophysiological methods and/or cognitive-behavioral and/or group therapy
- *Level 3:* Couple therapy, sex therapy, drug rehabilitation programs, etc.
- *Level 4:* Psychodynamic therapy

Psychoeducation

Effective treatment of the CPP patients begins with information. Most of my CPP patients receive a didactic on the psychophysiology of stress and emotions and the impact on pain. The patient learns the names and the bodily effects of neurochemicals associated with stress, anxiety, depression, and the consequent effect on nerves and muscles. For instance, I use the image of a shark when describing the scavenging, catabolic effect of cortisol release due to stress. CPP patients often report that they could *visualize* the release of the neurochemicals when *upset* (observe sweating due to anxiety, feel muscle tension when irritated, etc.) and could therefore reduce the effect.

We also spend time with anatomical information (e.g., anatomy book) to illuminate the nerves, muscles, and reproductive organs associated with their pelvic pain condition (McDonald & Elliott, 2001; Rogers, 1998). We discuss the development of pelvic trigger points by illustrating how muscles increasingly contract into a *crushing shield* around nerves when the nerve says "ouch" (e.g., cut and crushed). The increasing *shield* causes hypoxia and further pain. Understanding this *vicious circle* process helps my patients visualize and then manage affective states, muscle tension, and ultimately their

pain levels. I have found that CPP patients are more motivated and amenable to treatment when they understand the theory and concepts behind medical and psychological intervention.

Remember, the average CPP patient has become quite *well-informed* about his or her condition (similar to fibromyalgia patients) and may ask many questions. It is important that clinicians *do their homework* and develops a good working understanding of the pelvis and proven medical interventions. (For good references for background on the pelvic anatomy and pelvic pain, see McDonald & Elliott, 2001; Rogers, 1998). It is important to respond to the intensity and scope of questions with an open mind and not personalize this (sometimes) frustrating process. Many CPP patients are desperate. They are willing to try almost any *concoction* or treatment they read about. It is important to realistically evaluate their *finds* and sympathize with their desperate anxiety.

Homework

Homework is the cornerstone of an effective treatment program for patients with CPP and cognitive-behavioral treatment in general (see Turk, Chapter 7, this volume). Homework has the exceptional quality of being both diagnostic and therapeutic. Diagnostically, homework brings to the surface treatment *snags* that include areas of limited coping or significant psychological issues. Illuminated snags warrant additional practice and reinforcement or possibly a higher level of intervention (e.g., psychotherapy) if the problem continues unchanged. Homework is also therapeutic by providing and encouraging more adaptive skills to enhance efficacy in daily living and coping with pain.

Behavioral

As noted previously, there are numerous books and articles written on the topic of behavioral therapy for pain (e.g., Fordyce, 2001; see Sanders, Chapter 6, this volume, for more detailed information on behavioral techniques with chronic pain patients). There are no known behavioral articles specifically addressing CPP.

Activity Log

The "daily activity diary" can help facilitate a structured, adaptive behavioral plan to increase realistic activities of daily living (ADLs) as medical treatment unfolds. I have found two subsets of CPP patients regarding activity level. The first group feels guilty that they cannot pursue employment and/or domestic duties. Domestically, they try to *catch up* whenever they have reduced pain. They typically overcompensate and do too much. Consequently, pain is heightened causing a dramatic reduction in function and getting "behind" for the next 1 to 3 days. A behavioral treatment plan to break the repetitive cycle involves helping the patient understand the merit of smaller but consistent reinforcers. For example, she is shown that cleaning one room per day over 4 days with limited pain is more efficacious than cleaning all the rooms in 1 day and spending the next 3 days in bed due to severe pain. Repeated encouragement may be necessary because of the ego investment that many women (and society) place on accomplishing domestic duties. Maximum hourly levels are established in each therapy session.

The second group of CPP patients has difficulty initiating ADLs. Limited or absent activity usually results from spurious, superstitious correlations between activity and pain. CPP patients start tasks, have pain (probably from disuse or ignorance), and then do not press on to increased muscle tone and ultimately less pain. For example, women with CPP underestimate the extent to which abdominal and pelvic muscles are used in even the most basic ADLs (e.g., standing while washing dishes and vacuuming). Education with anatomy books can be helpful. The CPP patient must be informed that the correlation between emotions, activity, and pain may not always be contiguous. It may take up to 24 hours to manifest changes in tension or pain (increased and decreased). These patients need a behavioral approach that gives specific (minimum) goals for daily activity dependent on the degree of pain and physical limitations.

Behavioral Reinforcers

Even words can be positive or negative reinforcers when working with CPP patients.

For example, when working with vaginismus patients, it is important to eliminate the word "pain" from their descriptive vocabulary. In my experience, the word "pain" causes negative expectations and exacerbates the reflexive spasm of the introital musculature. I have the patient convert "pain" to other focal sensory descriptors such as "stretching," "pulling," or "burning." These words may have strong vocabulary value but usually have less emotional loading and therefore do not cause the same degree of muscle tension or spasm.

When working with the CPP patient, the clinician must be cautious in using sexual activity as a reinforcer or as encouragement for behavioral intervention. Many CPP patients are at best ambivalent regarding the resumption of sexuality—even if the pelvic pain or dyspareunia can be resolved. Conflicts and resentments in couples managing CPP frequently can spill to the bedroom. Some patients feel like an *object*, or as one patient reported, a *receptacle*. In her relationship, sex was frequently pursued with little consideration of her pain. Because she had no "evidence" of pathology, her husband would treat her unavailability as an *excuse*. The woman with CPP may need, at minimum, more effective communication and closeness with the partner before resuming sexual activity, even after her pain is reduced or resolved. Thus connecting pain reduction with resumption of sexual activity may alter the woman's motivation and compliance with treatment.

Behavioral therapy can also help family members develop reinforcement patterns that decrease pain or secondary gain behaviors, which might include family members providing a supportive understanding environment to help an interstitial cystitis patient plan, problem-solve, and then execute brief, but increasing, social visits from friends as well as designing and accompanying her on trips to locations with easily accessible restrooms along the way.

Psychophysiological Interventions

The use of progressive relaxation training (PRT), guided imagery, self-hypnosis, breathing exercises, and biofeedback is well-known for the treatment of patients with pain (see Arena & Blanchard, Chapter

8, and Syrjala & Abrams, Chapter 9, this volume). There is limited literature regarding the specific use of these techniques with CPP patients.

Patients with chronic pain dwell on signs and symptoms of their condition. This is especially true for CPP patient who also have a preoccupation with somatic *cues* about their pelvis and abdomen. Psychophysiological techniques can be effective in helping CPP patients recondition and relabel aspects of their somatic focus. For instance, pain from bending over to pick up a toy from the floor (bending pain) can be redirected to "tense abdominal muscles/fascia that need relaxing." Practicing a relaxation tool can decrease impotence (e.g., feeling like a victim) and increase self-efficacy (e.g., controlling muscle tension in specific body parts). Furthermore, all these techniques can *force* the CPP patient to take time during her day and rest. This is important because many CPP patients do not give themselves permission for *downtime* as it is not productive.

I use combinations of each psychophysiological technique with the exception of hypnosis. Patients are given a handout of scripts for PRT, guided imagery, and breathing exercises and a prerecorded audiotape of a staff member reading different scripts. The purpose and outcome of these techniques are quite similar. The choice of one relaxation, distraction technique over another is primarily individualistic (patient and clinician).

The use of psychophysiological techniques concomitant with trigger point injections can be especially helpful for CPP patients with abdominal or pelvic muscle tension. The use of PRT before and after medical intervention can mutually enhance the relaxation of muscles and the return of oxygen to the compressed, hypoxic nerve.

I know of only one study showing the efficacy of biofeedback with CPP patients. Glazer, Rodke, Swenscionis, Hertz, and Young (1995) used portable EMG biofeedback with women suffering with painful intercourse due to vulvar vestibulitis. After 16 weeks of pelvic floor retraining, 83% reported a reduction of pain and 79% were able to resume intercourse.

When implemented by a well-trained professional, hypnosis can help with the management of pelvic pain (see Barber, 2001).

Weisberg (2000) presents an excellent (and quite typical) clinical example of a woman experiencing CPP. A multifactorial treatment approach that included hypnosis, cognitive-behavioral therapy, and family systems therapy was reported to be helpful in decreasing this patient's pelvic and psychological symptoms (see Kerns, Otis, & Wise, Chapter 12, this volume). Weisberg (2000) hypothesizes that hypnosis can enhance stabilization of the autonomic and endocrine dysregulation caused by stress and historical trauma (see also Elliott, 1996a; Heim, Ehlert, Hanker, & Hellhammer, 1998). He believes that some patients with CPP have organic symptoms that are "maintained or exacerbated by unresolved developmental conflicts and current stressors in a state-dependent manner" (Weisberg, 2000. p. 124). The treatment by hypnosis can help CPP patients "view physical symptoms as useful sources of state-encoded information rather than through an anxiety-base, 'organic versus psychogenic' lens" (Weisberg, 2000, p. 126).

Patients with a history of sexual or physical trauma may have paradoxical reactions when using relaxation techniques. A rare, but good, example is a patient who presented with multiple body location complaints including pelvic pain. Her pain location drawing was almost completely covered in various colors—each indicating a different level and frequency of pain. Because of numerous trigger points, the treatment team recommended that she receive biofeedback and a relaxation tape to be used at home. During biofeedback provided in the clinic, she reported an overwhelming influx of emotions and demonstrated characteristics of dissociation. She described intrusive, traumatic memories as her body began to relax and muscle tension decreased. She had a history of multiple traumatic childhood events, including sexual abuse. (The patient had been afraid to tell us of her history for fear that we would not believe her pain reports.) She reported being *uptight* all her life with considerable difficult *sitting still* long enough to even read a book. She had not worked on her childhood abuse because she was afraid that a professional would punitively disbelieve her reports, similar to her own mother. This patient was referred for psychotherapy to decrease the psychological sequelae and somatic manifestations of her abuse in a supportive environment.

Cognitive-Behavioral Techniques

Resources for developing cognitive-behavioral techniques with pain patients are numerous (see Turk, Chapter 7, this volume) The purpose of cognitive-behavioral with CPP patients is to accomplish at least some of the following:

- Increase awareness of feelings and stress
- Increase awareness of nonadaptive beliefs
- Increase awareness of nonadaptive behavioral patterns
- Increase coping
- Enhance self-efficacy and decrease the victim role
- Provide an environment for creative problem solving

The way patients think about their pelvic pain can dramatically affect their experience of the pain and the efficacy of treatment. Chapman and Turner (2001) provide a good background on how pain can impair the cognitive process. I agree with Pincus, Pearce, and McCelland (1995) who state that "pain biases memory, and it may cause the patient to preferentially recall negative ideas and feelings." Research suggests that these negative, pessimistic beliefs (common to CPP patients) are nonadaptive and exacerbate the experience of pain (Gil, Williams, Keefe, & Beckman, 1990). Furthermore, when pessimism coalesces with rumination, *catastrophizing* results and further increases muscle tension and exacerbates *destructive* neurochemical release. Sadly, "pain becomes the theme around which the patient organizes thinking and action" (Mandler, 1979, cited in Chapman & Turner, 2001).

The way patients think and believe about their pain may also directly affect the outcome of treatment. Bandura, O'Leary, Taylor, Gauthier, and Gossard (1987) found that enhancing cognitive strategies for self-efficacy increased pain tolerance. The interesting part of this study is that the increased pain tolerance was secondary to neurochemical changes, not just increased efficacy, because the pain tolerance effect could be blocked with naloxone.

Homework

The first cognitive-behavioral homework increases the CPP patient's awareness of how she *predicts* and *prejudices* current situations with what has happened to them in the past (recent and earlier). The patient then challenges these (nonadaptive) predictions and prejudices by asking, "What *data* do I have *in the present* to draw these conclusions or assumptions?" Data only include an overt verbal expression from their partner or people in the world around them. Finally, the CPP patient inserts the word "might" into her sentence. For example, the patient would change the sentence "I *always* have increased pain when I clean house" to "I *might* hurt after I clean house." The use of the word "might" can result in decreased defensive behaviors due to preemptive anxiety and premature stress and therefore decreased muscle tension and pain. *Might* has a tendency to decrease nihilism and increase self-considered and efficacious possibilities.

Another homework series prescribes skills for the management of feelings and stress. I use a four-step approach that includes (1) acknowledgment of the feeling(s), (2) acceptance of the feeling(s)—independent of what it is, (3) verbalization of the feeling(s) to self and others (when appropriate), and (4) a conscious *choice* regarding what to do about the feeling(s). This process helps the patient feel less *victimized* by her feelings and develop a greater sense of self-efficacy. This creates psychological and physiological changes that can positively affect the experience of pain.

Parenthetically, CPP patients, most of whom are women, may have additional difficulty with this homework. Society often teaches (rewards) women for being self-sacrificing, especially related to their family. CPP patients often confuse self-efficacy with being selfish. I use the phrase "*consider* myself" as a daily mantra. With practice it helps patients develop a nice balance between self-care and caring for their families.

Cognitive-behavioral therapy can also help CPP patients increase awareness of dysfunctional and maladaptive pain behavior constellations, which then leads to pattern-specific problem solving. The patient then practices or rehearses the *antidote* plan(s). For example, a CPP patient with endometriosis was able to connect the visit of her (intrusive) mother-in-law with a significant increase in her abdominal and deep vaginal pain. She became aware of the increasing tension in her abdomen and consequent pain as the visit approached. Escalation of pain was common as the visit progressed. We were able to dissect both her belief system and previous lack of coping-skill options. We developed a series of *if–then* options. If the mother-in-law did X, then she could counter with Y. She created *signals* to be used with her husband that indicated different parts of the plan. For instance, if she rubbed her nose, she and her husband were to convene in the kitchen and discuss how to manage her increasing frustration and stress. Wiggling her ear meant "time to go to the grocery store to get milk." The patient was able to rehearse and role-play during therapy and at home with her husband. The increased sense of self-efficacy due to the plan and the increased intimacy in the marriage due to a *team approach* was able to ward off the usual negative, pain-escalating effects of the mother-in-law's visit.

Psychodynamic Therapy

The use of psychodynamic techniques for the treatment of pain disorders has been controversial at best (see, e.g., Tunks & Merskey, 2001; see also Basler, Grzesiak, & Dworkin, Chapter 5, this volume). However, with the continued awareness of childhood trauma/neglect in the history of pelvic pain patients, a more insight-oriented approach may become necessary for a subset of CPP patients.

Psychodynamic therapy is based on the premise that abuse or trauma causes "a unique template of expectations, autonomic nervous system responses, and behaviors" (Schofferman, Anderson, Hines, Smith, & White, 1992). This template then becomes *activated* throughout life when either physical (e.g., pain) or emotional stress (e.g., divorce), or both, is experienced. Behaviors adaptive to the child coping with trauma (e.g., dissociation) may be quite nonadaptive to the adult trying to function in the world or cope with CPP.

Insight-oriented intervention can help CPP patients make important connections between their pain condition, limited treatment efficacy, and (understandable) defenses or maladaptive behaviors created as *survival techniques* in the past. Therapy helps patients see how past traumas can still be affecting their current pain experience. Initially, patients are (need to be) skeptical about connections with the past; however, time, support, and continued connections help the patient explain confusing, *illogical* pain treatment *snags*. I have found that patients eventually become involved in the exploratory nature of the psychodynamic process and therefore make considerable gains in managing their pain.

When other psychological interventions have not worked, I begin to explore the possibility that the patient cannot afford to get better (give up her historical or preconscious defenses). For example, patients with sexual abuse may have strong trepidation regarding the resolution of their pelvic pain because of the fear that their husbands will try to *catch up for lost time* and treat them in an objectifying pressuring way similar to their abuse. Therefore, these CPP patients may have reflexive (preconscious) muscle contraction due to present and past anxiety and fears. Continued medical intervention is typically of little value until the defenses can be resolved.

A good example involves a patient who presented with lower left quadrant pain and severe dyspareunia. She had received numerous diagnostic, pharmacological, and surgical trials. Our pain team diagnosed her with ilio-hypogastric neuropathy of unknown etiology and myofascial trigger points exacerbated by a stressful job and poor coping skills. The patient was an active and motivated participant in our program, but she did not respond to medical treatments with any continuity. Attempts to decrease her overwhelming *work stress* with classic cognitive-behavioral techniques were mostly unsuccessful and seemingly sabotaged with episodic chaos. This led us to take a psychodynamic history that revealed a physically abusive, unpredictable alcoholic father, and a submissive mother who sacrificed the daughter to protect herself from the father's wrath.

During our second session, the patient began to cry and eventually added a description of repeated sexual abuse by her father. She had been afraid to tell us because a physician had told her that the pain was probably *all in her head* because of the abuse. The discussion revealed that most of the job stress was related to a new boss. She began to make connections that the boss looked like and acted like her father (e.g., unpredictable criticism and humiliating style). This revelation to the patient produced a number of strong emotional responses (sadness, anger, anxiety) over the next few sessions. The patient was able to mourn the heinous lack of sexual boundaries by her father and the abandonment by her mother. This historical connection and support from a *good parent* (the therapist) helped her observe and then manage the reflexive abdominal and pelvic *clenching* response every time her boss communicated with her. Luckily, the patient was able to change positions within her company. This change did not relinquish her pain condition, but, rather, it allowed our treatments to be more effective and, over a more typical course, reduce her pain.

Psychodynamic therapy may also help the efficacy of medical treatment when the patient has a history of trauma (Schofferman, Anderson, Hines, Smith, & White, 1992). These authors studied the impact of childhood trauma factors on surgical outcome for postlumbar surgery patients. These factors included (1) physical abuse, (2) sexual abuse, (3) alcohol/drug use in primary caregiver, (4) abandonment, and (5) "emotional neglect." When patients reported three to five of these factors, there was only a 27% chance of a successful surgical outcome but a 95% chance of success if none of these factors were endorsed. The authors reported that psychotherapy focused on abuse/neglect issues (e.g., limited capacity for interpersonal attachment and consoling) resulted in patients moving from surgical "failures" to surgical "successes." The authors posit that therapy helped the patients reduce preconscious roadblocks and fears of developing *healthy, secure attachments* allowing them to more effectively participate in treatment as well as life in general.

Group Therapy

Group therapy has proven to be a cost-effective modality for pain patients (Tunks & Merskey, 1990; see Keefe, Beaupre, Gil,

Rumble, & Aspnes, Chapter 11, this volume for more detailed desciption of using group therapy for chronic pain patients). Groups available to CPP patients are often peer led or facilitated by a professional. CPP patients can benefit from the understanding and discussion of other patients suffering from the same problems and treatment experiences. It is important to note, however, that clinicians should be prepared and available to address the collective questions and frustration, sometimes hostility, developed during a CPP peer group meeting.

Albert (1999) demonstrated the efficacy of group treatment for CPP patients. Each group consisted of up to six women with CPP and two physiotherapists. The focus of the groups were *development of self-knowledge* followed by *assuming self-responsibility for one's own life* and *performing self-activeness*. Participants were encouraged to enhance feelings of self-control and *personal mastery of their emotions*. At 1-year follow-up, 39% of the women who completed the program were pain free. Visual analog scale (VAS) scores on average decreased from 2.8 to 0.9 ($p < 0.01$) and analgesics usage reduced from 2.8 "units" per week to 0.9 units ($p < 0.01$).

I tend to mix CPP patients into a heterogeneous chronic pain group. We provided a 10-week group for up to eight patients led by two master's-level therapists. The group consisted of didactics (see earlier), exercise, and open discussion. At the end of the structured 10-week program, patients were given the option to join an ongoing open-ended group led by the same two therapists. The focus of the second group was more on interpersonal interaction, support, and skills with only a modicum of didactics.

National organizations are a good community resource to find peer-led groups for women with CPP. Most notable are the Endometriosis Society and the Vulvar Vestibulitis Society.

Couple Therapy

In my experience, marital distress can be a common and disturbing consequence of CPP. In patients with chronic pain, 56% were shown to have scores on the Locke–Wallace Marital Adjustment Test that were in the *impaired* range (Locke & Wallace,

1959, cited in Basford, 1998). The relationship problems (e.g., animosity, abandonment, hurt feelings, and limited communication) that develop during CPP often require a structured set of skills that facilitate relationship reacquaintance. I use the skills described in the cognitive-behavioral section to help couples manage accumulated negative feelings and to increase communication efficacy. Partners of CPP patients often need information from a professional who explains the physical, psychological, and sexual aspects of CPP. This meeting can sometimes reduce the perpetual distrust, anger, and distance caused by the absence of a specific diagnosis and the prior ineffectiveness of numerous intervention attempts.

Sex Therapy

Sexual problems have been shown to be quite common for women with CPP (Elliott, 1996a). For example, Peters and colleagues (1991) found that 71% of their patients experienced dyspareunia, 42% anorgasmia, and 27% postcoital pain. Harrop-Grifiths and colleagues (1988) compared the sexual dysfunction frequency of women with CPP and infertility controls. They found that 52% had dyspareunia (vs. 6.7% of controls), 28% reported inhibited sexual desire (vs. 6.7%), 16% reported inhibited orgasm (vs. 3.3%), and 28% reported inhibited sexual excitement (vs. 16.7%).

Sexual problems can be devastating to the self-esteem and relationship satisfaction of women with CPP. Fortunately, many of the sexual problems experienced by women with CPP can be successfully treated with sex therapy techniques provided by a trained clinician (Elliott, 1996b). In fact, the treatment of vaginismus, see later, has a 100% success rate when the woman is willing to complete the program. Conversely, organic dyspareunia (e.g., labia burns secondary to radiation therapy for cancer and deep dyspareunia secondary to endometriosis) can be recalcitrant to therapeutic resolution. Nevertheless, even these problem can be greatly helped by sex therapy when creative problem solving incorporates the realistic physical limitations and expands the couple's sexual repertoire (Anderson & Elliott, 1993). The CPP patient and her partner need to be given hope and a good refer-

ral if the pain psychologist is not adequately trained to treat sexual dysfunctions.

Most psychogenic sexual dysfunctions and disorders have been attributed to an increase in performance anxiety and *spectatoring* among healthy individuals (Masters & Johnson, 1970). These maladaptive cognitions (e.g., "Is this going to hurt again?" "Is my partner going to get mad or disappointed?" and "Am I ever going to have an orgasm again?") are quite disruptive to the psychological and neurochemical aspects of sexual function. Sexual problems are compounded by the CPP patients' acute awareness of cues and responses that *indicate* pain associated with sexual activity. Furthermore, the concomitant sensitivity to her partner's reaction/response (e.g., frustration and disappointment) is common but mutually exacerbates expectations and increases performance fears. The cumulative result is a significant increase in distractions from sexually enhancing bodily sensations and decreased physiological capacity to respond. Performance vigilance escalates, creating a vicious circle that results in diminished libido and limited sexual interaction with her partner.

Women with CPP often feel a *duty* to provide their partners with sexual interaction independent of their own sexual interest or painful consequence. It is common for women with CPP to be present in *body only*. During sexual activity done out of duty, thoughts are often nonsexual (e.g., making a shopping list, sorting the laundry, and reviewing a work project) or countersexual (e.g., negative aspects of the partner, monitoring body changes, and encouraging a quick completion). Therefore, women with CPP may pass time with distracting thoughts until the partner can *get it over with*. This culture makes some CPP patients terrified that their partner will leave them if they do not perform sexually and keep him happy. Many feel that their only choices are pain or being alone.

The treatment process must encourage an exploration of what is available versus what is missing or unavailable. The realistic limitations of her CPP provide direction for creative problem solving and treatment options. Women with CPP (and their partner) may need to redefine their views of sexuality. This may include greater exploration of unaffected body parts. For example, many couples (especially men) use intercourse as a primary source of expressing love in the relationship. The clinician, through sex therapy, can help the couple expand their sensual/sexual repertoire while broadening their resources for expressing love (e.g., communication skills). This is helpful for women who have intractable dyspareunia.

Masters and Johnson (1970) described sensate focus as a strategy to decrease performance anxiety and spectatoring. Sensate focus is most effective when prescribed as *touching for one's own interest* to decrease performance expectations and anxiety. The patient and partner are encouraged to focus on the sensations of temperature, texture, and pressure (TTP) and refocus from distractions (e.g., "Is he getting upset?" "Did I pack the kids lunch?"). Concerns of doing it *right* or for the other person are discouraged. Increased ability to focus on sensations is the goal, not pleasuring the partner (self), let alone trying to create arousal. Finally, valuable diagnostic information is gleaned from the couple's reactions and difficulties in completing the sensate focus assignments. When necessary, these snags can be used to develop specialized homework before proceeding to the next level of sensate focus.

Lack of sexual desire is a common secondary problem of women with CPP. Libido problems are rarely hormonal except in the case of pharmacological castration (e.g., gonadotropin-releasing hormone agonist). Problems with sexual desire almost always result from a fear of pain and distress or conflict in the relationship. The increasing frustration, distance, and petulance of the partner are not aphrodisiacs for the women with CPP. In fact, decreased libido may be a necessary protective limit and should be addressed in an open and supportive way. It is critical to educate partners on how pressure and even supportive attempts to get her *in the mood* (e.g., flowers and sex toys) are not helpful or effective. These attempts often cause her to become even more sexually withdrawn, which perpetuates the cycle. Sex therapy techniques can be helpful in creating a more conducive environment for a woman to develop, experience, and then act on her sexual feelings.

Fatigue, a common symptom of patients in pain, may need special problem-solving attention. Pelvic pain is physically draining even though the woman (and her partner) complain that she did "nothing all day" to warrant being "too exhausted" for sex. Therefore, time-management suggestions may be helpful (e.g., taking a nap before a sexual encounter and dividing more evenly the various household tasks). The touching homework assignments can be redesigned to involve limited physical effort but still provide an opportunity for sensual and sexual expression for the couple.

Sex therapy homework provides couples (or individual women) with a structured, boundary-inclusive process. The homework rebuilds the sexual relationship from scratch. For instance, breast and genitals are always *off limits* in the beginning and then we slowly (over weeks) progress back to intercourse. Therefore, neither partner has to interpret the intention or lack of intention of the other because the homework defines the maximum *on limit* behaviors. This process can greatly reduce the trepidation associated with a return to sexual expression common to women with CPP. It also decreases the pressure felt by both partners to quickly return to pre-CPP patterns of sexual interaction. The pace of assignments is determined by the woman's progress and comfort. This offers the women with CPP a sense of empowerment and safety concerning her body and sexuality that may have diminished since the onset of her pain.

Vaginismus, a common secondary problem for women with CPP, which is defined as the involuntary, reflexive spasm of the pubococcygeous muscle resulting from real or perceived threats of penetration, deserves a special treatment note (e.g., Elliott, 1996b). Treatment of vaginismus typically requires the use of progressive dilators. I use a box of four Young's adult dilators starting with the smallest. The patient is first taught to redefine her description from *pain* to other words (e.g., "stretching," "pinching," "stinging," and "burning"). She is also instructed to do Kegel exercises that involve contracting the pubococcygeous muscle and holding for 1 second and then releasing. The patient is asked to do 8–10 repetitions of this exercise two to three times per day. The first dilator is inserted with the help of an artificial lubricant twice per day for 15 minutes then once per day for 30 minutes. Over the next days to weeks, she progresses from 30 minutes to 1 hour to 2 hours, and finally she sleeps overnight with the dilator. After the second overnight insertion, she moves on to the second dilator. Each subsequent dilator follows exactly the same pattern. When the final dilator is started, a decision is made whether to include the partner to increase comfort with the transition from the dilator to the penis. Specific exercises are given regarding the female inserting the penis in the female astride position.

Concluding Comment

I have tried to encourage an interdisciplinary approach by illuminating the vast array of psychological, sexual, and medical symptoms experienced by patients with CPP. I hope that this chapter generates more interest in pelvic pain and increases the limited number of clinicians willing to get experience and then work with this important and challenging subset of chronic pain patients

References

Albert, H. (1999). Psychosomatic group treatment helps women with chronic pelvic pain. *Journal of Psychosomatic Obstetrics and Gynaecology, 20,* 216–225.

Andersen, B. L., & Elliott, M. L. (1993). Sexuality for women with cancer: Assessment, theory and treatment. *Journal of Sex and Disability, 11,* 7–37.

Bandura, A., O'Leary, A., Taylor, C. B., Gauthier, J., & Gossard, D. (1987). Perceived self-efficacy and pain control: Opioid and nonopioid mechanisms. *Journal of Personality and Social Psychology, 53,* 563–571

Barber, J. (2001). Hypnosis. In J. D. Loeser, S. D. Butler, C. R. Chapman, & D. C. Turk (Eds.), *Bonica's management of pain* (3rd ed., pp. 1768–1778). Baltimore: Williams & Wilkins.

Bashford, R. A. (1998). Psychiatric illness. In J. F. Steege, D. A. Metzger, & B. S. Levy (Eds.), *Chronic pelvic pain: An integrated approach* (pp. 267–282. Philadelphia: Saunders.

Beard, R. W., Belsey, E. M., Lieberman, M. B., & Wilkinson, J. C. M. (1977). Pelvic pain in women. *American Journal of Obstetrics and Gynecology, 128,* 566–570.

Beard, R. W., Reginald, P., & Pearce, S. (1988). Psychological and somatic factors in women with pain due to pelvic congestion. *Advances in Experimental Medicine and Biology, 245,* 413–421.

Chapman, C. R., & Turner, J. A. (2001). Psychological aspects of pain. In J. D. Loeser, S. D. Butler, C. R. Chapman, & D. C. Turk (Eds.), *Bonica's management of pain* (3rd ed., pp. 180–190). Baltimore: Williams & Wilkins.

Ehlret, U., Heim, D., & Hellhammer, D. H. (1998). Chronic pelvic pain as a somatoform disorder. *Psychotherapy and Psychosomatics, 68,* 87–94.

Elliott, M. L. (1996a). Chronic pelvic pain: What are the psychological considerations? *American Pain Society Bulletin, 6,* 1–4.

Elliott, M. L. (1996b). Chronic pelvic pain: Intervention strategies for psychological factors. *American Pain Society Bulletin, 6,* 10–16.

Fordyce, W. E. (2001). Operant or contingency therapies. In J. D. Loeser, S. D. Butler, C. R. Chapman, & D. C. Turk (Eds.), *Bonica's management of pain* (3rd ed., pp. 1745–1750). Baltimore: Williams & Wilkins.

Fry, R. P., Crisp, A. H., Beard, R. W., & McGuigan, S. (1993). Psychosocial aspects of chronic pelvic pain, with special reference to sexual abuse: A study of 164 women. *Postgraduate Medical Journal, 69,* 566–574.

Gambone, J. C., & Reiter, R. C. (1990). Nonsurgical management of chronic pelvic pain: A multidisciplinary approach. *Clinical Obstetrics and Gynecology, 33,* 205–211.

Gil, K. M., Williams, D. A., Keefe F. J., & Beckman J. L. (1990). The relationship of negative thoughts to pain and psychological distress. *Behavior Therapy, 21,* 349–362.

Glazer, H. I., Rodke, G., Swenscionis, C., Hertz, R., & Young, A. W. (1995). Treatment of vulvar vestibulitis syndrome with electromyographic biofeedback of pelvic floor musculature. *Journal of Reproductive Medicine, 40,* 283–290.

Grace, V. M. (1998). Mind/body dualism in medicine: The case of chronic pelvic pain without organic pathology. A critical review of the literature. *International Journal of Health Services, 28,* 127–151.

Gross, R. J., Doerr, H., Caldirola, D., Guzinski, G. M., & Ripley, H. S. (1980–1981). Borderline syndrome and incest in chronic pelvic pain patients. *International Journal of Psychiatric Medicine, 10,* 79–96.

Harrop-Griffiths, J., Katon, W., Walker, E., Holm, L., Russo, J., & Hickok, L. (1988). Association between CPP and psychiatric diagnosis and child sexual abuse. *Obstetrics and Gynecology, 71,* 589–594.

Heim, C., Ehlert, U., Hanker, J. P., & Hellhammer, D. H. (1999). Abuse-related posttraumatic stress disorder and alterations of the hypothalamic–pituitary–adrenal axis in women with chronic pelvic pain. *Psychosomatic Medicine, 60,* 309–318.

Jamieson, D. J., & Steege, J. F. (1996). The prevalence of dysmenorrhea, dyspareunia, pelvic pain, and irritable bowel syndrome in primary care practices. *Obstetrics and Gynecology, 87,* 55–58.

Kames, L. D., Rapkin, A. J., Naliboff, B. D., Afifi, S., & Ferrer-Brechner, T. (1990). Effectiveness of an interdisciplinary pain management program for the treatment of chronic pelvic pain. *Pain, 41,* 41–46.

Keller, L. S., & Butcher, J. N. (1991). *Assessment of chronic pain patients with the MMPI-2.* Minneapolis: University of Minnesota Press.

Locke, M. J., & Wallace, K. M. (1959). Short marital adjustment and prediction tests: Their reliability and validity. *Marriage and Family Living, 21,* 251.

Mandler, G. (1979). Thought processes, consciousness and stress. In V. Hamilton & D. M. Warburton (Eds.) *Human stress and cognition* (pp. 179–201). New York: Wiley.

Masters, W. H., & Johnson, V. E. (1970). *Human sexual inadequacy.* New York: Little, Brown.

Mathias, S. D., Kupperman, M., Liberman, R. F., Lipschutz, R. C., & Steege J. F. (1996). Chronic pelvic pain: Prevalence, health-related quality of life, and economic correlates. *Obstetrics and Gynecology, 87,* 321–327.

McDonald, J. S., & Elliott, M. L. (2001). Gynecological Pain Syndromes. In J. D. Loeser, S. D. Butler, C. R. Chapman, & D. C. Turk (Eds.), *Bonica's management of pain* (3rd ed., pp. 1415–1447). Baltimore: Williams & Wilkins.

McGowan, L., Pitts, M., & Clark, C. D. (1999). Chronic pelvic pain: The general practitioner's perspective. *Psychology, Health and Medicine, 4,* 303–317.

Peters, A. A. W., van Dorst, E., Jellis, B., van Zuuren, E., Hermans, J., & Trimbos, J. B. (1991). A randomized clinical trial to compare two different approaches in women with CPP. *Obstetrics and Gynecology, 7,* 740–744.

Pincus, T., Pearce, S., & McCelland, A. (1995). Endorsement and memory bias of self-referential pain stimuli in depressed patient. *British Journal of Clinical Psychology, 34,* 255–265.

Piotrowski, C. (1997). Assessment of pain: A survey of practicing clinicians. *Perceptual and Motor Skills, 86,* 181–182.

Rapkin, A. J., & Kames, L. D. (1987). The pain management approach to chronic pelvic pain. *Journal of Reproductive Medicine, 32,* 323–327.

Rapkin, A. J., Kames, L. D., Darke, L. L., Stampler, F. M., & Naliboff, B. D. (1990). History of physical and sexual abuse in women with chronic pelvic pain. *Obstetrics and Gynecology, 76,* 92–96.

Reiter, R. C., Shakerin, L. R., Gambone, J. C., & Milburn, A. K. (1991). Correlation between sexual abuse and somatization in women with somatic and nonsomatic chronic pelvic pain. *American Journal of Obstetrics and Gynecology, 165,* 104–109.

Rogers, R. M. (1998). Basic pelvic neuroanatomy. In J. F. Steege, D. A. Metzger, & B. S. Levy (Eds.), *Chronic pelvic pain: An integrated approach* (pp. 31–58). Philadelphia: Saunders.

Rosenthal, R. H., Ling, F. W., Rosenthal, T. L., & Stovall, T. G. (1991). Assessing chronic pelvic pain: Clinical use of the Eysenck Personality Questionnaire. *Journal of Psychosomatic Obstetrics and Gynaecology, 12,* 31–38.

Schei, B. (1991). Sexual factors in pelvic pain: A study of women living in physically abusive relationships and of randomly selected controls. *Psychosomatic Obstetrics and Gynaecology, 12*(Suppl.), 99–108.

Schofferman, J., Anderson, A., Hines, R., Smith, G., & White, A. (1992). Childhood psychological trauma correlates with unsuccessful lumbar spine surgery. *Spine, 17*(Suppl.), S138–S144.

Slocumb, J. C., Kellner, R., Rosenfeld, R. C., & Pathak, D. (1989). Anxiety and depression in patients with the abdominal pelvic pain syndrome. *General Hospital Psychiatry, 11,* 48–53.

Steege, J. F., Stout, A. L., & Somkuti, S. G. (1993). Chronic pelvic pain in women. *Obstetric and Gynecological Survey, 48,* 95–110.

Toomey, T. C., Hernandez, J. T., Gittelman, D. F., & Hulka, J. F. (1993). Relationship of sexual and physical abuse to pain and psychological assessment variables in chronic pain pelvic patients. *Pain, 53,* 105–109.

Tunks, E. R., & Merskey, H. (2001). Psychotherapy in the management of chronic pain. In J. D. Loeser, S. D. Butler, C. R. Chapman, & D. C. Turk (Eds.), *Bonica's management of pain* (3rd ed., pp. 1789–1795). Baltimore: Williams & Wilkins.

Turk, D. C., & Melzack, R. (Eds.). (2001). *Handbook of pain assessment* (2nd ed.). New York: Guilford Press.

VanLankveld, J. J. D. M., Weijenborg, P. T. M., & Kuile, M. M. T. (1996). Psychological profiles of and sexual function in women with vulvar vestibulitis and their partners. *Obstetrics and Gynecology, 88,* 65–69.

Walker, E. A., Katon, W. J., Hansom, J., Harrop-Griffiths, J., Holm, L., Jones, M. L., Hickok, L. R., & Russo, J. (1995). Psychiatric diagnoses and sexual victimization in women with chronic pelvic pain. *Psychosomatics, 36,* 531–540.

Walker, E. A., Katon, W. J., Neraas, K., Jemelka, R. P., & Massoth, D. (1992). Dissociation in women with chronic pelvic pain. *American Journal of Psychiatry, 149,* 534–537.

Weisberg, M. B. (2000). Chronic pelvic pain and hypnosis. In L. M. Hornyak & J. P. Green (Eds.), *Healing from within: The use of hypnosis in women's health care* (pp. 119–138) Washington, DC: American Psychological Association.

Wesselman, U. (2001). Chronic pelvic pain. In D. C. Turk & R. Melzack (Eds.), *Handbook of pain assessment* (2nd ed., pp. 567–578). New York: Guilford Press.

Wexler, B. D. (1995). Psychological factors associated with psychogenic chronic pelvic pain and participation or non-participation in a multidisciplinary treatment program. *Dissertation Abstracts International, 56*(6-B), 3470.

Wood, D. P., Wiesner, M. G., & Reiter, R. C. (1990). Psychogenic chronic pelvic pain: Diagnosis and management. *Clinical Obstetrics & Gynecology, 33,* 179–194.

Zondervan, K., & Barlow, D. H. (2000). Epidemiology of chronic pelvic pain. *Baillieres Clinical Obstetrics and Gynecology, 14,* 403–414.

23

Treating Patients with Complex Regional Pain Syndrome

David V. Nelson

It is difficult to provide valid treatment guidelines, psychological or otherwise, for a disorder that has little epidemiological information, lacks understanding of its natural course or basic pathophysiology, and lacks agreement even on its definition and diagnostic criteria. Such is the case for complex regional pain syndrome (CRPS). Indeed, CRPS is recognized as one of the most puzzling and enigmatic of the chronically painful disorders (Janig, 1996; Nelson & Novy, 1996).

Optimal treatment requires the clinician to be as thoroughly grounded as possible in terms of a basic understanding of relevant conceptual and taxonomic issues; what little is known about the epidemiology, hypotheses, and controversies regarding pathophysiology; and special issues for adaptation of pain management strategies to assist the patient with CRPS (Stanton-Hicks et al., 1998). This chapter provides an overview of these matters to orient clinical practice for psychological treatment of CRPS.

Evolution of Basic Concepts and Taxonomy

Historical Overview

Mitchell and his colleagues (Mitchell, 1872; Mitchell, Moorehouse, & Keen, 1864) are generally credited with providing the first clear descriptions of wartime peripheral nerve injuries involving persistent burning pain, although Paget in 1862 (cited in Galer, Schwartz, & Allen, 2001) described patients with "distressing" pains in the fingers after nerve injury with associated "nutritional changes." Rather than label the disorder simply "burning pain," Mitchell adopted the term "causalgia" (Michell, 1867, cited in Galer et al., 2001) and observed in some cases other associated localized changes, such as appearance and temperature of skin. Reports of wartime injuries continued to provide much of the basis of accumulating observations of related phenomena in cases of major nerve injuries to limbs, along with reports of diffuse burning pain and associated localized changes seen in various other conditions or injuries but without specifically identifiable nerve injuries (Bonica, 1953; Galer et al., 2001; Schwartzman & McLellan, 1987). In addition to spontaneous pain and pain frequently manifested as allodynia (i.e., pain due to a stimulus which does not normally provoke pain) or hyperalgesia (i.e., increased response to a stimulus that is normally painful), other features were often manifested, including edema, skin color and temperature changes; excessive sweating or dryness in the region of pain; dystrophy or atrophy of skin, nails, and other soft tissues; motor function disturbances; extreme behavioral responses such as excessive guarding appearing absurd to others; severe psychological distress; and frank psychiatric disturbances (Bonica, 1990).

The term "reflex sympathetic dystrophy" (RSD) was first used in 1946 by Evans (1946) to apply to this diverse array of similar conditions reported under different names. Indeed, in reviewing the nomenclature, Rizzi, Vissentin, and Mazzetti (1984) reported the use of at least 21 different labels for such conditions (e.g., algoneurodystrophy, reflex neurovascular dystrophy, posttraumatic vasomotor disorders, shoulder–hand syndrome, and Sudeck's atrophy). Bonica (1953), in his classical first textbook on pain management, proposed including in one all-inclusive term, RSD, these various symptom clusters. In 1986, Roberts proposed the term "sympathetically maintained pain" (SMP) to be used synonymously with RSD, based on evidence that treatment via interruption of the sympathetic nervous system (SNS) (e.g., through regional sympathetic anesthesiological blockade) often improved or resulted in remission of symptoms. Bonica (1990) elevated to almost dogma the role of SNS involvement and blockade as the first line treatment of choice, thereby further reinforcing the central role of SNS dysfunction in reflex *sympathetic* dystrophy. However, Campbell, Meyer, and Raja (1992) coined the term "sympathetically independent pain" (SIP) for apparent cases of causalgia or RSD that did not respond to sympathetic blockade. Furthermore, it became increasingly clear that not all symptoms were characteristically seen, dystrophy was not universally present, and attempts to explain symptoms from a "reflex arc" in the spinal cord and/or SNS were flawed (Livingstone, 1943; Stanton-Hicks et al., 1995). Ultimately, it became necessary to abandon the unequivocal presumption of a central role of SNS dysfunction in this syndrome or dystrophy as an inevitable feature, which led to a search for a different consensus label for such disorders (Stanton-Hicks et al., 1995).

Diagnostic Criteria and Taxonomy

The current definition of CRPS found in *Classification of Chronic Pain* (Merskey & Bogduk, 1994) reflects the evolution of the controversies of the concepts of RSD, SMP, and SIP and attempts to provide a working basis for clinical and research efforts to proceed more productively. The approach taken focused on description without any presumption as to underlying mechanisms. The word "complex" was chosen to denote the varied clinical phenomena found in addition to pain. *Regional* distribution of symptoms and features is a hallmark. While usually affecting the distal part of a limb, symptoms may occur on the face or torso and may spread to other body areas. *Pain* remains the cardinal symptom of the *syndrome*, although there are rare cases in which other characteristic features occur in the absence of pain, raising the question as to whether such cases should be included in this group of disorders (Stanton-Hicks et al., 1995).

Two types of disorders are set forth under the rubric of CRPS (Merskey & Bogduk, 1994). The more common (Type I) is that which has typically been known as RSD. The second (Type II) refers to the classical description of causalgia. The possibility of a third "not otherwise specified" type for those patients who do not fit either Type I or II, as well as the possibility of subgroups within each type that reflect the heterogeneity of disorders potentially lumped within CRPS, remain open considerations (Stanton-Hicks et al., 1995).

Diagnostic criteria for Type I are a syndrome that typically develops after an initiating noxious event, or a cause of immobilization, and must include the following essential features: continuing pain or allodynia or hyperalgesia, with pain disproportionate to any inciting event; evidence at some time of edema, changes in skin blood flow (e.g., color or temperature changes), or abnormal sudomotor activity (e.g., excessive sweating or dryness) in the region of the pain; and diagnosis excluded by the existence of conditions that would otherwise account for the degree of pain and dysfunction (e.g., diabetic peripheral neuropathy, Raynaud's disease, and thrombosis). Type II requires the same essential features noted for Type I but is distinguished by the presence of a known nerve injury, traditionally injuries involving the large named nerves, such as the median or sciatic nerve. The pain of Type II is not necessarily limited to the distribution of the injured nerve (Merskey & Bogduk, 1994; Stanton-Hicks et al., 1995). Classic symptoms and signs such as burning pain and some dystrophic signs/symptoms previously thought to be cardinal features were discarded, and there is some support to justify this (Galer, Bruehl, & Harden, 1998).

The adoption by the International Association for the Study of Pain (IASP) of these criteria has been only another marker in the dynamic evolution of controversy over CRPS. Since their inception, the criteria have been subjected to criticism as being too vague, allowing for the overdiagnosis of the syndrome, and also discarding some key signs and symptoms that many considered to be important defining findings (Galer et al., 2001). The criteria were written, though, with the expectation that they would be subjected to scrutiny and validation studies for further refinement (Stanton-Hicks et al., 1995). Indeed, a subsequent multisite study (Harden et al., 1999) examining the internal validity and comprehensiveness of the IASP criteria via principal components analysis (PCA) of a standardized sign/symptom checklist suggested a somewhat different grouping of important features. As in the original IASP criteria, a separate pain/sensation criterion was supported. However, unlike those criteria, the PCA indicated that vasomotor symptoms form a factor distinct from a sudomotor/ edema factor. A fourth distinct factor also emerged that was not included in the original IASP criteria, namely, changes in range of motion, motor dysfunction, and trophic changes. These and other related findings suggested that the IASP criteria could be improved by separating vasomotor signs and symptoms (i.e., temperature and skin color changes or asymmetry) from those reflecting sudomotor dysfunction (i.e., sweating changes or asymmetry) and edema; and, further, that motor (i.e., decreased range of motion and weakness, tremor, and dystonia) and trophic (hair, nail, skin) changes may be an important and distinct component of CRPS not presently incorporated as such (Harden et al., 1999). An experimental revision of the CRPS diagnostic criteria was accordingly proposed (Harden et al., 1999), and it is expected that with further evaluation and validation scrutiny, the evolution-

ary process of defining and understanding CRPS will continue (Galer et al., 2001).

For the time being, a general conceptual framework of CRPS can guide some understanding of the overlap in symptomatology of various related and overlapping disorders, while helping to maintain some potentially important distinctions. Figure 23.1 illustrates the conceptual overlap of signs and symptoms of related disorders. As Stanton-Hicks and colleagues (1995) note, CRPS may be viewed as overlapping with SMP, defined as pain that is maintained by sympathetic efferent innervation or by circulating catecholamines (or clinically as a patient reports good pain relief after a sympatholytic procedure, e.g., sympathetic block; Galer et al., 2001). SMP may be a feature of several different painful conditions and is not necessarily an essential requirement of any one condition. Further, given the demonstration of SIP in CRPS perhaps in the majority of cases, SMP and CRPS are then obviously not synonymous. SMP implies a presumed mechanism but is not a diagnosis per se. Hence, SMP may be an important mechanism for some but not necessarily all patients with clinical diagnosis of CRPS. Further, manifestations of SMP occur in other diagnoses considered to be distinct from CRPS (e.g., herpes zoster, diabetic neuropathy, and phantom pain). Each of these other conditions may include patients who respond to sympathetic blockade and so may be considered to share the presumed mechanisms of SMP. However, even this assumption of abnormal activity in the autonomic nervous system (ANS) in SMP is only hypothetical at present (Stanton-Hicks et al., 1995). Indeed, while the relief experienced after sympathetic block may be due to the anesthetic effect on sympathetic fibers, alternative explanations are quite possible and findings are challenging to reconcile. Galer and colleagues (2001) have summarized some of these, for example, local anesthetic may be absorbed onto adjacent nonsympathetic nerve fibers or alter other regions of the nervous system besides the SNS, the time of onset and duration of pain relief do not correlate with the timing of sympathetic block, there is a lack of correlation between affected limbs' catecholamine concentration (presumably an index of SNS activity) and pain relief after

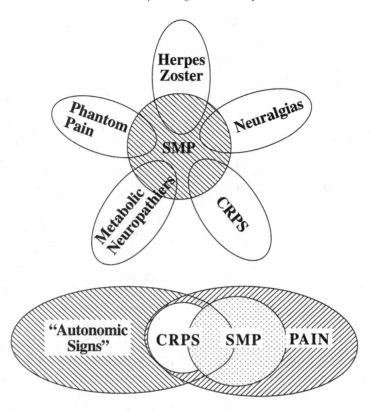

FIGURE 23.1. Relationship between SMP and selected painful conditions. This is meant to be a conceptual framework and the magnitude of the intersection between sets is not intended to represent a quantitative relationship. SMP may exist as an entity not associated with any other condition. The list of associated conditions is not meant to be exhaustive. From Stanton-Hicks et al. (1995). Copyright 1995, with permission from Elsevier Science.

sympathetic blockade, and so on. Hence, treatment guided by a strong reliance on a SNS dysfunction conceptualization may lead to erroneous and potentially unhelpful messages to patients as well as limit the range of therapeutic options considered.

Epidemiology and Natural Course

The few published reports on epidemiological information about CRPS (historically published about RSD, causalgia, or other terms in addition to CRPS) are typically quite small in numbers and suffer greatly from selection biases, such as often being based on restricted military or tertiary referral center clinic samples that may not accurately reflect the general population. Hence, the information that is available is incomplete.

The one prospective study that has been conducted was carried out before current IASP criteria were adopted. The study looked at 829 patients with RSD from a tertiary referral surgical clinic in the Netherlands (Veldman, Reynen, Arntz, & Goris, 1993). Information from this study was complemented by a retrospective chart review of 134 patients diagnosed with CRPS from a multidisciplinary pain center in the United States (Allen, Galer, & Schwartz, 1999). A few smaller-scale studies and those analyzing specific aspects of RSD, causalgia, CRPS, or similarly labeled conditions provide additional information (e.g., Pak, Martin, Magness, & Kavanaugh, 1970; Subbarao & Stillwell, 1981).

The incidence and prevalence of CRPS in the general population is unknown. In Sweden, population approximately 8.6 million, *International Classification of Diseases*

(ICD-9-CM; World Health Organization, 1978) codes for "causalgia" identified 27 cases in 1990, 40 cases in 1991, 38 cases in 1992, and 29 cases in 1993. The "RSD" code was reported in 67 cases in 1990, 44 in 1991, 40 in 1992, and 80 in 1993. The code for "pain in an extremity" was reported in 1,249 cases in 1990, 1,374 in 1991, 2,091 in 1992, and 2,458 in 1993. Given that these figures were obtained by searching for the main diagnoses of hospitalization records, it is probable that they represent only the most advanced cases. The primary implication is that CRPS is likely to be a constant, small, but significant medical condition (Stanton-Hicks et al., 1998).

Age

CRPS affects both adults and children. The Veldman and colleagues (1993) study in the Netherlands found an age range from 4 to 84 years, median age of 41 years, and mean duration of RSD of 405 days. The Allen and colleagues (1999) study in the United States examined patients ranging from 18 to 71 years with a mean age of 41.8, age at time of injury ranging from 14 to 64 (mean of 37.7) years, and mean duration of symptoms before pain clinic evaluation of 39 (range 2 to 168) months. A relatively recent review (Wilder, 1996) of several pediatric studies (typically in specialty clinics not necessarily representative of the general population) reporting in the aggregate on more than 395 pediatric patients found average age of onset to be 12.5 years with a range of 3 to 18 years.

Sex

In the selective samples examined thus far, there has generally been a higher female to male ratio. In the Netherlands study it was 3:1 and in the U.S. pain center study it was 2.3:1. Similarly, an analysis of 125 cases of management of RSD of the upper extremity in a rehabilitation facility found a 2.9:1 ratio (Subbarao & Stillwell, 1981). A review of the clinical manifestations and management of 140 patients with RSD at the Mayo Clinic during 1965 and 1966 found a 3:2 preponderance of females (Pak et al., 1970). The combined pediatric studies included in the review cited previously reported a female-to-male ratio of 4:1 (Wilder, 1996).

Location

A single limb is involved in the majority of cases of CRPS, with upper and lower extremity pain being reported fairly equally in adults (Allen et al., 1999; Veldman et al., 1993). In children and adolescents, there is a notable predominance of lower-extremity involvement with a computed lower-versus-upper-extremity ratio of 5.3:1 (Wilder, 1996). Much less frequently, the face or torso may be involved. Various patterns of spread have also been observed, for example, further ipsilaterally with gradual and significant enlargement of the area affected initially, "independent spread" or distant, noncontiguous spread (such as from first in a hand to then in a foot or vice versa), "mirror-image spread" to a homologous area of the contralateral limb, and rare cases of spreading total body CRPS (Maleki, LeBel, Bennett, & Schwartzman, 2000; Schwartzman & McLellan, 1987). It has been hypothesized that these various forms may suggest local spread of pathology (in instances of more contiguous spreading), consequences of generalized susceptibility (in instances of independent spread), possibly due to abnormal neural functioning spreading via the corpus callosum, and/or represent aberrant central nervous system (CNS) regulation of neurogenic inflammation (Maleki et al., 2000).

Precipitating Events

A variety of incidents have been linked to the onset of CRPS symptoms. The most common is trauma, often relatively minor or even trivial, most typically fracture, sprain, or strain, and often involving immobilization in a cast or splint and, to a somewhat lesser extent following surgery, contusion or crush injury, myocardial infarction, spinal cord injury, stroke or other head injury, and other sundry occurrences—for example, injections or intravenous infusions (Galer et al., 2001; Schwartzman & McLellan, 1987). Substantial minorities also identify no known precipitating causes in up to 10–23% (Allen et al., 1999; Galer et al., 2001; Veldman et al., 1993). In addition, sometimes a higher than expected occurrence of recent stressful life events has been reported by patients prior to the onset of their RSD (Van Houdenhove et al., 1992).

Related Environmental Factors

High rates of work-related injuries (e.g., 56% in Allen et al., 1999; 53% in DeGood, Cundiff, Adams, & Shutty, 1993; 67% in Nelson & Novy, 1996) have been reported in association with onset of CRPS, but it is difficult to determine the extent to which this is biased by the specialized clinical (typically tertiary pain clinic) samples studied. Reported extent of involvement in litigation has varied considerably (e.g., from 12% litigating in DeGood et al., 1993, to 95% either in or planning litigation related to pain in Nelson & Novy, 1996).

Although certain features stand out, such as occurrence in children even at young ages as well as adults in all age groups, the higher female-to-male preponderance, primary precipitating trigger of soft tissue injuries, and frequent association with work injuries, the overall picture of inferences to be drawn from these and other demographic, clinical, and environmental factors remains unclear given the degree of incomplete information and variability among specialized centers reporting data. Prospective studies of large cohorts are sorely needed to fill in gaps in knowledge about epidemiology of CRPS (Allen et al., 1999).

Natural Course

A related important issue involves the historically accepted view of the natural course of CRPS. Until recently, there was general acceptance of a three-stage progression of CRPS from acute to dystrophic to atrophic, each characterized by persistent and often burning or aching pain but accompanied by distinct changes in expression of skin color and temperature; sudomotor activity; and hair, nail, and skin tissue abnormalities, ultimately resulting in irreversible changes (Bonica, 1990; Schwartzman & McLellan, 1987). However, the Netherlands study of Veldman and colleagues (1993) found no evidence for invariable progression through these stages, and subsequent research has further confirmed this (Galer et al., 2001).

Hence, the variability in symptom manifestations and extent of irreversible damage appear to reflect yet another set of unexplained findings associated with the heterogeneity of expression of CRPS symptoms. What is clear is that CRPS may follow a chronic course, often with severe pain and other associated symptoms persisting in some individuals, whereas others experience reduction or remission of symptoms, subject to flaring under various circumstances in a sometimes rather unpredictable manner.

Pathophysiology

In recent years the investigation into potential pathophysiological mechanisms involved in CRPS has intensified (Janig & Stanton-Hicks, 1996). The general consensus is that the pathophysiology of CRPS is still not known (Galer et al., 2001). The complexity and puzzling nature of findings reported has not yet been cogently resolved (Janig, 1996).

Much more is known about the mechanisms of pain following peripheral nerve injuries, but the reasons that some peripheral injuries (or CNS or other physiological insults) evolve into CRPS is unknown (Galer et al., 2001). Galer and colleagues (2001) have provided a useful conceptual model for integrating the diverse possibilities consistent with known information about CRPS to explain the variability that is observed. Figure 23.2 depicts this model for understanding the hetereogeneity among possible pathophysiological processes and sites involved in the development and maintenance of CRPS.

The model takes note of the different contributing influences that have been suggested in the various branches of the nervous system, including the peripheral nervous system (PNS), CNS, and ANS. Furthermore, regional myofascial dysfunction (MD) has been observed and may well play an important (secondary or perhaps even primary) role in the development of CRPS. In individual cases, these potential sites of abnormality (PNS, CNS, ANS, MD) may reflect different degrees of contribution to the interaction of factors producing CRPS. This may also explain some of the heterogeneity of symptoms among individuals and

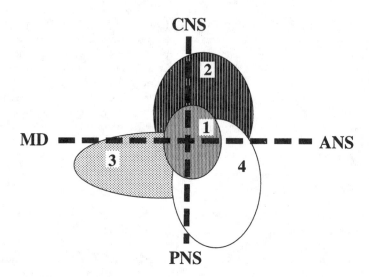

FIGURE 23.2. A model for understanding the heterogeneity among pathophysiologic processes and sites involved in the development and maintenance of complex regional pain syndrome (CRPS). Potential sites of abnormality among CRPS patients include the peripheral somatic nerves (PNS), the central nervous system (CNS), which includes spinal cord and all supratentorial events such as psychological processes, the autonomic nervous system (ANS), both its peripheral and central components, and myofascial dysfunction (MD), which may be primary or secondary. Four theoretical CRPS patients are depicted: Patient 1 has an equal degree of PNS, CNS, ANS, and MD abnormal function responsible for CRPS symptoms; patient 2 has mostly CNS, ANS, and MD dysfunction; patient 3's symptoms derive mostly from ANS and MD; and patient 4's CRPS symptoms develop from PNS and ANS pathophysiologic processes. From Galer, Schwartz, and Allen (2001). Copyright 2001 by Lippincott Williams & Wilkins. Reprinted by permission.

at any given time in the same person with CRPS. Also, as the model may incorporate psychological processes, stress, and other environmental and psychosocial factors relevant at the time of injury or onset of CRPS and subsequently over time, a more complete understanding may emerge regarding evolution of the interaction of these factors. This model may prove useful in helping patients better understand a multidimensional approach to treatment that has some rational basis for selecting the specific interventions that may be recommended.

Still, at this time, more questions remain unanswered than there are answers to basic questions regarding pathogenesis. Galer and colleagues (2001) have summarized some of these, including, to restate or modify a few, the following:

• Why do only a small number of patients develop CRPS after simple soft tissue injuries or even after well-defined nerve injuries?

• Why does the syndrome develop with this particular injury and not a similar injury the person may have previously experienced?

• Why do similar injuries in different people result in some manifesting signs of abnormal ANS activity and others do not?

• What are the differential roles of internal and environmental influences at the time of injury or onset of CRPS?

• To what extent is the SNS actually involved in the development or maintenance of CRPS?

• To what extent is a genetic predisposition involved?

• Why is there such significant variability among the different symptom classes of abnormalities seen in patients with CRPS? Are there distinct pathophysiological mechanisms that yield similar appearing clinical presentations?

• Might different treatments ultimately be devised that target the different underlying pathophysiological mechanisms?

Indeed, the list of questions is extensive and challenging.

Despite the lack of knowledge about the pathophysiology of CRPS, a number of hypotheses have been offered. The classical view that there is simply hyperactivity of the SNS in CRPS has been largely discredited over the past decade (1990s; cf. the authoritative reviews of Bonica, 1990, and Galer et al., 2001), although SNS manifestations are present and SMP or a role for SNS abnormality does appear to provide a partial explanatory mechanism for certain aspects of some individual presentations (Janig, 1996).

Although it is not possible here to review all the postulated mechanisms that have been discussed in the literature, there are some particularly salient hypotheses or issues worth mentioning. None are fully satisfactory and all have yet to reconcile conflicting findings. One of these hypotheses has focused on an exaggerated regional inflammatory response as an alternative to the primary focus on SNS abnormalities (Veldman et al., 1993). Furthermore, given the potential for input from the periphery to interact with the ANS and CNS, there may be changes that occur secondarily and that set in motion neuroplastic changes resulting in development of unusual symptom features of a spreading or progressive nature and/or the perpetuation of various combinations of puzzling clinical symptomatology (Bennett & Roberts, 1996; Coderre, Katz, Vaccarino, & Melzack, 1993). Moving beyond the focus simply on the SNS, and extrapolating from various findings in CRPS that suggest adaptive (i.e., neuroplastic) changes in the CNS, Galer, Butler, and Jensen (1995) hypothesized that an important functional neuroanatomical region involved in CRPS is the central ANS consisting of the amygdala, hypothalamus, insular cortex, and periaqueductal gray. Following this line of reasoning, it would be possible to conceptualize relations of various symptoms of CRPS with functional aspects of these structures.

Another set of hypotheses centers around the role of the protection and decreased use of the injured body part by the patient. As previously noted, there is a high rate of immobilization (including casting and splinting) reported with the onset of CRPS, typically around the time of fractures or soft tissue injuries. Furthermore, with any injury

there may be a natural tendency to protect and guard in order to prevent worse pain and to promote healing. However, extreme forms of guarding and protecting have been observed in patients with CRPS (Bonica, 1990). This has sometimes been associated with exquisite sensitivity to even slight touch, breezes, movement, or vibration and led historically to characterizations of rather bizarre behaviors routinely included in descriptions of patients with causalgia and RSD (Bonica, 1953, 1990). Bonica (1990) presumed that extreme guarding was due to the severe nature of the pain and other associated symptoms of CRPS and these seemed increasingly refractory to change with disease progression to advanced stages.

However, the classical teaching of volitional behavior in this regard has been challenged by alternative explanations suggesting neurological involvement. Indeed, recent reports of neglect-like symptoms (Galer et al., 1995; Galer & Jensen, 1999) similar to that seen in stroke patients and hemisensory impairment (sometimes distant from and/or ipsilateral to the affected limb) in patients with CRPS (Rommel et al., 1999) support hypotheses related to CNS dysfuction and possible neuroplastic changes in the CNS.

Galer and Jensen (1999) found that in a survey of neglect-like symptoms in patients with CRPS, 60% endorsed the statement, "My painful limb feels as though it is not part of my body." The majority of patients also endorsed the following: "I need to focus all of my attention on my painful limb to make it move the way I want it to." Other similar statements (e.g., "If I don't focus my attention on my painful limb it would lie still, like dead weight," "My painful limb feels as though it is not part of my body") were frequently endorsed. Respondents also reported the common practice of not discussing these experiences with health care providers or family members due to shame or fear of having signs of psychiatric disturbance. Interestingly, thalamic perfusion (positron emission tomography) and functional magnetic resonance imaging abnormalities indicating decreased activity in the side of the thalamus contralateral to the affected limb (and possibly linked to other CNS sites of abnormal functioning) that would be compatible with the mechanisms of a neglect syndrome have also been reported (Apkarian, 1996; Fukumoto, Ushida, Zinchuk, Yamamoto, & Yoshida, 1999; Iadarola et al., 1995).

The consequences of a neglect-like syndrome would include a greater tendency to disuse of the affected limb. Disuse may explain at least part of the signs and symptoms of CRPS, as disuse over time may result in edema, decreased blood flow and coldness, and thereby trophic changes in associated tissues (Galer et al., 2001). This may also suggest an important matter to focus on in rehabilitation of patients with CRPS, regardless of its etiological significance. For example, mobilization of a limb as early as medically feasible following injury might be emphasized in a preventive framework. With the onset of symptoms of CRPS, patients may benefit from open, supportive discussion of the nature of their perceptions to "normalize" the experience of different and unusual feelings. They may also benefit from regular and specific modeling and cuing of appropriate movements and use of affected body parts and appropriately targeted reinforcement of successive approximations of increasingly more functional use of affected body parts, as well as planned self-monitoring and self-reinforcement with cognitive-behavioral strategies (see Sanders, Chapter 6, and Turk, Chapter 7, this volume; see also Bandura, 1997; Fordyce, 1976; Kanfer & Goldstein, 1986; Turk, Meichenbaum, & Genest, 1983).

Another area of hypothesizing surrounds the documented incidence of MD in association with CRPS. Palpation of MD trigger points has been observed to reproduce CRPS pain and associated symptoms (Galer et al., 2001). Available evidence suggests that MD is more common in upper extremity than lower extremity cases, and a correlation exists between the presence of MD and motor neglect but not between duration of CRPS and MD (Rashiq & Galer, 1999). The extent to which MD is primary or secondary in subsets of patients with CRPS is not yet known, but anecdotal reports indicate that if it is present, pain and associated symptoms improve when MD trigger points resolve (Galer et al., 2001). Accordingly, treatment principles applied to MD are likely to have relevance for at least some patients with CRPS. For example, relaxation therapies may have particular relevance in

this process as well as neuromuscular retraining with specifically targeted surface electromyography biofeedback (Cram & Kasman, 1998; Donaldson, Nelson, & Schulz, 1998; Kasman, Cram, & Wolf, 1998).

Additional observations of abnormalities of motor function in patients with CRPS have led some to focus on hypotheses regarding CRPS as a movement disorder (Schwartzman & Kerrigan, 1990; Thimineur, Sood, Kravitz, Gudin, & Kitaj, 1998). Range-of-motion decreases are commonly observed (Galer et al., 2001). Furthermore, weakness, tremor, and dystonia, along with dystrophy or atrophy of muscles are commonly observed (Schwartzman & Kerrigan, 1990; Stanton-Hicks et al., 1995). Based on the factor-analytic findings reported previously on the standardized signs and symptoms checklist for CRPS (Harden et al., 1999), motor dysfunction may be a key feature for many patients, despite the lack of inclusion of it as a diagnostic criteria in the current IASP classification (Merskey & Bogduk, 1994). This, too, has some implications for targeting appropriate therapeutic interventions. Similar to suggestions offered previously for neglect-like symptoms, acknowledgement and open discussion of these features in a supportive context as well as specific operant-behavioral and cognitive-behavioral strategies (e.g., modeling, cuing, reinforcement of successive approximations of optimally adaptive functional movements, self-monitoring, and self-reinforcement) may be useful.

Psychological factors have also been proposed as potential pathophysiological influences. Historically, given the case reports of sometimes quite bizarre behavior of patients with causalgia and RSD, the lack of a defined pathophysiology, and other enigmatic features of the disorder, some authors have declared the primary pathology to lie in the psyche or personality of individuals thus afflicted (Lankford, 1982). An extreme view has challenged the legitimacy of the reality basis of the complaints of patients with CRPS and suggested that a "pseudoneurological" or "psychogenic pseudoneuropathy" exists in such persons (Ochoa, 1992). It has been proposed that such patients really have "a distinct, potentially treatable, neuropsychiatric cerebral disorder" (Ochoa,

1992, p. 365). Furthermore, such persons may be characterized as manifesting conversion, somaticizing, or even malingering (Ochoa, 1999). Clearly, such a position will significantly influence treatment recommendations. However, this is definitely a minority view, albeit a vocal one, and is not generally accepted (Galer et al., 2001, Stanton-Hicks et al., 1998).

Role of Psychological Factors

Psychological Etiology

There is general agreement that many patients with CRPS manifest important and often profound behavioral and emotional issues (Lynch, 1992). However, in an extensive review of the adult and pediatric literature from the late 1800s to the early 1990s, Lynch (1992) could find no clear substantiation of the claim that psychological factors or certain personality traits predispose to the development of CRPS. Concurrently, Bruehl and Carlson (1992) reviewed 20 articles in English-language journals that described psychological data on adult or pediatric patients diagnosed with RSD. They found the methodological quality of these studies to be generally poor, thus restricting conclusions to be drawn. However, their conclusions were that depression, anxiety, or life stressors (frequently reported as present by patients with RSD) might influence development of RSD through alpha-adrenergic (i.e., a type of SNS) activity, but the dearth of high-quality studies made it impossible to draw any definitive conclusions about etiological significance of these factors. Van Houdenhove and colleagues (1992) articulated a conceptualization suggesting the role of hyperarousal due to life stress or other factors preceding or around the time of injury or during the subsequent initial period of healing and personal inadequacies of stress-coping mechanisms. However, the lack of convincing evidence that SNS dysfunction is the primary problem in CRPS highlights the limitation of this hypothesis as a unifying conceptualization.

Still, the intriguing role of life stress continues to receive some attention. Geertzen and colleagues (1998) recently reported a comparison of 24 patients with upper extremity CRPS to 42 hand pathology patients waiting for elective hand surgery on a stressful life events scale. Significantly more patients in the CRPS versus the control group had experienced a stressful life event in the 3 months preceding onset of their symptoms, and they rated the degree of seriousness of the life events higher than the control group. The issue remains open as to the potential relevance of life stress and hyperarousal in explaining aspects of CRPS symptoms in subsets of patients (Galer et al., 2001; Geertzen, de Bruijn-Kofman, de Bruijn, van de Wiehl, & Dijkstra, 1998; Van Houdenhove et al., 1992).

Additional recent studies have cast further doubt on the presumed distinctiveness of a specific personality type or functioning on the development or maintenance of CRPS. For example, DeGood and colleagues (1993) compared patients with RSD, low back pain (LBP), and headache pain (HAP) on a variety of self-reported demographic, behavioral, pain, and mood measures. All three groups demonstrated elevations indicative of pain, emotional distress, and behavioral disturbance. The RSD group reported the highest level of pain intensity, the most employment disruption, and the highest percentage receiving pain-related financial compensation. However, the RSD group reported less emotional distress on the Symptom Checklist—90R than did LBP and HAP patients. DeGood and colleagues hypothesized that this paradox may be due to the lesser chronicity of the RSD patients as well as their apparently experiencing a more sympathetic response from doctors, employers, and insurance carriers than those with LBP and HAP. The data did not support the hypothesis that patients with RSD, relative to other patients with chronic pain, are uniquely disturbed in psychosocial functioning.

Similar conclusions were reached by Nelson and Novy (1996), who compared patients with RSD from a multidisciplinary pain center with those with myofascial pain syndromes on demographic and clinical characteristics, responses to a pain questionnaire, and responses to the Minnesota Multiphasic Personality Inventory (MMPI). With only a few minor exceptions, the two groups appeared comparable with respect to a wide range of demographic, clinical, and psychological functioning indices. The patients with RSD had shorter duration of pain, were taking fewer pain medications, were less likely to be working, and were more likely to be receiving workers' compensation payments, but both groups had comparable numbers of pain-related surgeries, pain intensity ratings, and perceived ability to cope. A wide range of functioning was in evidence for both groups on the MMPI scales, with only minor differences. Again, a specific psychological profile, uniquely neurotic or otherwise, was not demonstrated.

Monti, Herring, Schwartzman, and Marchese (1998) took a somewhat different approach by obtaining diagnoses based on the Structured Clinical Interview for the third edition, revised, of *Diagnostic and Statistical Manual of Mental Disorders* (DSM-III-R; American Psychiatric Association, 1987) in order to compare 25 patients with CRPS Type I to a control group of 25 patients with chronic LBP from disc-related radiculopathy. Both groups were similar in terms of pain intensity and duration. Both groups also showed a similar amount of major psychiatric comorbidity, in particular major depressive disorder, and a high incidence of personality disorders. However, the extent of psychiatric disturbance in both groups was present in similar proportions. The authors proposed that the high incidence of personality pathology in both groups might represent an exaggeration of maladaptive traits and coping styles due to a chronic, intense state of pain.

These and all other studies that have relied on statistical comparisons of patients with CRPS versus patients with other chronic pain conditions, instead of clinician observations or anecdotal case summaries only, have yet to find a definitive role for a unique set of personality factors or psychological disturbances to explain the etiology or maintenance of CRPS. All do find evidence for the important role of suffering and emotional and behavioral disturbances in many patients with CRPS, but the degree of disturbance is not necessarily more than is observed in other chronic pain states. On the other hand, this does not rule out the possibility that psychological factors may interact in ways as yet unidentified to explain the onset or progression of symptoms in subsets of patients with CRPS. It also

does not mean that there are no special or unique features of CRPS that are important in the management of the syndrome.

Treatment of CRPS

Principles of treatment have evolved considerably over the past decade from a primary reliance on sympathetic blockade or interruption (Bonica, 1990) supplemented with modalities of physical and psychological therapies to a more integrated multidimensional and multidisciplinary approach (Stanton-Hicks et al., 1998). This has been driven by the limitations practically as well as conceptually of the former approach. Matters have been improved by efforts to better describe and define the syndrome without presumption as to an underlying mechanism of SMP, to better understand relevant demographic and clinical characteristics, and to more fully explore the diversity of potential mechanisms contributing to the heterogeneity of expression of symptoms in CRPS. Some practitioners, though, may still rely on outdated notions for intervention, whether by choice because of vested interest in a particular treatment or through ignorance. This is a disservice and may contribute to unnecessary disability and suffering (Chapman, 2000).

Consensus Report Guidelines for Therapy

In the late 1990s, guidelines produced by an international consensus workshop attended by a number of leading basic scientists and physicians in the field were published to serve as a standard reference for the treatment of CRPS (Stanton-Hicks et al., 1998). It is important to note that the guidelines reflect the informed opinions of these experts while the research database of controlled or uncontrolled clinical trials remains sparse. With that caveat in mind, it is noteworthy that a coordinated approach is recommended that is built around a treatment algorithm emphasizing physical therapy for the normalization of function with other therapies (medications, analgesics including regional anesthesia, neuromodulation whether via peripheral nerve or spinal cord stimulation or other means, and psychotherapy) designed as agents to facilitate these goals. A biopsychosocial conceptualization and interdisciplinary team approach is considered fundamental to the delivery of treatment with the patient being a key member of the team. Self-management and low technological intervention are emphasized, with invasive and interventional therapies such as regional anesthesia or neuromodulation and neurostimulation reserved for times at which there is failure to achieve anticipated progress. Psychological interventions are key elements of the continuum of care offered throughout the rehabilitation process (cf. Covington, 1996). Consideration of the treatment algorithm with that in mind forms the basis for guiding psychological treatment of patients with CRPS.

Physical Therapy and Functional Rehabilitation

It is presumed that early intervention within the first 2 months following onset of CRPS symptoms may focus almost entirely on physical therapy, because it is believed that the dysphoric and other behavioral or emotional dysfunctions associated with CRPS are likely to be minimal during this period (Stanton-Hicks et al., 1998). There is some evidence to support this view, including reports of return to previously normal emotional functioning following successful treatment of CRPS (Lynch, 1992). Regardless, the first step involves the development of a therapeutic alliance and rapport. Specific physical therapy procedures early in treatment focus on motivation, mobilization, and desensitization (i.e., techniques to normalize sensibility of the affected region through means of tactile and proprioceptive input, such as gentle application of stimulation with cold, heat, massage, movement, pressure, vibration; cf. Oerlemans et al., 2000). The tendency to overprotect and guard the affected area and consequently corresponding disuse requires specific attention to begin to overcome any (extreme) fear of movement (understandable in part due to the exquisite sensitivity of the affected region to even typically benign stimuli) and to normalize use of the affected limb (Stanton-Hicks et al., 1998). Given the emerging evidence suggesting neglect-like symptoms that may have a CNS basis (Galer & Jensen, 1999), this may represent

a particular challenge, because the guarding and protective behaviors may reflect a more profound dysfunction than is the case with volitional guarding often seen in other chronic pain conditions (Keefe & Williams, 1992).

From a psychological standpoint, the approach in this early stage as well as subsequent stages of treatment would potentially benefit from specific application of operant behavioral principles. The consensus guidelines emphasize that a "measured pace" that is "time contingent" is considered optimal for attaining functional improvement (Stanton-Hicks et al., 1998). Accordingly, the incorporation of operant behavioral principles (see Sanders, Chapter 6, this volume; Fordyce, 1976) for structuring goal-based quota scheduling of therapy exercises and other activities is particularly salient. Individual flexibility is required to adapt to the "dynamic and unique nature of this disease entity" (Stanton-Hicks et al., 1998).

Galer and colleagues (2001) have suggested one particular structure for progressive restoration of motion, strength, and motor control and functional activities of standing, walking, and engagement in other activities of daily living based on operant principles. Their recommendations follow from the basic principles of such an approach originally discussed in detail by Fordyce (1976). The primary strategy is first to establish a baseline for each activity to the point of tolerance signaled by escalating pain, fatigue, or muscle weakness. These baselines are typically quantified in terms of number of repetitions, movement cycles, or elapsed time. Treatment then proceeds initially with a goal set for each activity at a level of 80% of baseline. This is done for a prescribed number of sessions per day. Sessions on subsequent days are increased by one repetition (or 5–10% for activities based on time elapsed) with the focus on attainment of the quota and not on the limit of endurance. The quotas are to be adhered to, with the patient performing no more and no less than the specified goals for the session. Various modifications are made in the quotas based on progressive increases in resistance for certain exercises or other factors specific to the activity at hand. Hence, the dosing of activity and exercise is likely to be optimally paced and endurance, strength, and other positive benefits achieved on a more steady and less frustrating course. All other physical therapy procedures, for example, progressive increases in range of motion, aerobic capacity and conditioning, and weight bearing, are handled according to similar principles. Specific activities, exercises, and so forth are discussed in greater detail in descriptions of various physical therapy procedure protocols (Oerlemans et al., 2000).

There is no protocol sufficiently empirically validated to suggest that it is better to follow than another in terms of a specific structure for physical therapy. On the other hand, there is a certain degree of convergence in some of the necessary tasks for such therapies. The consensus guidelines lay out a general pattern of increasing scope from gentle reactivation and desensitization to isometrics; greater movement and flexibility in range of motion; stress loading; and a focus on ergonomics, walking/swimming, and other movement therapies; aerobic conditioning; and ultimately work hardening and maximizing engagement in all other activities—for example, school, homemaking, and recreation (Stanton-Hicks et al., 1998). At each stage in the progression of treatment, operant principles are applicable, including quota-based increases, cuing and shaping with reinforcement of successive approximations of desired responses, modeling as needed, and the like. This approach also lends itself to objective monitoring of progress toward agreed-on goals and can have a self-sustaining positive aspect (Fordyce, 1976).

It is important to keep in mind that motor function disturbances, guarding, and other features of CRPS may have a strong basis in nervous system changes (whether CNS or PNS) that are not strictly volitional or even just simply reactive to pain. To a certain extent, the intense and unusual nature of the pain (e.g., allodynia and hyperalgesia) associated with CRPS makes it particularly difficult for patients to engage in physical-based therapies and activities. Hence, conveying to patients an understanding of this reality is important for maximizing rapport and motivation and providing the necessary support to overcome barriers to movement and use of affected body parts. Also, there may be an inherent limitation in the extent to which desensitization may occur or other features of the syndrome may respond to modification, but typically substantial progress can occur and result in significant reduction or even remission of symptoms (Stanton-Hicks et al., 1998). Indeed, although the motor function disturbances of CRPS may reflect CNS dysfunction, in addition to any PNS dysfunction and volitional protective movements, an operant approach will maximize potential for restoration of function (Galer et al., 2001).

Secondary myofascial pain syndromes are also to be addressed. Throughout this and all aspects of the physical focus on restoration of function, relaxation techniques (with or without electromyogram or temperature biofeedback) may be used to enhance the response to myofascial therapies. Surface electromyography may also be used to normalize associated muscle imbalance patterns with specific neuromuscular retraining, keeping in mind potential limiting factors such as joint or other musculoskeletal dysfunctions (Cram & Kasman, 1998; Donaldson et al., 1998; Kasman et al., 1998).

Medications

Most reported trials of medications used in the treatment of CRPS are small anecdotal studies. Guidance is frequently sought in the literature and clinical experience base for pharmacological treatment from what is known about other neuropathic pains (Stanton-Hicks et al., 1998). Indeed, for the broader class of neuropathic pain, there are few well-designed drug treatment trials (Kingery, 1997). Accordingly, there are no adequate predictors of choice of drug and the approach is largely one of an informed trial and error (Stanton-Hicks et al., 1998).

Informed opinion, though, does suggest that a variety of drugs may be useful for some patients to varying degrees (Galer et al., 2001; Stanton-Hicks et al., 1998). There is no set order for systematically approaching the pharmacotherapy of CRPS, and it is important to help patients understand that this lack of definitive knowledge does not prevent informed application and extrapolation of the limited findings. It is sometimes difficult, but possible, to convey to patients that they are not simply serving as a "guinea pig" for which there is no rationale for drug selection.

The consensus guidelines recommend attempting to attain maximum pain control to facilitate other functional rehabilitation efforts while balancing this with aggressiveness of drug options (Stanton-Hicks et al., 1998). There is a potential role for each of the following: nonsteroidal anti-inflammatory drugs for milder stages of syndrome severity and as an adjunct particularly when there is an associated inflammatory process such as in joint or tendon; tricylic (e.g., amitriptyline, desipramine, and doxepin) and other heterocyclic (e.g., maprotiline) antidepressants that have often demonstrated value for analgesia as well as for effects on mood and sleep in neuropathic pain syndromes such as diabetic neuropathy and postherpetic neuralgia (but not necessarily in CRPS); possibly selective serotonin reuptake inhibitors (e.g., fluoxetine and paroxetine) in cases in which depression and anxiety are prominent; "membrane stabilizing" and anticonvulsant drugs (e.g., carbemazepine, gabapentin, and valproic acid); local anesthestics (e.g., topical lidocaine); antiarrhythmics (e.g., mexilitine); corticosteroids; calcitonin biophosphonates; capsaicin topical cream for application to localized areas of hyperalgesia; alpha-adrenergic blocking agents (e.g., terazosin, prazosin, and phenoxybenzamine) and the topical transdermal application of alpha–2 agonists (e.g., clonidine); and opioids. Although the use of opioids is controversial, and they have been considered generally ineffective in neuropathic pain, they may be useful in selected patients (Galer et al., 2001; Stanton-Hicks et al., 1998). However, no controlled studies of opioid use in CRPS exist, and, as mentioned, most of the recommendations for other classes enumerated previously are extrapolated from the sparse clinical trials literature or informed opinion on neuropathic pain syndromes (Kingery, 1997). In any event, guidelines have been evolving for the management of opioid medications in chronic pain management (Portenoy, 1996), and operant principles of time-contingent in preference to pain-contingent or PRN dosing, as originally discussed by Fordyce (1976), form the most rational basis for psychological–behavioral management of such pharmacotherapy for CRPS.

Regional Anesthetic Techniques

Use of regional anesthestic techniques may be considered in the treatment of CRPS (Stanton-Hicks et al., 1998). The purpose would be to provide some analgesia to facilitate engagement in other therapies of functional restoration. If regional sympathetic blockade is effective, it is important to determine whether repeating the procedure can increase the duration of the effect. Some advocate more definitive chemical lysis or radiofrequency lesioning if there is sufficient demonstration of sustained effect. One of the problems with this approach is the unfortunate overreliance by some on an outmoded notion of SMP as the presumed underlying mechanism of CRPS, the emphasis on a curative model that has not demonstrated utility in CRPS, and the need to balance analgesia with appropriate functional capabilities to engage in the other more physically based therapies (Stanton-Hicks, Raj, & Racz, 1996).

Neuromodulation

Although spinal cord stimulation (SCS) was first proposed in 1967 as a pain management technique, overenthusiastic application led to substantial disappointment and less usage. However, recent years have witnessed a renaissance in the clinical practice of SCS. This has been fostered by more critical application of the technique, substantial refinements in the equipment and other aspects of the technology, and improved patient selection criteria (North, 1993; see Doleys, Chapter 16, this volume). SCS is now receiving increased attention as a potential treatment for CRPS. The consensus guidelines suggest that SCS may be considered, particularly in cases that are proving particularly refractory or not progressing satisfactorily (Stanton-Hicks et al., 1998). Recent reports suggest potentially good response in some patients (Kemler et al., 2000; Schwartzman, 2000). The literature on SCS has also become more sophisticated in incorporating psychological selection criteria for SCS. Provisional guidelines are detailed in an extensive review of the literature on SCS and include careful consideration of affective disturbances (e.g., untreated or poorly treated major depression or severe anxiety may impede optimal response); extent of suicidal or homicidal thinking; psychotic-like symptoms; alcohol or other drug dependence; compensation, litigation, or other potent environmental influences; lack of appropriate social support; severity of neurobehavioral cognitive deficits; unstable personality and interpersonal functioning; and so on (Nelson, Kennington, Novy, & Squitieri, 1996a). Multifactor weighting of criteria, timing of intervention, and ability to conceptualize SCS as one component within multidisciplinary rehabilitation are other important considerations (Nelson et al., 1996a, 1996b).

In addition, implantable spinal medication pump delivery systems are sometimes advocated in neuropathic pain states. The application of such implantable technology has limited empirical documentation for CRPS, but with various combinations of drugs in such systems (e.g., baclofen and opioid) is likewise considered for neuromodulation in cases not progressing satisfactorily or under conditions when it seems advisable to limit dose-related side effects of oral medications by providing far less medication targeted intraspinally (Stanton-Hicks et al., 1998; van Hilton, van de Beeck, Hoff, Voormolen, & Delhaas, 2000). Similar psychological selection criteria considerations apply in principle, although there is hardly any empirical literature to provide validated guidance (cf. Nelson et al., 1996a, 1996b).

Cognitive-Behavioral and Other Psychotherapies

The general guidelines for psychological treatment of CRPS emphasize principles and strategies that for the most part are those described in the treatment of chronic pain conditions in general. These have been well summarized in other reviews (see Turk, Chapter 7, this volume; see also Caudill, 2002; Turk et al., 1983). They include cognitive-behavioral therapy (CBT) for specific treatment of emotional disorders (Beck, 1976; Beck, Rush, Shaw, & Emery, 1979) and for specific pain management issues, in-

cluding developing acceptance or "ownership" of the chronic pain condition, goal setting, relaxation and related self-regulation training, appropriate pacing to optimize up- versus downtime, cognitive restructuring, communication expressiveness skills, problem solving, generalization, maintenance, and relapse prevention (Caudill, 2002; Sternbach, 1987; Turk et al., 1983). CBT fosters active self-management and aims to restore a sense of perceived control (Jensen, Turner, Romano, & Karoly, 1991).

Group therapy for psychoeducational interventions and for social support or social comparison are typically advocated as well (see Keefe, Beaupre, Gil, Rumble, & Aspnes, Chapter 11, this volume; see also Gentry & Owens, 1986; Jensen et al., 1991). In addition, family therapy in specific family or general group settings has been advocated (see Kerns, Otis, & Wise, Chapter 12, this volume; see also Kerns, 1999). There is substantial support for the importance of attending to and modifying as needed the potentially powerful influence of family reinforcement contingencies surrounding patients' pain behaviors (Fordyce, 1976; Romano et al., 1995) as well as to ensure optimal support for both patients and family members in coping and adjustment (Sternbach, 1987).

In addition to the general CBT approach to pain management, there is increasing interest in the application of other psychotherapies. For example, based on evidence from cluster analyses of multidimensional pain profiles in other chronic pain conditions, there is some support for more specifically targeting treatments, such as those that may aim to address specific aspects of interpersonal distress and dysfunction (Turk, Okifuji, Sinclair, & Starz, 1998; Turk & Rudy, 1990). Models exist for adapting interpersonal psychotherapies for such specifically targeted problems (Weissman, Markowitz, & Klerman, 2000). Other aspects of general psychotherapy have also been discussed and may be applicable (see Basler, Grzesik, & Dworkin, Chapter 5, this volume, on psychodynamic psychotherapy; see also Galer et al., 2001; Stanton-Hicks et al., 1998).

Fear of reinjury is a particularly difficult issue (Bonica, 1990). Patients with CRPS are often aware that their pain condition resulted from a seemingly minor or even trivial event. This, combined with the exquisite sensitivity and more intense pain so easily provoked, often results in patients manifesting great fear of reinjury and possibly self-limiting behaviors that further augment any guarding or protective maneuvers, whether volitional or CNS based (see Vlaeyen, de Jong, Sieben, & Crombez, Chapter 10, this volume). Hence, this issue requires an explicit focus for functional restoration and may be addressed with CBT (Galer et al., 2001; Stanton-Hicks et al., 1998).

Specific Symptom Psychological Treatments

Specific symptom therapies have been suggested throughout the history of treatment for CRPS. One of the most prominent of these has been temperature biofeedback. This modality was first suggested in large part because of the presumed basis of SNS dysfunction in CRPS. Temperature changes, with extreme coldness and cold sensitivity, were emphasized in early writings on CRPS (Bonica, 1953), leading to the suggestion that temperature biofeedback specifically targeting the temperature dysregulation of the affected limb might be useful for symptom amelioration. Case study reports gave some credence to this view (Alioto, 1981; Blanchard, 1979), as did one study of 20 patients who had been refractory to other forms of treatment but who did well with temperature biofeedback intervention, including substantial numbers returning to work (Grunert, Devine, Sanger, Matloub, & Green, 1990). However, this form of biofeedback has not been investigated with sufficient rigor to recommend it above other forms of biofeedback or self-regulation training. Further, the original conceptual basis of SNS dysfunction is fundamentally flawed. On the other hand, that does not discredit it as a form of symptom control in selected individuals. It is important to keep in mind, though, that the temperature dysregulation in evidence in CRPS is as or more often manifested in terms of heat and warmth of the affected body part as it is in coldness (Galer et al., 2001). This poses a problem for standard temperature biofeedback paradigms that encourage hand or foot warming as the primary goal. Still, the mechanism underlying success of temperature biofeedback is not known, but it has been suggested that a key aspect of biofeedback training may actually be the cognitive mechanisms that occur and sense of control that is learned (Holroyd et al., 1984). If so, learning temperature control theoretically could be beneficial in terms of an overall self-regulation process regardless of the mechanisms of disease.

Hypnosis has similarly been advocated as a potentially effective intervention for certain aspects of symptom reduction in CRPS. One case report documented hand warming and relief of some RSD symptoms (Gainer, 1992), but otherwise the technique has not been investigated extensively (Galer et al., 2001).

Treatment of Children

Some believe that children are generally more responsive to conservative treatment and intervention focused primarily on progressive desensitization, and an exercise therapy program may be sufficient if begun early in the disease (Sherry, Wallace, Kelley, Kidder, & Sapp, 1999; Stanton-Hicks et al., 1998). On the other hand, there are reports that some children (just as some adults) experience quite difficult treatment courses and may have persistent pain and dysfunction after completion of a treatment program (Anderson & Fallat, 1999; Greipp, Thomas, & Renkun, 1988; Murray, Cohen, Perkins, Davidson, & Sills, 2000). It is possible that with appropriate modifications, particularly focusing on family counseling in the treatment process and countering well-meaning but ill-advised recommendations by previous health care providers to restrict use of affected body parts, treatment may proceed largely along the consensus guidelines for adults. Furthermore, children may be particularly responsive to CBT for pain management (Stanton-Hicks et al., 1998; see McGrath & Hillier, Chapter 27, this volume).

Final Comments

The treatment of CRPS is based largely on consensus guidelines of informed opinion supplemented with a sparse literature of clinical trials. A thorough understanding of the phenomenology of CRPS, current conceptualization of multifactorial contributions to the expression of symptoms in CRPS, the unusual features often manifested, the controversies surrounding pathophysiology, and extrapolations from the general chronic pain management and specific, related neuropathic pain literature provide grounding for application of psychological principles in treatment. Ideally, future summaries of the state of the art in the psychological treatment of CRPS will be able to provide more solid evidence and validation for effective intervention strategies.

References

Alioto, J. T. (1981). Behavioral treatment of reflex sympathetic dystrophy. *Psychosomatics, 22,* 539–540.

Allen, G., Galer, B. S., & Schwartz, L. (1999). Epidemiology of complex regional pain syndrome: A retrospective chart review of 134 patients. *Pain, 80,* 539–544.

American Psychiatric Association. (1987). *Diagnostic and statistical manual of mental disorders* (3rd ed., rev.). Washington, DC: Author.

Anderson, D. J., & Fallat, L. M. (1999). Complex regional pain syndrome of the lower extremity: A retrospective study of 33 patients. *Journal of Foot and Ankle Surgery, 38,* 381–387.

Apkarian, A. V. (1996). Primary somatosensory cortex and pain. *Pain Forum, 5,* 188–191.

Bandura, A. (1997). *Self-efficacy: The exercise of control.* New York: Freeman.

Beck, A. T. (1976). *Cognitive therapy and the emotional disorders.* New York: New American Library.

Beck, A. T., Rush, A. J., Shaw, B. F., & Emery, G. (1979). *Cognitive therapy of depression.* New York: Guilford Press.

Bennett, G. J., & Roberts, W. J. (1996). Animal models and their contribution to our understanding of complex regional syndromes I and II. In W. Janig & M. Stanton-Hicks (Eds.), *Reflex sympathetic dystrophy: A reappraisal* (pp. 107–122). Seattle: IASP Press.

Blanchard, E. B. (1979). The use of temperature biofeedback in the treatment of chronic pain due to causalgia. *Biofeedback and Self-Regulation, 4,* 183–188.

Bonica, J. J. (1953). *The management of pain.* Philadelphia: Lea & Febiger.

Bonica, J. J. (1990). Causalgia and other reflex sympathetic dystrophies. In J. J. Bonica, J. D. Loeser, C. R. Chapman, & W. E. Fordyce (Eds.), *The management of pain* (2nd ed., Vol. 1, pp. 220–243). Philadelphia: Lea & Febiger.

Bruehl, S., & Carlson, C. R. (1992). Predisposing psychological factors in the development of reflex sympathetic dystrophy: A review of the empirical evidence. *Clinical Journal of Pain, 8,* 287–299.

Campbell, J. N., Meyer, R. A., & Raja, S. N. (1992). Is nociceptor activation by alpha–1 adrenoceptors the culprit in sympathetically-maintained pain? *APS Journal, 1,* 3–11.

Caudill, M. A. (2002). *Managing pain before it manages you* (Rev. ed.). New York: Guilford Press.

Chapman, S. L. (2000). Chronic pain rehabilitation: Lost in a sea of drugs and procedures? *APS Bulletin, 10, 1,* 8–9.

Coderre, T. J., Katz, J., Vaccarino, A. L., & Melzack, R. (1993). Contribution of central neuroplasticity to pathological pain. *Review of Clinical and Experimental Evidence, 52,* 259–285.

Covington, E. C. (1996). Psychological issues in reflex sympathetic dystrophy. In W. Janig & M. Stanton-Hicks (Eds.), *Reflex sympathetic dystrophy: A reappraisal* (pp. 191–215). Seattle, WA: IASP Press.

Cram, J. R., & Kasman, G. S. (1998). *Introduction to surface electromyography.* Gaithersburg, MD: Aspen.

DeGood, D. E., Cundiff, G. W., Adams, L. E., & Shutty, M. S., Jr. (1993). A psychosocial and behavioral comparison of reflex sympathetic dystrophy, low back pain, and headache patients. *Pain, 54,* 317–322.

Donaldson, C. C. S., Nelson, D. V., & Schulz, R. (1998). Disinhibition in the gamma motoneuron circuitry: A neglected mechanism for understanding myofascial pain syndromes? *Biofeedback and Self-Regulation, 23,* 43–57.

Evans, J. A. (1946). Reflex sympathetic dystrophy. *Surgical Gynecology and Obstetrics, 82,* 36–44.

Fordyce, W. E. (1976). *Behavioral methods for chronic pain and illness.* St. Louis, MO: Mosby.

Fukumoto, M., Ushida, T., Zinchuk, V. S., Yamamoto, H., & Yoshida, S. (1999). Contralateral thalamic perfusion in patients with reflex sympathetic dystrophy syndrome. *Lancet, 354,* 1790–1791.

Gainer, M. J. (1992). Hypnotherapy for reflex sympathetic dystrophy. *American Journal of Clinical Hypnosis, 34,* 227–232.

Galer, B. S., Bruehl, S., & Harden, R. N. (1998). IASP diagnostic criteria for complex regional pain syndrome: A preliminary empirical validation study. *Clinical Journal of Pain, 14,* 48–54.

Galer, B. S., Butler, S., & Jensen, M. P. (1995). Case reports and hypothesis: A neglect-like syndrome may be responsible for the motor disturbance in reflex sympathetic dystrophy (complex regional pain syndrome–1). *Journal of Pain and Symptom Management, 10,* 385–391.

Galer, B. S., & Jensen, M. (1999). Neglect-like symptoms in complex regional pain syndrome: Results of a self-administered survey. *Journal of Pain and Symptom Management, 18,* 213–217.

Galer, B. S., Schwartz, L., & Allen, R. J. (2001). Complex regional pain syndromes—Type I: Reflex sympathetic dystrophy, and Type II: Causalgia. In J. D. Loeser, S. H. Butler, C. R. Chapman, & D. C. Turk (Eds.), *Bonica's management of pain* (3rd ed., pp. 388–411). Philadelphia: Lippincott Williams & Wilkins.

Geertzen J. H. B., de Bruijn-Kofman, A. T., de Bruijn, H. P., van de Wiel, H. B. M., & Dijkstra, P. U. (1998). Stressful life events and psychological dysfunction in complex regional syndrome type I. *Clinical Journal of Pain, 14*, 143–147.

Gentry, W. D., & Owens, D. (1986). Pain groups. In A. D. Holzman & D. C. Turk (Eds.), *Pain management: A handbook of psychological treatment approaches* (pp. 100–112). New York: Pergamon Press.

Greipp, M. E., Thomas, A. F., & Renkun, C. (1988). Children and young adults with reflex sympathetic dystrophy syndrome. *Clinical Journal of Pain, 4*, 217–221.

Grunert, B. K., Devine, C. A., Sanger, J. R., Matloub, H. S., & Green, D. (1990). Thermal self-regulation for pain control in reflex sympathetic dystrophy syndrome. *Journal of Hand Surgery, 15A*, 615–618.

Harden, R. N., Bruehl, S., Galer, B. S., Saltz, S., Bertram, M., Backonja, M., Gayles, R., Rudin, N., Bhugra, M. K., & Stanton-Hicks, M. (1999). Complex regional pain syndrome: Are the IASP diagnostic criteria valid and sufficiently comprehensive? *Pain, 83*, 211–219.

Holroyd, K. A., Penzien, D. B., Hursey, K. G., Tobin, D. L., Rogers, L., Holm, J. E., Marcille, P. J., Hall, J. R., & Chila, A. G. (1984). Change mechanisms in EMG biofeedback training: Cognitive changes underlying improvement in tension headache. *Journal of Consulting and Clinical Psychology, 52*, 1039–1053.

Iadarola, M. J., Max, M. B., Berman, K. F., Byas-Smith, M. B., Coghill, R. C., Gracely, R. H., & Bennett, G. J. (1995). Unilateral decrease in thalamic activity observed with positron emission tomography in patients with chronic neuropathic pain. *Pain, 63*, 55–64.

Janig, W. (1996). The puzzle of "reflex sympathetic dystrophy": Mechanisms, hypotheses, open questions. In W. Janig & M. Stanton-Hicks (Eds.), *Reflex sympathetic dystrophy: A reappraisal* (pp. 1–24). Seattle, WA: IASP Press.

Janig, W., & Stanton-Hicks, M. (Eds.). (1996). *Reflex sympathetic dystrophy: A reappraisal.* Seattle: IASP Press.

Jensen, M. P., Turner, J. A., Romano, J. M., & Karoly, P. (1991). Coping with chronic pain: A critical review of the literature. *Pain, 47*, 249–283.

Kanfer, F. H., & Goldstein, A. P. (Eds.). (1986). *Helping people change: A textbook of methods* (3rd ed.). New York: Pergamon Press.

Kasman, G. S., Cram, J. R., & Wolf, S. L. (1998). *Clinical applications in surface electromyography: Chronic musculoskeletal pain.* Gaithersburg, MD: Aspen.

Keefe, F. J., & Williams, D. A. (1992). Assessment of pain behaviors. In D. C. Turk & R. Melzack (Eds.), *Handbook of pain assessment* (pp. 275–284). New York: Guilford Press.

Kemler, M. A., Barendse, G. A., van Kleef, M., de Vet, H. C., Rijks, C. P., Furnee, C. A., & van den Wildenberg, F. A. (2000). Spinal cord stimulation in patients with chronic reflex sympathetic dystrophy. *New England Journal of Medicine, 343*, 618–624.

Kerns, R. D. (1999). Family therapy for adults with chronic pain. In R. J. Gatchel & D. C. Turk (Eds.), *Psychosocial factors in pain: Critical perspectives* (pp. 445–456). New York: Guilford Press.

Kingery, W. S. (1997). A critical review of controlled clinical trials for peripheral neuropathic pain and complex regional pain syndromes. *Pain, 73*, 123–139.

Lankford, L. L. (1982). Reflex sympathetic dystrophy of the upper extremity. In J. E. Flynn (Ed.), *Hand surgery* (3rd ed., pp. 656–670). Baltimore: Williams & Wilkins.

Livingstone, W. K. (1943). *Pain mechanisms: A physiological interpretation of causalgia and its related states.* London: MacMillan.

Lynch, M. E. (1992). Psychological aspects of reflex sympathetic dystrophy: A review of the adult and paediatric literature. *Pain, 49*, 337–347.

Maleki, J., LeBel, A. A., Bennett, G. J., & Schwartzman, R. J. (2000). Patterns of spread in complex regional pain syndrome, type I (reflex sympathetic dystrophy). *Pain, 88*, 259–266.

Mersky, H., & Bogduk, N. (Eds.). (1994). *Classification of chronic pain: Descriptions of chronic pain syndromes and definitions of pain terms* (2nd ed.). Seattle, WA: IASP Press.

Mitchell, S. W. (1872). *Injuries of nerves and their consequences.* London: Smith Elder.

Mitchell, S. W., Morehouse, G. R., & Keen, W. W. (1864). *Gunshot wounds and other injuries of nerves.* New York: Lippincott.

Monti, D. A., Herring, C. L., Schwartzman, R. J., & Marchese, M. (1998). Personality assessment of patients with complex regional pain syndrome type 1. *Clinical Journal of Pain, 14*, 296–302.

Murray, C. S., Cohen, A., Perkins, T., Davidson, J. E., & Sills, J. A. (2000). Morbidity in reflex sympathetic dystrophy. *Archives of Diseases in Children, 82*, 231–233.

Nelson, D. V., Kennington, M., Novy, D. M., & Squitieri, P. (1996a). Psychological selection criteria for implantable spinal cord stimulators. *Pain Forum, 5*, 93–103.

Nelson, D. V., Kennington, M., Novy, D. M., & Squitieir, P. (1996b). Psychological considerations in implantable technology: Picking up where we left off. *Pain Forum, 5*, 121–126.

Nelson, D. V., & Novy, D. M. (1996). Psychological characteristics of reflex sympathetic dystrophy versus myofascial pain syndromes. *Regional Anesthesia, 21*, 202–208.

North, R. B. (1993). The role of spinal cord stimulation in contemporary pain management. *APS Journal, 2*, 91–99.

Ochoa, J. L. (1992). Reflex sympathetic dystrophy:

A disease of medical understanding. *Clinical Journal of Pain, 8*, 363–366.

Ochoa, J. L. (1999). Truths, errors, and lies around "reflex sympathetic dystrophy" and "complex regional pain syndrome." *Journal of Neurology, 246*, 875–879.

Oerlemans, H. M., Oostendorp, R. A., de Boo, T., van der Laan, L., Severens J. L., & Goris, J. A. (2000). Adjuvant physical therapy versus occupational therapy in patients with reflex sympathetic dystrophy/complex regional pain syndrome type I. *Archives of Physical Medicine and Rehabilitation, 81*, 49–56.

Pak, T. J., Martin, G. M., Magness, J. L., & Kavanaugh, G. J. (1970). Reflex sympathetic dystrophy: Review of 140 cases. *Minnesota Medicine, 53*, 507–512.

Portenoy, R. K. (1996). Opioid therapy for chronic nonmalignant pain: A review of the critical issues. *Journal of Pain and Symptom Management, 11*, 203–217.

Roberts, W. J. (1986). A hypothesis on the physiological basis for causalgia and related pains. *Pain, 124*, 297–311.

Rashiq, S., & Galer, B. S. (1999). Myofascial dysfunction in complex regional pain syndrome. *Clinical Journal of Pain, 15*, 151–153.

Rizzi, R., Visentin, M., & Mazzetti, G. (1984). Reflex sympathetic dystrophy. In C. Benedetti, C. R. Chapman, & G. Moricca (Eds.), *Recent advances in the management of pain* (pp. 451–464). New York: Raven Press.

Roberts, W. J. (1986). A hypothesis on the physiological basis for causalgia and related pains. *Pain, 124*, 297–311.

Romano, J. M., Turner, J. A., Jensen, M. P., Friedman, L. S., Bulcroft, R. A., Hops, H., & Wright, S. F. (1995). Chronic pain patient-spouse behavioral interactions predict patient disability. *Pain, 63*, 353–360.

Rommel, O., Gehling, M., Dertwinkel, R., Witscher, K., Zenz, M., Malin, J. P., & Janig, W. (1999). Hemisensory impairment in patients with complex regional pain syndrome. *Pain, 80*, 95–101.

Schwartzman, R. J. (2000). New treatments for reflex sympathetic dystrophy. *New England Journal of Medicine, 343*, 654–656.

Schwartzman, R. J., & Kerrigan, J. (1990). The movement disorder of reflex sympathetic dystrophy. *Neurology, 40*, 57–61.

Schwartzman, R. J., & McLellan, T. L. (1987). Reflex sympathetic dystrophy: A review. *Archives of Neurology, 44*, 555–561.

Sherry, D. D., Wallace, C. A., Kelley, C., Kidder, M., & Sapp, L. (1999). Short- and long-term outcomes of children with complex regional pain syndrome type I treated with exercise therapy. *Clinical Journal of Pain, 15*, 218–223.

Stanton-Hicks, M., Baron, R., Boas, R., Gordh, T., Harden, N., Hendler, N., Koltzenburg, M., Raj, P., & Wilder, R. (1998). Complex regional pain syndromes: Guidelines for therapy. *Clinical Journal of Pain, 14*, 155–166.

Stanton-Hicks, M., Janig, W., Hassenbusch, S.,

Haddox, J. D., Boas, R., & Wilson, P. (1995). Reflex sympathetic dystrophy: Changing concepts and taxonomy. *Pain, 63*, 127–133.

Stanton-Hicks, M., Raj, P. P., & Racz, G. B. (1996). Use of regional anesthetics for diagnosis of reflex sympathetic dystrophy and sympathetically maintained pain: A critical evaluation. In W. Janig & M. Stanton-Hicks (Eds.), *Reflex sympathetic dystrophy: A reappraisal* (pp. 217–237). Seattle: IASP Press.

Sternbach, R. A. (1987). *Mastering pain: A twelve-step program for coping with chronic pain.* New York: Ballantine Books.

Subbarao, J., & Stillwell, G. K. (1981). Reflex sympathetic dystrophy syndrome of the upper extremity: Analysis of total outcome of management of 125 cases. *Archives of Physical Medicine and Rehabilitation, 62*, 549–554.

Thimineur, M., Sood, P., Kravitz, E., Gudin, J., & Kitaj, M. (1998). Central nervous system abnormalities in complex regional pain syndrome (CRPS): Clinical and quantitative evidence of medullary dysfunction. *Clinical Journal of Pain, 14*, 256–267.

Turk, D. C., Meichenbaum, D., & Genest, M. (1983). *Pain and behavioral medicine: A cognitive-behavioral perspective.* New York: Guilford Press.

Turk, D. C., Okifuji, A., Sinclair, J. D., & Starz, T. W. (1998). Differential responses by subgroups of fibromyalgia syndrome patients to an interdisciplinary treatment. *Arthritis Care and Research, 11*, 397–404.

Turk, D. C., & Rudy, T. E. (1990). Robustness of an empirically derived taxonomy of chronic pain patients. *Pain, 43*, 27–36.

van Hilten, B. J., van de Beeck, W.-J. T., Hoff, J. I., Voormolen, J. H. C., & Delhaas, E. M. (2000). Intrathecal baclofen for the treatment of dystonia in patients with reflex sympathetic dystrophy. *New England Journal of Medicine, 343*, 625–630.

Van Houdenhove, B., Vasquez, G., Onghena, P., Stans, L., Vandeput, C., Vermaut, G., Vervaeke, G., Igodt, P., & Vertommen H. (1992). Eiopathogeneis of reflex sympathetic dystrophy: A review and biopsychosocial hypothesis. *Clinical Journal of Pain, 82*, 300–306.

Veldman, P. H. J. M., Reynen, H. M., Arntz, I. E., & Goris, R. J. A. (1993). Signs and symptoms of reflex sympathetic dystrophy: Prospective study of 829 patients. *Lancet, 342*, 1012–1016.

Weissman, M., Markowitz, J. C., & Klerman, G. (2000). *Comprehensive guide to interpersonal psychotherapy.* New York: Basic Books.

Wilder, R. T. (1996). Reflex sympathetic dystrophy in children and adolescents: Differences from adults. In W. Janig & M. Stanton-Hicks (Eds.), *Reflex sympathetic dystrophy: A reappraisal* (pp. 67–77). Seattle, WA: IASP Press.

World Health Organization. (1978). *International classification of diseases ninth revision basic tabulation list with alphabetic index.* Geneva: Author.

24

Treating Patients with Noncardiac Chest Pain and Functional Gastrointestinal Pain Syndromes

Richard Mayou

General Principles

This chapter is concerned with some of the most common presenting problems in primary care and with their treatment in nonspecialist as well as specialist settings. It differs from most other chapters in this book in that it is substantially devoted to early treatment to minimize distress and disability and to prevent the misunderstandings and uncertainties that often exacerbate and maintain problems.

Epidemiology

The World Health Organization's international study of primary care found "unexplained" symptoms to be common, troublesome, and disabling in all countries and cultures they investigated. Up to half will remain disabled by the symptoms at 12-month follow-up. Outcome is worse for patients who go on to secondary and tertiary care (Simon, 2000). In primary care only a small proportion ever receive a specific physical diagnosis (Kroenke & Mangelsdorff, 1989). There is no evidence to support the validity of the many overlapping syndromes described by different specialties that show

marked national and cultural variation (Aaron & Buchwald, 2001; Wessely, Nimnuan, & Sharpe, 1999). However, operationally defined groupings (such as those discussed in this chapter) are useful in everyday clinical practice.

Etiology

In understanding management it is helpful to begin by considering etiology (Mayou, Bass, & Sharpe, 1995). Medically unexplained symptoms are often put down to either hidden physical or psychological causes, but this separation of mind and body causes is unhelpful; it is also generally unacceptable to patients. An alternative approach focuses on an interactive model in which physical, psychological, behavioral, and social factors all contribute to symptom formation. This approach suggests that unexplained symptoms arise from minor physiological or pathological bodily sensations that are perceived as symptoms of illness and then result in physical disability. The extent to which these bodily sensations are noticed and the *interpretation* that is placed on them depends on the understanding (attribution, cognitive interpretation) and mood of an individual patient. These factors include (1) personality, emotional distress; (2) illness experience, beliefs, and understanding; and (3) social circumstances.

Once established, symptoms may be maintained by cognitive, behavioral, emotional, or social variables. A patient perceiving family or doctors to be anxious or uncertain (e.g., through receiving contradictory or ambiguous advice) may experience further concern (Kouyanou, Pither, & Wessely, 1997). Inadequate medical care is a major cause of chronic disability.

Classification

We believe that in clinical practice it is best to take a multidimensional approach to describe the symptom or pattern of symptoms, underlying physical processes, and any associated psychiatric disorder (Mayou et al., 1995).

Treatment

Because of the heterogeneity of clinical presentation and course we propose a "stepped" approach to management (Mayou et al., 2000). This approach should provide simple reassurance and help to all newly consulting patients. Those who fail to improve should be offered more intensive assessment and treatment and the small proportion who do not respond to what is available in primary or secondary medical care may benefit from referral to psychologists or psychiatrists.

There is good evidence (O' Malley et al., 1999) that antidepressant medication is valuable when there are clear symptoms of depressive illness. They are also valuable for some pain syndromes whether or not depressive symptoms are prominent. Systematic reviews have concluded that cognitive-behavioral methods (Kroenke & Swindle, 2000; Morley, Eccleston, & Williams, 1999) can be effective in a wide range of syndromes. Other useful interventions include assistance in dealing with major personal family or social difficulties, involving a close relative in management.

NEWLY PRESENTING SYMPTOMS

Within a consultation (Table 24.1), the tasks include the need to define the reasons

TABLE 24.1. Principles of Assessment

- Appropriate physical investigation
- Identify patient's concerns and beliefs
- Review previous history of "unexplained" symptoms
- Questions about the ways in which patient reacts to and copes with symptoms
- Screening questions for psychiatric and social problems
- Consider interviewing relatives

for a patient's attendance (including the nature and history of the problem), to choose an appropriate action for the problem (Table 24.2), and to achieve a shared understanding of the problem (Price, 2000).

Establishing a shared model of the etiology of symptoms enables the patient to feel that the symptoms are being taken seriously—as real and deserving of medical attention. In this way it is possible to avoid an anxious, disabled patient being treated by a bewildered doctor.

SPECIALIST REFERRAL

There is a temptation to refer difficult patients to another specialist, but this can result in greater long-term difficulties without achieving an effective treatment plan. When there is a clear reason for further medical or psychiatric referral, a clear explanation to

TABLE 24.2. Principles of Treatment

General principles
- Consider symptoms as real and familiar
- Identify and treat psychiatric disorder
- Introduce significance of behavioral and psychological factors
- Provide explanation—including a credible linkage of behavioral and psychological factors with physical symptoms
- Offer opportunity for discussion of patient's and family's worries
- Provide practical advice on coping with symptoms
- Provide practical advice on return to normal activity

Specific treatments
- Discuss and agree treatment plan
- Follow up review

the patient and a clear referral letter are essential.

Components of Treatment

• *Investigation.* Examination and further medically indicated investigation are essential. Thereafter, further investigation or referral should be resisted, with explanation, unless there are specific indications.

• *Reassurance and explanation.* Most patients are reassured by being told that (1) their illness is common and (2) their doctor is familiar with it. However, such explanations increase anxiety if they do not address an individual's own personal unexpressed worries about underlying illnesses (Table 24.3).

• *Communication.* Misunderstandings between patients and their families and friends, and between doctors and others involved in treatment, frequently reinforce erroneous beliefs and maladaptive behavior. Discussion needs to be accompanied by written information for patients, relatives, and all those involved in care. It is often helpful to circulate the agreed treatment plan.

• *Specific psychological treatments.* A minority of patients need more than antidepressant medication or specific psychological treatment (Tables 24.4 and 24.5). The latter should aim at modifying beliefs, dealing with anxiety, and providing a graded return to normal activity. This may include discussion of how anxiety can increase vigilance for physical symptoms, which in turn generates further distress. Simple advice about inappropriate negative thoughts and controlling thoughts can be offered in combination with encouragement to use physical relaxation techniques.

TABLE 24.3. Effective Reassurance

• Accept reality of symptoms
• Explanation of causes
• Explain that symptoms are common, well recognized, and have a good prognosis
• Understand patient and family beliefs and worries
• Plan and agree simple self-help
• Provide written information and plans
• Offer to see the partner or other close relative
• Offer follow-up if required

TABLE 24.4. Nonspecialist Treatments

• Providing sympathetic treatment of underlying problems
• Agreeing to simple behavioral plans with patient and family
• Giving advice about anxiety management
• Encouraging the use of diaries
• Advising regarding graded increase in activities
• Suggesting antidepressant medication if clear depressive disorder
• Referring to self-help programs

Noncardiac Chest Pain

Epidemiology

Chest pain is frequent in the general population and is one of the most common reasons for consultation in primary care, with an estimated prevalence of approximately 12% in primary care. Symptoms are usually mild and have a transient course (Chambers, Bass, & Mayou, 1999). A minority present more clinical difficulty of two types: acute severe pain and persistent pain associated with distress and limitation (Potts & Bass, 1995).

Acute central chest pain accounts for 20–30% of emergency medical admissions; more chronic chest pain is the most common reason for referral to cardiac outpatient clinics. They pose one of the most important and difficult diagnostic problems in medicine—the recognition of ischemic heart disease (Lee & Goldman, 2000). At least half of those referred to cardiac outpatient clinics and around two-thirds of emergency admissions have a noncardiac cause of chest pain (Chambers et al., 1999). As few as 11–44% of patients referred for routine cardiac outpatient assessment have evidence of organic disease.

Unfortunately increasing emphasis on the diagnosis and early treatment of ischemic

TABLE 24.5. Specialist Treatments

• Anxiety management
• Cognitive therapy to modify beliefs
• Diary monitoring
• Program of graded increase in activity
• Antidepressant medication
• Illness-specific interventions (e.g., treating physical deconditioning in chronic fatigue)

heart disease has not been accompanied by similar advances either in longer-term care or in the management of the noncardiac causes of pain. Although these patients have a good outcome in terms of mortality, over two-thirds continue to report symptoms and many remain dissatisfied with their care. A proportion remain on cardiac medication and continue to attend emergency departments, primary care, and outpatient clinics. It is clinically desirable to make an early and confident diagnosis of noncardiac chest pain, because appropriate management in primary care is likely to have considerable benefits (Chambers et al., 1999).

Etiology

Unitary causal explanations are rarely helpful, and there is evidence of subtle interactions between (often multiple) physical, psychological, and social factors that often overlap (Cooke, Smeeton, & Chambers, 1997). In many cases there will be an interaction between physiological and minor pathological processes (Table 24.6) (e.g., extrasystoles, esophageal spasm or reflux, and costochondral discomfort), psychological factors (i.e., the way in which the somatic sensations are perceived, interpreted—or misinterpreted—and acted on), and the behavior and reactions of doctors and others (Thurston, Keefe, Bradley, Krishnan, & Caldwell, 2001). Once established, symptoms such as chest pain may be *maintained* by a variety of factors such as the patient's selective focusing on his or her heart, the reaction of friends and family, or the behavior of doctors—for example, inappropriate pre-

TABLE 24.6. Common Causes of Noncardiac Chest Pain

Esophageal disorders
- Gastroesophageal reflux
- Esophageal dysmotility

Musculoskeletal disorders
- Costochondritis
- Increased muscular tension

Referred pain from thoracic spine

Hyperventilation

Psychological disorders
- Panic attacks
- Depression

TABLE 24.7. Iatrogenic Factors Maintaining Noncardiac Symptoms and Disabilities

- Giving "probable angina" diagnosis before investigation
- Immediate prescription without explanation of possible causes before investigation
- Lack of explanation for distressing and continuing symptoms
- Inconsistent/ambiguous information
- Reassurance contradicted by continued antianginal medication or other indications of uncertainty
- Lack of communication with all involved in care leading to contradictory and conflicting advice

scribing of cardiac medication (Mayou, Bass, Hart, Tyndel, & Bryant, 2000) (Table 24.7).

Treatment

Symptomatic treatments—for example, for oesophageal spasm and reflux (Achem et al., 1997; Chambers, Cooke, Angiannsah, & Owen, 1998)—have an important role in the treatment of some patients; they rarely provide a complete cure for those who are anxious and who are worried about heart disease. Symptomatic treatment should be a part of a wider overall management plan. For patients with continuing symptoms and disability, often with coexisting psychological problems such as abnormal health beliefs, depressed mood, panic attacks, or other symptoms such as fatigue or palpitations, psychological or psychopharmacological treatments play a role (Thurston et al., 2001).

Selective serotonin reuptake inhibitors (SSRIs) have been shown to be effective in these patients (Varia et al., 2000) and tricyclic antidepressants are helpful in reducing reports of pain in patients with chest pain and normal coronary arteries (Achem et al., 1997; Cannon et al., 1994; Varia et al., 2000), especially if there are accompanying depressive symptoms.

Cognitive-behavioral therapy (CBT) is also effective (Chambers et al., 1999). Two studies have shown the effectiveness of specialist cognitive-behavioral techniques. The first (Klimes, Mayou, Pearce, Coles, & Fagg, 1990) was a study of 31 patients with persistent noncardiac chest pain refereed by general practitioners; the second replicated the findings within the setting of normal outpatient care (Mayou et al., 1997). In both trials the intervention groups had a substantially better outcome in terms of symptoms, mood, quality of life, and reduced concern about heart disease. Recently, similar findings have been reported in a randomized trial (Van Peski-Oosterbaan et al., 1999) and for a study of cognitive-behavioral treatment delivered on a group basis (Potts, Lewis, Fox, & Johnstone, 1999). However, a further evaluation (Sanders et al., 1997) of a brief intervention based on cognitive-behavioral principles immediately after negative coronary angiography was ineffective and was thought to be inappropriate and unacceptable by a significant proportion of patients.

It is apparent that recruitment for these trials was difficult in that some logical treatment was not seen as being required or acceptable. It is clearly necessary that the psychological treatment should be fully integrated with medical care, rather than seen as separate implying that symptoms are not cardiologically real (Mayou et al., 2000). A further recent study of patients referred to cardiologists and diagnosed as suffering from benign palpitation indicates that an early intervention by a cardiac nurse immediately after cardiological assessment is welcomed by patients and is also effective (Mayou, Sprigings, Birkhead, & Price, 2002).

Assessment

The key to establishing a positive diagnosis of noncardiac chest pain, in both primary care and the cardiac clinic, is to consider the pattern of chest pain symptoms and also address possible physical and psychosocial causes.

QUALITY OF CHEST PAIN

Recent attempts to determine whether certain chest pain clinical characteristics can help to establish a positive diagnosis of noncardiac chest pain (NCCP) have been encouraging. For example, three questions have been shown to help to differentiate patients with chest pain but normal coronary arteries from those with coronary heart disease (Chambers et al., 1999).

EVIDENCE FOR COMMON SPECIFIC CAUSES

Gastroesophageal reflux is an important cause of atypical chest pain, but there is no convincing evidence that chest pain of uncertain origin is often related to disturbances of esophageal motility (Wu, Cooke, Anggiansah, Owen, & Chambers, 2000).

Only a minority of patients who present to family doctors with NCCP are suffering from conspicuous anxiety or depressive disorders (Chambers et al., 1999), although rates are higher among those referred for specialist assessment. Nevertheless, it is important to identify depression, panic, and phobic anxiety.

PATIENT BELIEFS AND WORRIES

Even if there is no formal psychiatric illness, it is essential to ask about the patient's *thoughts* when the patient presents with chest pain, because during an episode of chest pain patients with coronary heart disease are *less* likely to report frightening thoughts, and if they do, these are rarely the predominant experience. Patients with panic attacks, however, frequently have frightening thoughts that usually predominate during the chest pain.

STRESSFUL LIFE EVENTS

Distressing life events can precipitate not only anxiety and depressive disorders but also medically unexplained symptoms. Events signifying loss, threat, and rejection are of particular importance. Open questions are useful (e.g., "Tell me about any changes or setbacks that occurred in the months before your chest pain began").

Management

The need for early and effective intervention is crucial, but how should this best be provided? Because patients vary not only in the terms of the frequency and severity of symptoms and associated disability but also in their needs for explanation and treatment of their physical and psychological problems, management needs to be *flexible* (Mayou,

TABLE 24.8. Assessment and Early
Management in Primary Care of
Noncardiac Chest Pain

History of pain and other symptoms; risk factors

If high risk of ischemic heart disease, refer for
specialist assessment

If low risk:
- Identify noncardiac causes
- Give explanation
- Advise regarding coping with symptoms
  and return to normal activity
- Discuss worries
- Offer review if persistent

Bass, & Bryant, 1999) (Tables 24.8 and
24.9).

- *Patients with a low risk of coronary
disease* (e.g., young, female with no cardiac
risk factors) and atypical pain do not usually need cardiac investigation. Many patients, especially those with family histories
of heart disease or obvious risk factors, are
concerned that they have heart disease.
There is a need for clear explanation of the
noncardiac cause, together with advice
about coping with symptoms and maintaining activities. Worries should be discussed.

- *Patients with an intermediate or high
risk* (e.g., middle-age male who smokes)
should normally have noninvasive investigations even if the chest pain is "not typical" of ischemic pain. This will usually require referral to a cardiology outpatient

TABLE 24.9. Management of Noncardiac
Chest Pain

Initial
- Explanation of the diagnosis
- Reassurance that it is a real, common, and
  well-recognized problem
- Advice on any specific treatment
- Advice on behavior (e.g., do not avoid
  exercise)
- Discussion of concerns
- Written and audiovisual information
- Information and discussion with relatives

Follow-up review

Specialist treatments
- Cognitive-behavioral therapy
- Antidepressant medication
- Psychosocial intervention for associated
  psychological family and social difficulties

clinic or an emergency assessment. When referring patients, it is important to indicate
that there are many causes of chest pain and
to avoid prescribing treatments in a manner
that appears to confirm a cardiac diagnosis.

- *Avoiding iatrogenic worries.* Consultation for chest pain is worrisome, and inevitably many patients assume that they
have severe heart disease, which is likely to
have a major adverse effect on their life.
These concerns may be greatly increased by
delays in investigation, comments, or behaviors by doctors, which inadvertently appear to reinforce beliefs about heart disease,
and by contradictory and inconsistent comments (Mayou et al., 2000).

- *Effective reassurance.* Those with mild
symptoms or symptoms of shorter duration
may improve following negative investigation and simple reassurance. Further hospital attendance may be unnecessary. Others
with more severe symptoms and illness concerns would benefit from a follow-up visit
4–6 weeks after the cardiac clinic visit (or
emergency room visit).

- *Symptomatic treatment.* In some patients obvious musculoskeletal problems
can be treated—for example, with nonsteroidal anti-inflammatory agents. Proton-
pump inhibitors are effective in providing
relief of the symptoms typical of gastroesophageal reflux, even in those with an essentially normal esophageal mucosa (Chambers et al., 1998). In some cases esophageal
function testing may reveal a motility disorder or acid reflux unresponsive to first-line
medication. These may require specialist
gastroenterological referral.

- *Communication.* Problems in the care
of both angina and noncardiac chest pain
often arise from failures in communication
between primary and secondary care. The
increasing use of computerized exchange of
key information is part of the answer (Ray
et al., 1998).

Specialist Treatments

Antidepressant medication is valuable when
symptoms of major depression are prominent; otherwise cognitive-behavioral treatment is to be preferred. Table 24.10 shows
the main components of such treatment,
which usually requires between 4 and 10
sessions.

TABLE 24.10. Cognitive-Behavioral Treatment of Noncardiac Chest Pain

1. Functional analysis of complaints, an explanation of the rationale for psychological treatment, an introduction to progressive muscular relaxation.
2. Discuss the role of breathing; forced voluntary breathing to demonstrate how easily "real" unpleasant sensations can be induced; learning of slow-paced breathing control.
3. An introduction to distraction (focusing attention away from symptoms and associated worry) and to monitoring the relationship between chest pain and physical activity.
4. Learn to apply skills (relaxation, slow-paced breathing, and distraction) and to monitor effects on pain.
5. Review and management of any maintaining factors (e.g., morbid health beliefs). Use of exposure to counteract avoidance of exertion, response prevention methods to counterchecking (e.g., repeated pulse taking) and other reassurance-seeking behaviors, pacing activities to control unrealistic expectations, cognitive challenge of any persistent beliefs about organic illness, and problem solving of social problems.

Functional Gastrointestinal Pain

In primary care about half of patients presenting with gastrointestinal pain have functional disorders (Table 24.11). The most common is irritable bowel syndrome (IBS), which is the subject of the remainder of this chapter. Similar general principles apply to the management of other functional disorders—for example, dyspepsia (Bytzer & Talley, 2001)—although there has been considerably less research on etiology or management. IBS is a disorder producing abdominal pain, bloating, and disturbances of bowel function. Lack of diagnostic precision, uncertainties about etiology, and the absence of specific treatments have caused considerable difficulties to developing effective clinical care. Clinical practice and research are based on symptom-based criteria developed from epidemiological study, the best known being the Rome criteria for IBS and other functional disorders.

Epidemiology

Evidence from the United States and Britain indicates that IBS is prevalent at 14–24% among women and 5–19% among men. First presentation is usually between 30 and 50 years and prevalence decreases after the age of 60. The course is characteristically fluctuating (Drossman, Whitehead, & Camilleri, 1997; Goldberg & Davidson, 1997).

Up to 70% of people with IBS symptoms do not seek medical attention, and consultation appears to be affected by cultural practice, the severity of the symptoms, and evidence of psychological disturbance. Only a minority of those who consult in primary care are referred to gastroenterology specialists (Thompson, Heaton, Smyth, & Smyth, 2000). However, IBS is the commonest disorder seen in specialist gastroenterology practice. In a U.S. survey, functional disorders as a whole accounted for 35% of attenders, of which most (19%) were IBS (Russo, Gaynes, & Drossman, 1999).

Prevalence of psychological disorder varies according to the treatment setting. In the general population and general practice it is about 10–20%, similar to general population rates. In the specialist outpatient setting it is between 30 and 40% and is even higher for patients with chronic "treatment-resistant" symptoms. A number of studies have reported high rates of adverse previous events, including sexual and emotional

TABLE 24.11. Functional Gastrointestinal Disorders

- Functional dyspepsia
  Ulcer-like dyspepsia
  Dysmotility-like dyspepsia
  Unspecified dyspepsia
- Irritable bowel syndrome
- Functional abdominal bloating
- Functional constipation
- Functional diarrhea
- Unspecified functional bowel disorder
- Functional abdominal pain syndrome
- Unspecified functional abdominal pain syndrome

abuse in early life (Drossman et al., 1997; Katon, Sullivan, & Walker, 2001). Abdominal pain in childhood can be a precursor to adult IBS (Hotopf, Carr, Mayou, Wadsworth, & Wessely, 1998; Walker, Guite, Duke, Barnard, & Greene, 1998).

Patients with IBS symptoms are more likely to report other symptoms and consult about them than those without bowel symptoms. The small minority of subjects who are frequent attenders with complaints of IBS are more likely to consult for a wide range of other unexplained symptoms, such as fatigue and gynecological complaints (Bass, Bond, Gill, & Sharpe, 1999). There is considerable overlap with other functional syndromes such as chronic fatigue syndrome and fibromyalgia.

Etiology

No specific pathophysiological basis is evident, but a variety of physiological processes that are also associated with abdominal pain in those without IBS have been identified (Drossman et al., 1997; Goldberg & Davidson, 1997; Horwitz & Fisher, 2001; Ringel & Drossman, 1999). These include abnormal bowel motility, enhanced visceral sensitivity, autonomic dysfunction, and central nervous system modulation.

The interaction of peripheral and central neuromuscular mechanisms conflicts and clearly interacts with psychological and behavioral factors, which include exacerbation of symptoms at times of stress, importance of beliefs, and variations in illness behavior.

Treatment

MEDICAL TREATMENTS

Systematic review suggests that a number of widely used physical treatments are beneficial in providing symptomatic relief. These treatments include muscle relaxants for abdominal pain and loperamide for diarrhoea (Horowitz & Fisher, 2001; Jailwala, Imeriale, & Kroenke, 2000)

PSYCHOLOGICAL TREATMENT

It is difficult to design and carry out high-quality randomized controlled trials as patients cannot be blinded to the treatment

they are receiving and because of the wide differences in psychological disorder between patients in different treatment settings (Talley, Owen, Boyce, & Paterson, 1996). Studies should be considered according to whether the patients are recruited from—primary care or outpatient clinics—or were focused upon treatment-resistant patients. The most convincing evidence for the efficacy of psychological treatments is for patients with chronic pain or abdominal symptoms.

Blanchard (2001) has reviewed psychological treatments of several types: Brief psychodynamic psychotherapy (Guthrie, Creed, Dawson, & Tomenson, 1991), hypnotherapy (Whorwell, Prior, & Faragher, 1984), cognitive-behavioral treatment, and biofeedback. He concludes that there is strong evidence for brief psychodynamic psychotherapy and hypnotherapy and less methodologically impressive but more cumulatively persuasive evidence for various CBT treatments (Blanchard, 2001; Toner et al., 1998).

ANTIDEPRESSANT MEDICATION

Antidepressant medication is indicated when there is clear evidence of a depressive disorder, but there is also evidence that antidepressants may help to reduce pain in the absence of significant overt psychopathology. The best evidence is for tricyclic antidepressants, as there have been few studies that have evaluated newer antidepressants (Jailwala et al., 2000).

Assessment

Assessment follows the general principles discussed in earlier sections of this chapter and is summarized in Table 24.12. Blanchard (2001) provides detailed information about the procedures and instruments used in the extensive research to develop effective psychological treatment.

Clinical Management

Treatment should be positive and reassuring and should provide an explanation and advice and meet patients' individual needs (Blanchard, 2001; Drossman, 1995; Drossman et al., 1997). Treatment follows a

TABLE 24.12. Assessment of Functional Gastrointestinal Pain

- Is the pain acute or chronic?
- Is there a pain history?
- Is the pain associated with disturbed physiology?
- What is the patient's understanding of the illness?
- Does the patient accept that stress may play a role?
- Is there abnormal illness behavior?
- What is the family's involvement?
- How does the disorder affect daily function?
- What is the reason for the consultation?
- Is there a concurrent psychiatric diagnosis?
- Is there a history of psychological trauma?
- What are the patient's psychosocial resources?

Note. Data from Drossman (1995); Drossman et al. (1997); and Guthrie and Thompson (2001).

stepped and multidisciplinary approach as outlined by Drossman (1995) and by Guthrie and Thompson (in press). Tables 24.13 and 24.14 summarize these approaches.

An adequate first stage of treatment depends on setting aside adequate time so that there is no feeling of rush and there is an opportunity to deal with the patient's concerns. Investigations are limited to those indicated by the history and examination. The discussion of the explanation of the symptoms includes discussion of physiological and psychological factors and emphasizes the role the patient can play in relieving the pain and disability by participating in agreed-on strategies or exercise. It may be helpful to encourage membership in a self-help group.

Treatment should be consistent and needs to allow for repeated requests for explanation and queries about the management approach. It is sensible to emphasize that the main goals of treatment are improved function and decreased disability rather than

TABLE 24.13. Primary Care of Functional Gastrointestinal Pain

- Explain and advise
- Reassure regarding cancer, stressors, etc.
- Explain exacerbation by psychological factors
- Treat depression
- Refer if symptoms persistent or atypical

TABLE 24.14. Specialist Care of Functional Gastrointestinal Pain

- Detailed assessment
- Limited investigation
- Clear explanation
- Standardized medical care
- Consideration of psychological treatment if no improvement
- Consideration of antidepressant medication

complete abolition of symptoms. The combination of such general measures with widely accepted more specific medical care is effective in a high proportion of cases. It is clinical experience that over 70% of patients with IBS who are referred for secondary care experience improvement in their symptoms or are able to cope with them better.

Management of more persistent problems can be improved by incorporating brief psychological management strategies and by giving further attention to patients' understanding of these symptoms and particularly to their fears about cancer. It may be possible for the physician or a nurse colleague to incorporate simple psychological treatments into management in the gastroenterolgy clinic. This is especially so if there is access to a consultation–liaison psychiatrist or to a psychologist who has special experience with these problems and who can advise on less demanding forms of treatment.

Each of the four main psychological treatment approaches—cognitive therapies, behavioral therapies, interpersonal therapies, and hypnotherapies—can be standardized using treatment protocols (Blanchard, 2001). Most are delivered on a one-to-one basis, once weekly, over a period of 8 to 16 weeks. Tables 24.15 and 24.16 summarize the key elements of cognitive-behavioral and interpersonal therapies, respectively.

Antidepressant treatment should be considered if there is clear evidence of depressive disorder. There is also evidence that antidepressants may help to reduce pain in the absence of depression.

Patients with Chronic Symptoms

Patients who are severely disabled by chronic abdominal pain and other IBS symptoms

TABLE 24.15. Cognitive-Behavioral Therapy of Functional Gastrointestinal Pain

1. Diaries to monitor pain and other symptoms and associated thoughts and behavior.
2. Identify underlying beliefs or fears about the pain.
3. Therapeutic work is directed at:
   a. Self-understanding (in which subjects explore idiosyncratic beliefs and fears and their relation to their pain).
   b. Decentering (in which subjects gain distance from their selves and identify their repetitive, instinctive thoughts).
   c. Disconfirmation experiments in which patients challenge their fears or irrational beliefs.
4. Graded experience in leisure, social, and physical activities.
5. Educational packages to increase understanding of the condition.
6. Progressive muscle relaxation and anxiety management strategies.

are unlikely to respond to simpler psychological interventions, whatever form they take. More intensive treatments have been devised for use in day, or even inpatient, settings over a period of weeks or months (Table 24.17). These interventions are difficult to evaluate; the particular components vary from one center to another, but most

TABLE 24.16. Interpersonal Therapies for Functional Gastrointestinal Pain

- Focus on resolving difficulties or problems in interpersonal relationships, which underlie or exacerbate abdominal symptoms.
- Key problem areas include unresolved grief or loss, role transitions, and relationship discord.
- Initial focus on the person's abdominal symptoms, which are explored in great detail.
- Identification of emotional distress and abnormal feelings or linked to physical symptoms.
- Understanding key problem areas in relationships and their link to physical and psychological symptoms.
- Identification of maladaptive relationship patterns that may have developed following key childhood experiences (e.g., childhood sexual abuse).
- Solutions to interpersonal difficulties are tested out in the therapy and implemented in

TABLE 24.17. Treatment of Patients with Chronic Abdominal Pain

- Collaborative care
- Extended cognitive-behavioral therapy
- Treatment of associated psychiatric disorders and social problems
- Consideration of interpersonal therapy

are based on cognitive-behavioral principles together with a variety of other strategies, including family and cultural interventions. Pain programs can also be involved in significant improvement in physical and work activity and reductions in analgesic consumption.

Conclusion

In this chapter I have emphasized the need for small changes in everyday practice in primary care and in specialist cardiology and gastroenterology practice to make initial medical assessment more effective as treatment, together with early recognition of more severe and persistent problems that require more intensive intervention. Such changes in delivery could be cost-effective and could mean that specialist psychological and psychiatric expertise can be directed to the management of a small minority of patients as well as to the training and supervision of nonspecialists. In the most complicated cases, adaptation of the procedures described in other chapters of this book will be necessary.

References

Aaron, L. A., & Buchwald, D. (2001). A review of the evidence for overlap among unexplained clinical conditions. *Annals of Internal Medicine, 134,* 868–881.

Achem, S. R., Kolts, B. E., MacMath, T., Richter, J., Mohr, D., Burton, L., & Castell, D. O. (1997). Effects of omeprazole versus placebo in treatment of noncardiac chest pain and gastroesophageal reflux. *Digestive Diseases and Sciences, 42,* 2138–2145.

Bass, C., Bond, A., Gill, D., & Sharpe, M. (1999). Frequent attenders without organic disease in a gastroenterology clinic. Patient characteristics and health care use. *General Hospital Psychiatry, 21,* 30–38.

Blanchard, E. B. (2001). *Irritable bowel syndrome.*

Psychosocial assessment and treatment. Washington, DC: American Psychological Association.

Bytzer, P., & Talley, N. J. (2001). Investigating selected symptoms: Dyspepsia. *Annals of Internal Medicine, 134*, 815–822.

Cannon, R. O., Quyyumi, A. A., Mincemoyer, R., Stine, A. M., Gracely, R. H., Smith, W. B., Geraci, M. F., Black, B. C., Uhde, T. W., Waclawiw, M. A., Maher, K., & Benjamin, S. B. (1994). Imipramine in patients with chest pain despite normal coronary angiograms. *New England Journal of Medicine, 330*, 1411–1417.

Chambers, J., Bass, C., & Mayou, R. (1999). Editorial. Non-cardiac chest pain: Assessment and management. *Heart, 82*, 656–657.

Chambers, J., Cooke, R., Angiannsah, A., & Owen, W. (1998). Beneficial effects of omeprazole in patients with chest pain and normal coronary anatomy: Preliminary findings. *International Journal of Cardiology, 65*, 51–55.

Cooke, R. A., Smeeton, N., & Chambers, J. B. (1997). A comparative study of chest pain characteristics in patients with normal and abnormal coronary angiograms. *Heart, 78*, 142–146.

Drossman, D. A. (1995). Diagnosing and treating patients with refractory functional gastrointestinal disorders. *Annals of Internal Medicine, 123*, 688–697.

Drossman, D. A., Whitehead, W. E., & Camilleri, M. (1997). Irritable bowel syndrome: A technical review for practice guideline development. *American Gastroenterological Association, 112*, 2120–2137.

Goldberg, J., & Davidson, P. (1997). A biopsychosocial understanding of the irritable bowel syndrome: A review. *Canadian Journal of Psychiatry, 42*, 835–40.

Guthrie, E., Creed, F., Dawson, D., & Tomenson, B. (1991). A randomized controlled trial of psychotherapy in patients with refractory irritable bowel syndrome. *Gastroenterology, 100*, 450–457.

Guthrie, E., & Thompson, D. (in press). Psychological management of patients with abdominal pain. *British Medical Journal*.

Horowitz, B.J., & Fisher, R.S. (2001). The irritable bowel syndrome. *New England Journal of Medicine, 344*, 1846–1850.

Hotopf, M., Carr, S., Mayou, R., Wadsworth, M., & Wessely, S. (1998). Why do children have chronic abdominal pain, and what happens to them when they grow up? Population based cohort study. *British Medical Journal, 316*, 1196–1200.

Jailwala, J., Imeriale, T. F., & Kroenke, K. (2000). Pharmacologic treatment of the irritable bowel syndrome: A systematic review of randomized, controlled trials. *Annals of Internal Medicine, 133*, 136–147.

Katon, W., Sullivan, M., & Walker, E. (2001). Medical symptoms without identified pathology: Relationship to psychiatric disorders, childhood and adult trauma, and personality traits. *Annals of Internal Medicine, 134*, 917–25.

Klimes, I., Mayou, R. A., Pearce, M. J., Coles, L., & Fagg, J. R. (1990). Psychological treatment for atypical non-cardiac chest pain: A controlled evaluation. *Psychological Medicine, 20*, 605–611.

Kouyanou, K., Pither, C. E., & Wessely, S. (1997). Iatrogenic factors and chronic pain. *Psychosomatic Medicine, 59*, 597–604.

Kroenke, K., & Mangelsdorff, D. (1989). Common symptoms in ambulatory care: Incidence, evaluation, therapy and outcome. *American Journal of Medicine, 86*, 262–266.

Kroenke, K., & Swindle, R. (2000). Cognitive-behavioral therapy for somatization and symptom syndromes: A critical review of controlled clinical trials. *Psychotherapy and Psychosomatics, 69*, 205–215.

Lee, T. H., & Goldman, L. (2000). Evaluation of the patient with acute chest pain. *New England Journal of Medicine, 342*, 1187–1195.

Mayou, R., Bass, C., & Bryant, B. (1999). Management of non-cardiac chest pain: From research to clinical practice. *Heart, 81*, 387–392.

Mayou, R. A., Bass, C., Hart, G., Tyndel, S., & Bryant, B. (2000). Can clinical assessment of chest pain be made more therapeutic? *Quarterly Journal of Medicine, 93*, 805–811.

Mayou, R., Bass, C., & Sharpe, M. (1995). *Treatment of functional somatic symptoms*. Oxford, UK: Oxford University Press.

Mayou, R., Bryant, B., Sanders, D., Bass, C., Klimes, I., & Forfar, C. (1997). A controlled trial of cognitive behavioural therapy for non-cardiac chest pain. *Psychological Medicine, 27*, 1021–1032.

Mayou, R., Sprigings, D., Birkhead, J., & Price, J. (2002). A randomized controlled trail of a brief educational and psychological intervention for patients presenting to a cardiac clinic with palpitation. *Psychological Medicine, 32*, 699–706.

Morley, S., Eccleston, C., & Williams, A. (1999). Systematic review and meta-analysis of randomized controlled trials of cognitive-behaviour therapy and behaviour therapy for chronic pain in adults, excluding headache. *Pain, 80*, 1–13.

O'Malley, P. G., Jackson, J. L., Santoro, J., Tomkins, G., Balden, E., & Kroenke, K. (1999). Antidepressant therapy for unexplained symptoms and symptom syndromes. *Journal of Family Practice, 48*, 980–90.

Potts, S. G., & Bass, C. M. (1995). Psychological morbidity in patients with chest pain and normal or near-normal coronary arteries: A long-term follow- up study. *Psychological Medicine, 25*, 339–347.

Potts, S. G., Lewin, R., Fox, K. A. A., & Johnstone, E.C. (1999). Group psychological treatment for chest pain with normal coronary arteries. *Quarterly Journal of Medicine, 92*, 81–56.

Price, J. R. (2000). Managing physical symptoms: The clinical assessment as treatment. *Journal of Psychosomatic Research, 48*, 1–10.

Ray, S., Archbold, R. A., Preston, S., Ranjadayalan, K., Suliman, A., & Timmis, A. D. (1998). Computer-generated correspondence for patients attending an open-access chest pain clinic. *Journal of Royal College of Physicians, 32*, 420–421.

Ringel, Y., & Drossman, D. A. (1999). From gut to

brain and back—a new perspective into functional gastrointestinal disorders. *Journal of Psychosomatic Research, 47,* 205–10.

Russo, M. W., Gaynes, B. N., & Drossman, D. A. (1999). A national survey of practice patterns of gastroenterologists with comparison to the past two decades. *Journal of Clinical Gastroenterology, 29,* 339–343.

Sanders, D., Bass, C., Mayou, R., Goodwin, S., Bryant, B., & Tyndel, S. (1997). Non-cardiac chest pain: Why was a brief intervention apparently ineffective? *Psychological Medicine, 27,* 1033–1040.

Simon, G. (2000). Epidemiology of somatoform disorders and other causes of unexplained medical symptoms. In M. G. Gelder, J. J. Lopez-Ibor, & N. Andreasen (Eds.), *New Oxford textbook of psychiatry* (pp. 1076–1080). Oxford, UK: Oxford University Press.

Talley, N. J., Owen, B. K. O., Boyce, P., & Paterson, K. (1996). Psychological treatments for irritable bowel syndrome: A critique of controlled treatment trials. *American Journal of Gastroenterology, 91,* 277–286.

Thompson, W. G., Heaton, K. W., Smyth, G. T., & Smyth, C. (2000). Irritable bowel syndrome in general practice: Prevalence, characteristics, and referral. *Gut, 46,* 78–82.

Thurston, R. C., Keefe, F. J., Bradley, L., Krishnan, K. R. R., & Caldwell, D. S. (2001). Chest pain in the absence of coronary artery disease: A biopsychosocial perspective. *Pain, 93,* 95–100.

Toner, B. B., Segal, Z. V., Emmott, S., Myran, D.,

Ali, A., Digasbarro, J., & Stuckless, N. (1998). Cognitive behavioural group therapy for patients with irritable bowel syndrome. *International Journal of Group Psychotherapy, 48,* 215–243.

Van Peski-Oosterbaan, A. S., Spinhoven, P., van Rood, Y., Van der Does, J.W., Bruschke, A. V., & Rooijmans, H.G. (1999). Cognitive-behavioural therapy for noncardiac chest pain: A randomized trial. *American Journal of Medicine, 106,* 424–429.

Varia, I., Logue, E., O'connor, C., Newby, K., Wagner, H. R., Davenport, C., Rathey, K., & Krishnan, K. R. (2000). Randomized trial of sertraline in patients with unexplained chest pain of noncardiac origin. *American Heart Journal, 140,* 367–372.

Walker, L. S., Guite, J. W., Duke, M., Barnard, J. A., & Greene, J. W. (1998). Recurrent abdominal pain: A potential precursor of irritable bowel syndrome in adolescents and young adults. *Journal of Pediatrics, 132,* 1010–1015.

Wessely, S., Nimnuan, C., & Sharpe, M. (1999). Functional somatic symptoms; one or many? *Lancet, 354,* 936–939.

Whorwell, P. J., Prior, A., & Faragher, E. B. (1984). Controlled trial of hypnotherapy in the treatment of severe refractory irritable bowel syndrome. *Lancet, 2,* 1232–1244.

Wu, E. B., Cooke, R., Anggiansah, A., Owen, W., & Chambers, J.B. (2000). Are oesophageal disorders a common cause of chest pain despite normal coronary anatomy? *Quarterly Journal of Medicine, 93,* 543–550.

25

Treating Pain in Cancer Patients

Paul Crichton
Stirling Moorey

Pain is a significant and common problem in patients with cancer, especially those with advanced disease. Patients who are afraid of dying frequently turn out, on closer questioning, to be afraid of dying *in great pain*. Uncontrolled pain is also a factor that increases suicide risk in patients with cancer. The prevalence of pain varies in different types of cancer, with relatively little pain reported by patients with leukemia compared with cancers affecting internal organs, especially the lungs, gastrointestinal, and genitourinary tracts. Patients with bone involvement and cervical cancer have the highest prevalence of pain (Breitbart & Payne, 1998).

Pain can also occur as a consequence of treatment. Surgery can lead to pain because of damage to tissue directly affected by the operation or by the indirect consequences of surgery (e.g., lymphoedema in the arm after ipsilateral breast surgery and lymphadenectomy). Chemotherapy can cause pain (e.g., peripheral neuropathy with vincristine). Radiotherapy can also result in pain if it damages nerves (e.g., fibrosis of the bracchial plexus), although of course it is often useful in reducing certain kinds of pain (e.g., pain caused by vertebral metastases) (Breitbart & Payne, 1998).

Multifactorial Model of Pain in Cancer

A multifactorial model of pain stresses the interaction between physical, emotional, cognitive, behavioral, and interpersonal responses to internal and environmental stress.

Emotions and Pain

More than perhaps any other sensory system, pain has an emotional quality. Emotional distress can be a consequence of pain, a cause of pain, or a concurrent problem with independent sources (Craig, 1994). In chronic pain, which is more common in cancer, it may be that the majority of emotional disturbances are caused by pain rather than the other way round (Gamsa, 1990). Anxiety can exacerbate pain through the effect of increased autonomic nervous system activity on muscle tension, vasoconstriction, and gastrointestinal motility. Depression is also associated with pain. Derogatis and colleagues (1983) found that 39% of patients who received a psychiatric diagnosis, usually adjustment disorder or major depression, had significant pain, compared with 19% of those who did not receive a psychiatric diagnosis. A recent study found that cancer patients who are depressed are more likely to report pain than those who are not depressed (Ciaramella & Poli, 2001). In patients with advanced cancer, emotional disturbance has been associated with increased pain (Bond & Pearson, 1969; McKegney, Bailey, & Yates, 1981). Syrjala and Chapko (1995) found in a prospective study that maladaptive coping strategies, lower levels of self-efficacy, and distress caused by the treatment or disease progression were predictive of pain intensity. Conversely, positive emotional states can diminish pain (see "Special Considerations in the Psychological Management of Cancer Pain" section).

Cognition and Pain

Cognitive factors have a strong influence on how pain is experienced and interpreted and may mediate between mood and pain. Maxwell, Gatchel, and Mayer (1998) examined the interaction between depression, pain, and disability and three cognitive factors (cognitive distortion, perception of control over symptoms, and interference with activities). When these three variables were held constant, pain and disability did not have a significant association with reported depression. Cognitive distortions are biases in our thinking that lead us to misinterpret or skew information about ourselves, the world, or other people.

One significant cognitive distortion shown to be associated with pain is catastrophizing. "Catastrophizing" is the tendency to assume that the most pessimistic outcome is the most likely to occur. It has been associated with pain in rheumatoid arthritis (Keefe, Brown, Wallston, & Caldwell, 1989) and the tendency to experience more intense pain following a variety of surgical procedures (Butler, Damarin, Beaulieu, Schwebel, & Thorn, 1989). Women who are undergoing surgery for breast cancer experience more pain postoperatively and require more analgesia if they catastrophize (Jacobsen & Butler, 1996). In cancer, the thought that pain may signify disease progression is present in 61% of patients (Ahles, Ruckdeschel, & Blanchard, 1984). Spiegel and Bloom (1983) reported that women with breast cancer were likely to ex-

perience their pain as more severe if they thought that it was caused by spread of their cancer and if they were depressed. Conversely, Daut and Cleeland (1983) demonstrated that patients with cancer were less likely to report that pain interfered with pleasurable activities if they thought the pain was caused by something unrelated to their cancer rather than if they thought that it was caused by disease progression. Catastrophizing is therefore an important reaction to cancer pain. The assumption that pain inevitably means the cancer is worsening closes off other possible outcomes and makes the person feel helpless and hopeless.

Perceived control is a second important cognitive factor. Patients who have adopted a fatalistic attitude toward their lives in general are more likely to adopt maladaptive strategies for coping with their pain and report greater psychological distress than those who feel they can exert greater control over their lives (Crisson & Keefe, 1998). A third cognitive factor is perceived interference with activities. The extent to which a patient believes that cancer interferes with his or her ability to get on with life has a marked effect on coping with pain. Turk and colleagues (1998) found that cancer patients experiencing difficulties in coping with pain were more likely to report that it significantly interfered with their activities compared to patients who were experiencing pain but coping more effectively. From a cognitive perspective it is not the pain itself but the meaning of the pain that determines how we adjust to it. Pain is not a neutral sensation but may be associated with anger if there is a sense that it is unjust, or may be associated with guilt. Both adults and children sometimes experience guilt about their pain and interpret it as punishment (Eisendrath, Way, Ostroff, & Johanson, 1986; Gaffney & Dunne, 1987).

The meaning given to pain will influence the extent to which we attend to or ignore it. Selective attention refers to the degree to which we focus on painful sensations. If pain signifies disease progression, it is likely we will notice any twinge or ache. Once this becomes the focus of attention the sensation can become magnified, creating a vicious circle of pain and catastrophic thinking. The thresholds for a stimulus to be perceived as painful vary enormously from person to person depending on the importance given to the perception. They also vary from one time to another within the same individual and from one part of the body to another within people (compare the effect of a grain of sand below an eyelid and thousands of grains of sand beneath one's feet) (Hendry, 1999).

Behavioral Factors and Pain

What we do when in pain can have a profound effect on our experience of pain. Fear of pain or of making the physical disability worse can lead to avoidance of exercise or activity of any kind (Asmundsen, 1999). Again a vicious circle is created in which inactivity allows more time for focusing on pain and thinking negatively about it. As the patient does less, the consequent deconditioning may mean that when exercise is attempted it causes more pain and so confirms the belief that it is safer not to do things because being active only causes more suffering.

Social Factors and Pain

Social factors have a significant influence on pain experience. This influence can be understood from a developmental perspective (Craig, 1994). Newborn babies cry and grimace with pain, which can be seen as a reflex with social communication value on which, as the baby grows up, social influences are superimposed. Thus, children and adults who have witnessed others exposed to intense and persistent pain may themselves come to exhibit abnormal pain behavior. In the context of cancer, this exposure may be the experience of seeing a relative slowly dying of cancer in considerable pain. When patients behave in ways that communicate their pain to their family, for example, through sighing, groaning, and grimacing, they may be treated in overly supportive ways that reinforce their sense of vulnerability and dependence. Conversely, lack of social support can exacerbate pain. Turk and Rudy (1990) found that patients with chronic pain who perceived their family and friends as unsupportive suffered emotional distress as a consequence.

Environmental Factors and Pain

Stressful events can increase and prolong pain and reduce the ability to tolerate pain (Sternbach, 1974; Weisenberg, 1977). Stressors can range from the trauma of divorce or bereavement to daily "hassles" at work and at home (Sternbach, 1986). Patients with cancer are often exposed to stressors (e.g., looking after young children while having to attend frequent hospital appointments).

Physical Factors and Pain

Physical treatments of pain will have an impact at the level of pain receptors and perhaps at other levels of the sensory system, but this impact can be mediated by nonphysical factors, such as expectations from the specific type of physical treatment and/or previous experience of it (Melzack & Wall, 1965). Psychotropic drugs, such as antidepressants, may influence pain receptors directly, but may also have an indirect effect on pain by improving depressed mood. Psychological treatments of pain may influence the cognition and mood of the sufferer and hence both the perception of and the reaction to pain.

A related concept to that of pain is suffering, which can be regarded as a negative response induced not only by pain but by anxiety, depression, the loss of loved ones, and other psychological stressors of various kinds. Thus not all suffering is caused by pain, but in a medicalized culture, such as our own, it is often described in the language of pain (Loeser & Melzack, 1999). Cassell (1982) has remarked that suffering occurs when the physical or psychological integrity of the person is threatened. It is arguable that the stigma still associated with cancer increases suffering.

Pain and Suicide in Patients with Cancer

Fear of pain and a painful death is common in patients with cancer. In some cases this fear may be related to the experience of seeing friends or relatives who were not given adequate pain control decades ago when modern analgesics were not available or in circumstances in which care of patients with cancer was generally inadequate. Severe pain that is difficult to control has, it is hoped, become less common today but still occurs, and when it does, it probably increases the risk of suicide. A number of studies have reported that most patients who committed suicide had inadequately controlled, severe pain (Hietanen, Lonnquist, Henriksson, & Jallinoja, 1994; Massie, Gagnon, & Holland, 1994; Owen, Tenant, Levi, & Jones, 1992). This has been found in other studies. Although only a small percentage of patients with cancer commit suicide, the incidence is higher than in the general population (Bolund, 1985; Farberow, Schneidman, & Leonard, 1963).

Patients with advanced disease have the highest suicide risk among patients with cancer and are more likely to have pain, depression, delirium, and deficit symptoms. The suffering caused by the disease and its treatment, often over many years, is now exacerbated by uncontrolled pain, a combination that can easily generate a sense of profound hopelessness. It may be that it is pain, not on its own but associated with psychological disorder, especially one which affects mood, which increases suicide risk in these patients (Breitbart & Payne, 1998). Other factors, besides pain, which are thought to be associated with increased suicide risk, include advanced illness and poor prognosis, depression and hopelessness, delirium, impaired sense of control and helplessness, exhaustion, history of psychological disorder, previous suicide attempts, and family history of suicide (Breitbart & Payne, 1998).

Assessment of Suicide Risk in Patients with Cancer

Patients are frequently referred for psychiatric assessment of suicide risk when they are demonstrating signs of acute distress, especially sudden tearfulness, or mention suicide or euthanasia. This may occur in the context of receiving bad news about the initial diagnosis or evidence of a relapse after a lengthy period of remission, but it may also occur for no obvious reason. On more detailed specialist assessment, most of these patients turn out not to pose a significant suicide risk. Nursing and medical staff who are sometimes themselves inadequately trained or inexperienced in dealing with situations of this kind often seek specialist help. The psychiatric assessment, which should be carried out as soon as possible, should be followed by a conversation with the referrer, which not only can offer reassurance (when appropriate) but also can have an educational function. In addition, psycho-oncology teaching sessions for nonpsychiatric staff looking after patients with cancer should include advice about the assessment of suicide risk. This advice should include the caveat that staff should err on the side of caution and that if any doubt remains about the suicide risk in an individual patient, a referral to specialist services should be made.

An assessment of suicide risk should include two checklists of questions:

1. *A graded hierarchy of questions about current suicidal ideas and intent.* These might begin with a question such as "Have you ever felt in the last few days or weeks that you would just like to go to sleep and not wake up?" If the answer is positive, then "Do you think you might ever do anything to harm yourself?" Further questions, if appropriate, would explore intent and plans, including method, measures to prevent being discovered while still alive, messages for relatives and friends, and so forth, in an attempt to form an opinion about the seriousness of the intent.

2. *Questions about the aforementioned suicide risk factors.* Fleeting suicidal thoughts are extremely common in patients with cancer and do not on their own (without other evidence to suggest the possibility of suicide) indicate a significant suicide risk. However, if for other reasons a patient is thought to pose a serious suicide risk, transferring that patient to an acute psychiatric ward without his or her consent, possibly under a section of the Mental Health Act (in the United Kingdom), might actually further increase the suicide risk. The patient's already diminished sense of control may, under these circumstances, become a sense of complete loss of control (perceived loss of control being itself a suicide risk factor).

Acute psychiatric wards, populated often by young men with florid psychotic symptoms, are not always therapeutic environments and overworked staff may not have the time and energy to devote to a suicidal patient. Moreover, a patient with cancer may require physical treatments that psychiatric staff is not trained to administer. Often it may be a better option for the suicidal patient with cancer to remain on a medical ward or even at home—provided he or she can be continuously supervised (in hospital by a trained psychiatric nurse). Appropriate measures should be considered to reduce the impact of relevant risk factors, whenever possible, for example, improving pain control, antidepressant therapy (some antidepressants have an analgesic effect), investigation and treatment of delirium, and giving patients the opportunity to ventilate their feelings of helplessness and hopelessness. And, in most of these cases, the patient would need to remain in hospital.

Special Considerations in the Psychological Management of Cancer Pain

As Turk and Fernandez (1990) observed over a decade ago, the contribution of psychological factors to cancer pain has tended to be ignored or played down. Although there have been changes in clinical attitudes, there is perhaps still an assumption that cancer pain has a clear physical origin and therefore should be managed solely by physical means, as if it were disrespectful to a patient who is already suffering from a life-threatening illness to suggest that psychological factors might be playing a part in his or her suffering.

It is only relatively recently that the similarities between pain in cancer and pain in other chronic conditions have been demonstrated. Turk and colleagues (1998) compared patients with cancer who were experiencing pain with patients with noncancer chronic pain. They found that both groups had similar levels of pain severity, but the cancer patients had higher levels of perceived disability and lower levels of activity. As might be expected, the cancer patients received higher levels of support and solicitous behavior from others, particularly if they had metastatic disease. The two groups could not be differentiated in a number of important areas. The vast majority of cancer patients could be allocated to

one of the same three groupings previously identified with chronic pain patients: dysfunctional, interpersonally distressed, and adaptive copers. The "dysfunctional" group had high levels of pain, high mood disturbance, and low perceived control, and they saw pain as seriously interfering with their lives. The interpersonally distressed group had high mood disturbance associated with a perception of low social support and negative responses from others. The adaptive copers had low distress and a sense of personal control and did not see the pain as significantly interfering with their lives.

These similarities between cancer pain and pain in other chronic conditions are encouraging because they suggest that the treatment techniques used with other pain syndromes can also be applied to cancer sufferers. Nevertheless, there are still some important differences between chronic pain syndromes and cancer.

Chronic pain in cancer is usually the result of a disease- or treatment-related nociceptive stimulus that may progress as the disease progresses. It is essential that pain be monitored because it may indicate disease progression. As Turk and Fernandez (1990) observed, there may be problems distinguishing appropriate from maladaptive pain in cancer. Physical disability from treatment (e.g., chemotherapy) or the disease itself in its later stages may limit the proactive behaviors available to the cancer patient in a way that does not apply in other pain syndromes (e.g., chronic back pain). Socializing the cancer patient to a biopsychosocial model of pain control is challenging when family, professionals, and society may be encouraging a purely medical model of pain.

Assessment of Pain

The person carrying out the assessment requires knowledge of the potential causes of pain in cancer and the treatment of cancer, must be able to recognize typical pain syndromes (see below), and must be well informed about appropriate modes of physical and psychological treatment.

A thorough assessment should include questions about the following points.

1. Location of the pain
   - Superficial, deep
   - Segmental (within the territory of spinal cord segments)
   - In the area innervated by a single nerve or cluster of nerves (plexus)
2. Factors that can exacerbate and relieve the pain (these questions can be highly informative both for the diagnosis and treatment of the pain)
   - Provoked by breathing (respiratory tract?)
   - Provoked by swallowing (esophagus?)
   - Provoked by exercise and relieved by rest (ischaemic?)
   - Provoked and relieved by certain movements or postures (musculoskeletal?)
3. Quality of the pain
   - Steady, fluctuating
   - Rhythmic and cramping (obstruction of a hollow viscus?)
   - Deep pains tend to have an aching quality
   - Throbbing (arterial pulsation)
   - Sharp stabs of pain (nerve root, sensory nerve ganglion?)
   - Dull pain exacerbated by coughing, sneezing (nerve root?)
4. Temporal characteristics: onset, pattern, course
5. Severity of pain as rated by the patient (e.g., as mild, moderate, or severe or on a 0–10 scale), supplemented by assessment of the effect the pain has on the patient's behavior (e.g., wakens the patient up at night and makes it impossible for the patient to continue working)
6. Mechanisms that reproduce and relieve the pain. These can be not only of diagnostic value but may even have a therapeutic effect. Asking a patient to hyperventilate may induce chest pain; then, asking him or her to hypoventilate may relieve it. Anxious patients can learn from this and increase their sense of control when they realize it is something they can do on their own (e.g., to abort an episode of acute anxiety).

Cancer Pain Syndromes

1. Tumor-related nociceptive pain syndromes (nociceptive = caused by tissue injury, e.g., to bone, joints, or muscles such as back pain from spinal metastases). Analgesic medication can prevent nociception from giving rise to pain, but so too can downstream modulation from the brain, as suggested by Melzack and Wall (1965) in their gate control theory.
2. Tumor-related neuropathic pain syndromes (neuropathic = caused by damage to nerve tissue either due to local or distant effects of the primary tumor; e.g., tumor infiltration or compression of nerve tissue). Damage to peripheral nerves can cause pain or abnormal sensations, such as burning, in the dermatome innervated by the nerves.
3. Treatment-related syndromes (e.g., radiation fibrosis can damage peripheral nerves and cause chronic pain [Portenoy & Lesage, 1999]).

Further Points to be Borne in Mind by the Assessor

1. Not all pain is pathological. The brief pain on movement of a joint, the "stitch" in the side from diaphragmatic cramp, and a more persistent ache in the shoulder or neck are all examples of "normal pains," which are usually of short duration, come and go for no obvious reason, and are not associated with disease. Patients with cancer can become anxiously preoccupied with their own body and observe it, sometimes with obsessional checking rituals, for possible signs of a relapse of their illness. Such patients can misinterpret normal pains for something much more sinister. Reassurance by an oncologist or general practitioner tends to have only a temporary effect because the anxiety often returns, and with it the anxious self-monitoring. In these circumstances the underlying anxiety may need to be explored and treated appropriately.
2. The multifactorial model of pain just described makes it clear that an essential part of an assessment of pain is a careful exploration of the cognitive, emotional, and sociocultural factors that may influence the pain in the individual patient, even if there is a fairly obvious organic cause of the pain. Back pain might be mildly annoying for many of us but could have a more sinister significance

for a woman with breast cancer. It would not be surprising if a patient with cancer who had recently lost a loved parent became depressed—and also more distressed by preexisting cancer-associated pain or more likely to misinterpret normal pains as symptoms of relapse.

Rating Scales Used with Cancer Patients

These include:

1. Memorial Pain Assessment Card (MPAC) has visual analog scales for pain intensity, pain relief, and mood. MPAC can be filled in by patients in under 30 seconds (Fishman, Pasternak, & Wallenstein, 1987)
2. Brief Pain Inventory (BPI) has numeric scales for pain intensity and a percentage scale for pain relief after treatment. Patients can shade in parts of a figure of a body to indicate localization of pain, and the BPI includes seven questions on the effects of pain (Daut, Cleeland, & Flanery, 1983)

Psychological Treatment of Pain in Patients with Cancer

Psychological Barriers to Adequate Pain Treatment

Patients may experience a number of problems in getting professional help with their pain. They need to receive information about the signs and symptoms that indicate that the pain is out of control and requires urgent attention. It is helpful for them to be made aware in advance of the sorts of facts about the pain they should try to communicate to professional staff whom they would like to help them. They should be informed about possible side effects, symptoms of overdose, and allergic reactions. It is useful for patients to know the sort of symptoms that do not constitute an emergency but should be reported nonetheless. Finally, they should receive some instruction in how to make the best use of their pain medication (Houts, 1994).

Fear of dependence on the part of the oncologist and the patient can lead to inadequate doses of analgesics. There is evidence (Macaluso, Weinberg, & Foley, 1988) that patients with cancer who have a history of drug dependence can develop tolerance and physical dependence but are unlikely to become psychologically dependent. Increasing doses of opioid analgesics occur usually in the context of disease progression or tolerance. Although tolerance and physical dependence often go hand in hand, they are both different from psychological dependence, which is marked by intense craving for the drug and accompanied by strenuous and unremitting efforts to obtain it (Breitbart & Payne, 1998).

Doctors and nurses are often afraid of colluding with what they perceive as the excessive demands of the small number of patients who have a history of drug dependence. In the management of drug-dependent patients who do not have cancer, the setting of and adherence to strict boundaries are widely regarded as essential to successful treatment. In the case of patients with cancer, this situation can result in undermedication. It is probably good to set limits and to try to maintain them, but it may be counterproductive if the whole staff–patient relationship is allowed to revolve around the single issue of the most appropriate doses of analgesics. In cases of doubt it is probably better to believe the patients' reports about their pain (Breitbart & Payne, 1998).

There is also an ethical dimension to pain control (Ventafridda, 1994). Other things being equal, adequate pain control is preferable to inadequate pain control, and inadequately controlled pain can be seen as intrinsically wrong in that it causes unnecessary suffering, with no obvious benefit to the sufferer. Withholding drugs to lower the risk of later dependence is not necessarily always the right thing to do, because the decision depends on a careful consideration of the pros and cons of withholding versus granting adequate pain control. There is also a strong moral case for involving the patient in the decision-making process and in some circumstances permitting the patient to self-administer the drug. In patients with advanced cancer and a poor prognosis, the risk of later dependence may be of far lesser importance, or even of no importance, with regard to decisions about adequate doses of analgesics (Breitbart & Payne, 1998).

Multidisciplinary Pain Clinic

The multifactorial nature of pain requires diverse skills not usually found in a single individual. This suggests that a team whose members collectively possess all the relevant skills can be a useful approach to the assessment and treatment of cancer patients with pain. The members of such a clinic might be:

- An anaesthetist, preferably with experience in administering acupuncture
- A psychologist/psychiatrist
- A nurse
- A physiotherapist

As well as providing a clinical service, such a team could audit the effectiveness of various treatment modalities and carry out research into various aspects of pain and pain therapies.

Psychological Treatments of Pain

Psychotherapy will focus on the pain caused by the illness and will employ a number of techniques, including active and empathic listening, reinforcement and mobilization of the patient's strengths, and already tested coping mechanisms and the development of new ones, which may include relaxation techniques, distraction, and activity scheduling. Psychotherapy will also include some education about the use of analgesics and advice about communicating more effectively with medical and nursing staff. In the terminal stages of the illness the patient may become increasingly fatigued and may be sedated to some extent by analgesic medication. As a consequence, sessions will be shorter and additional time may well be required to support relatives. Concomitant anxiety and depression can increase the sensitivity to pain and may have to be treated in addition to the pain itself.

Cognitive-Behavioral Therapy

It has been observed that "more has been written about cognitive-behavioral aspects of chronic pain and cognitive-behavioral therapy (CBT) than any other chronic medical problem" (White, 2001, p. 123). Morley, Eccleston, and Williams (1999) reviewed 25 trials of CBT for chronic pain. The treatment was consistently found to be more effective than waiting-list controls. Compared with alternative treatments, CBT produced significantly greater change on measures of pain, positive measures of cognitive coping, and reduced behavioral expression of pain. CBT, however, was not significantly more effective than other treatments on measures of mood, negative cognitive coping (e.g., catastrophizing), or social role functioning. Cancer patients can have similar reactions to pain to those of chronic pain patients (Turk et al., 1998), which means that the same techniques can be applied. The general principles of CBT for pain are described by Turk (Chapter 7, this volume). Here we describe how some of these techniques may be applied in people with cancer.

Engaging the Patient

CBT seeks to help patients become effective problem-solvers, taking as much responsibility for their pain control as possible and exploring methods they can use themselves in conjunction with their medical treatment. Some people take to this approach straight away, because it fits their view of themselves and the way they like to cope with stress. For others, however, this approach may not be immediately appealing. They may not see themselves as "copers" and may not believe they have the capacity to solve problems.

Beliefs about the nature of pain (e.g., "No matter what I do, if I am going to be in pain, I will be in pain.") or about cancer pain (e.g., "Cancer pain cannot be controlled in the same way as other types of pain") can affect a patient's motivation to use pain control strategies. The aim with these patients is to establish rapport by listening empathically to their description of the pain and its impact on their life, and to begin to explore the possibility that they can exert some control over the pain.

Allowing the patient to acknowledge and express their feelings and to validate them (Moorey & Greer, 1992) is an important part of the process of engagement of the cancer patient, and it is essential that the patient does not get the impression that the therapist is implying the pain is "all in the mind." The emphasis is on the way in which things we think and do can make the pain better or worse. Gentle questioning may identify situations in which the person has been actively caught up in doing something and not been so preoccupied with pain, or other situations in which they may dwell on their physical symptoms with consequent increase in pain. Developing an idiosyncratic cognitive-behavioral model of the pain can help to suggest that there is an alternative to the view that cancer pain is exclusively influenced by physical factors. Often the therapy is presented as an experiment in discovering whether or not pain control strategies can be helpful.

Cognitive-Behavioral Analysis

The therapist can use a simple model linking pain, environmental factors, thoughts, feelings, behaviors, and selective attention. Tracing the sequence from trigger (e.g., seeing a program about someone dying from cancer) to thoughts ("That could happen to me!") to emotions (fear) and exacerbation of pain demonstrates how all the systems interact with each other. The behavioral final consequence might be that the patient cancels a social engagement and so allows the pain to control his or her life, rather than being in control of his or her life. The role of selective attention can also be highlighted in this model—the negative thoughts lead patients to attend to their pain more, while the avoidance of the social event means that there is more time to focus on the pain. Figure 25.1 shows how this conceptualization can be shared in diagrammatic form with the patient.

Self-Monitoring

One of the primary tools of the cognitive-behavioral approach to pain is self-monitoring, often with the aid of a pain diary in which not only the pain and its intensity are recorded but also possible triggers of the pain and, crucially, the negative thoughts associated with the pain. Information is gathered about external factors that might make the pain better or worse, and also internal factors such as mood and thoughts. Pain diaries can help to challenge beliefs that the person is helpless in the face of the pain by establishing that pain changes depending on what the person thinks or does.

Cognitive Restructuring and Behavioral Experiments

Once people have begun to identify some of their negative automatic thoughts with a

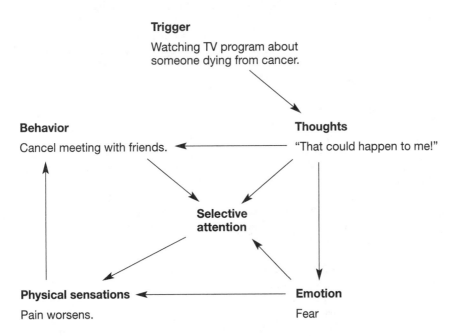

FIGURE 25.1. Cognitive-behavioral analysis of a cancer patient's pain.

pain diary, they can start to question the helpfulness and the reasonableness of such thoughts. Typical negative automatic thoughts might be: "This pain is only going to get worse," "This pain is making it hard for me to get up. If it gets worse, I won't be able to do anything at all," or "This pain in my chest means that the cancer has spread here as well and that I am going to die soon." Sternbach (1974) observed that patients often anticipate that increases in pain will accelerate with time, although the evidence suggests that this does not happen. But patients can come to realize that the pain is not always continuous and severe but variable and may depend on certain factors which they can influence. By modifying these factors, they may be able, indirectly, to modify the pain. They may also come to realize that the disability caused by the pain is not total and that there are certain things they can still do despite the disability.

Discussion with the therapist using the data from the pain diary can help to challenge maladaptive thoughts and beliefs. Patients can then work between sessions to challenge the negative thoughts themselves and to evaluate the effects of using coping strategies or changing their behavior. CBT was originally developed for the treatment of depression and anxiety, and these techniques can be effective with the mood disturbance associated with cancer pain (Greer et al., 1992; Moorey & Greer, 1992; Moorey et al., 1994, Moorey, Greer, Bliss, & Law, 1998)

Patients are encouraged to challenge their negative thoughts by trying to think of alternative cognitive responses to the same situation (e.g., instead of the negative automatic thought, "I can't do this because of the pain I'm in," the alternative thought, "It's going to hurt as much whether I do it or not, so I might as well do it"). The pain diary can now be used to record both negative thoughts and alternative thoughts. By recognizing some of their negative thoughts and considering alternative responses, patients may acquire a sense of enhanced control of what previously appeared to them to be a completely hopeless situation. Many of the beliefs about pain lend themselves to behavioral experiments. For instance, a belief that the pain is constant and unbearable can be tested by grading it using the diary.

Grading can help the patient to recognize the variable nature and differing patterns of many pains. A belief that the pain will accelerate with time can be tested by examining the dosage of pain-relieving drugs used and the pain scores in the diary over a series of weeks.

The idea that nothing can be done once one is in pain can be evaluated by spending a week selectively attending to pain whenever it occurs and then a second week trying distraction tasks. Once the person can see that excessive focusing on physical symptoms exacerbates the pain and that distraction can lessen it, he or she feels less helpless and more motivated to use pain-control techniques. Some people reduce their activities to guard against pain, but this may lead to increased depression and pain. Activity scheduling with a series of graded tasks can increase the range and duration of activities and demonstrate that mood and pain improve. If the patient is avoiding tasks that are perceived as likely to cause significant pain, he or she may be helped to rehearse these tasks in imagery and use relaxation as a means of reducing the anticipatory anxiety.

Coping Strategies

A variety of coping strategies have been used with chronic pain. These can be used in their own right or within the context of a cognitive-behavioral approach (see also Syrjala & Abrams, Chapter 9, this volume).

RELAXATION TECHNIQUES

Relaxation techniques can reduce the sensory and affective dimensions of pain (Philips, 1988). But relaxation techniques are useful not only because they often are effective but because patients can administer them to themselves and thus enhance their own sense of control in a situation which may initially appear to be beyond their control. Perhaps the greatest obstacle to acquiring a mastery of relaxation techniques is to underestimate the time it takes to learn them. They are probably best learned under the direct supervision of a trained professional. Once this has been accomplished, relaxation tapes can be helpful in reinforcing and facilitating what has already been learned.

Simple breathing exercises can be effective in reducing the anxiety pain can provoke. The benefit of breathing exercises can be increased by progressive muscle relaxation, in which the patient learns to contract and relax certain muscle groups in a systematic way while concentrating on the subjective experience of increased tension followed by relaxation. Once a relaxed state has been achieved, imagery and distraction can be used to reach an even deeper state of relaxation.

IMAGERY

The imagination is a powerful cognitive faculty that has played a role in spells and charms in times past and has now been rediscovered and used in the technique known as imagery or guided imagery. This is best done when a state of relaxation has been achieved. The context of the pain can be transformed (e.g., by imagining that one is taking part in a game of football or tennis rather than lying in hospital). Some patients can experience pain relief by imagining that the part of the body that is painful is detached from the rest of their body (disassociated somatization).

Often it is best to let the patient chose the particular setting. The patient is asked to close his or her eyes and imagine a place where he or she feels completely safe and at ease. The patient is asked to provide some basic details (e.g., about the time of day, the season, and the weather) and the therapist uses this information to describe the scene in greater detail and invites the patient to use all the sensory modalities to experience in imagination what it might be like to be there in reality (e.g,, breathe in the salty sea air, let the sand run through your fingers, listen to the rhythmical crashing of the waves on the shore, watch the seagull drifting on a current of warm air).

HYPNOSIS

Hypnosis has been shown on electroencephalographic (EEG) analysis to be a heightened form of concentration rather than a kind of sleep (the word "hypnosis" is derived from "hypnos," the ancient Greek word for sleep). The intense concentration that results from hypnosis can be used to al-

ter the perception of pain. Hypnosis is usually effective for about two-thirds of the general population (Breitbart & Payne, 1998), although the extent to which responders are hypnotizable varies greatly. This also applies to patients with cancer. Hypnotizability does not require a good imagination and is not correlated with personality measures. It has been suggested (Barber & Gitelson, 1980) that patients should use self-hypnosis and should try not to resist the pain but use mental filters to reduce it. Some can reduce pain by sensory transformation (e.g., changing the temperature sensation in the painful body part); others can experience pain relief by concentrating on a particular sensation in another part of the body or by imagining themselves in a relaxing scene.

BIOFEEDBACK

EMG and temperature biofeedback techniques have been employed successfully to learn how to control pain with relaxation (Loscalzo & Jacobsen, 1990; see also Arena & Blanchard, Chapter 8, this volume). Fotopoulos, Graham, and Cook (1979) found that cancer patients who had used electromyographic and EEG biofeedback techniques could significantly reduce their pain during the period of treatment, but that only 2 of the 17 were able to sustain this reduction after the end of treatment.

OTHER STRATEGIES FOR REFOCUSING ATTENTION

Both music (Munro & Mount, 1978) and art therapy (Connell, 1998) can focus the attention in a particularly intense way and thus distract from pain. Active rather than passive engagement will require greater concentration and will have a more powerful analgesic effect. In the case of music, patients can be strongly engaged on an emotional level. In the case of art therapy, patients may actually depict their experience of pain in a pictorial representation that, by putting the pain in a particular context, may alter the experience of the pain itself. The expression of pain in a piece of music played by the patient or in a painting by the patient may also have a cathartic effect. Creativity can be a powerful way for patients to regain some of the control they have lost and thus enhance their well-being and reduce their vulnerability to the ravages of pain.

Pain Control in Advanced Disease

In the final stages of the illness patients may be debilitated and also less alert because they are taking considerable doses of analgesics. Here the focus shifts from recovery to accommodation. Patients need to be as comfortable as possible so that they are still capable of having some positive experiences. An important consideration is then how to make the best use of whatever time is left (e.g., to complete important tasks so far left undone, to make a record of important things from their own lives, and to say farewell to loved ones).

Efficacy of Psychological Interventions in Cancer Pain

Most studies of psychological interventions in cancer pain have focused on the acute pain associated with medical or surgical interventions. A number of trials have investigated the effectiveness of various strategies in coping with the pain of bone marrow aspiration in children with leukemia (e.g., Jay, Elliott, Fitzgibbon, Wood, & Siegel, 1995; Liossi & Hatira, 1999; Zeltzer & LeBaron, 1982). Hypnosis has been the most studied intervention. It seems to be more effective than treatment as usual. Compared with hypnosis, cognitive and behavioral coping strategies were found to be equally effective in one study (Liossi & Hatiri, 1999). In another study, a cognitive intervention reduced distress less around the time of the operation than conventional anesthesia but had a more beneficial effect on adjustment 24 hours later (Jay et al., 1995). Studies of bone marrow transplantation procedures in adults have supported the effectiveness of hypnosis (Syrjala, Cummings, & Donaldson, 1992, Syrjala, Donaldson, Davis, Kippes, & Carr, 1995). In a recent review, Redd, Montgomery, and DuHamel (2001) concluded that although a variety of behavioral methods have been shown to reduce acute treatment-related pain, there is increasing evidence that these methods are not

equally effective. Hypnotic-like methods, involving relaxation, suggestion, and distracting imagery, hold the greatest promise for pain management. Unfortunately, research is scant on the use of behavioral intervention to control prolonged pain associated with invasive medical procedures (Sellick & Zara, 1998).

The psychologist or psychiatrist working in this area is more likely to see cancer patients who are suffering from chronic pain problems. There have been fewer outcome studies with this patient group. Sloman, Brown, Aldana, and Chee (1994) taught relaxation to oncology inpatients. Both relaxation from an audiotape and relaxation taught directly to the patient by a clinician proved equally effective in controlling pain and more effective than treatment as usual. Arathuzik (1994) compared relaxation and imagery training with and without other cognitive and behavioral techniques in 24 women with breast cancer. Both treatments were equally effective.

The evidence so far confirms the effectiveness of psychological methods of pain control in cancer, particularly simple techniques such as hypnosis and relaxation. The addition of other cognitive and behavioral strategies has yet to be shown to add to the effect of these methods. It is likely that CBT will prove most effective in cases of complex chronic pain, where the sort of psychological factors described previously play an important role in exacerbating the already distressing pain from the cancer. CBT and other psychological interventions seem to be most helpful in people who are at high risk for psychological distress (Sheard & Maguire, 1999), and the same may apply to pain. Further controlled trials of psychological treatments are therefore needed to evaluate the strong clinical impression that these treatments can make a major contribution to the overall management of pain in people with cancer.

References

Ahles, T. A., Ruckdeschel, J. C., & Blanchard, E. B. (1984). Cancer-related pain—I. Prevalence in an outpatient setting as a function of stage of disease and type of cancer. *Journal of Psychosomatic Research, 28,* 115–119.

Arathuzik, D. (1994). Effects of cognitive-behavioral strategies on pain in cancer patients. *Cancer Nursing, 17,* 207–214.

Asmundsen, G. J. G. (1999). Beyond pain: The role of fear and avoidance in chronicity. *Clinical Psychology Review, 19,* 97–119.

Barber, J., & Gitelson, J. (1980). Cancer pain: Psychological management using hypnosis. *CA—A Cancer Journal for Clinicians, 3,* 130–136

Bolund, C. (1985). Suicide and cancer: 11 medical and care factors in suicide by cancer patients in Sweden, 1973–1976. *Journal of Psychosocial Oncology, 3,* 17–30.

Bond, M. R., & Pearson, I. B. (1969). Psychological aspects of pain in women with advanced cancer of the cervix. *Journal of Psychosomatic Research, 13,* 13–19.

Breitbart, W. (1987). Suicide in cancer patients. *Oncology, 1,* 49–54.

Breitbart, W., & Payne, D. K. (1998). Pain. In J. Holland (Ed.), *Psycho-oncology* (pp. 450–467). New York: Oxford University Press.

Butler, R. W., Damarin, F. L., Beaulieu, C., Schwebel, A. I., & Thorn, B. E. (1989). Assessing cognitive coping strategies for acute postsurgical pain. *Psychological Assessment, 1,* 41–45.

Cassell, E. J. (1982). The nature of suffering and the goals of medicine. *New England Journal of Medicine, 306,* 639–645.

Ciaramella, A., & Poli, P. (2001) Assessment of depression among cancer patients: The role of pain, cancer type and treatment. *Psycho-oncology, 10,* 156–165.

Connell, C. (1998), *Something understood: Art therapy in cancer care.* London: Wrexham.

Craig, K. D. (1994). Emotional aspects of pain. In P. D. Wall & R. Melzack (Eds.), *Textbook of pain* (3rd ed., pp. 261–274). Edinburgh: Churchill Livingstone.

Crisson, J. E., & Keefe, F. J. (1998). The relationship of locus of control to pain coping strategies and psychological distress in chronic pain patients. *Pain, 35,* 147–154.

Daut, R. L., & Cleeland, C. (1983). The prevalence and severity of pain in cancer. *Cancer, 50,* 1913–1918.

Daut, R. L., Cleeland, C. S., & Flanery, R. C. (1983). Development of the Wisconsin Brief Pain Questionnaire to assess pain in cancer and other diseases. *Pain, 17,* 197–210.

Derogatis, L. R., Morrow, G. R. Fetting, J., Penman, D., Piasetsky, S., Schmale, A. M., Henricks, M., & Carnicke, C. (1983). The prevalence of psychiatric disorders among cancer patients. *Journal of the American Medical Association, 249,* 751–757.

Eisendrath, S. J., Way, L. W., Ostroff, J. W., & Johanson, C. A. (1986). Identification of psychogenic abdominal pain. *Psychosomatics, 27,* 705–712.

Farberow, N. L., Schneidman, E. S., & Leonard, C. V. (1963). Suicide among general medical and surgical hospital patients with malignant neoplasms. *Medical Bulletin, 9.* Washington, DC: U.S. Veterans Administration.

Fishman, B., Pasternak, S., & Wallenstein, S. L. (1987). The Memorial Pain Assessment Card: A valid instrument for the evaluation of cancer pain. *Cancer, 60,* 1151–1158.

Fotopoulos, S. S., Graham, C., & Cook, M. R. (1979). Psychophysiological control of cancer Pain. In J. J. Bonica & V. Ventafridda (Eds.), *Advances in pain research and therapy* (Vol. 2, pp. 231–244). New York: Raven Press.

Gaffney, A., & Dunne, E. A. (1987). Children's understanding of the causality of pain. *Pain, 29,* 91–104.

Gamsa, A. (1990). Is emotional disturbance a precipitator or a consequence of chronic pain? *Pain, 42,* 183–195.

Greer, S., Moorey, S., Baruch, J. D. R., Watson, M., Robertson, B. M., Mason, A., Rowden, L., Law, M., & Bliss, J. M. M (1992). Adjuvant psychological therapy for patients with cancer: A prospective randomised trial. *British Medical Journal, 304,* 675–680.

Hendry, S. (1999). Pain. In R. A. Wilson & F. C. Keil (Eds.), *MIT encyclopedia of the cognitive sciences* (pp. 622–624) Cambridge: MIT Press.

Hietanen, P., Lonnquist, J., Henriksson, M., & Jallinoja, P. (1994). Do cancer suicides differ from others? *Psycho-oncology, 3,* 189–195.

Houts, P. S. (Ed.). (1994). *Home care guide for cancer.* Philadelphia: American College of Physicians.

Jacobsen, P. B., & Butler, R. W. (1996). Relation of cognitive coping and catastrophizing to acute pain and analgesic use following breast cancer surgery. *Journal of Behavioral Medicine, 19,* 17–29.

Jay, S., Elliott, C. H., Fitzgibbons, I., Woody, P., & Siegel, S. (1995). A comparative study of cognitive behavior therapy versus general anesthesia for painful medical procedures in children. *Pain, 62,* 3–9.

Keefe, F. J., Brown, G. K., Wallston, K. A., & Caldwell, D. S. (1989). Coping with rheumatoid arthritis pain: Catastrophizing as a maladaptive strategy. *Pain, 37,* 51–56.

Liossi, C., & Hatira, P. (1999). Clinical hypnosis versus cognitive behavioral training for pain management with pediatric cancer patients undergoing bone marrow aspirations. *International Journal of Clinical and Experimental Hypnosis, 47,* 104–116.

Loscalzo, M., & Jacobsen, P. B. (1990). Practical behavioral approaches to the management of pain and distress. *Journal of Psychosocial Oncology, 8,* 139–169.

Loeser, J. D., & Melzack, R. (1999, May 8). Pain: An overview. *Lancet, 353,* 1607–1609.

Macaluso, C., Weinberg, D., & Foley, K. M. (1988, July 14–17). *Opioid abuse and misuse in a cancer pain population* [Abstract]. Paper presented at the 2nd International Congress on Cancer Pain, Rye, NY.

McKegney, F. P., Bailey, C. R., & Yates, J. W. (1981). Prediction and management of pain in patients with advanced cancer. *General Hospital Psychiatry, 3,* 95–101.

Massie, M., Gagnon, P., & Holland, J. (1994). Depression and suicide in patients with cancer. *Journal of Pain and Symptom Management, 9,* 325–331.

Maxwell, T. D., Gatchel, R. J., & Mayer, T. G. (1998). Cognitive predictors of depression in chronic low back pain: Toward an inclusive model. *Journal of Behavioral Medicine, 21,* 131–143.

Melzack. R., & Wall, P. D. (1965). Pain mechanisms: A new theory. *Science, 165,* 971–979.

Moorey, S., & Greer, S. (1992). *Cognitive behaviour therapy for people with cancer.* Oxford, UK: Oxford University Press.

Moorey, S., Greer, S., Bliss, J., & Law, M. (1998). A comparison of adjuvant psychological therapy and supportive counselling in patients with cancer. *Psycho-oncology,7,* 218–228.

Moorey, S., Greer, S., Watson, M., Baruch, J. D. R., Robertson, B. M., Mason, A., Rowden, L., Tunmore, R., Law, M., & Bliss J. M. (1994). Adjuvant psychological therapy for patients with cancer: Outcome at one year. *Psycho-oncology, 3,* 39–46.

Morley, S., Eccleston, C., & Williams, A. (1999). Systematic review and meta-analysis of randomised controlled trials of cognitive behaviour therapy and behaviour therapy for chronic pain in adults, excluding headache. *Pain, 80,* 1–13.

Munroe, S. M., & Mount, B. (1978). Music therapy in palliative care. *Canadian Medical Association Journal. 119,* 1029–1034.

Owen, C., Tenant, C., Levi, J., & Jones, M. (1992). Suicide and euthanasia: Patient attitudes in the context of cancer. *Psycho-oncology, 1,* 79–88.

Philips, H. C. (1988). Changing chronic pain experience. *Pain, 32,* 165–172.

Portenoy, R. K., & Lesage, P. (1999, May 15). Management of cancer pain. *Lancet, 353,* 1695–1700

Redd, W. H., Montgomery, G. H., & DuHamel. K. N. (2001). Behavioral intervention for cancer treatment side effects. *Journal of the National Cancer Institute, 93,* 810–823.

Sellick, S. M., & Zaza, C. (1998). Critical review of 5 nonpharmacologic strategies for managing cancer pain. *Cancer Prevention and Control, 2,* 7–14.

Sheard, T., & Maguire, P. (1999). The effect of psychological interventions on anxiety and depression in cancer patients: Results of two meta-analyses. *British Journal of Cancer, 80,* 1770–1780.

Sloman R., Brown, P., Aldana, E., & Chee, E. (1994). The use of relaxation for the promotion of comfort and pain relief in persons with advanced cancer. *Contemporary Nursing, 3,* 6–12.

Spiegel, D., & Bloom, J. R. (1983). Pain in metastatic breast cancer. *Cancer, 52,* 341–345.

Sternbach, R. (1974). *Pain patients: Traits and treatment.* New York: Academic Press.

Sternbach, R. (1986). Pain and "hassles" in the United States: Findings of the Nuprin pain report. *Pain, 27,* 69–80.

Syrjala, K. L., & Chapko, M. (1995) Evidence for a biophysical model of cancer treatment-related pain. *Pain, 61,* 69–79.

Syrjala, K. L., Cummings, C., & Donaldson, G. W. (1992). Hypnosis or cognitive behavioral training for the reduction of pain and nausea during cancer treatment: A controlled clinical trial. *Pain, 48,*137–146.

Syrjala, K. L., Donaldson, G. W., Davis, M. W., Kippes, M. E., & Carr, J. E. (1995). Relaxation and imagery and cognitive-behavioral training reduce pain during cancer treatment: A controlled clinical trial. *Pain, 63,* 189–198.

Turk, D. C., & Fernandez, E. (1990). On the putative uniqueness of cancer pain: Do psychological principles apply? *Behaviour Research and Therapy, 28,* 1–13.

Turk, D. C., & Rudy, T. E. (1990). The robustness of an empirically derived taxonomy of chronic pain patients. *Pain, 43,* 27–35.

Turk, D. C., Sist, T. C., Okifuji, A., Milner, M. F., Florio, G., Harrison, P., Massey, J., Lema, M. L., & Zevon, M. A (1998). Adaptation to metastatic cancer pain, regional/local cancer pain and noncancer pain: Role of psychological and behavioral factors. *Pain, 74,* 247–256.

Ventafridda, V. (1994). The ethical dimensions of undermedication of pain. *Psycho-oncology, 3,* 35–37.

Weisenberg, M. (1977). Pain and pain control. *Psychological Bulletin, 84,* 1008–1044.

White, C. A. (2001). *Cognitive behaviour therapy for chronic medical problems: A guide to assessment and treatment in practice.* Chichester, UK: Wiley.

Zeltzer, L., & LeBaron, S. (1982). Hypnosis and nonhypnotic techniques for reduction of pain and anxiety during painful procedures in children and adolescents with cancer. *Journal of Pediatrics, 101,* 1032–1035.

26

Treating Patients with Somatoform Pain Disorder and Hypochondriasis

Michael Sharpe
Amanda C. de C. Williams

In this chapter we aim to guide the reader through the important though confusing interface of pain and psychiatry with particular reference to so-called somatoform pain disorder and hypochondriasis. We begin by outlining the fourth edition of the *Diagnostic and Statistical Manual of Mental Disorders* (DSM-IV; American Psychiatric Association, 1994), within which the somatoform disorders are a category.

Somatoform Disorders as Defined in DSM-IV

The essence of the concept of somatoform disorders is the occurrence of physical symptoms that are not explained by a medical condition or by alternative psychiatric diagnoses. According to DSM-IV, the somatoform disorders, which include pain disorder and hypochondriasis among other categories, are unified by: "the presence of physical symptoms that suggest a medical condition (hence the term 'somatoform,' meaning in somatic form) yet after assessment are found not to be fully explained by a general medical condition, by the direct effect of a substance or by another mental disorder"

(American Psychiatric Association, 1994, p. 445). It is further specified that the symptoms must be clinically significant by virtue of causing distress or impairment of functioning and that, in contrast to factitious disorder and malingering, they are not deliberately or intentionally produced. The specific diagnoses in question are defined as follows:

- *Somatoform pain disorder* (previously referred to as psychogenic pain disorder) is used to describe complaints of pain where psychological factors are judged to have an important role.
- *Hypochondriasis* is the term used for a presentation in which the salient feature is not the symptoms per se but rather the patient's interpretation of them as evidence of a serious often life-threatening illness, and that they persist despite medical assessment and reassurance.

Other somatoform diagnoses in which pain may feature are:

- *Somatization disorder* (historically referred to as hysteria or Briquet's syndrome) is defined as the presentation to doctors with multiple symptoms including pain, un-explained by disease, that have occurred over a long period and that began before age 30.

• *Undifferentiated somatoform disorder* is a "catch-all" category for patients who have multiple unexplained physical com-plaints that have lasted at least 6 months but do not meet criteria for somatization.

Problems with the Somatoform Disorder Concept

The category of somatoform disorder has been strongly criticized on several grounds (Martin, 1999). Several of the problems are relevant to our consideration of pain.

MIND–BODY DUALISM

The concept of somatoform disorder is in-herently dualistic. It implies that the prob-lem is "psychological" rather then "physi-cal" in nature. This dichotomization of illness is an unhelpful and sometimes dan-gerous oversimplification of a problem that is better understood from a broader biopsy-chosocial (Engel, 1980) perspective. Many so-called psychologial symptoms can be found to have physiological correlates (Sharpe & Bass, 1992).

MISLEADING CATEGORIES

Even within the psychological domain, the impression of separate disorders given by a categorical classification is misleading. Most patients who have pain that is judged to be inadequately explained by disease will have features of all these diagnoses to some degree. That is, the problem in reality is a dimensional one. The diagnosis the patient receives depends on how *much* of these fea-tures they have—not on their presence or absence.

UNACCEPTABLE LABELS

One of the functions of a diagnosis is to provide a "label" for patients that gives co-herence to their disparate symptoms. It also allows patients to explain their inability to function to others, but neither somatoform pain disorder nor hypochondriasis scores well on these counts. They are (not entirely

incorrectly) perceived by many patients as offensively implying that they are imagining their pain or "putting it on," which limits their usefulness to the clinician.

OVERSIMPLIFICATION

The treatment of chronic pain problems is multifaceted. Effective management re-quires a more detailed understanding of the range of factors perpetuating the pain than that offered by a simple diagnosis.

An Alternative to the Somatoform Concept

We suggest that as an alternative to these DSM-IV diagnoses, a simple formulation of the physiological, psychological, and social factors relevant to the patient's pain prob-lem is preferable. This argument is elaborat-ed herein, with examples. We also advocate a multiaxial summary of the pain problem as follows:

Biological
1. Pain: Site, nature, and severity of pain complaint.
2. Physiology: Physiological factors and/or medical conditions.

Psychological
3. Cognitions: Nature and intensity of ill-ness fears and concerns.
4. Emotion: Anxiety and depression.
5. Behavior: Degree of avoidance and reas-surance seeking.

Social
6. Social context: Stress, responses of oth-ers and obstacles to regaining function.
7. Medical care: Interaction with the med-ical system.

We first consider the general case of so-matoform pain, which is pain judged to be disproportionate to identifiable disease. We then address hypochondriasis as a special case of somatoform pain in which the pa-tient's fears and beliefs about underlying disease are predominant.

Somatoform Pain Disorder

Table 26.1 shows the operational criteria for somatoform pain disorder as defined in

TABLE 26.1. DSM-IV Diagnostic Criteria for Somatoform Pain Disorder

A. Pain in one or more anatomical sites is the predominant focus of the clinical presentation and is of sufficient severity to warrant clinical attention.

B. The pain causes clinically significant distress or impairment in social, occupational, or other important areas of functioning.

C. Psychological factors are judged to have an important role in the onset, severity, exacerbation, or maintenance of the pain.

D. The symptom or deficit is not intentionally produced or feigned.

E. The pain is not better accounted for by a mood, anxiety, or psychotic disorder and does not meet criteria for dyspareunia.

Subclassification

Pain disorder associated with psychological factors. Psychological factors are judged to have the major role in the onset, severity, exacerbation, or maintenance of the pain. (If a general medical condition is present, it does not have a major role in the onset, severity, exacerbation, or maintenance of the pain.)

Pain disorder associated with both psychological factors and a general medical condition. Both psychological factors and a general medical condition are judged to have important roles in the onset, severity, exacerbation, or maintenance of the pain. The associated general medical condition or anatomical site of the pain is coded on Axis III.

Pain disorder associated with a general medical condition. This "is not considered to be a mental disorder and is included here to facilitate differential diagnosis." A general medical condition has a major role in the onset, severity, exacerbation, or maintenance of the pain. (If psychological factors are present, they are not judged to have a major role in the onset, severity, exacerbation, or maintenance of the pain.) The diagnostic code for the pain is selected based on the associated general medical condition if one has been established or on the anatomical location of the pain if the underlying general medical condition is not yet clearly established.

Note. From American Psychiatric Association (1994). Copyright 1994 by the American Psychiatric Association. Adapted by permission.

DSM-IV (American Psychiatric Association, 1994).

Conceptual Limitations of Somatoform Pain Disorder

It is important to be aware of the conceptual limitations of these criteria. Diagnostic Criteria A and B describe the symptoms and disability of the pain problem. They draw on the patient's definition of pain and account of its impact on daily life. The latter is particularly important for a full assessment, because psychological variables play an crucial part in exacerbating the distress and disability of patients with chronic pain (Keefe, Dunsmore, & Burnett, 1992; Vlaeyen & Linton, 2000; Von Korff & Simon, 1996). Criterion C, concerning the role of psychological factors, is more problematic. First, our current scientific understanding of pain does not support the attribution of pain and its impact entirely to psychological origins; second, it requires a difficult judgment about the role of psychological factors; and third, making the role of psychological factors explicit to the patient risks damage to the therapeutic relationship. Furthermore, the suggested solution of using the Axis III of the DSM classification, which codes associated medical conditions, is unsatisfactory for pain problems (Wall, 1999; Woolf et al., 1998) and therefore offers little help.

As with other symptoms that may be classified as "somatoform," pain is a particularly challenging clinical problem for several reasons. First, it is a subjective sensory and emotional experience[1], second, there is no simple relationship between the severity of pain expressed by the patient and identifiable pathology; and third, the diagnosis of a somatoform disorder depends on establishing or presuming the inadequacy of medical explanations for the pain (Kirmayer, Robbins, & Paris, 1994).

A Case Example

A 38-year-old man presented with severe constant pain in his neck, shoulders, arms, and upper back and unilaterally in his low back, right buttock, and leg; he also had frequent headaches accompanied by nausea. He described weakness in his arms and hands, a sense that his head was too heavy for his neck, intermittent dizziness, and tingling in arms and right foot. He was afraid of falling when dizzy and walked with the support of his wife out of doors; using a cane was too painful for either arm or neck. The pain had started with a "whiplash" accident while he was driving a van for work, which he had since lost. A court case was proceeding. The patient's treatment was initially the provision of a neck support from orthopedic surgery, mobilization maneuvers in physiotherapy (which he abandoned as too painful), and advice to rest until the pain resolved. However, the pain worsened and spread over the subsequent 2 years, during which time compound opioids and low-dose antidepressants were prescribed for his pain and benzodiazepines for muscle tension. He reported negligible analgesic effects from these drugs. The orthopedic department discharged him, saying it could do no more, and the patient's general practitioner was perplexed by the degree of disability (and associated family problems), which had resulted from a relatively minor injury. Of the two medicolegal reports, one described X-ray changes to cervical vertebrae; the other suggested that "unconscious mechanisms" associated with secondary gain were maintaining the pain in the absence of any significant lesion.

The crux of the matter in this case is the judgment that the pain is caused by "psychological" rather than "medical" factors. This judgment presents a general problem for diagnosing all somatoform symptoms and is predicated on the thorny issue of when a pain has a medical explanation and when it does not. Although this judgment may be relatively easy to make when a patient has major disease, it is much harder when no or minimal disease is apparent. This is not simply because the clinician (and patient) may continue to wonder if disease is causing the pain but has simply not been identified but also because the absence of pathology as conventionally defined does not logically lead to the conclusion that the symptom is entirely "psychological" in origin. The more that so-called "medically unexplained symptoms" are studied, the more evidence accrues that pathophysiological mechanisms as well as psychological mechanisms are involved (Sharpe & Carson, 2001). For these reasons, we propose that chronic pain is better understood from a biopsychosocial perspective than from a categorical "medical" or "psychological" classification.

A Biopsychosocial Perspective

BIOLOGICAL PAIN MECHANISMS

The most common general medical conditions associated with the symptoms of chronic pain are musculoskeletal problems, neuropathies, and malignancies. Malignant conditions are not discussed further here, but the pain associated with other conditions is not infrequently considered to merit a somatoform diagnosis.

Pain not apparently associated with a medical condition can be associated with a known biological mechanism. We now know that peripheral noxious stimulation including tissue damage can initiate short- and long-term changes in the nervous system. These occur at all levels from the peripheral nerves to the cortex (Loeser & Melzack, 1999; Wall, 1994). Although pain usually resolves with healing of damaged tissue, this does not always occur. Chronic pain can consequently be described as a failure of physiological homeostatic regulation (Loeser & Melzack, 1999; Wall, 1994; Woolf & Mannion, 1999). "Normal sensory function is the product of an actively maintained equilibrium between neurons and their environment. Any disruption of this equilibrium that results from changes in sensitivity, excitability, transmission, growth status, and survival can initiate profound changes in sensory function, which explains why diverse diseases can manifest as pain" (Woolf & Mannion, 1999, p. 1960).

Neuropathic pain is hard to diagnose, except peripherally, but may constitute part of many common chronic pain complaints such as low back pain (Woolf & Mannion, 1999). It shows a variable and unstable relationship between mechanisms and patients' symptoms: One patient may have more than one mechanism, and each may vary over time; two patients presenting with the same symptom may nevertheless have different mechanisms (Woolf & Mannion, 1999). Two characteristics of neuropathic pain, which are particularly relevant to somatoform diagnoses, are hyperalgesia, the increased ("excessive" or "exaggerated") response to a standard noxious stimulus, and allodynia, pain in response to what is normally a nonnoxious stimulus.

Pain can also originate entirely in the brain, as it does in many phantom pain phenomena, in pain in paraplegics below the level of spinal cord transection (Loeser & Melzack, 1999), in poststroke pain, and in some thalamic disorders.

Like neuropathic pain, visceral pain often occurs in the absence of identifiable injury. Mechanisms of contraction, torsion, hypoxia, and inflammation are more important than trauma (Cervero & Laird, 1999). Again of particular relevance in the context of somatoform concepts is that visceral pain is often diffuse and poorly localized (or somatically referred), and its boundaries may not coincide with those of organ systems.

Other pain mechanisms, which are partly understood, may be labeled somatoform pain disorder and may result from less well-understood neural mechanisms. For example, the influence of sympathetic nervous system activity on pain and pain-associated phenomena may be widespread and is evident in disorders such as chronic regional pain syndrome where hair, skin, and nail growth and temperature regulation are also affected. Pains subject to sympathetic influence do not fit segmental patterns of sensory inervation and can produce "glove or stocking distributions," meaning an area of pain covering the extremities of the limbs (Veldman, Reynen, Arntz, & Goris, 1993). Furthermore, central pain mechanisms may play a part in bodily pains that apparently lack a basis in tissue pathology such as fibromyalgia syndrome (Staud, Vierck, Cannon, Mauderli, & Price, 2001), which is commonly regarded as a somatoform disorder.

The presence of other symptoms such as numbness and tingling with the pain may increase the likelihood that it is considered "psychological." However, even a few weeks of sedentary behavior and bedrest in healthy subjects leads to decrements in physical and mental condition and performance, including symptoms of fatigue, stiffness, vestibular and balance problems, and gastrointestinal problems (Lamb, Stevens, & Johnson, 1965). These problems are arguably better understood as part of the development and maintenance of chronic pain problems rather than as independent symptoms whose report indicates abnormal symptom reporting in the patient. In summary, the diagnosis of somatoform pain based purely on the absence of obvious physical findings to substantiate the complaint is logically and scientifically unsatisfactory.

PSYCHOLOGICAL PAIN MECHANISMS

If we discard the notion of a purely psychogenic pain, what approach can usefully be taken to understanding the psychological component of these complex clinical phenomena? A number of psychological factors can be discerned. In fact, there is positive evidence for role of psychological factors in the etiology of chronic pain.

Depressed Mood. Higher scores on mood measures are commonly associated with reports of pain (Hotopf, Mayou, Wadsworth, & Wessely, 1999; Von Korff, Le Resche, & Dworkin, 1993). The notes in DSM-IV state that chronic pain is often associated with depressive disorders. The question of the causal direction between pain and depression has generated much controversy, but if pain is accepted as a sensory and emotional experience, as in the International Association for the Study of Pain (IASP) definition, linear causation is unlikely to be a productive model. Various models have been proposed to try to elucidate this relationship between pain and depression. Influential models of depression and pain include those of Rudy, Kerns, and Turk (1988), based on empirical work that demonstrated the mediation of the relationship by the impact of pain on the patient's life and on his or her sense of control; and of Banks and Kerns (1996), who posited both diathesis and stress, emphasizing the particular characteristics of chronic pain in that it was constant, inherently aversive, inescapable, potentially pervasive in its impact, and associated with significant losses. McCracken (1998) noted that the processes of acceptance and adaptation to pain require a clear starting point, unavailable to the patient whose chronic pain remains undiagnosed, unexplained, and doubted by family, friends, and medical authorities.

Both anxiety and depression share processes of selective or narrowed attention and specific belief-based interpretation, often described in pain as catastrophic thinking (Sullivan et al., 2001). The identification of cognitive and behavioural mechanisms, which span diagnoses, is more useful than simply seeking to subsume one diagnosis under another (Costello, 1993; Pincus & Williams, 1999). In both there is a narrowed focus of attention and selective memory; thoughts about the pain may include catastrophic and pessimistic predictions; attributional patterns tend to undermine the sense of control. Behaviorally, there is also a disinclination to be physically active (including sexually), fatigue, disturbed sleep, and weight gain, and those symptoms may be attributed by a diagnostician to pain, to mood (as "vegetative" symptoms), or to both, causing difficulties for the diagnosis of depression.

Many chronic pain patients who otherwise seem depressed attribute their symptoms to pain rather than to the self (Chapman & Gavrin, 1999; Skevington, 1995). That is, chronic pain patients who are unhappy, relatively inactive, and gloomy about the future, and who describe themselves as failures, may still attribute all those to pain, believing that with sufficient pain relief they would return to their "normal selves," active and satisfied with their lifestyle and prospects. There is, therefore, a phenomenological overlap between chronic pain and depression: Both represent conservation of scarce resources and withdrawal from any risk of further damage. It is likely that several pathways link pain and depression and the relationship is most unlikely to be straightforward.

Fear and Avoidance. In their cognitive and behavioral model of pain, Vlaeyen and Linton (2000; see also Vlaeyen, de Jong, Sieben, & Crombez, Chapter 10, this volume) described the role of fear and of avoidance. Fears of what is causing the pain, or of exacerbating pain and damage, may be based on personal experience or may be acquired from medical or paramedical information and advice (Barsky & Borus, 1999). Such fears may not be irrational but simply based on false premises. Unfortunately, they are easily established and hard to extinguish (Marks & Nesse, 1994). The patient who understands an authoritative doctor to have told him that his spine is "degenerating," that nerves are "trapped," or discs "crushed," as a cause of his pain, will understandably set a high priority on avoiding further damage, which is incorrectly assumed to be signaled by increased pain.

To continue activity as normal would appear to risk imminent serious disability. However, avoidance of specific activities or movements (attempts to protect the body include behaviors such as guarding or distorted gait) in fact worsens the situation and becomes self-maintaining, because it (1) minimizes pain and anxiety, which is inherently reinforcing (Fordyce, 1976), and (2) prevents the associated fears of harm from activity being disconfirmed (Philips, 1987).

Focusing of Attention and Catastrophic Thinking. Associated with fear is hypervigilance to symptoms. The level of anxiety about pain predicts the extent to which other nonspecific symptoms are reported (McCracken, Faber, & Janeck, 1998). The tendency to catastrophic thinking is a strong predictor in the early stages of acute low back pain of having disabling continued pain a year later (Burton, Tillotson, Main, & Hollis, 1995). Earlier roots may lie in childhood experience, family patterns of dealing with illness, and experience of professional health care (Craig, Boardman, Mills, Daly, & Drake, 1993; Hotopf et al., 1999).

SOCIAL PAIN MECHANISMS

Social and interpersonal factors are also undoubtedly relevant to the aetiology of chronic pain. However, there has been an unhelpful focus on solely social factors and on the putative benefits of being disabled, often archaically termed "secondary gain," an important aspect of which is solicitous attention from a partner. Although the evidence for secondary gain as a major factor causing pain-associated disability is limited (Newton-John & Williams, 2000), the behavior of others is likely to be important in either enabling or fostering helplessness.

Another important interpersonal factor concerns the interaction of the patient and doctor (Sullivan, 2001). Doctors are often more comfortable with and usually more knowledgeable about "medical" symptoms than about psychological problems (Dworkin, Wilson, & Massoth 1994). Barsky and Borus (1995) have emphasized the increasing medicalization of physical distress, fueling unrealistic expectations of patients and physicians, and the investment of health professionals and others in promoting symptoms as diseases and the part played by systems of medical certification of work disability and the compensation in raising the likelihood of the patient presenting physical symptoms.

SUMMARY AND IMPLICATIONS

The biological, psychological, and social factors described previously are all relevant to an understanding of chronic pain. However, the fact that one of these factors can be identified does not justify defining the pain as a "psychological phenomenon." It is always tempting to resort to single-factor explanations. But the challenge of maintaining complex biopsychosocial understanding is worth pursuing because in our opinion it is more likely to lead to effective treatment.

Practical Management

ASSESSMENT

Pain and Its Meaning. Successful assessment requires first that the pain patient feels believed. Patients who feel disbelieved, or who think that the clinician is searching primarily for evidence of psychopathology or deliberate deception, are likely to deny and conceal psychological experiences associated with the pain. Paradoxically, therefore, an excessive emphasis on psychological factors may make them less apparent. It can help if the clinician uses examples such as stress-related headache and phantom limb pain to develop a shared understanding that pain is neither a simple peripheral physical problem nor merely "imagined."

The patient should be asked to describe where the pain is, what it feels like (which may elicit disturbing images such as "barbed wire being pulled up and down my spine," "electric shocks," and "something hard growing inside my stomach," which are important to address in treatment), what makes it worse and better, and what the patient believes to be causing the pain and exacerbations in pain. Patients may feel embarrassed at revealing to a doctor an inaccurate model of how the body works and what is wrong. However, questions about what has been explained in previous consultations, whether they have read anything about their symptoms (including on websites), and what they think of this information will help to build a picture of their personal understanding. Verbatim excerpts can also be useful later in treatment, as they may demonstrate catastrophic misinterpretation of harmless phenomena (for instance, numbness and tingling are often interpreted as indicating a risk of paralysis; a weak knee "giving way" as imminent loss of function). Questions about whether the pain is thought to be stable or to be worsening over time also offer the opportunity to understand the patient's model of pathological process, and his or her expectations about the future. It is common for patients to fear "ending up in a wheelchair," or even becoming bed bound, and to see this as incompatible with worthwhile existence.

Impact of Pain on Lifestyle. Next, it is important to assess the restrictions suffered by the patient. What activities are avoided because of the pain, and which activities are pursued but are difficult or no longer enjoyable because of pain? As the patient explains each, reference can be made to the reported pains and to the movements or conditions that precipitate them. DSM-IV notes include as examples of impairment the inability to work or attend school; the areas of domestic activity, leisure pursuits, family life, social life, and intimate relationships should also be sampled.

Chronic pain is widely appreciated as having an impact on the patient's family and close associates (Flor, Turk, & Scholz, 1987; Roy, 1992), who often report feeling frustrated, at a loss over how to help, and confused by the lack of diagnosis or contradictory information. A shared sense of failure about the pain can lead to a complicit silence on the subject, and to a failure either to problem-solve or to provide mutual comfort. Useful questions to explore the behavior of others include whether others can detect the pain without the patient telling them, how they do so, how they respond and the effects of their response on the patient, whether patient and close other(s) discuss how best to manage the pain, and in whom, if anyone, the patient confides his or her difficulties.

Medical Help Seeking. Frequent use of health services and the substantial use of medication can be seen as evidence that the pain is the expression of a psychological problem. However, it may also reflect medical behavior with multiple referrals and prescriptions. The patient's relationship with his or her own doctor and specialists should be addressed. Questions such as "do you think your doctor understands your pain," or "how does/could he or she help" usually clarify the role played, wittingly or unwittingly, by the doctor in question. Repeated reassurance seeking and giving is addressed in the section on hypochondriasis.

The patient described above presented as angry, distressed, and ashamed. He felt he was "on the scrap heap"; his wife was having to work as well as running the house and family while he had become dependent on her; he felt that "there must be an answer" available from medical resources, suspected that such an answer was being withheld because of doubts about the authenticity of his pain in the absence of an identifiable origin, and felt deeply wronged by this as the accident had not been his fault. On questioning, he felt that he had sustained some serious damage to his neck vertebrae (as suggested by one of the medicolegal reports), which were pressing on nerves, producing pains all over his body. Further questioning elicited the belief that his neck was unstable and that therefore further movement of vertebrae might easily result in paralysis; the intermittent tingling he interpreted as a confirmation that this process was likely to occur. He therefore put as few demands as possible on his neck, kept it stiff and supported, and avoided most activity. In an effort to avoid addiction to opioids and benzodiazepines, he did not use them regularly as prescribed

but, rather, kept them until the pain was unmanageable and then used them in a large combined dose, after which he slept for some time.

Multidimensional Summary. The assessment may be summarized on a multiaxial scheme such as the one below

Biological
1. Pain: Chronic severe neck pain—generalized.
2. Physiology: Presumed neurophysiological sensitization, secondary muscle weakness, and distorted use.

Psychological
3. Cognitions: Fear about paralysis, despondency.
4. Emotion: Anxiety and depression.
5. Behavior: Marked avoidance.

Social
6. Social context: Family distress, blame and litigation.
7. Medical care: Misinformation and conflicting information, inappropriate treatments.

TREATMENT

Treatment Goals. The goals of treatment are (1) gaining increased control over the pain by physical, pharmacological, or psychological means; (2) the recovery as far as possible of the patient's normal function; (3) the reduction of distress associated with pain; and (4) the increase in the patient's independence in managing the pain and the consequent reduction of reliance on health care personnel and resources.

Management properly addresses all these goals. It should be noted that the last three unfortunately do not automatically follow from a partial pain reduction. The establishment of understanding and a shared model between patient and doctor underpin effective treatment by whatever modality. McQuay and Moore (1998) summarize the evidence for the effectiveness of many pain treatments. However, for other treatments in current use, such as spinal cord stimulation or spinal implantation of morphine pumps, too little empirical work exists to provide clear guidelines. Overall, the patient should be encouraged in a robustly critical outlook toward claims of miracle cures, whether from orthodox or complementary medicine.

Psychological Treatments. If psychological treatment is agreed on, it is best achieved using cognitive-behavioral methods (Morley, Eccleston, & Williams, 1999). However, that is not to say that components of such treatment cannot be appropriately used singly, or that they cannot be used alongside physical or pharmacological treatments. It is essential, however, that if several treatment modalities are used at the same time, they share common goals. For example, patients are understandably unwilling to exert themselves under the guidance of one clinician to achieve self-management of pain when another holds out the possibility of abolishing the pain.

Although psychodynamic psychotherapy has been recommended for chronic pain patients with complex problems (Grzesiak, Ury, & Dworkin, 1996; see Basler, Grzesiak, & Dworkin, Chapter 5, this volume), there is insufficient evidence to judge its efficacy. Nonetheless, the treatment described by Grzesiak and colleagues approximates thoughtful individual cognitive therapy with a particular focus on issues in the doctor–patient relationship. These include unrealistic expectations of the doctor's power and nihilism about the patient's own role.

Education and Information. A necessary precondition for engaging patients in increased activity, or movement that they may believe to be hazardous, is their positive collaboration. This is best achieved by "providing patients with information relevant to their condition and care, by avoiding pejorative labels or categories, by supporting and encouraging patients' coping efforts, and by generally showing respect and compassion for each patient's unique experience of pain." (Keefe, Jacobs, & Underwood-Gordon, 1997, p. 93).

Overpsychologizing the patient's problem is likely to make him or her feel misunderstood and therefore skeptical of the value of advice or treatment given in that context (Dworkin et al., 1994). Adequate understanding of the physiological aspect of the

patient's symptoms, shared as far as possible with the patient, underpins a joint approach to treatment and long-term management. The patient often requires information that is not easy either to access from available sources or to integrate with his or her experience. New information that offers nonthreatening alternative explanations for the patient's experience, including the pain-related fear model shown in Figure 26.1, can powerfully help in reconstruction of past, present, and future narrative, so the patient feels free to undertake previously avoided activities.

Setting Appropriate and Explicit Goals. DSM-IV observes that recovery may be aided by regularly scheduled activities that are undertaken despite pain; excellent advice, but rarely given, even in well-educated primary care practices (Turner, LeResche, Von Korff, & Ehrlich, 1998). Such advice moves the focus of doctor–patient interaction from relieving symptoms to achieving goal-directed activity. It is not uncommon for patients to list chores to restart but to find little pleasure in their performance. The clinician can usefully ensure that the plans include activities that are inherently satisfying and that therefore rapidly become self-sustaining. Goals often include adopting some regular exercise and stretch routines to counteract the effects of local or general disuse; these are better maintained if they involve social contact.

Working toward Goals. Following the recognition that it is fear of pain rather than pain itself that is disabling, the fear is addressed by a graded exposure program. This is akin to that used in the treatment of phobias (Vlaeyen & Linton, 2000). Graded exposure also serves the purpose of keeping the new activity within safe limits, as each step is carefully planned and does not exceed reasonable demands on patients' physical capacity and tolerance of acute anxiety. This is also important in addressing fears of the supervising clinician that the patient will damage him- or herself. Undertaking graded exposure with the clinician can be a useful part of treatment, not least for eliciting the "hot cognitions" that often sustain fears. However, generalization to the patient's

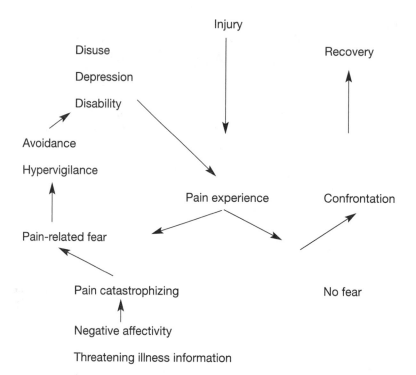

FIGURE 26.1 The factors that interact in the maintenance of chronic pain and routes of recovery. From Vlaeyen and Linton (2000). Copyright 2000 by the International Association for the Study of Pain. Adapted by permission.

own environment must be incorporated in the schedule if the benefit is to be sustained.

Cognitive Challenges. Patients' fears about pain center on damage, increased pain, and their short- and long-term consequences (Philips, 1987). It is worth (1) asking patients to explain what they mean by "not being able to cope" if the pain worsens (which may elicit fears about pain destroying the patient's sanity), (2) asking for the worst that can happen in terms of damage or pain, and (3) requiring the patient to estimate the risk before and after undertaking graded steps in the exposure program. Patients can then be helped to develop more accurate and helpful self-statements in response to catastrophic predictions, self-denigratory judgments ("I'm on the scrap heap"), misinterpretation of feelings as facts ("I feel helpless—I am helpless"), and other evidence of biased thinking. This applies also to difficulties eliciting or accepting help from others: Patients can usefully reflect on how they express pain and needs related to it, challenge unhelpful thoughts about being

diminished by being helped, and improve their negotiation skills.

Promoting Self-Management over the Longer Term. The ultimate goal of treatment is that the patient becomes self-managing and ceases to re-present with the chronic symptoms in the remote hope that a cure will be forthcoming. The need for confiding and understanding is generally better met within the patient's social and family circles, and it is worth remembering that treatment methods and principles are not the exclusive property of medical or psychological professionals (Von Korff et al., 1998). The anticipation of "bad patches" should be addressed so that the patient can better prepare him- or herself. Enabling the patient to be open-mindedly skeptical about promises of cure can help the patient to make better decisions about treatment.

It was explained to the patient in the case described that constant use of the orthopedic collar had weakened his neck muscles, adding to his sense of instability; that keeping his head relatively still had affected his

March 26

Dear MAC students,

Most of you know that the full time faculty here are on the standard 9 ½ month academic contract, the rest of the time is on academic leave for writing, conferences, and personal vacations, etc. I have taken only a bit of my academic leave for this academic year (July 1 2007 – June 30, 2008), so I am going to be away quite a bit between now and July.

This email is to let you know my schedule so that you can plan to consult with me as you need.

Week of March 31 (Spring Break): I am here as usual (Mondays I am generally not on campus as it is my clinical practice day, and I cannot respond to emails or phone calls usually).
Week of April 7: I am at a conference at U. Arizona Tucson. I will be able to occasionally track emails.
Week of April 14: I leave for San Diego for the faculty symposium on Wednesday and am gone for the rest of the week. I will be able to occasionally track emails.
Week of April 21: I am on academic leave and will not be on campus or available for consultation with students. I will be unable to respond to emails.
Week of April 28: On campus as usual.
Month of May, May 5 – May 30. I am teaching Psy 631a TuTh as an overload. In addition, I will be on campus one day a week to keep oversight on the BA and MAC programs. That day will be Tuesdays (May 6, 13, 20, 27). Some Wednesdays I will be here W 3-5 for Group Supervision (Psy 631b). Please hold all but emergency consultations for Tuesdays.
Weeks of June 2 and June 9. On campus as usual.
Weeks of June 16 and June 23 – on Academic leave. I will not be able to respond to emails.

1. Dr. Dalene Forester will be providing group supervision for me on dates I am gone. All Psy 631b students have been informed in person and with a calendar.
2. My MAC faculty backup just in case is Dr. Charles Powell, statewide lead faculty for the MAC, or Dr. Henry Venter, at the Fresno campus (emails cpowell@nu.edu and hventer@nu.edu, but most of the time you should be able to reach me by cell phone if there is a need for emergency consultation. Only consult with them if (a) I am not available and (b) you have discussed your concern with your academic advisor.

So, if you have consultation needs next week will be a good time and after that I will be gone most of two weeks.

Dr. Gregory White

Professor of Psychology
Regional Lead Faculty in Psychology
National University
Redding Academic Center
2195 Larkspur Lane
Redding, CA 96002
530-226-4007

balance; that he had lost physical condition through inactivity; and that opioids and benzodiazepines contributed to his dizziness. A model of chronic pain was explained that did not hinge on whether or not there was evidence of damage but that referred to changes in pain signaling in the nervous system. He was encouraged to view exacerbation of pain after activity not as evidence of further damage but as the predictable result of pushing himself to be active (crediting him with making the effort), but with an unfit body, excessive tension and postural distortions associated with protecting his neck, and worry that (in his words) "opened all the communication channels" to attend to pains and other symptoms.

Over time, the patient was encouraged to work toward modest goals, carefully pacing his activity as he gained strength and flexibility from specific exercises prescribed by a physiotherapist, particularly for his neck and including some for balance. The collar was gradually withdrawn, and his posture and gait were corrected, improving his standing, sitting, and walking tolerances. He was particularly satisfied with finding activities to do with his children and opted to take adult education classes both to help his children with their homework and to extend his work skills. Taking responsibility for their children gave his wife a break, his family life improved, his social circles enlarged, and he started to look for voluntary work. He stopped his daily use of opioids and benzodiazepines, managing flare-ups with nonsteroidal anti-inflammatory drugs, but stayed on an antidepressant at night to help his sleep. He developed a personal model of his pain, such that he no longer became anxious at the worsening of or changes in symptoms, and he shared this model with his primary care doctor so that she could remind him of it when he consulted her in a crisis.

ORGANIZATION OF MEDICAL CARE

Optimal care is based on regular rather than complaint-contingent scheduling of appointments and a clear self-management plan shared by a limited number of health professionals who liase effectively (Dworkin et al., 1994). Explicit recognition of the pa-

tient's achievements despite continued pain can be a powerful reinforcement and a boost to confidence. Conversely, apparent anxiety on the doctor's part about the safety of the plan, or mixed messages such as continuing to order investigations while recommending self-management, will undermine the patient's activity and confidence.

Summary

The judicious use of cognitive and behavioral pain management methods, guided by patients' predominant concerns and needs, and building on patients' strengths and resources in their environments, are the best option for treatment.

Hypochondriasis

The essential defining feature of hypochondriasis as defined in DSM-IV is a preoccupation with the fear of having or the idea one has a "serious disease." It is further specified that this belief be based on misinterpretation of one or more bodily signs or symptoms. This concern is unfounded as far as a thorough medical evaluation does not identify the condition and the patient's fear or preoccupation persists despite medical reassurance. Important exclusions are that the patient's belief is not so completely fixed that it meets criteria for a delusion and the symptoms are no better explained by another diagnosis such as depression.

To set a threshold for "caseness" as with other disorders, it is specified that the preoccupation with bodily symptoms causes clinically significant distress or impairment in social, occupational, or other important areas of functioning and lasts at least 6 months (American Psychiatric Association, 1994; see Table 26.2).

Conceptual Limitations of Hypochondriasis

DUALISM

As described for somatoform pain disorder, the main conceptual limitation with hypochondriasis is that the clinician has to make a judgment about whether the patient's complaints are explained by disease. There is a potential here for unhelpful disagreement;

TABLE 26.2. DSM-IV Diagnostic Criteria for Hypochondriasis

A. Preoccupation with fears of having, or the idea one has, a serious disease based on the person's misinterpretation of bodily symptoms.

B. The preoccupation persists despite appropriate medical evaluation and reassurance.

C. The belief in Criterion A is not a delusional intensity (as in Delusional Disorder, Somatic Type) and is not restricted to a circumscribed concern about appearance (as in Body Dysmorphic Disorder).

D. The preoccupation causes clinically significant distress or impairment in social, occupational, or other important areas of function.

E. The duration of the disturbance is at least 6 months.

F. The preoccupation is not better accounted for by Generalized Anxiety Disorder, Obsessive–Compulsive Disorder, Panic Disorder, a Major Depressive Episode, Separation Anxiety, or another Somatoform Disorder.

Note. From American Psychiatric Association (1994). Copyright 1994 by the American Psychiatric Association. Adapted by permission.

the clinician insisting that the patient's symptoms are "entirely psychological" and the patient insisting that they are "real."

ADEQUATE INVESTIGATION

There is also the question of what "adequate investigation" is to exclude disease. Again, patients may feel that they require a further investigation (such as an MRI scan) whereas the clinician may feel it is not indicated. In both these cases, it is important that differences in opinion about the nature of the pain are not resolved simply by labeling the patient as hypochondriacal but, rather, by trying to attain a shared understanding. As with somatoform pain disorder, this shared understanding is the basis of effective management.

APPROPRIATE REASSURANCE

The diagnosis of hypochondriasis can only be made when the person who fears disease has received "appropriate medical reassurance" that he or she is not suffering from disease. There are two potential difficulties here. The first is that adequate reassurance is not defined. In practice, reassurance may vary from simply telling the patient, "if you don't hear from us you can assume we didn't find anything," to a detailed review, explanation of test results, and exposition of a biopsychosocial model of symptoms. The second problem is that reassurance may actually make hypochondriasis worse. This

has even led to the suggestion that the second criterion should be rewritten as "the preoccupation persists *because of* (rather than despite) medical reassurance" (Warwick & Salkovskis, 1985).

Hypochondriasis or Health Anxiety

It has been argued that hypochondriasis would be better categorized as an anxiety disorder focusing around worry about health rather than as a somatoform disorder (Salkovskis & Warwick, 1986). There would appear to be some merit in this argument in that the core of hypochondriasis is anxiety about health (or rather about disease). The DSM-IV category is, however, broader as it also includes patients who have a *belief* that there is something wrong with them without necessarily being anxious as well as those who have predominantly anxiety. Restricting the category of hypochondriasis to health anxiety and regarding it as an anxiety disorder may therefore not capture the whole of the currently defined phenomena.

Somatoform Pain Disorder versus Hypochondriasis

The somatoform disorder classification places patients who present primarily with somatic symptoms in different categories from patients who present primarily with beliefs and fears about disease. Although this is an apparently tidy arrangement, it does not reflect clinical reality. Practicing clinicians rather tend to regard somatization (the presentation with unexplained somatic symptoms) and hypochondriasis (the presentation with fear or belief about disease) as separate dimensions. That is, the majority of patients present with concern about both symptoms and disease.

Hypochondriasis Disorder or Anxiety and Depression

There has been a lengthy and somewhat sterile debate about whether hypochondriasis should be regarded as a disorder in its own right or whether it is always a manifestation of depression and/or anxiety (Appleby, 1987). This problem can be most readily resolved by taking a dimensional approach (discussed later). The issue does, however, serve to remind us that it is important to seek evidence of anxiety disorders, including panic disorder, and depressive disorders in patients who present with pain associated hypochondriasis, as treatment of these may be important in the overall management of the condition.

Clinical Utility

A diagnosis has a number of functions. One is to predict prognosis and response to treatment and another is as a label to give to patients to "explain" their suffering.

A diagnosis of hypochondriasis or severe health anxiety tells us that the patient is likely to get multiple medical opinions to get reassurance. If not adequately managed, patients with hypochondriasis can cause mayhem in medical systems. Their repeated demands for reassurance and their infectious anxiety can lead to their having extensive multiple and unproductive investigations and treatments. Patients can also be made worse. There is evidence that repeated reassurance and investigation rather than reducing their anxiety in fact produce a rebound of increased anxiety (Warwick & Salkovskis, 1990). The patient and the doctor can then become locked in a spiral of investigation, anxiety, and further investigation based on a shared anxiety about missed disease (Howard & Wessely, 1996). Iatrogenic harm from inappropriate drug treatment or even

surgery may result (Kouyanou, Pither, & Wessely, 1997).

A Biopsychosocial Perspective

The factors relevant to a biopsychosocial perspective of pain-associated hypochondriasis are the same as those outlined previously for somatoform pain disorder. However, in this case the psychological factors of catastrophic thinking and focusing of attention are paramount. They are associated with social factors of reassurance seeking and psychological iatrogenesis.

A Case Example

Ms. A is a 25-year-old college graduate who presented repeatedly to her primary care doctors with head pain. She has expressed a great fear that there might be some serious cause. She was observed systematically to make appointments with each of the six doctors working in the health center. She explained this as maximizing the number of opinions she obtained on what was wrong with her in order to get to the truth. She was eventually sent to the hospital neurological department as an emergency. When seen by the assessing neurologist, he said that he did not believe there was a serious neurological cause for her head pain, but in response to her anxiety rather than medical indication he ordered a CT brain scan to provide "reassurance." The CT scan was normal. However, the patient expressed even greater anxiety that something had "been missed" and requested an MRI scan.

She was then referred to neuropsychiatry for further assessment again as an emergency. More detailed assessment revealed that the patient had a strong belief that she had a vascular tumor of the brain, which could hemorrhage *at any time and kill her.* Whenever she experienced head pain, she interpreted this as evidence that the tumor was about to burst and understandably became anxious. When she became anxious she started overbreathing and developed feelings of dizziness and paraesthesiae on her hands and mouth. She interpreted these physiological symptoms of hypocapnia as further evidence of impending neurological catastrophe and became even more anxious.

She reported having taken many medical books out of the library and to be studying these in detail to gain more information about cerebral bleeds. She also admitted to repeatedly checking her pulse to see if there was any evidence of tachycardia, "suggesting hemorrhage," and to seeking reassurance that she was not about to die, not only from each of her primary care doctors but also from friends and family. She said that she found the hospital neurological assessment and CT scan reassuring for a period of only about 1 day but that her concerns had subsequently returned even more strongly than before. This was her reason for requesting an MRI scan.

Practical Management

ASSESSMENT

The clinician who knows how to recognize and manage this condition can often produce a dramatic resolution to the problem. The predominant features that should alert the clinician to a hypochondriacal patient are urgency of presentation and of referral, strongly expressed anxiety about what is wrong at the beginning of the consultation (often with a phone call for reassurance preceding the consultation), a history of repeated negative medical assessments, and the repeated overt or covert seeking of reassurance during the assessment consultation. After the consultation, the patient may again telephone the assessing clinician to seek further reassurance about disease.

Appropriate Assessment. Once a patient who presents with a pain complaint is suspected of having a significant degree of hypochondriasis or health anxiety, a further assessment is important. Table 26.2 shows the elements to include in this assessment.

1. Detailed exploration of the person's beliefs and concerns about his or her health, including concerns about catastrophic and fatal developments and how these might be prevented.
2. A check that the patient's beliefs are at least briefly alterable and that they are not delusional (i.e., fixed), suggesting psychosis.
3. Assessment of the reasons that the person has these concerns (e.g., a history of

premature death and/or misplaced medical reassurance given to friends or relatives).
4. Detailed assessment of behaviors, including the frequency of self-checking behavior, reassurance seeking, and the reading of medical books and/or use of the Internet.
5. A careful assessment for the presence of anxiety disorder (including panic attacks) and for depressive disorder.

Assessment of Fears and Beliefs. Taking time and providing an empathic approach are essential prerequisites to exploring fears or beliefs that the patients themselves may find embarrassing to reveal. It is essential for clinicians to listen to the patient's concerns without providing premature information or reassurance. The patient should be told that you want to hear about all his or her concerns, however ridiculous they may seem. Useful questions may include the following: "What do you think is wrong with you?" "Do you think the doctors might have missed something?" "What is the worst you think could happen?" "What do you think you could do to prevent this happening?"

Having elicited the patient's beliefs and checking that he or she has understood them correctly, it is helpful for the clinician to explore how these beliefs have developed. Frequently the patient reports that a friend or relative has had a serious or fatal illness and that this illness was "missed" by the assessing physician. Useful questions are, "Why do you think you might have this problem?", "Have you known anyone else who has had a similar problem?", and "What makes you think the doctor may have missed something?"

Further history from our case example revealed that the patient's father had died the previous year of a stroke, after being seen by his primary care doctor the previous day and reassured that his headaches were not a sign of serious disease.

Understanding the background to the patient's beliefs is helpful in (1) seeing them as an understandable rather than totally irrational misinterpretation of symptoms; (2) providing the patient with an empathic understanding of his or her predicament; and (3) providing material for a cognitive-behavioral approach in which the beliefs and behavior are reviewed and modified.

Occasionally patients with hypochondriacal concerns have a psychotic illness. Delusional beliefs are fixed and would not be amenable even briefly to reassurance. They are also out of keeping with the patient's cultural context—a point that may be worth the clinician's checking on by making sure that he or she asks informants. Furthermore, the psychotic patient may have other evidence of psychosis such as delusions and hallucinations.

Assessment of Checking Reassurance and Information Seeking. Patients' strategies to obtain reassurance can be varied and sometimes covert. It is important to explore this sensitively with the patient. Patients may check their body in a variety of ways "to make sure that the worst is not happening." Overt reassurance seeking may involve making consultations with doctors, but more covert reassurance seeking may involve dropping hints in conversations with questions such as, "How do you think I look today?" Useful questions are, "How do you reassure yourself that the worst is not about to happen?", "How much does that help?", and "How long does the effect last." This question often elicits the account that the effective reassurance was temporary. This again provides a basis for a treatment program, which involves the patient voluntarily restricting reassurance seeking.

Patients' preoccupation with illness may also lead them to "surfing the net" and reading medical books to try to seek reassurance and gain more and more information about their condition. Unfortunately, much of the information can be unhelpful and may even give rise to greater fears. Again, the clinician should inquire about this.

Anxiety and Depression. Anxiety is usually obvious. Commonly the symptoms are accompanied by attacks of panic, and it is useful to identify these. Panic is treatable and provides an alternative explanation of symptoms that can be offered to the patient. It is also important to seek evidence of depression and worth remembering that hypochondriasis can develop into depression.

For the patient described previously, careful assessment revealed that many of her symptoms were due to panic. She did not have clear evidence of depression although it was difficult to distinguish the loss of interest related to a preoccupation with illness from a loss of interest reflecting depression. Follow-up over several weeks, however, revealed increasing evidence of depressive symptoms with tearfulness, loss of appetite, and social withdrawal.

Multidimensional Summary. The assessment may be summarized on a multiaxial scheme such as the one that follows:

Biological
1. Pain: Headache intermittent.
2. Physiology: Presumed muscle tension and hyperventilation.

Psychological
3. Cognitions: Severe fear about stroke.
4. Emotion: Marked anxiety and depression.
5. Behavior: Frequent reassurance seeking.

Social
6. Social context: Family concern about stroke and medical mistakes.
7. Medical care: Repeated reassurance.

TREATMENT

Both pharmacological and nonpharmacological interventions can be helpful. The important general management is to establish an empathic and collaborative approach with the patient. It is important for the clinician to show that he or she takes the patient's concerns seriously and does not believe they are "stupid" or "ridiculous." This does not mean agreeing with the patient's concerns but simply accepting them as legitimate and anxiety provoking.

It is also important to explain to the patient a model of hypochondriasis. In particular, it may be useful to draw a diagram for patients, which shows a vicious circle between fear of illness, anxiety, somatic symptoms, and further belief and a similar circle for reassurance seeking. An example is shown in Figure 26.2.

Specific management includes the use of antidepressant medication, the use of psychological treatment, and overall management of the patient's medical care. Antide-

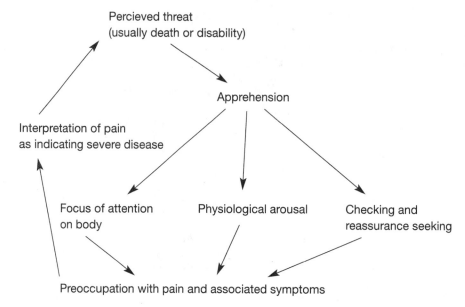

FIGURE 26.2 Cognitive-behavioral model of hypochondriasis. From Warwick and Salkovskis (1990). Copyright 1990 by Elsevier. Adapted by permission.

pressant medication including selective serotonin reuptake inhibitors (SSRIs) can be helpful. This is particularly the case when the patient is suffering from panic and/or a depressive disorder.

Ms. A, the patient described previously, was able to entertain the idea that her problem was fear about a stroke rather than an actual stroke. She agreed to stop seeking reassurance. She also accepted treatment with an SSRI antidepressant over a period of 1 month and her symptoms gradually resolved. When she stopped taking the SSRI antidepressant, however, she relapsed. The relapse responded to a brief psychological intervention consisting of a collaborative review of the lack of evidence for her fears.

The mainstay of psychological treatment is a cognitive-behavioral approach. The cognitive-behavioral model can be readily shared with patients and provides an alternative explanation to the possibility that they have a serious disease. Indeed the possibility of serious disease and the vicious circle model can be presented to the patient as competing alternatives that the clinician and patient must distinguish between.

Although found to be more effective than waiting-list treatment in a randomized trial

(Warwick, Clark, Cobb, & Salkovskis, 1996) a more recent trial in which cognitive-behavioral therapy (CBT) was compared with behavioral stress management found no substantial difference in their long-term effectiveness (Clark et al., 1998). It is these authors' view that forming an empathic collaborative relationship, providing the patient with an alternative explanation, and limiting reassurance seeking are essential ingredients of effective treatment.

ORGANIZATION OF MEDICAL CARE

An important part in the management of such patients is to limit reassurance seeking and further investigation, ideally by a self-imposed reduction in such activities by the patient. However, with the patient's permission it may also be helpful to ensure that those doctors involved in his or her care are aware of the problem and do not engage in further assessment or investigation unless it is clearly warranted by new evidence (Todd, 1984). What is sufficiently compelling new evidence is, of course, not entirely straightforward and must rely on the individual clinician's judgment. Suffice to say that symptoms should not automatically be met with further investigation: The probability of a new diagnosis emerging should be balanced against the known psychological harm of further tests. For doctors to be effective in addressing patients' anxieties, they may have to address their own. Otherwise they may tend to give mixed messages by, for example, telling the patient there is nothing wrong or to worry about while referring them for investigation or prescribing treatment "just in case." The construction and rehearsal of a positive biopsychosocial formulation of the pain problem can consequently help the doctor as well as the patient.

Although physicians may be skeptical about being told they should not simply reassure a patient, they are usually receptive to the explanation that new information is good and may require repetition, but that continuous repetition of information should be a warning sign that the patient is locked into a vicious circle of anxiety and reassurance, which is counterproductive. Rather, the patient can be told something like the following: "It appears to me that you are now repeatedly seeking reassurance. I understand that this is not going to be helpful for you in the long term so I would prefer not to do it. It will be more helpful if you can learn to manage these fears yourself. We can help you do that."

Conclusions and Synthesis

In this chapter we have attempted to address pain from the perspective of the somatoform disorders as described in DSM-IV. We regard the somatoform disorder classification as unhelpfully dualistic and potentially hazardous to effective patient care. Rather, we have emphasized that both a scientifically sounder and practically more helpful approach is to accept that the patient's complaint of pain is a biopsychosocial phenomenon in every case. We have rejected the notion that pain complaints can be comfortably dichotomized into "medical pain" and "psychiatric pain." This unhelpful and inaccurate dichotomization carries the dual dangers of overemphasizing the role of psychological factors where the physical basis of the pain is obscure and conversely underestimating the importance

of psychological factors in the patient who has obvious disease.

We have briefly reviewed the evidence for biological, psychological, and social factors in chronic pain. We regard psychological factors as important but do not regard their identification as meaning that physiological factors are absent. We have outlined principles of cognitive-behavioral management both for chronic "somatoform" pain in general and for hypochondriasis with pain as a symptom in particular.

In summary, therefore, we wish to urge clinicians to approach the symptom of pain from a biopsychosocial perspective and to avoid leaping to simplistic understandings of causation be they biological, psychological, or social. Holding a broad biological perspective and then focusing management on those factors that are most amenable to change is not always easy. It is, however, our strong belief that it is the best way effectively to manage patients suffering from pain.

Note

1. The International Association for the Study of Pain describes pain as a sensory and emotional experience, and does not require any identifiable tissue damage to verify the complaint of pain. An alternative definition by Chapman and Gavrin (1999) focuses on the meaning to the patient, which underlies his or her presentation: "Pain is a perceived threat or damage to one's biological integrity" (p. 2233).

References

American Psychiatric Association. (1994). *Diagnostic and statistical manual of mental disorders* (4th ed.). Washington, DC: Author.

Appleby, L. (1987). Hypochondriasis: An acceptable diagnosis? *British Medical Journal 294,* 857.

Banks, S. M., & Kerns, R. D. (1996). Explaining high rates of depression in chronic pain: A diathesis-stress framework. *Psychological Bulletin, 199,* 95–110.

Barsky, A. J., & Borus, J. F. (1995). Somatization and medicalization in the era of managed care. *Journal of the American Medical Association, 274,* 1931–1934.

Barsky, A. J., & Borus, J. F. (1999). Functional somatic syndromes. *Annals of Internal Medicine, 130,* 910–921.

Burton, A. K., Tillotson, K. M., Main, C. J., & Hollis, S. (1995). Psychosocial predictors of outcome in acute and subchronic low back trouble. *Spine, 20,* 722–728.

Cervero, F., & Laird, J. M. A. (1999). Visceral pain. *Lancet, 353,* 2145–2148.

Chapman, C. R., & Gavrin, J. (1999). Suffering: The contributions of persistent pain. *Lancet, 353,* 2233–2237.

Clark, D. M., Salkovskis, P. M., Hackmann, A., Wells, A., Fennell, M., Ludgate, J., Ahmad, S., Richards, H. C., & Gelder, M. (1998). Two psychological treatments for hypochondriasis. A randomised controlled trial. *British Journal of Psychiatry, 173,* 218–225

Costello, C. G. (1993). From symptoms of depression to syndromes of depression. In C. G. Costello (Ed.), *Symptoms of depression* (pp. 291–302). New York: Wiley.

Craig, T. K. J., Boardman, A. P., Mills, K., Daly-Jones, O., & Drake, H. (1993). The South London somatisation study. 1. Longitudinal course and the influence of early life experiences. *British Journal of Psychiatry, 163,* 579–588.

Dworkin, S. F., Wilson, L., & Massoth, D. L. (1994). Somatizing as a risk factor for chronic pain. In R. C. Grzesiak & D. S. Ciccone (Eds.), *Psychological vulnerability to chronic pain* (pp. 28–54). New York: Springer.

Engel, G. L. (1980). The clinical application of the biopsychosocial model. *American Journal of Psychiatry, 137,* 535–544

Flor, H., Turk, D. C., & Scholz, O. B. (1987). Impact of chronic pain on the spouse: Marital, emotional and physical consequences. *Journal of Psychosomatic Research, 31,* 63–71.

Fordyce, W. E. (1976). *Behavioral methods for chronic pain and illness.* St. Louis, MO: Mosby.

Grzesiak, R. C., Ury, G. M., & Dworkin, R. H. (1996) Psychodynamic psychotherapy with chronic pain patients. In R. J. Gatchel & D. C. Turk (Eds.), *Psychological approaches to pain management: A practitioner's handbook* (pp. 148–178). New York: Guilford Press.

Hotopf, M., Mayou, R., Wadsworth, M., & Wessely, S. (1999). Psychosocial and developmental antecedents of chest pain in young adults. *Psychosomatic Medicine, 61,* 861–867.

Howard, L. M., & Wessely, S. (1996). Reappraising reassurance—the role of investigations. *Journal of Psychosomatic Research, 41,* 307–311.

Keefe, F. J., Dunsmore, J., & Burnett, R. (1992). Behavioral and cognitive-behavioral approaches to chronic pain: Recent advances and future directions. *Journal of Consulting and Clinical Psychology, 60,* 528–536.

Keefe, F. J., Jacobs, M., & Underwood-Gordon, L. (1997). Biobehavioral pain research: A multi-institute assessment of cross-cutting issues and research needs. *Clinical Journal of Pain, 13,* 91–103.

Kirmayer, L. J., Robbins, J. M., & Paris, J. (1994). Somatoform disorders: Personality and the social matrix of somatic distress. *Journal of Abnormal Psychology, 103,* 125–136.

Kouyanou, K., Pither, C. E., & Wessely, S. (1997). Iatrogenic factors and chronic pain. *Psychosomatic Medicine, 59,* 597–604.

Lamb, L. E., Stevens, P. M., & Johnson, R. L. (1965). Hypokinesia secondary to chair rest from 4 to 10 days. *Aerospace Medicine, 36,* 755–763.

Loeser, J. D., & Melzack, R. (1999). Pain: An overview. *Lancet, 353,* 1607–1609.

Marks, I. M., & Nesse, R. M. (1994), Fear and fitness: An evolutionary analysis of anxiety disorders. *Ethology and Sociobiology, 15,* 247–261.

Martin, R. D. (1999). The somatoform conundrum: A question of nosological values. *General Hospital Psychiatry, 21*(3), 177–186.

McCracken, L. M. (1998). Learning to live with the pain: Acceptance of pain predicts adjustment in persons with chronic pain. *Pain, 74,* 21–27.

McCracken, L. M., Faber, S. D., & Janeck, A. S. (1998). Pain-related anxiety predicts non-specific physical complaints in persons with chronic pain. *Behaviour Research and Therapy, 36,* 621–630

McQuay, H., & Moore, A. (1998). *An evidence-based resource for pain relief.* Oxford, UK: Oxford University Press.

Morley, S. J., Eccleston, C., & Williams, A. C. de C. (1999). Systematic review and meta-analysis of randomised controlled trials of cognitive behaviour therapy and behaviour therapy for chronic pain in adults, excluding headache. *Pain, 80,* 1–13.

Newton-John, T. O., & Williams, A. C. (2000). Solicitousness revisited: A qualitative analysis of spouse responses to pain behaviours. In M. Devor, M. Rowbotham, & Z. Wiesenfeld-Hallin (Eds.), *Proceedings of the 9th World Congress in Pain* (pp. 1113–1122). Seattle, WA: IASP Press

Philips, H. C. (1987). Avoidance behaviour and its role in sustaining chronic pain. *Behaviour Research and Therapy, 25,* 273–279.

Pincus, T., & Williams, A. C. (1999). Models and measurements of depression in chronic pain. *Journal of Psychosomatic Research, 47,* 211–219.

Roy, R. (1992). *The social context of the chronic pain sufferer.* Toronto: University of Toronto Press.

Rudy, T. E., Kerns, R. D., & Turk, D. C. (1988). Chronic pain and depression: Toward a cognitive-behavioral mediation model. *Pain, 35,* 129–140.

Salkovskis, P. M., & Warwick, H. M. (1986). Morbid preoccupations, health anxiety and reassurance: A cognitive-behavioural approach to hypochondriasis. *Behaviour Research and Therapy, 24,* 597–602.

Sharpe, M., & Bass, C. (1992). Pathophysiological models in somatization. *International Review of Psychiatry, 4,* 81–97.

Sharpe, M., & Carson, A. J. (2001). "Unexplained" somatic symptoms, functional syndromes, and somatization: Do we need a paradigm shift? *Annals of Internal Medicine, 134*(9), Suppl. (Part 2), S926.

Skevington, S. M. (1995). *Psychology of pain.* Chichester, UK: Wiley.

Staud, R., Vierck, C. J., Cannon, R. L., Mauderli, A. P., & Price, D. D. (2001). Abnormal sensitization and temporal summation of second pain (wind-up) in patients with fibromyalgia syndrome. *Pain, 91,* 165–175.

Sullivan, M. D. (2001). Finding pain between minds and bodies. *Clinical Journal of Pain, 17,* 146–156.

Sullivan, M. J. L., Thorn, B., Haythornthwaite, J. A., Keefe, F., Martin, M., Bradley, L. A., & Lefevre, J. C. (2001). Theoretical perspectives on the relation between catastrophizing and pain. *Clinical Journal of Pain, 17,* 53–61.

Todd, J. W. (1984). Investigations. *Lancet, ii,* 1146–1147.

Turner, J. A., LeResche, L., Von Korff, M., & Ehrlich, K. (1998). Back pain in primary care. Patient characteristics, content of initial visit, and short-term outcomes. *Spine, 23,* 463–469.

Veldman, H. J. M., Reynen, H. M., Arntz, I. E., & Goris, R. J. A. (1993). Signs and symptoms of reflex sympathetic dystrophy: A prospective study of 829 patients. *Lancet, 342,* 1012–1016.

Vlaeyen, J. W. S., & Linton, S. J. (2000). Fear–avoidance and its consequences in chronic musculoskeletal pain: A state of the art. *Pain, 85,* 317–332.

Von Korff, M., Le Resche, L., & Dworkin, S. F. (1993). First onset of common pain symptoms: A prospective study of depression as a risk factor. *Pain, 55,* 251–258.

Von Korff, M., Moore, J. E., Lorig, K., Cherkin, D. C., Saunders, K., Gonzalez, V. M., Laurent, D., Rutter, C., & Comite, F. (1998). A randomized trial of a lay person-led self-management group intervention for back pain patients in primary care. *Spine, 23*(23), 2608–2615.

Von Korff, M., & Simon, G. (1996). The relationship between pain and depression. *British Journal of Psychiatry, 168*(Suppl. 30), 101–108.

Wall, P. D. (1994). Introduction. In P. D. Wall & R. Melzack (Eds.), *Textbook of pain* (3rd ed., pp. 1–7). Edinburgh: Churchill Livingstone.

Wall, P. D. (1999). *Pain: The science of suffering.* London: Weidenfeld & Nicolson.

Warwick, H. M., Clark, D. M., Cobb, A. M., & Salkovskis, P. M. (1996). A controlled trial of cognitive-behavioural treatment of hypochondriasis. *British Journal of Psychiatry, 169,* 189–195.

Warwick, H. M., & Salkovskis, P. M. (1985). Reassurance. *British Medical Journal, 290,* 1028–1028.

Warwick, H. M., & Salkovskis, P. M. (1990). Hypochondriasis. *Behaviour Research and Therapy, 28,* 105–117.

Woolf , C. J., Bennett, G. J., Doherty, M., Dubner, R., Kidd, B., Koltzenburg, M., Lipton, R., Loeser, J. D., Payne, R., & Torebjork, E. (1998). Towards a mechanism-based classification of pain? *Pain, 77,* 227–229.

Woolf, C. J., & Mannion, R. J. (1999). Neuropathic pain: Aetiology, symptoms, mechanisms, and management. *Lancet, 353,* 1959–1964.

27

A Practical Cognitive-Behavioral Approach for Treating Children's Pain

Patricia A. McGrath
Loretta M. Hillier

Interest in the special pain problems of infants, children, and adolescents has increased at an unprecedented rate during the past 20 years. As a consequence of intensive research, our knowledge of how children perceive pain and how we can alleviate their suffering has dramatically improved. In particular, we now recognize that children's pain is not simply and directly related to the extent of their physical injuries or the severity of their disease. We have learned that many psychological factors can modify the neural signals for pain and increase a child's pain and distress. As for adults, children's pain perception depends on complex neural interactions, where impulses generated by tissue damage are modified by ascending systems activated by innocuous stimuli and descending pain-suppressing systems activated by various situational and psychological factors (for review, see Loeser, 2001; P. A. McGrath, 1990; Price, 1999). However, children's pain seems more plastic than that of adults, so that environmental and psychological factors may exert an even more powerful influence on children's pain perception than on adults'.

Our increasing appreciation of the plasticity and complexity of children's pain has profound implications for psychological approaches to pain management. Because a child's pain is not wholly determined by the level of tissue damage, we cannot completely control pain by gearing our interventions solely to the putative source of tissue damage. Instead, we must also identify the situational and psychological factors that affect nociceptive processing and target our interventions accordingly.

Controlling children's pain requires a dual emphasis on administering appropriate analgesics or anesthetics and on selectively modifying the factors that exacerbate their pain. Our treatment emphasis should shift from an exclusive disease-centered focus to a more child-centered focus. In this chapter we describe the varied psychological aspects of children's pain, and the common factors that modify their pain perception. Case studies are presented to illustrate a practical approach for obtaining accurate information about the sensory characteristics of children's pain, for identifying causative and contributing factors, and for modifying the factors responsible for increasing pain, exacerbating distress, prolonging pain-related disability, and triggering pain episodes using psychological approaches.

Psychological Aspects of Children's Pain

Like adults, children experience a wide variety of acute, recurrent, and chronic pains. Acute pain, relatively brief pain caused by disease and trauma, is the most common type and forms the basis for how children learn about pain and how to treat it. Many otherwise healthy and pain-free children experience repeated episodes of headache, abdominal pain, or limb pain. These pains are not symptoms of an underlying organic disease that requires medical treatment. Instead, environmental and psychological factors are responsible for triggering episodes and prolonging disability. In addition, children can experience chronic pain due to disease, trauma, emotional distress, and unknown etiology.

Regardless of the type of pain, several factors can modify a child's pain perception and should be controlled to treat pain optimally. The model illustrated in Figure 27.1 provides a framework for assessing these causative and contributing factors, based on our knowledge of the plasticity and complexity of children's pain. Some factors are relatively stable for a child, such as gender, temperament, and cultural background, whereas other factors change progressively, such as age, cognitive level, previous pain experience, and family learning (shown in the open box in the figure). These child characteristics shape how children generally interpret the various sensations caused by tissue damage. In contrast, the cognitive, behavioral, and emotional factors (shown in the shaded boxes) are not stable. These situational factors represent a unique interaction between the child and the situation in which the pain is experienced (P. A. McGrath, 1990; P. A. McGrath & Hillier, 2001a; Ross & Ross, 1988).

Situational Factors

Situational factors can vary dynamically, depending on the specific circumstances in which children experience pain. For example, a child receiving treatment for cancer will have repeated injections, portacatheter access, and lumbar punctures—all of which may cause some pain (depending on the analgesics, anaesthetics, or sedatives used). Even though the tissue damage from these procedures is the same each time, the particular set of situational factors for each treatment is unique for a child—depending on a child's (and parent's expectations), a child's (and parent's *and* staff's behaviors), and a child's (and family's) emotional state. Although the causal relationship between an injury and a consequent pain seems direct and obvious, what children understand, what they do, and how they feel all affect their pain. Cognitive factors include parents' and children's understanding of the pain problem, their knowledge of effective therapies, and their expectations for the future. Behavioral factors refer to the specific behaviors of children, parents, and staff during pain episodes and also encompass parents' and children's wider behaviors in response to a recurrent or chronic pain problem. Emotional factors include parents' and children's feelings about the painful episodes or condition, the subsequent impact of pain and illness on the family, and the anxiety or depression that may underlie certain chronic conditions.

Complex and dynamic interactions occur among cognitive, behavioral, and emotional factors. Certain factors can intensify pain and distress, whereas others can eventually trigger pain episodes, prolong pain-related disability, or maintain the cycle of repeated pain episodes for children with recurrent pain syndrome (P. A. McGrath & Hillier, 2001b). Health care providers can modify situational factors and lessen a child's pain and minimize his or her disability. Because the extent to which a specific cognitive, behavioral, or emotional factor represents a primary underlying cause or secondary contributing factor varies among children and may vary over time for the same child, we must ascertain which factors are relevant for which children so we can select the most appropriate therapy for each child.

Child Characteristics

There is a complex interrelationship among age, cognitive level, gender, temperament, previous pain experience, family learning, and culture in shaping children's pain perception. Children's understanding of pain, the words they use to describe pain and how they evaluate new pain experiences is influenced by all these factors (e.g., Bijtte-

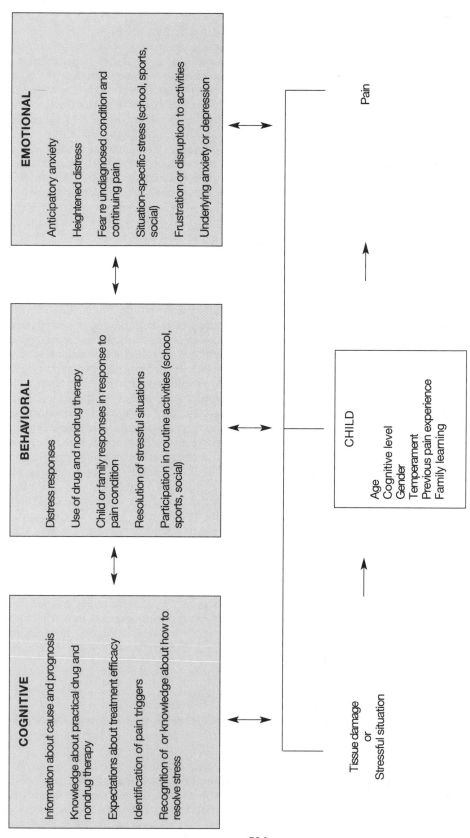

FIGURE 27.1. A model of the factors that can cause and contribute to children's pain. From McGrath and Hillier (in press). Copyright by Lippincott Williams & Wilkins. Reprinted by permission.

bier & Vertommen, 1998; Bournaki, 1997; Broome, Rehwaldt, & Fogg, 1998; Gaffney, 1993; P. A. McGrath, 1990; P. A. McGrath, Speechley, Seifert, & Gorodzinsky, 1997; P. J. McGrath & Unruh, 1987; Peterson, Harbeck, Farmer, & Zink, 1991; Ross & Ross, 1988). Children's pain intensity ratings and their overt distress (e.g., crying and resisting) during invasive medical procedures generally decrease with age (Bachanas & Roberts, 1995; Bijttebier & Vertommen, 1998; Bournaki, 1997; Fanurik, Zeltzer, Roberts, & Blount, 1993; LaMontagne, Wells, Hepworth, Johnson, & Manes, 1999). However, the effect of age most likely varies depending on the type of pain children experience and the nature of their previous pain experiences (i.e., positive experiences with similar painful experiences). For example, Bennett-Branson and Craig (1993) showed that postoperative pain (minor surgery) increased with age, while other studies have reported age-related decreases in postoperative pain (inpatient surgery; Palermo & Drotar, 1996), or no age-related differences in postoperative pain (oral surgery; Gidron, McGrath, & Goodday, 1995).

Children evaluate any new pain—the sensory features, its meaning or relevance, and their possible responses in accordance with their previous pain experiences. "Previous pain experience" encompasses several aspects—the number of pains, the type of pain, the strength of pain, and the positive or negative quality of the experience (P. A. McGrath & Hillier, in press). Each aspect may have a different, but equally important, impact on children's pain perception. As children mature, they experience a wider variety of pains that differ in quality, intensity, location, and duration (P. A. McGrath et al., 2000). They also learn new methods for lessening pain and gradually develop flexible repertoires of strategies to cope with different types of pain. Thus, children's previous pain experiences shape their understanding, influence their perceptions, and affect their emotional reactions.

The nature of children's previous pain experiences and their temperament influences how they respond to new painful stimuli. Children who approach new situations well or who seek information about the situation generally are less distressed during aversive or potentially threatening situations. As an example, children who have difficulty adapting to new situations, were more distressed during immunizations than were other children (Schechter, Berstein, Beck, Hart, & Scherzer, 1991). The similarity of a new pain to some prior experience (i.e., the particular type of pain), its sensory attributes, and the physical setting is probably the most salient feature for children in signaling the aversive significance of the pain and in shaping how they respond. Children with negative prior experience will undoubtedly expect a continuing negative experience, display more anxiety and distress, and be at risk for heightened pain (Bijttebier & Vertommen, 1998).

What children learn about pain, how they express pain, and how they cope with different types of pain are shaped by their family and culture. The pain language children use to describe pain naturally develops as they mature and develops through their culture from the words and expressions used by their families and peers, and from characters depicted in books, videos, and movies. Parents may provide younger children with more attention for pain reports than older children, who are encouraged to cope more independently. Boys may be encouraged to be stoic, whereas girls may be subtly reinforced to express discomfort. Parents may be more anxious, overtly protective, and concerned about the routine bumps and scrapes of childhood for their first-born children than for later children. Differences in parental responses may account for the higher pain sensitivity reported for first-born children (Vernon, 1974).

The family and society, in addition to being the primary models for the development of children's pain attitudes and behaviors, may also influence children's actual pain experiences. Schanberg, Keefe, Lefebvre, Kredich, and Gil (1998) demonstrated that parental pain history and family environment were related to the functional status and pain reports of children with juvenile primary fibromyalgia. Parents who reported multiple chronic pain conditions were more likely to have children with higher impairment and disability. Moreover, the presence of pain models within the family can increase pain complaints, reduce effective coping, and increase disability and impairment (Edwards, O'Neill, Zeichner, & Kucz-mierczyk, 1985; Edwards, Zeichner, Kuczierczyk, & Boczkowski, 1985; Schanberg et al., 1998).

An Integrated Approach for Treating Children's Pain

Controlling children's pain requires an integrated approach, because many factors are responsible, no matter how seemingly clear-cut the etiology. Adequate analgesic prescriptions administered at regular dosing intervals must be complemented by a practical cognitive-behavioral approach to ensure optimal relief. Psychologists who specialize in treating children's pain should have a working knowledge of the main categories of analgesic and adjuvant drugs administered to children, as well as the major types of anesthetic techniques available for children. Data about what types of drugs children receive, how much, and how often are essential components of their pain assessment, particularly for children with chronic pain. (For review of analgesic and anesthetic recommendations for different types of pain in infants, children, and adolescents, see Schechter, Berde, & Yaster, in press.)

Treating Children's Acute Pain

SITUATIONAL FACTORS THAT MODIFY ACUTE PAIN

Acute pains caused by trauma and disease are the most common pains children report (P. A. McGrath et al., 2000). These pains provide a warning signal to children about physical injury so that the pain has an adaptive biological significance. Children typically do not experience any prolonged emotional distress because the pain lessens progressively as their injuries heal. They quickly learn that the cause of their pain is physical damage, often easily visible, that their pain is relatively brief, and that many interventions can alleviate their discomfort. Thus, children usually have accurate age-appropriate information about the pain source and positive expectations for pain relief. They perceive that they have some control and have developed some pain-reducing strategies, such as seeking a parent for a special hug, cleansing and bandaging an in-

jured area, or taking medication. The aversive significance is determined more by the actual pain intensity and by any disruption in children's normal activities than by fears of continued pain and disability. As a result, children perceive acute pain more as the occasional inevitable result of daily activities than as something to fear.

In contrast, a different set of cognitive factors is typically present when children experience acute pain during invasive medical and dental procedures. Children may feel that they have no control in the situation; they may be uncertain about what to expect; they may not understand the need for a treatment that will hurt, particularly if they do not feel sick; they many not be offered any choices or participate in their treatment; and they may not know any simple pain-reducing strategies that they can use during the procedure. In fact, children may be told how to cope during a painful procedure in a manner that makes it easier for the adult administering the procedure but not necessarily better for the child. Lack of understanding about the pain, expectations for continuing pain, the aversive relevance of the procedure, and lack of simple pain control methods that children can use independently are all factors that can intensify children's pain and distress, even when children receive anxiolytics and analgesics.

Children, who require multiple invasive procedures throughout a prolonged period, are at risk for developing increasing anxiety about these procedures (Kellerman, Zeltzer, Ellenberg, & Dash, 1983). Children are often visibly distressed during procedures and may show more subtle emotional distress in their interactions with others (e.g., becoming more aggressive toward peers) or daily activities (e.g., withdrawing from hobbies they had enjoyed). Generally, the more distressed children are, the greater their pain (Bournaki, 1997; Fowler-Kerry & Lander, 1987; Jay, Elliott, Ozolins, Olson, & Pruitt, 1985). Some distress behaviors may reflect a child's underlying emotional distress, while other behaviors, particularly stalling, may represent a simple conditioned response. These responses develop when parents or health care providers inadvertently reinforce children by delaying the start of treatment or by inconsistently coaching, reassuring, or coercing children to cooperate.

Some inconsistencies in how procedures are conducted are common in clinical practice. The more procedures children have, the more likely that they will experience a difficult procedure—more pain, more nausea, and so forth. Children then become fearful and expect that another difficult procedure is inevitable. Children can also experience much anxiety about their health condition. The dynamics within a family change when a child is diagnosed with a major disease and the broader impact of the disease on the lives of the entire family can affect children's pain. Parents, siblings, and extended family members must adjust to an altered life wherein the family schedule is determined by the schedule of medical treatments and their impact on the ill child. Parents are distressed by the disease and its implications—the life-threatening potential (if any), pain, physical symptoms, and accompanying disability. Parents' heightened anxiety may affect how they behave toward the ill child (Blount et al., 1989; Blount, Sturges, & Powers, 1990; Bush, Melamed, Sheras, & Greenbaum, 1986). They may become too protective, inadvertently encouraging children to become overly dependent on them and to become passive sufferers during procedures rather than active copers. Physical disability, inaccurate expectations, social isolation, and loss of control over events will heighten children's distress and can exacerbate their pain. Yet, health care providers can easily modify most of the factors that contribute to children's acute pain by adopting a consistent cognitive-behavioral approach within their routine clinical practice.

A COGNITIVE-BEHAVIORAL APPROACH FOR
ACUTE TREATMENT-RELATED PAIN

In general, children's pain can be lessened by providing accurate age-appropriate information about pain, increasing control by giving children simple choices, explaining the rationale for what is happening and what can be done to reduce pain, and teaching children pain control methods that they can use independently. Many cognitive-behavioral interventions have been designed to incorporate these principles (e.g., Barrera, 2000; Ellis & Spanos 1994; Hilgard & LeBaron, 1984; Kazak, Penati, Brophy, &

Himelstein, 1998). Health care providers often teach children concrete methods to use during procedures such as how to breathe deeply, count slowly and regularly, and follow progressive muscle relaxation exercises. These methods combine principles of attention and distraction, whereby children's full attention is absorbed in an activity, with concrete physical tasks. Most health care providers use some type of cognitive-behavioral intervention. However, the specific interventions usually are different depending on the particular staff person, so that children receiving repeated procedures are exposed to varying versions of several interventions and children may not develop sufficient practice, confidence, or effectiveness with any one intervention.

Health care providers should adopt a more consistent approach using a few strategies in a systematic manner, so that children have predictability and acquire confidence in their ability to lessen their pain and distress. They can distribute guidelines for parents to assist children in preparing for invasive procedures, so that parents can begin to address the situational factors that could have an adverse impact on their children's pain experience. As an example, Table 27.1 shows a set of general guidelines for parents of children with cancer. Children who are anxious and distressed by scheduled treatments should be assessed by a psychologist or pain therapist to determine the specific sources of their anxiety and to develop an appropriate treatment program, as described in the following case study.

CASE STUDY: ACUTE TREATMENT-RELATED PAIN

A 6-year-old boy, John, was referred to the pain clinic because he began to experience severe pain and exhibit extreme behavioral distress during the finger pricks, venous blood sampling, and injections he required to manage his diabetes. John had been diagnosed with juvenile diabetes when he was 2 years old; his pain during treatments had increased gradually since then, and he was exhibiting numerous distress behaviors (stalling, crying, screaming, kicking, etc.). John's pain assessment included structured individual interviews with him and his parents at the clinic and a home visit to observe

TABLE 27.1 Guidelines for Preparing Children for Invasive Procedures

---

Be honest with your child about what will happen.

Explain the procedure in age-appropriate language so he or she can understand the whys and whats and whos—with respect to the rationale for the procedure, the equipment that will be used, and who will be present. (For young children, analogies with a pet are often beneficial. If your child has a pet and can understand that it needs injections and examinations, he or she may be less frightened when you explain what will happen as if the pet needed it. Ask the child how he or she could make it easier for the pet. In this way, your child may focus more on actively coping on being frightened.)

Emphasize the qualitative sensations he or she may experience such as cold, tingling, or pressure so that children focus on what they are feeling, not just on a hurting aspect.

If the procedure will cause some pain, describe the pain that the child may feel in familiar terms that he or she will understand. For instance, use examples of pains that he or she has experienced already during play or pains that he or she may have observed other family members experience without distress.

Focus attention on what you and your child can do to make the procedure less distressing and less painful. Have a game plan of simple things that he or she can do such as taking slow deep breaths while you pace the rhythm, becoming immersed in a distracting image, or attending to the various stages of the procedure (depending on his or her preference for being involved or being distracted).

Choice, control, and predictability are important for children receiving invasive treatments. Allow your child as much choice as possible such as which arm (for injections), whether to watch or look away, and which pain-reducing tool to use.

Remember that you and your child may have different preferences for coping with invasive procedures. You might prefer to be distracted while your child might prefer to be involved. It is important to follow your child's preferences rather than unintentionally require him or her to follow your preferences. You should know which is your child's preference from his or her past experiences—for example, does he or she watch or look away if you remove a sliver from his finger, does he or she like to remove bandages independently or prefer that you do it.

After the procedure is over, praise your child for coping and following the plan that you both chose. Even if your child showed some distress, praise him or her for trying and explain that you will work on the plan to make it better. Your child may need practice as with any other activity he or she has tried (e.g., riding a bike, roller-blading, and skating). Be careful to not praise your child for just getting through it—because you might be rewarding him or her for enduring it as a victim and inadvertently make the child more frightened or distressed for future procedures.

Note. From McGrath and Hillier (in press). Copyright by Lippincott Williams & Wilkins. Reprinted by permission.

how his finger pricks and injections were conducted.

Although much attention has been focused on pain problems for children who require repeated medical treatments, the emphasis has been primarily on children receiving treatments in hospitals. The unique problems parents experience when administering painful treatments to their children have not been documented fully. Thus, when possible, our pain therapists conduct home visits analogous to their observations of children receiving invasive treatments in the hospital. These visits enable therapists to directly observe children and their families and to assess the situational factors that contribute to the children's pain problems. When a home visit is not possible, the therapist must, in a clinical interview, emphasize that he or she needs to

know exactly what happens at home with the same richness and detail as if he or she were actually present. Because what parents and children believe happens during treatment is not always what actually happens, therapists must interview parents and children in a thorough manner. Subtle but relevant information may be overlooked unless a therapist carefully obtains information about all the situational factors that can affect pain.

John's mother usually prepared all the equipment in the kitchen near dinnertime and then called him for his finger prick, but the time of the procedure varied substantially. Usually John stalled and his mother needed to coerce him. However, when John's mother called him during the therapist's visit, he responded immediately and did not resist or cry. As his mother always did, she chose the finger for his prick, operated the glucose monitor, and evaluated the results. John returned to the playroom while she waited for his glucose reading. Approximately 3 minutes later, John was called back to the kitchen for his "boo-boo," the term used for his injections; again, he responded immediately. His mother prepared he syringe, and she selected and prepared the site for injection. John stayed calm throughout the injection and then returned to the playroom.

Although John's calm behavior at home was atypical, the therapist observed treatment aspects that could have had an adverse effect on John. The procedures were not consistently timed, either according to the clock or according to John's activities. Thus, he had no regular preparation time for himself before treatment and was generally anxious throughout a 2-hour period near dinnertime. The dramatic change in his demeanor and coping behavior during the home visit indicated that his typical behaviors reflected "bad habits" more than underlying emotional distress—suggesting that he would benefit greatly from relatively simple changes in how the procedure was conducted. In addition, the interviews revealed that John did not have a clear rationale for his treatments, their procedural aspects, and the equipment; he had inadequate control and lacked effective pain control methods; and his parents conducted the procedure differently and responded differently when he stalled. Thus, the therapist recommended a simple cognitive-behavioral treatment program consisting of four, 45-minute weekly sessions.

The focus of John's first session was educational. Although he had a good understanding about diabetes and why he required insulin injections, John did not understand the need for daily injections. He believed that injections were just one available treatment option, and that if he had a "new pancreas," he would not need insulin injections. Because John naturally preferred this "painless" option, the therapist focused on helping him understand that the only treatment available was insulin injections, and a pancreas transplant was only a possible future treatment option. Because John seemed frightened by the equipment used, he actively participated in practice sessions

during which he injected puppets. He also reviewed a photo album detailing treatment equipment, with pictures of children of various ages receiving finger pricks and injections. Some photographs were of children prior to their pain management programs, when they were very distressed; others showed the same children after their programs, when they used pain control methods and were not visibly distressed. Initially, John demonstrated his anxiety by trying to change the subject and distract his therapist. His therapist persisted and taught John about his pain-gating system. She also told him about methods to "close his gate," including selecting a finger for his finger prick; assisting his mother by opening the alcohol swab packet; rubbing the injection site before and after the injection; and distracting himself by counting, singing, talking to his brother, or squeezing his brother's hand. To encourage John to use these strategies, a behavioral program was designed in which he earned a sticker for each treatment during which he assisted his mother with the preparations and used a strategy from his list. (Note: Many behavioral programs are not effective because the emphasis is solely on minimizing the child's distress behavior rather than on increasing his or her active pain control. For example, children earn a sticker when they do not show distress rather than when they try to reduce their pain.)

At his second session, John had already earned a sticker for most of the injections he had received. His stalling, resisting, and screaming had lessened considerably. However, his parents were frustrated because John would often cooperate and remain calm during one treatment but then would be distressed during the next treatment. They did not know what to do and required assistance to develop some consistent methods of responding to John, regardless of how inconsistently he behaved or who conducted the procedure. For example, there was a delay of 3 minutes after John's finger prick until his glucose levels were ready. John's mother often forced him to remain with her throughout this time, even though he argued with her about returning to the playroom. In contrast, John's father allowed him to return to the playroom, but he had great difficulty getting John to return for his injection. After a discussion of alternative approaches, both parents were asked to encourage John to participate actively during the interim period. The emphasis was shifted from his parents forcing treatments onto John (as a passive recipient) to John's and his parents' working as an active team to treat his diabetes. He helped his parents to read the glucose monitor results, to determine how much insulin was required, and to prepare the syringe. Even when he felt anxious, attempted to leave the room, or tried to distract his parents, they were asked to continue the preparations while engaging John in conversation about upcoming events (e.g., what was for dinner and what was on TV). In addition, they agreed to stop calling John's injections "boo-boos" and to begin using the phrase "getting insulin." After injections, he helped to store the equipment and discard the swabs.

John also began to select the sites for his injections. The selection of injection sites is a common problem for children with diabetes who are referred to our clinic. Children often develop favorite sites while excluding others (particularly the abdomen site). Yet, children eventually must use all sites. There are simple methods for choosing all sites, while improving children's control without increasing their anxiety. For example, the therapist can mark all the required sites for injections with the child on a body outline. The outline is photocopied and the child cuts the copies into the different body regions (injection sites), so that there is a sufficient number of each injection site to provide a week's treatment sites. Before an injection, children pull a cutout from an envelope and use the site they selected. We have found that children are much less anxious because the focus switches from an almost continual parental pressuring to use the aversive site to an almost continual praise for the child assuming control each day. The child should first practice how to respond during injections the same way—regardless of the injection site; otherwise, he or she will not have the confidence to cope with the situation. After a short time of randomly selecting cutouts, children usually begin to rotate their injection sites independently. Another effective approach is to have children select stickers (representing the different sites) and place them on calendars or in a diabetes diary ahead of the scheduled treatments, so that on the day of treatment, the calendar dictates site selection. In this way, site selection does not lead to major confrontations between parents and children. John chose a sticker for his treatment calendar each day, to ensure that he was alternating sites appropriately.

Within 1 month (by John's fourth session) John had earned a sticker for all his injections. He used simple attention and distraction strategies from his pain control list. He no longer screamed, cried, or refused his injections. He actively participated in all procedures. As a result, his parents were no longer frustrated or anxious; they felt confident that they could be consistent even if he had a difficult day.

Treating Children's Recurrent Pain

SITUATIONAL FACTORS THAT MODIFY
RECURRENT PAIN AND PROLONG DISABILITY

Many children and adolescents experience repeated episodes of headache, abdominal pain, or limb pain. Unlike acute pain, these recurrent pains are not correlating symptoms of an injury that will lessen as the injury heals; they may have several interrelated environmental or psychological causes (Apley, MacKeith, & Meadow, 1978; Holden, Bachanas, Kullgren, & Gladstein, 2001; P. A. McGrath & Hillier, 2001a; Rappaport & Leichtner, 1993; Walker, 1999). Nevertheless, parents usually try to understand recurrent pain from an acute pain perspective, where pain is due to a single cause and can be relieved by a single treatment. They do not understand that these pains, unlike most of the pains their children have experienced, need a different treatment approach. As a consequence, there is usually much uncertainty about the cause and prognosis for these recurrent pains.

Parent's understanding of recurrent pain syndrome guides their behaviors toward children and shapes children's emotional responses to the particular pain problem. We will describe the interplay of cognitive, behavioral, and emotional factors that can potentially trigger pain episodes and prolong pain-related disability for recurrent headache. (For a review of the factors relevant for recurrent abdominal pain, see Walker,

1999.) Parents of children with recurrent migraine or tension headache often hold inaccurate beliefs about the etiology of the pain, effective drug and nondrug therapies, and the role of environmental versus stress triggers, as listed in Table 27.2 (P. A. Mc-

TABLE 27.2 Common Situational Factors for Children with Recurrent Headache

Misbeliefs about etiology
 Single, as yet undiagnosed, cause
 "Presumed" environmental triggers

Misbeliefs about pain control
 Poor knowledge of effective drug and
  nondrug therapies
 Reliance on one ineffective method
 Belief that no treatment will be effective

Beliefs about the role of stress
 Limited understanding that stress can cause
  pain (especially headache)
 Little knowledge about the situations that are
  continuing stressors for children
 Little understanding of the impact of
  children's high expectations for achievement

Child and parent behaviors during pain episodes
 Inconsistent parental responses
 Ineffective use of analgesic drugs and
  independent nondrug therapies
 Children withdrawn from school, sports, or
  social activities

*Parent behaviors in response to painful
  condition*
 Primary focus on additional medical
  consultations and diagnostic investigations
 Persistent search for environmental triggers
 Failure to resolve continuing sources of stress

Emotional factors
 Child's situation-specific stress
 Child's emotional suppression or denial
 Child or parental anxiety re high expectations
  for achievement
 Fear re an undiagnosed condition
 Fear re the likelihood of increasing pain and
  disability
 Frustration re the unpredictability of painful
  episodes and interruption of family activities
 Anger toward health care providers for failing
  to cure the pain
 Underlying depression or anxiety (for some
  children)

Note. From McGrath and Hillier (2001). Copyright 2001b by the International Association for the Study of Pain (www.painbooks.org). Adapted by permission.

Grath & Hillier, 2001b). Children typically share their parents' erroneous beliefs and expectations. In addition, some children have unrealistic expectations for achievement or set unattainable goals.

When children first develop headache, parents seek medical attention. They often receive reassurance that the pains are not caused by disease, or by a physical disorder, but they usually do not receive a firm diagnosis, recommendations for identifying potential pain triggers, treatment recommendations, or a clear prognosis. As the pains, continue, parents remain worried about the cause for pain and continue to seek additional tests out of fear that their child has an undiagnosed medical problem. Parent interpret their child's pain from an outdated disease model—where pain is due to a single cause (usually injury) and can be relieved by a single treatment.

Parents expect that they will eventually find one treatment that will immediately stop the recurrent attacks. Thus, they may reject potentially effective treatments after only one attempt, even though the treatment would address some of the causes and might help to lessen headache severity over time.

Parents (and children) usually do not receive an explanation for how recurrent pains can be triggered by many different factors, particularly stressful events. When parents realize that their child is prone to repeated episodes they usually search the child's immediate environment for the causes and tentatively identify certain foods, weather conditions, and physical activities as pain triggers. Some parents, convinced that these environmental stimuli are the only causes, unduly emphasize their importance. Children then become increasingly anxious about these suspected triggers. When they cannot avoid them, children become so anxious that they actually develop headache—not from the environmental stimulus but from their anxiety. The pain episodes become a conditioned response to certain environmental stimuli (Andrasik, Blake, & McCarran, 1986; P. A. McGrath & Hillier, 2001a). The longer children endure the apparently unpredictable pain episodes and the more their parents search for environmental causes, the greater is the risk that children will develop "learned" pain triggers.

Moreover, many parents lack a clear rationale for how to select drug and nondrug therapies and how to use them appropriately, so that children lack a predictable plan for pain control. Children often do not know how to use practical and independent strategies to lessen pain during episodes. Children may adopt an increasingly passive role—depending primarily on parents, rest, or medication—rather than learning how to actively lessen pain and modify the factors that trigger recurrent episodes.

Although parents generally acknowledge the role of stress in provoking some types of adult headache, they often have difficulty in accepting that stress is a relevant factor for their children. Parents do not understand that stress related only to major life events such as marital discord, job loss, illness, death, or moving to a different city is not the typical source of stress for children with recurrent headache. Instead, the primary source is continuing stress associated with normal childhood activities: school, sports, and social relationships (P. A. McGrath & Hillier, 2001a; Hillier & McGrath, 2001). Children are unable to fully resolve the stress they experience. Either they cannot recognize their true feelings or their feelings have been minimized because they seem trivial from their parents' adult perspective.

Various behaviors are critical to the development of the different recurrent pain syndromes, as shown for recurrent headache in Table 27.2. Typically, a child presents several of these behaviors, with all contributing equally to the pain syndrome. Parents' uncertainty about how to control pain can lead them to respond to children's headache complaints in a manner that inadvertently increases children's distress, pain, and disability. Moreover, when parents seek additional diagnostic tests, attribute headaches solely to environmental triggers, and fail to identify and resolve relevant stress triggers, their behaviors directly maintain the cycle of repeated headache attacks (P. A. McGrath & Hillier, 2001a).

Many children are distressed by their inability to adequately relieve pain. They often do not follow a consistent pain control plan—either medication or psychological therapies. Parents may reinforce pain-related disability when they allow children to stay home from school, encourage them to

withdraw from potentially stressful sports or social activities, and relieve them from routine family responsibilities without helping children to address the underlying causes for painful episodes. Similarly, parents' responses to their children's recurring pains can prolong or intensify the children's pain and disability. Parents may respond inconsistently to children's repeated pain complaints—providing excessive emotional and physical support during some pain episodes, expressing frustration that the pain is interfering with the family's plans during some episodes, and suggesting that children should manage independently during other episodes. As a result, these children may gradually exaggerate their complaints or develop new symptoms to convince their parents they need support. When a parent is disabled by a similar pain or a chronic pain problem, his or her pain coping has a major influence on children. Children may not understand that their pain is different and does not have to be disabling.

Children (and parents) are usually extremely anxious about the true etiology for their pain, the effectiveness of different drugs for alleviating painful episodes, and the future implications for living normally without unpredictable episodes of debilitating pain. Anxiety is especially strong when parents do not understand their child's diagnosis. The continuing pain episodes cause worry that the child has an underlying medical condition. In addition, many children with recurrent pains have not learned effective and practical responses that truly alleviate the source of anxiety. Instead, their anxiety is suppressed and eventually released in real pain episodes. As children learn to recognize and express their feelings, the frequency and intensity of their recurrent pain episodes decrease (P. A. McGrath & Hillier, 2001a; P. A. McGrath, Hinton, & Boone, 1993; Osterhaus et al., 1993).

A COGNITIVE-BEHAVIORAL APPROACH FOR TREATING RECURRENT HEADACHE

Although analgesic drugs can relieve the pain of individual headache attacks, drug therapy alone does not alleviate the cycle of recurrent attacks. Effective treatment requires a multimodal approach with cognitive-behavioral therapy in addition to abortive drug therapy. Strong and consistent evidence supports the efficacy of most cognitive and behavioral therapies for relieving children's headache (for review, see Duckro & Cantwell-Simmons, 1989; Hermann, Kim, & Blanchard, 1995; Holden, Deichman, & Levy, 1999; P. A. McGrath, Stewart, & Koster, 2001). Child-centered treatment recognizes that certain causative factors are relevant for all children with recurrent headache, but that the extent to which they are primary causes or secondary contributing factors varies among children. Thus, the specific components of the cognitive-behavioral program are based on the results of a pain assessment wherein a therapist identifies the relevant factors for a child and selects the components that should modify the specific factors that trigger attacks and those that exacerbate pain and disability (Hillier & McGrath, 2001).

Parents and children should understand that this treatment directly contrasts with the "single cause and single treatment" approach normally adequate for relieving acute pain. Parents and children should understand that each causative factor must be treated and that the most effective treatment includes education, basic drug and nondrug pain management techniques, and resolution of the stressful situations that provoke headache.

Children with relatively recent onset of headache or a mild problem may benefit from a brief educational intervention that can be delivered within the child's primary medical setting. Treatment components include (1) accurate diagnostic information—causes and true headache triggers; (2) explicit pain management recommendations— analgesics and nondrug methods to use during headache attacks; (3) guidelines for alleviating the syndrome—how to identify stressors through prospective monitoring, how to modify causes and contributing factors, and how to minimize disability behaviors. This brief educational intervention can significantly lessen headache attacks, decrease pain, and minimize disability for many children with recurrent migraine and tension-type headache. (For a full description of this intervention, see P. A. McGrath & Hillier, 2001c).

School- and home-based treatment programs can effectively reduce headache activity for children (Burke & Andrasik, 1989; Griffiths & Martin, 1996; Guarnieri & Blanchard, 1990; Larsson & Melin, 1989; P. J. McGrath et al., 1992). However, some children also require individualized cognitive-behavioral programs in which therapists teach children how to lessen pain during headache attacks and guide families to identify and modify relevant causative and contributing factors. Individualized programs are potentially the optimal and most practical interventions because they match treatments to the particular needs of each child. Programs are based on the common factors that contribute to recurrent headache (as listed in Table 27.2), but the primary emphasis and the specific treatment components (e.g., the type of nondrug pain control method, the use of a behavioral contingency program to encourage children to attend school, and the use of biofeedback) may vary depending on the results of the pain assessment and in consideration of a child's sex, age, and cognitive level.

Our program begins with a comprehensive pain assessment to provide a concise history of the headache problem, a descriptive profile of the headache characteristics, and an appraisal of whether the usual causative and contributing factors are relevant for children (Hillier & McGrath, 2001; P. A. McGrath & Koster, 2001). The therapist provides feedback to parents and children about the responsible factors and assists parents and children to understand the multifactorial etiology of recurrent headache, to follow a practical treatment plan for reducing pain during headache attacks, and to modify the responsible factors so as to lessen headache attacks and headache-related disability, as illustrated in the following case study (Hillier & McGrath, 2001).

CASE STUDY: RECURRENT HEADACHE

Kendra, an 8-year-old girl, had had occasional headaches since she was 3 years old. During the past 2 years, they increased in frequency and length, so that Kendra became more disabled. At the time of her pain assessment, Kendra had approximately two headaches per week; the headaches usually began at school. The pain was unilateral and localized to her left or right eye and corresponding temporal region. She described the pain as "strong" with a numerical rating of 8 (0–10 Colored Analogue Scale); the quality was "pushing" and aching. Kendra reported that severe headaches were preceded by a visual aura. She was nauseous during many headaches, missed much classtime, and was often bedridden. Kendra lacked effective pain control methods, preferring to withdraw from activities, rest, and occasionally use acetaminophen. She and her parents attributed the headache attacks to multiple environmental triggers including various foods and drinks, humidity, bright sun, and change in barometric pressure.

Kendra lives at home with her parents and older brother Scott. Kendra reported that she and Scott fight continually and that she does not like to play with him. Both her parents suffer from chronic pain: her mother from debilitating migraine headache and her father severe chronic back pain. Her father's disability confines him to home where he requires much assistance. Kendra perceives that he is constantly nagging her about helping around the house. Kendra is in the third grade and has average grades. She is frequently disruptive in class and freely admits that she does not like to work but prefers to socialize with her classmates. Her teachers informed Mrs. K that they are constantly reminding Kendra to listen to them and that she is frequently disturbing other children. (A previous assessment indicated that she did not have a learning disability.)

Kendra enjoys swimming lessons and Karate lessons regularly, where she receives individual coaching. However, she has a history of disruptive behaviors in sports and activities that require teamwork. Kendra presents as a happy, personable, and talkative child. Although she readily discusses her life, she tends to deny all typical problems children encounter and any specific problems related to her activities and relationships. In the interview, she demonstrated poor problem-solving ability. Her mother reported that Kendra attempted to solve her problems independently but usually eventually needed her mother's assistance. When her mother helps her, Kendra usually spends most of the time justifying her actions and opinions rather than learning how to think out the solution.

The results of the assessment indicated that although several factors were maintaining Kendra's headaches, they were caused primarily by underlying emotional distress, possibly anxiety or low self-esteem. This distress was reflected in her difficulty in maintaining peer relationships and resolving conflicts with classmates and teammates. Her father's pain and disability cause significant family stress. Her mother's belief that the headaches were caused only by environmental triggers and her tendency to deny the existence of any familial stress or school stress prevents her from assisting Kendra to resolve the true headache triggers. Moreover, her mother's own migraine-related disability provides a salient role model for headache disability and suffering.

Kendra enrolled in a cognitive-behavioral program (for a description of the full program, see Hillier & McGrath, 2001). A therapist assisted her to identify and resolve the true headache triggers and to develop more effective stress management and problem-solving skills, especially in her peer relationships. The therapist taught Kendra some active and independent pain control methods and helped her mother to differentiate her headaches from those of Kendra so that she could respond to Kendra's pain complaints in a manner that encourages Kendra to relieve her headache and minimize disability. Kendra's headaches and disability improved significantly throughout the program, with headache frequency reduced to one mild attack per month.

Treating Children's Chronic Pain

SITUATIONAL FACTORS THAT MODIFY CHRONIC PAIN

Children can experience a diverse array of chronic pain related to disease, trauma, and psychological factors, as well as pain of unknown etiology (Bush & Harkins, 1991; P. A. McGrath, 1999; P. J. McGrath & Finley, 1999; Schechter, Berde, & Yaster, 1993). Many of the cognitive, behavioral, and emotional factors described previously for acute treatment-related pain and recurrent pain are relevant factors for children with chronic pain. However, the most salient situational factor is probably the relevance or aversive significance of the prolonged pain and any accompanying disability. All aspects of children's and their families' lives are adversely affected by the pain. Children may endure a prolonged period of physical disability, continuing pain, and varied medical treatments. The family must adjust to the child's illness and any accompanying physical limitations. Parents are distressed by the pain itself, its implications for their children's future, its life-threatening potential (if any), and the prospect of continuing pain and progressive disability. The dynamics within the family (both for siblings and extended family members) inevitably change as chronic pain prevents children from pursuing their normal activities and as each family member adjusts to the altered circumstances.

The emotional impact is intensified when pain is related to progressive disease. Parents' grief is generally proportional to the severity of the disease, particularly when it may be fatal, the extent of accompanying symptoms, the number of invasive medical treatments required, the aversive side effects of treatments, the nature of disability, and the intensity of children's pain.

Although most families receive accurate information about their disease or condition and required medical treatments, the initial emphasis is naturally on disease management so that few families receive concrete information about their pain, the environmental factors that intensify it, and effective nondrug therapies to complement the primary analgesic or anesthetic treatment regimen. Most families do not receive any information about the plasticity and complexity of pain so that they try to understand their child's chronic pain from an erroneous acute pain model—wherein there is a single cause and single treatment. As for recurrent pain, parents often adopt an "acute pain" perspective as they care for children so that they become increasingly anxious or frustrated when single treatment modalities do not fully relieve pain. When pain has multiple sources, with varied nociceptive and neuropathic components, children will undergo sophisticated investigations by different specialists and families may receive contradictory messages as to the probable responsible physical mechanisms.

Health care providers may inadvertently foster a "try and see" treatment approach so that parents are adopting a "wait until it fails" attitude about treatment alternatives. Moreover, they are not given clear criteria for evaluating the efficacy of drug and nondrug interventions so that the first instance of breakthrough pain is considered evidence of treatment failure. They rarely receive a consistent message that the best treatment course is a balance of drug and nondrug therapies, that the course is dynamic with the varied therapies selected according to what is currently happening for the child, and that children can also use some simple pain control methods to augment the medical regimen. Thus, families become increasingly anxious and distressed. The unpredictability of pain, the uncertainty of eventual pain relief, a progressive tendency to assume a passive patient role, and an increasing number of conditioned pain triggers create ideal circumstances for exacerbating pain intensity and increasing children's disability.

Many children with chronic pain have behavioral limitations due to weakness or pain. Yet, their disability may be larger than their pain. For example, some children with complex regional pain syndrome (formerly labeled "reflex sympathetic dystrophy") progressively limit activities because of pain. Over time their disability steadily increases. But their behavioral restrictions do not prevent further pain; instead, their disability becomes a separate problem. This problem can be confounded by the responses of parents, siblings, and health care providers. They may inadvertently encourage children to adopt passive patient roles, to behave differently from other children, and to depend primarily on others for pain control. As children become increasingly disabled, they withdraw from their usual school, social, and physical activities. Children with chronic pain may become so preoccupied with somatic complaints that they are unable to participate fully in any activity. Instead, they are continuously monitoring their bodies for new signs and symptoms of illness or for evidence that any activity is increasing their pain. As children's general physical activity and normal exercise decrease, abnormal sensory input may increase, producing concomitant increases in pain.

Children may feel angry, frightened, and depressed. However, they may suppress feelings of anger and depression in a sincere effort to cope well so that they please their worried parents. Continued emotional suppression can create serious problems as they mature. Older children and adolescents may be more emotionally distressed (depressed and anxious) because they are more aware of the consequences of their disease. Some children and adolescents experience almost continuous pain due to underlying anxiety, depression, or emotional suppression. These emotions are not the effects of the pain but its main cause. Children need psychotherapy and medication to discover and remove the source of emotional distress.

A COGNITIVE-BEHAVIORAL APPROACH FOR CHRONIC PAIN

Effective treatment of chronic pain requires a cognitive-behavioral approach, in addition to drug and physical therapies, because multiple factors affect a child's pain and disability. Treatment begins with a thorough assessment of these factors, using structured interviews and standardized measures (for review of the pain measures used in clinical practice with children, see Finley & McGrath, 1998; P. A. McGrath & Gillespie, 2001; P. A. McGrath & Koster, 2001). Cognitive-behavioral strategies must be incorporated into a flexible and versatile intervention program. Individualized child-centered programs are typically developed in specialized pain clinics, where different health care staff providers contribute to both the assessment and treatment protocols. Specific interventions, such as those listed in Table 27.3, are selected according to the main contributing factors, in relation to a child's cognitive level, temperament, and interests.

Children and parents should always receive specific feedback on causes and contributing factors and a rationale for the treatments selected, as outlined in the following case study. Treatment includes evaluating children's pain regularly, determining treatment efficacy, and revising the treatment plan as needed to adjust to changes in children's physical condition and to the dynamic factors that influence their pain and suffering. Parents should be informed about the rationale for a particular dosing regimen, the difference between neuropathic and nociceptive pain and why different drugs are needed to control them, how to

TABLE 27.3 Components of Cognitive-Behavioral Program

Cognitive
  Age-appropriate information—multifactorial etiology and treatment rationale
  Action plan—increased choices, control, and participation
  Practical pain control methods—attention and distraction, imagery, hypnosis
  Counseling—stress and life management
  Psychotherapy

Physical
  Deep rubbing and massage
  Physiotherapy and thermal stimulation
  TENS
  Acupuncture

Behavioral
  Simple exercises and resumption of activities
  Relaxation therapy
  Biofeedback
  Behavioral management
  Operant conditioning

encourage children to use nondrug pain control methods to augment their drug therapy, and how to encourage children to participate in social and peer activities as fully as possible. Health care providers should address parents' questions about opioid use, especially any fears related to dependency, tolerance, and addiction. When children are enrolled in individualized treatment programs, they should develop (with the therapist's assistance) clear and achievable treatment goals. In addition to the overall goals, usually less pain and less disability, the therapist should guide children to have subgoals that when resolved will lead to the achievement of the overall goal. These latter goals form the specific treatment objectives for the individual sessions (P. A. McGrath 1990; P. A. McGrath & Hillier, 1996).

CASE STUDY: CHRONIC PAIN

Sally, a 15-year-old girl, had chronic pain associated with fibromyalgia and also suffered from frequent headache. Her chronic pain had increased gradually despite no overt progression of her condition. Her mother and another relative were very disabled by fibromyalgia. At the time of her pain assessment, Sally was trying to continue a busy schedule of school, social, and sporting activities. She was extremely frightened that the increasing pain foreshadowed increasing disability and that she would soon be unable to maintain her lifestyle. Sally pushed herself and tried to ignore her condition, denying any physical limitations.

The therapist concluded from the assessment results that Sally's pain had increased as a result of her excessive emotional distress, failure to set realistic limits for her physical involvement, and an extremely busy schedule that prevented any true periods of relaxation and restoration. In fact, Sally's activities were intensifying her pain, but her level of involvement was much higher than that for other adolescents. Thus, even if Sally limited some activities, she would not be considered disabled. The therapist assisted Sally to express her fears and reassured her that the disability she saw in other family members would not necessarily develop. It was critical to manage the condition while minimizing its impact on her life. By monitoring Sally's activities, the therapist assisted her to listen to her body cues and develop more realistic expectations for what she could do. Sally learned that either extreme—too much or too little—in physical activity would exacerbate her pain.

Initially Sally needed concrete reminders to pace herself, but she was motivated and quickly learned to develop a more appropriate balance between physical exertion and relaxation periods. She also developed more appropriate criteria for when to use medication and how to augment medication with practical nondrug pain control methods. Sally accomplished her treatment goals within six sessions. Her almost continual pain decreased to occasional "flare-ups"; her headache attacks decreased from ~ 5 each week to occurring coincident with the flare-ups. Sally had maintained her treatment benefits at our 1-year follow-up. (For additional examples of how to use cognitive-behavioral techniques with children with recurrent and chronic pain, see P. A. McGrath & Hillier, 1996, 2001a.)

Summary

Children's pain is plastic and complex. The neural responses initiated by tissue damage can be modified by a diverse array of situational factors, so that children can experience very different pains from the same type of tissue damage. We cannot completely control a child's pain by gearing our interventions solely to the source of tissue damage; instead, we must also control the factors that modify pain and prolong disability. Pain management begins with a thorough assessment to determine the causes (sources of noxious stimulation) and to identify the primary and secondary contributing factors that are affecting the pain. A consistent treatment program can then be developed by selecting the appropriate treatments for modifying not only nociceptive input but also relevant situational factors.

Health care providers should adopt a consistent cognitive-behavioral approach wherein they carefully integrate the practical strategies that have been shown to lessen a child's pain, emotional distress, and disability into their routine clinical practice. Children who have pain problems (whether treatment related, recurrent pain, or chronic pain) require more intensive and individualized programs, where psychologists or pain specialists can assist children and families to understand the complexity of the problem; to use prescribed therapies (drug or physical); to learn effective nondrug strategies selected according to the child's age, interests, and abilities; and to modify their lives so as to minimize pain and consequent disability. Individual differences among children and their families, as well as relevant situational factors, necessitate that all pain programs be flexible so that they can be adapted to the unique needs of each child, family, and pain problem.

References

Andrasik, F., Blake, D. D., & McCarran, M. S. (1986). A biobehavioral analysis of pediatric headache. In N. A. Krasnegor, J. D. Arasteh, & M. F. Cataldo (Eds.), *Child health behavior: A behavioral pediatrics perspective* (pp. 394–434). New York: Wiley Interscience.

Apley, J., MacKeith, R., & Meadow, R. (1978). *The child and his symptoms: A comprehensive approach.* Oxford, UK: Blackwell Scientific.

Bachanas, P. J., & Roberts, M. C. (1995). Factors affecting children's attitudes toward health care and responses to stressful medical procedures. *Journal of Pediatric Psychology, 20,* 261–275.

Barrera M. (2000). Brief clinical report: Procedural pain and anxiety management with mother and sibling as co-therapists. *Journal of Pediatric Psychology, 25,* 117–121.

Bennett-Branson, S. M., & Craig, K. D. (1993). Post-operative pain in children: Developmental and family influences on spontaneous coping strategies. *Canadian Journal of Behavioural Science, 25,* 355–383.

Bijttebier, P., & Vertommen, H. (1998). The impact of previous experience on children's reactions to venipunctures. *Journal of Health Psychology, 3,* 39–46.

Blount, R. L., Corbin, S. M., Sturges, J. W., Wolfe, V. V., Prater, J. M., & James, J. D. (1989). The relationship between adults' behavior and child coping and distress during BMA/LP procedures: A sequential analysis. *Behavior Therapy, 20,* 585–601.

Blount, R. L., Sturges, J. W., & Powers, S. W. (1990). Analysis of child and adult behavioral variations by phase of medical procedure. *Behavior Therapy, 21,* 33–48.

Bournaki, M. C. (1997). Correlates of pain-related responses to venipunctures in school-age children. *Nursing Research, 46,* 147–154.

Broome, M. E., Rehwaldt, M., & Fogg, L. (1998). Relationships between cognitive behavioral techniques, temperament, observed distress, and pain reports in children and adolescents during lumbar puncture. *Journal of Pediatric Nursing, 13,* 48–54.

Burke, E. J., & Andrasik, F. (1989). Home- vs. clinical-based biofeedback treatment for pediatric migraine: Results of treatment through one-year follow-up. *Headache, 29,* 434–440.

Bush, J. P., Melamed, B. G., Sheras, P. L., & Greenbaum, P. E. (1986). Mother-child patterns of coping with anticipatory medical stress. *Health Psychology, 5,* 137–157.

Bush, J. P., & Harkins, S. W. (Eds.). (1991). *Children in pain: Clinical and research issues from a developmental perspective.* New York: Springer-Verlag.

Duckro, P. N., & Cantwell-Simmons, E. (1989). A review of studies evaluating biofeedback and relaxation training in the management of pediatric headache. *Headache, 29,* 428–433.

Edwards, P. W., O'Neill, G. W., Zeichner, A., & Kuczmierczyk, A. R. (1985). Effects of familial pain models on pain complaints and coping strategies. *Perceptual and Motor Skills, 61,* 1053–1054.

Edwards, P. W., Zeichner, A., Kuczmierczyk, A. R., & Boczkowski, J. (1985). Familial pain models: The relationship between family history of pain and current pain experience. *Pain, 21,* 379–384.

Ellis J. A., & Spanos, N. P. (1994). Cognitive-behavioral interventions for children's distress during bone marrow aspirations and lumbar punctures: A critical review. *Journal of Pain and Symptom Management, 9,* 96–108.

Fanurik, D., Zeltzer, L. K., Roberts, M. C., &

Blount, R. L. (1993). The relationship between children's coping styles and psychological interventions for cold pressor pain. *Pain, 53,* 213–222.

Finley, G. A., & McGrath, P. J. (Eds.). (1998). *Measurement of pain in infants and children.* Seattle, WA: IASP Press.

Fowler-Kerry, S., & Lander, J. R. (1987). Management of injection pain in children. *Pain, 30,* 169–175.

Gaffney A. (1993). Cognitive developmental aspects of pain in school-age children. In N. L. Schechter, C. B. Berde, & M. Yaster (Eds.). *Pain in infants, children, and adolescents* (pp. 75–85). Baltimore: Williams & Wilkins.

Gidron, Y., McGrath, P. J., & Goodday, R. (1995). The physical and psychosocial predictors of adolescents' recovery from oral surgery. *Journal of Behavioral Medicine, 18,* 385–399.

Griffiths, J. D., & Martin, P. R. (1996). Clinical- versus home-based treatment formats for children with chronic headache. *British Journal of Health Psychology, 1,* 151–166.

Guarnieri, P., & Blanchard, E. B. (1990). Evaluation of home-based thermal biofeedback treatment of pediatric migraine headache. *Biofeedback and Self-Regulation, 15,* 179–184.

Hermann, C., Kim, M., & Blanchard, E. B. (1995). Behavioral and prophylactic pharmacological intervention studies of pediatric migraine: An exploratory meta-analysis. *Pain, 60,* 239–256.

Hilgard, J. R., & LeBaron, S. (1984). *Hypnotherapy of pain in children with cancer.* Los Altos, CA: William Kaufman.

Hillier, L. M., & McGrath, P. A. (2001). A cognitive-behavioral program for treating recurrent headache. In P. A. McGrath & L. M. Hillier (Eds.), *The child with headache: Diagnosis and treatment* (pp. 183–220). Seattle, WA: IASP Press.

Holden, E. W., Bachanas, P., Kullgren, K., & Gladstein, J. (2001). Chronic daily headache in children and adolescents. In P. A. McGrath & L. M. Hillier (Eds.), *The child with headache: Diagnosis and treatment* (pp. 221–241). Seattle, WA: IASP Press.

Holden, E. W., Deichmann, M. M., & Levy, J. D. (1999). Empirically supported treatments in pediatric psychology: Recurrent pediatric headache. *Journal of Pediatric Psychology, 24,* 99–109.

Jay, S. M., Elliott, C. H., Ozolins, M., Olson, R. A., & Pruitt, S. D. (1985). Behavioural management of children's distress during painful medical procedures. *Behaviour Research and Therapy, 23,* 513–552.

Kazak, A. E., Penati, B., Brophy, P., & Himelstein, B. (1998). Pharmacologic and psychologic interventions for procedural pain. *Pediatrics, 102,* 59–66.

Kellerman, J., Zeltzer, L., Ellenberg, L., & Dash, J. (1983). Adolescents with cancer: Hypnosis for the reduction of the acute pain and anxiety associated with medical procedures. *Journal of Adolescent Health Care, 4,* 85–90.

LaMontagne, L. L., Wells, N., Hepworth, J. T.,

Johnson, B. D., & Manes, R. (1999). Parent coping and child distress behaviors during invasive procedures for childhood cancer. *Journal of Pediatric Oncology Nursing, 16,* 3–12.

Larsson, B., & Melin, L. (1989). Follow-up on behavioral treatment of recurrent headache in adolescents. *Headache, 29,* 250–254.

Loeser, J. D., Butler, S. D., Chapman, C. R., & Turk, D. C. (Eds.). (2001). *Bonica's management of pain* (3rd ed.). Philadelphia: Lippincott Williams & Wilkins.

McGrath, P. A. (1990). *Pain in children: Nature, assessment, and treatment.* New York: Guilford Press.

McGrath, P. A. (1999). Chronic pain in children. In I. K. Crombie, P. R. Croft, S. J. Linton, L. LeResche, & M. Von Korff (Eds.), *Epidemiology of pain* (pp. 81–101). Seattle, WA: IASP Press.

McGrath, P. A., & Gillespie, J. (2001). Pain assessment in children and adolescents. In D. C. Turk & R. Melzack (Eds.), *Handbook of pain assessment* (2nd ed., pp. 97–118). New York: Guilford Press.

McGrath, P. A., & Hillier, L. M. (1996). Controlling children's pain. In R. Gatchel & D. Turk (Eds.), *Psychological treatment for pain: A practitioner's handbook* (pp. 331–370). New York: Guilford Press.

McGrath, P. A., & Hillier, L. M. (Eds.). (2001a). *The child with headache: Diagnosis and treatment.* Seattle, WA: IASP Press.

McGrath, P. A., & Hillier, L. M. (2001b). Recurrent headache: Triggers, causes, and contributing factors. In P. A. McGrath & L. M. Hillier (Eds.), *The child with headache: Diagnosis and treatment* (pp. 77–107). Seattle, WA: IASP Press.

McGrath, P. A., & Hillier, L. M. (2001c). Treating recurrent headache: An effective strategy for primary care providers. In P. A. McGrath & L. M. Hillier (Eds.), *The child with headache: Diagnosis and treatment.* (pp. 77–107). Seattle, WA: IASP Press.

McGrath, P. A., & Hillier, L. M. (in press). Modifying the psychological factors that intensify children's pain and prolong disability. In N. L. Schechter, C. B. Berde, & M. Yaster (Eds.), *Pain in infants, children, and adolescents* (2nd ed.). Philadelphia: Lippincott Williams & Wilkins.

McGrath, P. A., Hinton, G. G., & Boone, J. E. (1993). Management of recurrent headaches in children. *Abstracts: 7th World Congress on Pain.* Seattle, WA: IASP Press.

McGrath, P. A., & Koster, A. L. (2001). Headache measures for children: A practical approach. In P. A. McGrath & L. M. Hillier (Eds.), *The child with headache: Diagnosis and treatment* (pp. 77–107). Seattle, WA: IASP Press.

McGrath, P. A., Speechley, K. N., Seifert, C. E., Biehn, J. T., Cairney, A. E. L., Gorodzinsky, F. P., Dickie, G. L., McCusker, P. J., & Morrisy, J. R. (2000). A survey of children's acute, recurrent, and chronic pain: Validation of the Pain Experience Interview. *Pain, 87,* 59–73.

McGrath, P. A., Speechley, K. N., Seifert, C. E., & Gorodzinsky, F. P. (1997). A survey of children's pain experience and knowledge—Phase 1. In T. S. Jensen, J. A. Turner, & Z. Wiesenfeld-Hallin (Eds.), *Proceedings of the 8th World Congress on Pain: Progress in pain research and management* (pp. 903–916). Seattle, WA: IASP Press.

McGrath, P. A., Stewart, D., & Koster, A. L. (2001). Nondrug therapies for childhood headache. In P. A. McGrath & L. M. Hillier (Eds.), *The child with headache: Diagnosis and treatment* (pp. 129–158). Seattle, WA: IASP Press.

McGrath, P. J., & Finley, G. A. (Eds.) (1999). *Chronic and recurrent pain in children and adolescents.* Seattle, WA: IASP Press.

McGrath, P. J., Humphreys, P., Keene, D., Goodman, J. T., Lascelles, M. A., Cunningham, S. J., & Firestone, P. (1992). The efficacy and efficiency of a self-administered treatment for adolescent migraine. *Pain, 49,* 321–324.

McGrath, P. J., & Unruh, A. (1987). *Pain in children and adolescents.* Amsterdam: Elsevier.

Osterhaus, S. O., Passchier, J., Helm-Hylkema, H., de Jong, K. T., Orlebeke, J. F., de Grauw, A. J., & Dekker, P. H. (1993). Effects of behavioral psychophysiological treatment on schoolchildren with migraine in a nonclinical setting: Predictors and process variables. *Journal of Pediatric Psychology, 18,* 697–715.

Palermo, T. M., & Drotar, D. (1996). Prediction of children's postoperative pain: The role of presurgical expectations and anticipatory emotions. *Journal of Pediatric Psychology, 21,* 683–698.

Peterson , L., Harbeck, C., Farmer, J., & Zink, M. (1991). Developmental contributions to the assessment of children's pain: Conceptual and methodological implications. In J. P. Bush & S. W. Harkins (Eds.), *Children in pain: Clinical and research issues from a developmental perspective* (pp. 33–58). New York: Springer-Verlag.

Price, D.D. (1999). *Psychological mechanisms of pain and analgesia.* Seattle, WA: IASP Press.

Rappaport, L.A., & Leichtner, A.M. (1993) Recurrent abdominal pain. In N. L. Schechter, C. B. Berbe, & M. Yaster (Eds.), *Pain in infants, children, and adolescents.* Baltimore: Williams & Wilkins.

Ross, D. M., & Ross, S. A. (1988). *Childhood pain: Current issues, research, and management.* Baltimore: Urban & Schwarzenberg.

Schanberg, L. E., Keefe, F. J., Lefebvre, J. C., Kredich, D. W., & Gil, K. M. (1998). Social context of pain in children with juvenile primary fibromyalgia syndrome: Parental pain history and family environment. *Clinical Journal of Pain, 14,* 107–115.

Schechter, N. L., Berde, C. B., & Yaster, M. (Eds.). (1993). *Pain in infants, children, and adolescents.* Baltimore: Williams & Wilkins.

Schechter, N. L., Berde, C. B., & Yaster, M. (Eds.). (in press). *Pain in infants, children, and adoles-*

cents (2nd ed.). Philadelphia: Lippincott Williams & Wilkins.

Schechter, N. L., Bernstein, B. A., Beck, A., Hart, L., & Scherzer, L. (1991). Individual differences in children's responses to pain: Role of temperament and parental characteristics. *Pediatrics, 87,* 171–177.

Vernon, D. T. A. (1974). Modeling and birth order in responses to painful stimuli. *Journal of Personality and Social Psychology, 29,* 794–799.

Walker, L. S. (1999). The evolution of research on recurrent abdominal pain: History, assumptions, and a conceptual model. In P. J. McGrath & G. A. Finley (Eds.), *Chronic and recurrent pain in children and adolescents* (pp. 141–172). Seattle, WA: IASP Press.

28

Persistent Pain in the Older Patient

Kim Pawlick
Susan J. Middaugh

The proportion of the population over the age of 65 years is increasing, and the older population itself is aging. Currently, there are nearly 35 million people age 65 or older in the United States (12.4% of the total population) (U.S. Census Bureau, 2001). Approximately 20% of the U.S. population is projected to be 65 years or older by the year 2030 (U.S. Census Bureau, 2000), and by 2050, 5% of the population is expected to be 85 years of age or older (U.S. Census Bureau, 2001). Awareness of these population trends has led to increased concern about wellness and health care among older adults. Subsequently, the relative quantity of both medical and psychologic studies devoted to the study of persistent pain in older people has increased significantly in recent years (Norton, Asmundson, Norton, & Craig, 1999). The new information published on geriatric pain is in keeping with the biopsychosocial model (Norton et al., 1999). Assessment and treatment of psychosocial factors are considered essential to pain management by the American Geriatrics Society (AGS) Panel on Chronic Pain in Older Persons (1998).

Problems associated with persistent pain in older adults include psychological distress (see, e.g., Casten, Parmelee, Kleban, Lawton, & Katz, 1995; Livingston, Watkin, Milne, Manela, & Katona, 2000), disability (see, e.g., Guccione et al., 1994; Leveille et al., 1999), changes in social relationships (Roy, Thomas, & Cook, 1996), poor physical health, (Nahit, Silman, & MacFarlance, 1998), and increased health care utilization and costs (Lavsky-Shulan et al., 1985). Although, the problems faced by older adults are similar to the problems faced by younger adults with persistent pain, there are aspects of pain (Gibson & Helme, 1995; Lansbury, 2000; Turk, Okifuji, & Scharff, 1995), disability (Corran, Gibson, Farrell, & Helme, 1994; Cutler, Fishbain, Rosomoff, & Rosomoff, 1994), and psychosocial distress (Gatz & Hurwicz, 1990; Geerlings, Beekman, Deeg, & van Tilburg, 2000) that are unique to or more common among older adults.

Ageism can influence the older adult's pain experience. Both older adults (Ferrell, 1991) and health professionals (Weiner, Peterson, & Keefe, 1999) are vulnerable to mistaken beliefs about pain and aging. Ageism is common within medical settings and can affect health care in a variety of ways (Schaie, 1993).

1. *Assumption that age is related to the presenting complaint.* Pain in the older adult is often wrongly assumed to be the direct result of aging. Pain results from specific injuries or diseases, not from aging per se. Although the prevalence of some causes of pain, such as osteoarthritis and hip fractures, increase with age, there is no reason to expect or accept pain as a consequence of aging. Similarly, psychological symptoms can be misperceived as consequences of aging rather than perceived as treatable symptoms. Gloominess is not a normal or necessary consequence of aging, yet both the general and medical communities tend to associate aging with greater unhappiness (Gatz, 2000).

2. *Preconceptions regarding age-related behavioral limitations.* Older adults are sometimes mistakenly perceived as less flexible and are viewed as less likely to benefit from treatments involving behavioral change. In general, older patients are likely to accept and benefit from nonpharmacological interventions for pain (Helme et al., 1996; Sorkin, Rudy, Hanlon, Turk, & Stieg, 1990) and psychological distress (Dorfman et al., 1995; Rokke & Scogin, 1995; Walker & Clarke, 2001). The assumption that once depressed the older adult is destined to remain depressed is false (Zarit, Femia, Gatz, & Johansson, 1999).

3. *Myths and stereotypes.* The myth that pain sensitivity and perception diminish with age in much the same way that hearing and visual acuity diminish is false (Harkins, 1996). The qualitative properties of pain (e.g., sensations of burning, aching, and stabbing) are similar in older and younger adults (Harkins & Price, 1997).

An assortment of stereotypes relates to older adults with pain. One such stereotype is the older woman who complains incessantly about pain because she is attention seeking and complaining fills a void in her life. Although a subset of older women tends to "catastrophize" about pain (Keefe et al., 2000), the majority of older adults are reluctant to complain about pain (Gibson & Helme, 1995; Lansbury, 2000). Another stereotype is the passive older adult who is resigned to suffer and thus is reluctant to participate in potentially helpful interventions. Again, most older adults welcome the opportunity to participate in potentially

helpful treatments (Helme et al., 1996; Middaugh, Levin, Kee, Barchiesi, & Roberts, 1988; Sorkin et al., 1990).

4. *Generalization of experience with specific groups of older patients to different patient groups.* Experiences with specific individuals or groups of older adults may not be applicable to other dissimilar older adults. Participants in specialized pain clinics seem to differ from older adults who are not involved in specialty treatment (Roy et al., 1996). The "oldest old" are different from the "young old." For example, among a sample of older Swedes, those who reported greater resignation and dependency and less knowledge about their condition tended to be among the older old (mean age = 86 years vs. 78 years) (Hall-Lord, Larsson, & Steen, 1999). Living environment is another relevant distinguishing variable. Living in a nursing home is associated with greater risk for persistent pain (Ferrell, Ferrell, & Osterweil, 1990; Roy & Thomas, 1986), and pain seems to have a different impact on the older person living independently than on the person living in a nursing home (Williamson & Schulz, 1992). Gender is yet another distinguishing variable. Older women and men have different rates of pain problems and their responses to pain differ (Brattberg, Parker, & Thorslund, 1997; Keefe et al., 2000). Finally, generational differences should be considered. Findings from current research may not be applicable to future generations, because most of the current data on pain and aging has been obtained using cross-sectional methodology.

Age-related biases are found in the assessment and treatment of persistent pain. Although older individuals are likely to participate in pain treatment when offered, they are at risk for not expecting or requesting treatment for their pain (Nahit et al., 1998; Ruzicka, 1998). Ageism can bias the health professional's treatment approach. Kee, Middaugh, Redpath, and Hargadon (1998) found that while none of the 96 pain programs queried actively excluded older patients, almost one-third had admitted no geriatric patients, or limited admissions to the youngest members of the geriatric age range. Similarly, when provided with vignettes describing older patients and younger patients with the same medical problem, older patients were 15% less likely to be recommended for treatment than younger. Older patients seen in pain treatment centers are offered less treatment and fewer treatment options than their younger counterparts (Kaplan & Kepes, 1989; Melding, 1991).

Scope of the Problem

Surveys of the general population indicate that 24–50% of seniors report pain problems (see, e.g., Brattberg et al., 1997; Kendig, Browning, & Young, 2000). When nursing home residents are queried, this figure rises to 45–83% (Ferrell et al., 1990; Weiner, Peterson, Ladd, McConnell, & Keefe, 1999). The wide range of estimates is partly related to the fact that some studies include pain of relatively mild severity in their results. Among a sample of community dwelling older adults, the majority (83%) reported pain, but only 26% reported pain that nearly always interfered with functioning (Lansbury, 2000). The distinction between acute, recurrent, and persistent pain is frequently blurred, thus making it difficult to determine the extent of persistent pain. However, even the lowest estimates indicate that persistent pain is a problem for many older adults. Some older persons struggle with more than one painful condition, and those with more than one problem area of pain have greater difficulty than those with only one pain problem (Leveille et al., 1999).

As people age, the risk for some diseases known to cause persistent pain, such as osteoarthritis, cardiovascular disease, and herpes zoster, increases (Harkins, Kwentus, & Price, 1990; Kramarow, Lentzner, Rooks, Weeks, & Saydah, 1999). However, the prevalence of some other pain problems, such as headaches, decline in later life (Harkins et al., 1990; Tibblin, Bengtsson, Furunes, & Lapidus, 1990). Some specific pain problems, such as back pain, appear more prevalent among the younger old (65–74 years) than the older old 85+ years (Leveille et al., 1999).

Although many older adults have the same persistent pain for the remainder of life, improvement and recovery are possible. A Swedish longitudinal study which followed middle-age adults into older adulthood (Brattberg et al., 1997) found that not all study participants reported increased pain with age, and a small proportion of participants reported decreased pain with age. Among seniors with a disability, progressive deterioration is not the only course. Mendes de Leon, Seeman, Baker, Richardson, and Tinetti (1997) found that 10% of persons 65+ years report a new episode of disability each year, but 20–25% of these people later report full recovery of functioning.

Compared to younger adults, the older adult's persistent pain is more likely to have a gradual onset and a longer duration (Corran et al., 1994; Thomas & Roy, 1988). The pain experience of the older adult with circumstances similar to those more commonly found in younger patients (e.g., pain related to recent accident or work injury) may be different from the older patient with pain related to a progressive disease generally associated with old age. If a 25-year-old student and a 70-year-old retiree experience the same back pain sensation, much of their pain experience will be similar. However, age-related differences in physical, psychological, and social variables lead to differences in experiences of and responses to pain. Family members, health care providers, and others are apt to respond differently to the 25-year-old with persistent pain than to the 70-year-old with similar pain.

Human development is associated with both and continuity. Similarly, there are both change and continuity in the experience of pain across the lifespan. The focus of this chapter is to examine how change and continuity across the lifespan affect the assessment and treatment of the older adult with persistent pain.

Assessment

Pain (Nahit et al., 1998; Ruzicka, 1998) and distress (Dorfman et al., 1995) are often overlooked in older adults. One reason may be that symptoms are less conspicuous in older compared to younger adults. The long-drawn-out onset and ubiquitous nature of the older person's pain may increase the likelihood that pain will be readily accepted and less noticeable. Pain, disability, and low mood are often expected aspects of aging, and expected symptoms are generally less noticeable than unexpected symptoms.

The possible impact of stoicism on assessment of older adults has been considered. Research examining general defensiveness and social desirability bias finds that older adults are no more likely than younger adults to bias responses in a defensive manner (Harper, Kotick-Harper, & Kirby, 1990; Kee, Middaugh, & Pawlick, 1996). When asked, older adults appear as likely as younger to report symptoms of emotional distress and pain. However, without prompting, older adults may be reluctant to express concerns about pain or emotional distress (Gibson & Helme, 1995; Lansbury, 2000). Feelings of alienation, fears of dependency, and concerns about disappointing others with poor treatment outcome are some of the reasons given by older adults for not seeking treatment for pain (Lansbury, 2000). Although older adults appear less likely to report pain without prompting, they do not seem to label pain differently than younger adults when prompted (Harkins & Price, 1997). Regardless of initial presentation, assessment should include direct inquiry about undesirable symptoms such as pain, disability, and psychological distress.

When using common assessment tools in this special population, one needs to consider the possibility of compromised validity. In addition, the possibility that standard assessment tools may not address issues that are especially relevant or unique to older adults should be considered.

Pain Assessment

The common, simple, subjective measures of pain, such as the Visual Analog Scale (VAS) or numeric rating scales, appear valid when used by older adults (Bergh, Sjöström, Odon, & Steen, 2000). When VAS, graphic, and numeric rating scales were compared, the majority of geriatric patients were able to complete all the pain scales successfully (Bergh et al., 2000). Only 5% of patients were unable to use any of the three scales. Those who had difficulty using the pain scales tended to be among the older old. The Geriatric Pain Questionnaire, a quick, easy questionnaire, specifically designed for

pain assessment in older people, has good validity and reliability (Ferrell, Stein, & Beck, 2000). However, using this age-specific measure makes comparisons with other age groups difficult.

Behavioral observation is a key component of pain assessment. In general, level of agreement between the older person's self-reported pain and care provider's reports (family and nurse) is usually low to moderate (Weiner et al., 1999). One possible reason for the differences is that older adults with pain tend to identify "pain behaviors" as those behaviors that reduce pain, but caregivers tend to identify pain behaviors as those behaviors that "communicate" pain. Observation of pain-reducing behaviors such as moving slowly, taking medications, and lying down can provide important information about pain (Weiner et al., 1999). Sometimes, such behaviors are not noticed by others because they are viewed as "normal." In addition, the older person may limit activities so that pain-producing behaviors are not performed and thus not observed. Asking the individual to perform functional activities not normally observed may provide important additional information about pain (Weiner et al., 1999). Structured measures are available to assess pain behavior in older adults, but they may be too complex and time consuming to be used in a busy setting (Miller et al., 1996).

Assessment usually includes information about both current and past pain. Often, patients are expected to report pain over the past weeks, months, or even years. Memory for pain has been shown to be poor in the general population (Erskine, Morley, & Pearce 1990). Memory, especially contextual memory, generally declines with age (Spencer & Raz, 1995). Although the memory decline is generally slight, reduced memory for temporal and contextual information can negatively affect pain assessment. Thomas (1999) suggests that the older adult's memory for chronic pain is less accurate than memory for acute pain, because chronic pain is less discrete and specific. Guiding the patient in the use of specific, personally relevant memory cues can be helpful. For example, for the patient having difficulty recalling when his pain changed from moderate to severe, prompting him to recall when he stopped attending church because of increased pain can provide helpful information. Because current pain is known to bias reports of past pain (Eich, Reeves, Jaeger, & Graff-Radford 1985), reports of past pain should be judged with present pain ratings in mind. Most older adults are able to use simple pain diaries to record information about pain and interventions between assessment points.

Pain Assessment and Cognitive Impairment

Those with cognitive impairments tend to report slightly less pain than those without cognitive impairment (Parmelee, Smith, & Katz, 1993; Sengstaken & King, 1993). Patients with cognitive and communication deficits are at risk for undertreatment of pain (Kaasalainen, Robinson, Hartley, Knezacek, & Ife, 1998). Patients with mild to moderate cognitive impairment are usually able to use standard assessment scales (Ferrell, Ferrell, & Rivera, 1995; Parmelee et al., 1993). Ferrell and colleagues (1995) compared five pain scales and found that 83% of the cognitively impaired nursing home participants were able to complete at least one of the scales. In another study, approximately two-thirds of 156 cognitively impaired older adults were able to complete at least one of three standard pain self-assessment tools (Krulewitch et al., 2000). Inability to complete the self-assessment tools was associated with greater cognitive impairment. Measures with verbal anchors appear less problematic than purely visual measures. Allowing sufficient time for the patient to process and communicate pain information, providing visual cues, and amplifying visual and auditory information when appropriate can improve success with pain assessment (Ferrell et al., 1995). Level of cognitive impairment does not seem to influence the agreement between patients' and care providers' assessments of pain (Weiner et al., 1999).

Behavioral observation is the most reliable method of assessing pain in the nonverbal or severely cognitively impaired patient (Kaasalainen et al., 1998). Agitation, aggression, withdrawal, crying, grimacing, and guarding a body part are all examples of behaviors that can signal pain. Differentiating pain behaviors from behavioral disturbances due to other causes can be difficult. A change in a person's baseline behavior may be a sign of new or increased pain. Sometimes effective pain treatment will reduce behavioral disturbance. Some patients with "difficult behavior" improve when placed on pain medications such as acetaminophen (Douzjian et al., 1998). The relationship between behavioral disturbance and pain is blurry, and erring on the side of increased pain management may help to reduce some types of behavioral disturbance.

Disability and Functional Status

Longer life expectancy may result in a longer period of well-being following retirement (Birren, 2000), or extension of life may result in greater opportunity for pain and disability (Kaplan, Haan, & Wallace, 1999). The rate of disability among seniors is expected to drop slightly over time, but the absolute number of seniors with disabilities is expected to increase (Manton & Gu, 2001). In addition to physical factors, psychosocial factors such as lack of companionship, financial limitations, and transportation difficulties can limit functioning and activity involvement (Satariano, Haight, & Tager, 2000). Erroneous beliefs regarding abilities and physical decline may affect decisions regarding activity involvement and can lead to inactivity and deconditioning (O'Brien Cousins, 2000). Not all disabilities are associated with pain, but nonpainful conditions such as sensory loss or cardiopulmonary disease can cause added limitations and stress.

Although some people may prefer to reduce activity levels in later years, others may prefer to maintain previous activity levels. It is important to assess not only achieved functioning and activity involvement but also relevant beliefs, attitudes, and satisfaction with functioning and activity involvement. Pain, disability, and psychological distress are distinct but interrelated. In a recent study, Scudds and Robertson (2000) found that pain severity, pain frequency, taking pain medications, number of pain locations, number of chronic conditions, sleep quality, and age were all related to level of self-reported disability in community-dwelling older adults. Pain contributes to disability independent of physical condition in older adults (Guccione et al., 1994; Leveille et al., 1999). Level of activity restriction has been found to mediate the relationship between pain and depression in community-dwelling older adults (Williamson & Schulz, 1992). On the other hand, the relationship of pain to depression remains significant even after controlling for health and functional status among older adults living in institutions (Parmelee, Katz, & Lawton, 1992). Williamson and Schulz (1992) suggest that activity restriction is related more directly to depression in community-dwelling elderly as compared with institutional-dwelling elderly. Community dwellers are more responsible for their daily living activities and leisure activities and therefore may experience greater loss when faced with functional limitations. However, among community dwellers, illness severity and pain only account for 25% of the variance in activity restriction, suggesting that other psychosocial factors play important roles in activity restriction.

Disability Measures

MEASURES OF ACTIVITIES OF DAILY LIVING

Measures of activities of daily living (ADLs) assess basic self-care skills such as bathing, feeding, and dressing. Either the patient or an important other (nurse, family member, etc.) rates the patient's capabilities. The subjective nature of these instruments makes them vulnerable to bias (Ostir et al., 1999). ADL measures focus on fundamental abilities; thus they tend to have low ceilings. An older adult with pain may score within the normal range but have functional limitations that interfere with quality of life and independent living (for a review of ADL measures, refer to Cohen & Marino, 2000).

INSTRUMENTAL ACTIVITIES OF DAILY LIVING

Instrumental activities of daily living (IADLs) are self-report measures that assess involvement in complex activities required for independent living such as shopping and housekeeping. IADL measures have also been criticized for being vulnerable to report bias and being insensitive to mild to moderate levels of impairment (Ostir et al., 1999). Both ADL and IADL measures identify the individual's "inabilities." They do not take into account those tasks that a person accomplishes with great effort or difficulty. Among a group of older women, severity of back pain was associated with self-reported difficulty with daily activities but not with inability to perform tasks (Leveille et al., 1999). Changes in IADLs are likely to occur earlier in the chronic disease process than changes in ADLs.

PERFORMANCE MEASURES

Performance measures assess actual performance on a variety of physical tasks such as lifting and bending. Although these measures can be affected by psychological factors such as poor motivation and anxiety, they are less vulnerable to subjective bias than ADL and IADL measures. Among community-dwelling disabled older women, severity of reported back pain was significantly associated with scores on physical performance measures (Leveille et al., 1999).

IMPACT SCALES

Impact scales measure perceived levels of activity restriction and symptom interference with daily life. As these instruments tend to focus on the person's perceptions of impairment, they can be helpful in identifying those limitations that the person finds distressing. Impact scales identify problems early in the disease process and may be especially relevant to emotional adjustment. Standard impact scales such as the Sickness Impact Profile (SIP; Gilson et al., 1975) appear valid for use in older adults (Fletcher, Dickenson, & Philp, 1992). However, some measures include items related to vocational restriction that may be inappropriate for retirees.

Emotional Distress

Aging is associated with a decrease in negative affect, but decreased positive affect is also associated with aging (Charles, Reynolds, & Gatz, 2001). Older adults are more prone to experiencing a lack of positive feelings than excessive negative feelings (Gatz & Hurwicz, 1990). Anxiety disorders are the most common disorder among older adults, but the prevalence of anxiety disorders in the elderly is slightly lower than in the general population (Blazer, George, & Hughes, 1991). Rates of depressive symptoms vary among the various subgroups of elderly. Community samples report the lowest levels and nursing home residents report the highest (Blazer, 1994). In a recent community survey, 9.1% of the older respondents met the criteria for depression and 9.9% reported subthreshold depression (Hybels, Blazer, & Pieper, 2001). This figure is slightly higher than the National Institute of Mental Health's (NIMH) estimated 6% prevalence of depression among older Americans (NIMH, 2001). The older old appear slightly more likely to experience depressive symptoms than the younger old (Zarit et al., 1999). Older women are more likely than older men to be diagnosed with a depressive disorder (Hybels et al., 2001). Depressive (Geerlings et al., 2000) and anxiety (Fisher & Noll, 1996) symptoms that do not meet the disorder criteria according to the fourth edition of *Diagnostic and Statistical Manual of Mental Disorders* (DSM-IV; American Psychiatric Association, 1994) are relatively common among older adults.

Subclinical depressive symptoms have been shown to have negative consequences on the health and well-being of older adults (Gatz & Hurwicz, 1990; Geerlings et al., 2000). Nondysphoric depression in older adults is associated with increased risk of death, functional impairment, cognitive impairment, and psychological distress (Gallo, Rabins, Lyketsos, Tien, & Anthony, 1997). Older white men have the highest rates of suicide (NIMH, 2001), and poorly controlled pain and emotional distress places the older person at greater risk for suicide (Stenager, Stenager, & Jensen, 1994).

Both pain (Roy & Thomas, 1986; Williamson & Schulz, 1992) and disability (Livingston et al., 2000) are associated with depression among older adults. Prospective studies indicate that poor physical health (Aneshensel, Frerichs, & Huba, 1984; Geerlings et al., 2000) and pain (Livingston et al., 2000) can lead to depression. Conversely, depression can lead to poor health and increased pain (Parmelee et al., 1992). The relationship between pain and depression appears weaker among nursing home patients in part because both pain and depression are relatively common in this population (Ferrell, Ferrell, & Osterweil, 1990). Among institutionalized older adults, higher anxiety is associated with higher pain (Casten et al., 1995; Parmelee et al., 1992). Although, the relationship between anger and pain in older adults has not been explored, anger may be an important emotional component of pain in older adults, as it is in other populations (Okifuji, Turk, & Curran, 1999).

Among older adults receiving treatment for pain, rates of depression vary from 17% (Helme et al., 1996) to 58% (Corran et al., 1994). These rates of depression clearly exceed the rates of depression found in the older general population, but they are similar to or less than the rates of depression found in younger pain patients (see, e.g., Kee et al., 1996; Turk et al., 1995). Older pain patients tend to report less anxiety than younger pain patients (Corran et al., 1994; Kee et al., 1996). The relationship between pain intensity and depression was found to be stronger in older pain patients compared to younger pain patients, and perceived life interference was related to depression in younger but not older patients (Turk et al., 1995).

Psychological Assessment

The Geriatric Depression Scale (GDS; Yesavage et al., 1983) is designed specifically for evaluating older adults. The GDS is a useful screening tool, but it does not allow for comparisons with other age groups. Screening tools such as the Beck Depression Inventory (BDI; Beck & Steer, 1987) and Center for Epidemiological Studies— Depression Scale have acceptable reliability and validity in older adults (Lewinsohn, Seeley, Roberts, & Allen, 1997; Olin, Schneider, Eaton, & Zemansky, 1992). However, concern has been raised that endorsement of somatic items related to illness or aging may bias scores on depression measures (Gatz, 2000). Endorsement of items related to effort, sleep, or energy could be associated to physical illness, aging, or depression. Inventories that eliminate or reduce somatic symptoms can be used, but there is an associated risk of underestimating depression. Modifying criteria to lessen the reliance on somatic symptoms does not significantly improve diagnostic accuracy (Gatz, 2000). Employing standard screening tools while examining individual items or core "affective" subscales is a good compromise (Grayson, Mackinnon, Jorm, Creasey, & Broe, 2000).

Most of the psychological tests commonly used in the assessment of pain patients are valid when used by older adults. The sample used to develop norms for the Minnesota Multiphasic Personality Inventory (MMPI-2) included older individuals (17.4% ages 60+ years), and an examination of subgroups based on age found that separate norms are not needed for different age groups (Graham, 1990; Keller & Butcher, 1991). Standard self-report anxiety measures can also be used with older adults (Stanley, Novy, Bourland, Beck, & Averill, 2001).

Assessment should include examination of problems secondary to alcohol and/or drugs. Older adults are generally more susceptible to the effects of alcohol (Center for Substance Abuse Treatment, 1998) and medications (Forman, 1996; Popp & Portenoy, 1996). Alcohol abuse is not uncommon in older adults and is associated with reduced physical strength, increased fall risk, and poor cognitive functioning (Fingerhood, 2000). Polypharmacy and use of psychotherapeutic drugs for pain, emotional distress, and insomnia are relatively common among older people, especially among those receiving pain treatment (Redpath, Middaugh, Kee, & Levin, 1992). Although many older adults are able to take these medications without complications, complications such as cognitive impairment, sedation, and poor physical function are more common in older adults than in younger (Forman, 1996; Popp & Portenoy, 1996). Deliberate opioid abuse is relatively rare among older adults (Popp & Portenoy, 1996), but the possibility of unintentional misuse and noncompliance should be explored.

If the psychological interview suggests problems with mental status, further information can be obtained through interview of a significant other in conjunction with mental status testing. The assessment of cognitive status should consider transient, reversible factors that can impair mental function. Depression (LaRue, Goodman, &

Spar, 1992), problems related to medications (Rummans, Davis, Morse, & Ivnik, 1993), or substance abuse (Fingerhood, 2000) can present as cognitive impairment. For instance, older persons with benzodiazepine dependence show significant deficits in ability to learn and remember new material 6–10 days after detoxification (Rummans et al., 1993). Withdrawal from alcohol can present as confusion beginning several days after the cessation (Fingerhood, 2000).

Pain and fatigue, aggravated by the rigors of the evaluation process itself, can make accurate evaluation of cognitive status difficult. When this is the case, and the patient is otherwise an appropriate candidate for pain rehabilitation, an effective approach is to admit the patient for a 1-week treatment trial. The members of the pain team are then able to provide detailed information regarding the patient's ability to learn new information and put behavioral changes into practice. The questionable older pain patient often performs surprisingly well once ancillary problems, such as inappropriate medications and inadequate sleep, are addressed.

Bruce and colleagues (1992) examined the cognitive profiles of 36 older patients who were treated in a chronic pain rehabilitation program at the Mayo Clinic. Although 28% of the older pain group tested as mildly cognitively impaired and 11% tested as moderately impaired, most of these patients were able to complete, and benefit from, the program. Cognitive impairment alone is not sufficient cause to exclude patients from treatment.

Beliefs and Coping

Some older Americans believe that their best years are "yet to come," but a smaller group views life ahead as ominous and responds by "just trying to hold on" (Birren, 2000). A person with optimistic expectations about aging will respond differently to pain and disability than does a person expecting decline. Assessment should include discussion about beliefs and expectations related to the aging process.

Beliefs affect the older adult's appraisal of and response to pain (Keefe et al., 2000) and disability (Zarit et al., 1999). Coping strategies, the thoughts and/or behaviors used in an effort to manage or moderate pain, also affect the older adult's appraisal of and response to pain (Keefe & Williams, 1990). Maladaptive beliefs and coping strategies can lead to increased disability and chronicity in older adults (Hopman-Rock, Kraaimaat, Odding, & Bijlsma, 1998; Keefe & Williams, 1990). Older pain patients who are confident in their ability to control and decrease pain and who deny maladaptive response tendencies such as catastrophizing, tend to report less pain and distress (Gibson & Helme, 2000; Keefe et al., 2000)

Older adults referred to specialty pain clinics appear less likely to report adaptive beliefs and coping compared to non-treatment-seeking adults. In a recent Australian study, community-dwelling older adults favored self-directed, self-developed, convenient, and relatively easy pain management strategies (Lansbury, 2000). The participants expressed dislike for physical therapy, exercise, and pain medications. The majority used cognitive coping strategies such as distraction and reframing despite not having received formal training in these strategies. In comparison, older adults referred to pain clinics have been found to be relatively passive and at risk for maladaptive pain beliefs and coping strategies (Buckelew et al., 1990; Gibson & Helme, 2000; Turk et al., 1995).

Among patients referred to specialty pain clinics, older and younger appear fairly similar in their coping approaches (Kee et al., 1996; Keefe & Williams, 1990; Turk et al., 1995), but some age-related differences have been found. Sorkin and colleagues (1990) did not find significant age group differences in coping efficacy or adaptation, but older patients reported proportionately fewer cognitive coping strategies than did younger patients. Turk and colleagues (1995) found that the proportion of "adaptive copers" among older pain patients (37%) did not differ significantly from the proportion of adaptive copers (22%) among younger pain patients. However, they did find indications of age-related differences in cognitive appraisal. Compared to younger patients, older patients seemed more likely to view an increase in pain as permanent and inevitable. This difference in

appraisal seemed to affect the strength of association between pain severity and depression. Furthermore, a different study showed that older and younger patients referred for treatment were equally likely to hold an internal locus of control (LOC) orientation toward pain (Gibson & Helme, 2000). However, older were more likely than younger patients to consider pain to be related to chance and controlled by powerful others. Belief in powerful others was found to be associated with increased use of prayer and hope for coping with pain. These findings are consistent with previous research that found that older patients are more inclined to use prayer and hope in response to pain (Keefe & Williams, 1990) and older are more likely to believe that pain is related to chance than younger pain patients (Buckelew et al., 1990).

Among older adults, beliefs and coping are associated with outcome differences. Older pain patients with internal LOC tend to use more active, self-directed coping strategies than do those with external LOC (Gibson & Helme, 2000). A "chance orientation" is associated with less effective coping and greater distress (Gibson & Helme, 2000). Older patients who elect to complete multidisciplinary treatment tend to have a relatively strong belief in powerful others, and patients who reject such treatment tend to have a relatively strong belief in pain related to chance (Gibson & Helme, 2000). Among older patients, multidisciplinary treatment is associated with positive changes in internal LOC, but treatment is not associated with change in belief in powerful others or chance. The lack of change in powerful others and chance is different from the outcomes generally associated with multidisciplinary treatment (Lipchik, Milles, & Covington, 1993). Advancing age may be associated with greater acceptance of the uncontrollable aspects of health, which in turn may lead to a stronger inclination among older pain patients to view pain as partially controlled by powerful others and chance. Treatment of the older patient may lead to increased sense of personal control, but the belief that pain is also related to other factors outside personal control may be age related and less responsive to treatment.

Catastrophizing appears to be more common in older women than in older men. Keefe and colleagues (2000) examined the relationship of catastrophizing to pain and disability in a sample primarily consisting of older patients (mean age = 61 years) with osteoarthritis. Compared to men, women had higher levels of reported pain, disability, and pain behavior. The tendency to catastrophize mediated the relationship between gender and pain-related outcomes.

COPING MEASURES

In addition to discussing beliefs and coping during the clinical interview, assessment can include standardized self-report measures such as the Pain Locus of Control questionnaire (PLOC; Toomey, Mann, Abashian, & Thompson-Pope, 1991), the Coping Strategies Questionnaire (CSQ; Rosentiel & Keefe, 1983), and the Multidimensional Pain Inventory (MPI; Kerns et al., 1985). The reliability and validity of these measures have not been tested specifically in older adults, but all of these measures have been used successfully with older adults (Gibson & Helme, 2000; Herr, Mobily, & Smith, 1993; Keefe et al., 2000; Keefe & Williams, 1990; Sorkin et al., 1990; Turk et al., 1995).

Social Environment

WORK STATUS AND RETIREMENT

Successful adjustment to retirement is associated with multiple factors including reasons for retirement, financial impact, and activity involvement (Floyd, Haynes, Doll, Winemiller, & Lemsky, 1992). Pain and/or health problems can precipitate retirement. In such cases, people are faced with unexpected, and perhaps unwelcome, retirement. Simultaneous adaptation to retirement and pain may be especially stressful (Thomas, 1999). For those already retired, the onset of pain poses a threat to plans of enjoying the "golden years." Discussing the individual's expectations and beliefs about retirement will provide a more thorough understanding of the patient's experience. Although retirement and pain do not necessarily strain family relationships, both can cause added stress, particularly in relation-

ships with preexisting difficulties (Thomas, 1999). Therefore, the family's adjustment to the individual's retirement should also be discussed.

SOCIAL SUPPORT

Compared to younger pain patients, older pain patients are more likely to be widowed, to be retired, and to live alone or with nonfamily others (Sorkin et al., 1990; Turk et al., 1995). Both pain (Roy et al., 1996) and aging (see, e.g., Carstensen, 1992; Lang & Carstensen, 1994) are associated with decreased size in the support system and reduced frequency of social contact. Although a reduction in quantity of social support is normative and not necessarily problematic, one cannot assume that a reduction reported by a particular older person is age related. Older pain clinic patients are at greater risk for deficits in social and recreational activity than are community-dwelling older adults with relatively mild pain (Roy et al., 1996). If the quantity of social support drops below a critical level, social isolation and loneliness develop. Socially isolated older adults with persistent pain are at greater risk for depression and poor adaptation than are nonisolated older adults (Roy et al., 1996; Turk, Kerns, & Rosenberg, 1992).

The quantity of social support tends to decrease with age, but the quality and importance of social support remain stable and important across the lifespan (Carstensen, 1992; Lang & Carstensen, 1994). Both older and younger adults referred to pain clinics tend to report satisfaction with social support (Kee et al., 1996; Turk et al., 1995). Older community-dwelling adults with persistent pain report similar levels of satisfaction to older adults without pain (Cook & Thomas, 1994).

The effect of social support on pain and adjustment is related more closely to the type of support received than to satisfaction with support. Satisfaction with support has been found to be positively associated with poor adaptation among pain patients (Turk et al., 1992). Supportive family members can reinforce and encourage maladaptive behaviors. Support can lead to dependence or provide scaffolding for increased independence. A longitudinal study of older adults found that having extensive social ties and contact reduced the risk of developing a disability and enhanced recovery from an existing disability (Mendes de Leon et al., 1999). However, high levels of instrumental support were associated with greater risk of developing a disability, but instrumental support was also associated with enhanced recovery from disability. Although supportive, well-meaning family members sometimes promote the development of disability by taking over tasks and responsibilities, they can be helpful in providing the support needed to regain independence and functioning.

Unsupportive or punishing communications can be distressing. Noxious interactions can serve as punishers of pain behavior and result in fewer pain behaviors, but hostile and unsupportive interactions can also contribute to low mood (Turk et al., 1992). Among a group of patients receiving treatment for rheumatoid arthritis, hostile and disharmonious problematic social interactions were positively associated with psychological distress (Riemsma et al., 2000). Problematic social support was more strongly related to depression, functional limitations, and pain than was positive support (Riemsma et al., 2000).

Social Support Measures. A discussion about social relationships and activities is an important aspect of assessment. Observing of the interactions between the patient and significant other(s) can be helpful. There are various standardized social support measures available. The Social Provisions Scales (SPS; Cutrona & Russell, 1987) and the Social Support Questionnaire (SSQ; Sarason, Levine, Basham, & Sarason, 1983) are used most often and both have been shown to be reliable and valid among older populations (Victor, Henderson, & Lamping, 1999). The MPI, Part II (Kerns, Turk, & Rudy, 1985) is a pain-related social support measure. The patient provides information regarding the responses of significant others to the patient's pain behaviors. An alternative version of the MPI provides family members with the opportunity to rate their perception of their responses

to the patients' pain behaviors (Kerns & Rosenberg, 1995).

Treatment

Multidisciplinary Treatment

The efficacy of multidisciplinary treatment for chronic nonmalignant musculoskeletal pain is well supported (e.g., Deardorff, Rubin, & Scott, 1991; Flor, Fydrich, & Turk, 1992). Such programs combine cognitive behavioral psychology and physical rehabilitation therapies with medical management. Although some early preliminary studies seemed to indicate that older patients benefited less from multidisciplinary programs than younger patients did (e.g., Aronoff & Evans, 1982; Kaplan & Kepes, 1989), subsequent, better-designed studies provided evidence that older pain patients do benefit from multidisciplinary treatment. In a literature review, Gibson, Farrell, Katz, and Helme (1996) found that 10 of 13 known investigations of multidisciplinary treatment of older pain patients reported benefits associated with treatment.

A more recent study provides further evidence that older patients with persistent pain benefit from multidisciplinary treatment. Helme and colleagues (1996) collected data on 117 patients (mean age = 74 years) who participated in a multidisciplinary geriatric pain clinic. Patients varied considerably in pain diagnoses (musculoskeletal = 35%; neurological = 28%; other = 37%). Pain improved in 72% of participants. Psychological distress improved in 65% of participants while physical and psychosocial impairment were reduced in 53% of participants.

A study completed at our multidisciplinary pain clinic (Medical University of South Carolina) compared 23 older and 23 younger patients with chronic musculoskeletal pain who were similar in gender, diagnosis, and major treatment variables (inpatient vs. outpatient format, treatment time, and treatment content). All patients were treated in the same rehabilitation program. Both older and younger patients showed statistically significant and clinically relevant improvements with treatment. Both age groups showed decreased pain, improved physical functioning, and improved psychological well-being. The older patients not only showed improvements at discharge but continued to show long-term benefits at 1-year follow-up. On most measures, the gains for older subjects were similar in nature and extent to gains for younger patients, and age was not a statistically significant predictor of treatment success. Both the patients themselves and their clinicians judged the older group's response to treatment as positive and beneficial. The results of this study were presented in greater detail in the previous edition of this book chapter (Kee et al., 1996).

In their discussion of the few studies that did not show benefits, Gibson and colleagues (1996) suggest that "we must also consider whether it is the treatment program that fails the patient, rather than the patient who fails the treatment" (p. 98). Treatment can fail the older patient for a variety of reasons. Age bias may limit the therapies offered to the patient. An age-comparison, retrospective chart review showed that opioid therapy was prescribed most often for older patients, whereas physical therapy and biofeedback were considered "less suitable" for this age group (Kaplan & Kepes, 1989). Despite these differences in treatment approaches, the authors of this study concluded that the older patients showed a "less favorable outcome."

Older patients will appear unsuccessful if the success criteria chosen are not age appropriate. For example, 55 years is a reasonable age for retirement or semiretirement. If success is based disproportionately on achievement of "return to work," older patients will appear inordinately unsuccessful. Likewise, using health care utilization as a marker of treatment success can be inappropriate. Older patients show significant reductions in health care utilization that are equivalent or greater to the levels of reductions found among younger pain patients (Kee et al., 1996; Middaugh et al., 1988), but the utilization rates prior to treatment may be higher for some groups of older pain patients (Middaugh et al., 1988).

Although the efficacy of multidisciplinary pain treatment for older adults is established, the following questions and issues still face those involved in the treatment of the older adult.

SPECIALIZED GERIATRIC VERSUS AGE-HETEROGENEOUS PROGRAMS

The milieu of an exclusively geriatric clinic may be more supportive and comforting for the older patient than a clinic with mixed ages (Gibson et al., 1996). Older patients may benefit from sharing thoughts and feelings with peers who share similar outlooks, goals, and life experiences. No research has directly compared outcomes between specialized geriatric and age-heterogeneous programs. However, research indicates that the majority of older patients do benefit from treatment in age-heterogeneous clinics.

ARE OLDER PATIENTS MORE TIME-CONSUMING AND DIFFICULT?

Clinicians judge older patients as no more difficult or time-consuming to treat than younger patients (Kee et al., 1996). In fact, the time and energy invested in multidisciplinary treatment result in an overall decrease in health care utilization (Kee et al., 1996). Concurrent problems, such as major psychiatric disorders or severe medical problems, can complicate treatment in either older or younger patients. Referring the patient for treatment of the concurrent problem is often appropriate. If treatment is successful, the patient can then be offered treatment in the multidisciplinary program. If the problem is not treatable, sometimes offering a limited or adjusted treatment program is appropriate. For the patient with severe memory deficits, providing added structure and repetition and simplifying the strategies and techniques presented can be helpful. Enlisting a family member to assist the patient in pain management techniques can also bolster treatment. For the patient with hearing loss, hearing problems can usually be circumvented with minor adaptations (sitting close, making good eye contact, speaking slowly) and a little extra time early in the course of treatment. Providing these patients with written scripts to follow while listening to the instructional, progressive muscle relaxation tapes can be helpful. In most cases, once the patient becomes familiar with the script, he or she can hear the tape sufficiently well to carry out homework practice.

INPATIENT VERSUS OUTPATIENT TREATMENT

Older patients who received outpatient treatment were found to achieve the same end points as those treated as inpatients (Kee et al., 1996). These data should not be interpreted as an indication that all patients can be treated as outpatients and improve. Rather, if the appropriate treatment format is selected based on the patients' needs, treatment will be effective. In our clinic, we try to treat as many patients as possible on an outpatient basis. Despite this, the older patients at our clinic were found to be 1.7 times more likely to receive inpatient treatment than were younger patients. The best predictor of inpatient treatment was the patient's medication use. Patients taking high levels of medications require more intensive medical supervision. The relatively high use of medications in older patients seems to contribute to the increased likelihood of the older patients requiring inpatient care. Programs that offer only outpatient treatment are likely to disproportionately reject or provide inadequate treatment for older patients. This is particularly disconcerting due to the national trend in reduction of inpatient care.

Pain Management Skill Training

Nonpharmacological self-administered pain management strategies such as physical exercise, heat, cold, massage, and relaxation are recommended for older adults with pain (American Geriatrics Society Panel on Chronic Pain in Older Persons, 1998). Ferrell (1996) describes an effective pain education program for older adults that includes information about many nondrug interventions.

Biofeedback and related physiological self-regulation therapies can be used effectively with older pain populations (Middaugh, Kee, King, Peters, & Herman, 1992; Middaugh, Woods, Kee, Harden, & Peters, 1991). The biofeedback component generally consists of progressive muscle relaxation with electromyography (EMG) and skin temperature monitoring, diaphragmatic breathing, and EMG biofeedback training to teach improved control of muscles in the areas of pain. Problems, when they arise, may indicate a need for appropriate modification of treatment protocols.

Although many older adults benefit from learning pain-reduction behaviors, some may be reluctant to use the recommended interventions. Mistaken beliefs about the potential harm or risk associated with interventions can result in reluctance or fear. Misbeliefs about possible negative outcomes of physical exercise are fairly common among older women (O'Brien Cousins, 2000). Patients should be encouraged to discuss their fears and concerns so that inaccurate beliefs can be corrected. Some patients may believe that they will dislike interventions such as physical therapy or exercise (Lansbury, 2000). These patients may need extra encouragement and reinforcement related to these potentially helpful behaviors. Poor self-efficacy or practical barriers can also interfere with performance of potentially helpful behaviors. Some older patients are concerned about bothering or taking up too much of the treatment provider's time. The patient may not feel competent to use a suggested intervention but may be uncomfortable asking for additional instruction. Some patients may be unable to afford the materials recommended. Be certain that the person has the both the means and knowledge necessary to use the intervention(s). For example, if the patient is provided with a relaxation tape, confirm that a tape player is available and the person is comfortable operating the equipment.

Psychological Treatment

In general, older adults benefit from the same sorts of psychological interventions as do younger adults, and the benefits associated with treatment are comparable (Karel & Hinrichsen, 2000). Some concerns and problems are unique to, or more prevalent among, older adults, but the basic therapeutic processes and principles do not vary with age. Psychological treatment can be offered as part of a multidisciplinary treatment or separately. Sessions can be conducted on an individual basis or in a small-group format. Regardless of the type of psychological treatment provided, the provider needs to be mindful of countertransference issues such as concerns about one's own or another's aging, death, and loss of independence (Karel & Hinrichsen, 2000).

An estimated 63% of older adults with a

psychological disorder do not receive treatment (Rabins, 1996). Many older adults who could benefit from psychological treatment are not offered help, but when treatment is offered, the majority of older adults accept help (Dorfman et al., 1995). Among cognitive-behavior therapy participants, older adults were found to have higher attendance rates and lower dropout rates than younger adults (Walker & Clarke, 2001). Older adults are likely to prefer behavioral treatments to psychopharmacological interventions (Rokke & Scogin, 1995). Much of the research regarding psychological interventions for pain in older adults has been conducted in multidisciplinary treatment settings. In the few studies that examined stand-alone psychological treatment, treatment was associated with improvements in pain and well-being (Fry & Wong, 1991; Miller & LeLievre, 1982; Puder, 1988).

Cognitive-Behavioral Treatment

Cognitive-behavioral therapy is specifically recommended as part of geriatric pain treatment by the AGS (1998). The goals of behavioral interventions are to decrease maladaptive pain behaviors while increasing productive/beneficial behaviors. For older adults, activities targeted for *increase* often include IADLs, recreational/leisure activities, volunteer work, grandparenting, and so on. Some older adults easily identify behavioral goals, but for others identifying goals requires discussion and experimentation. For older adults simultaneously coping with other life changes such as retirement or widowhood, adaptive/rewarding activities may be less established and therefore more difficult to identify and initiate. Sometimes a patient experiences a medical event, such as a stroke, that causes both pain and non-pain disability. It may be difficult for the patient to differentiate the limitations that are due to pain from those that are due to the other problem(s). For example, a patient who has significant leg weakness due to a stroke may have the expectation that successful pain treatment will allow him to return to tennis. If playing tennis is unrealistic regardless of pain level, the clinician needs to assist the individual in setting goals that take the leg weakness into consideration.

The problematic behaviors identified for *decrease* among the elderly tend to be the same sorts of behaviors generally targeted in behavioral treatment. The goals of reducing reliance on medications, reducing health care utilization, and reducing pain behaviors are as appropriate for older as well as younger adults.

Treatment that specifically targets pain coping skills has been shown to be helpful for older adults (Fry & Wong, 1991; Keefe et al., 1999). Interventions that reduce catastrophizing are associated with reduced pain and disability (Keefe et al., 1999). The recent increased emphasis on increasing positive beliefs and coping strategies (in addition to reducing maladaptive beliefs) has carried over into the treatment of older adults (James, Kendell, & Reichelt, 1999). Some older adults may need assistance in developing and/or identifying positive beliefs related to worthiness and control. Developing an appreciation for the contributions made to others and society may be helpful for older adults facing role loss. Emphasizing those tasks that the patient completes without assistance may be helpful for those concerned about autonomy. Because older adults appear especially vulnerable to believing that increased pain is permanent and inevitable (Turk et al., 1995), and pain is controlled by external factors such as chance and powerful others, clinicians may need to spend extra time discussing and emphasizing the aspects of pain and health that are within the individual's control.

Communication Skills and Interpersonal Relationships

Including the spouse, family member, or care provider in psychologically oriented pain treatment is generally helpful (Keefe et al., 1999). The therapies commonly used to improve social and interpersonal relationships are generally effective with older adults and require little modification (Hinrichsen, 1997). The specific topics addressed in treatment vary with life stage (Thomas, 1999), but key concerns such as the need for autonomy and relatedness are essential to well-being across the lifespan (Ryan & La Guardia, 2000). Ryan and La-Guardia (2000) suggest well-being is related to the individual's ability to experience volitional reliance on others. Therefore, it is helpful to determine what factors will allow the older person to rely on others while maintaining autonomy.

Misbeliefs about aging can contribute to problematic support. For example, the belief that the older person is on an irreversible course of deterioration can contribute to oversolicitous behavior and unnecessary worry. Discussing misbeliefs with support providers may lead to more appropriate support and reduced worry. Providing the patient with assertive communication training can also be helpful. Some older adults are reluctant to ask for assistance because of concerns about "burdening" others. In such cases, supportive others may provide "unhelpful" assistance because they do not have enough information to know what would be helpful. The medical care provider should also be alert for the tendency to be a "good patient" in order to please the provider. The pain team may overlook the "good" patient's needs because he or she reports doing so well.

Intervention is needed for patients experiencing excessive negative interactions, such as explicit expressions of anger and blame. In some cases, these expressions of anger and blame may be part of the extended history of relationship, and in such cases non-pain-related issues should be addressed in therapy. In other cases, interpersonal conflicts are related to changing roles, circumstances, and/or pain-related stress, and the conflict will resolve when these stressors are clarified and addressed.

For the socially isolated patient, the social support provided by the treatment environment may improve the patient's mood and outlook. In such cases, assisting the patient in making this association and exploring alternative ways of increasing social involvement can help maintain improvements. Participation in a seniors' group can help with both pain and depression in older adults (Roy et al., 1996).

Conclusion

Review of the literature provides solid evidence that older adults are at risk for persistent pain and associated problems. However, if managed appropriately pain and associated problems are generally preventable and/or responsive to treatment. In many respects, the psychosocial aspects of assessment and treatment of pain in the older adult do not differ from those in young or middle-age adults. The primary challenge is understanding and acknowledging age-related differences without overgeneralizing and allowing ageism to interfere with appropriate care.

References

American Geriatrics Society Panel on Chronic Pain in Older Persons. (1998). The management of chronic pain in older persons. *Journal of the American Geriatric Society, 46,* 635–651.

American Psychiatric Association. (1994). *Diagnostic and statistical manual of mental disorders* (4th ed.). Washington, DC: Author.

Aneshensel, C. S., Frerichs, R. R., & Huba, G. J. (1984). Depression and physical illness: A multiwave, nonrecursive causal model. *Journal of Health and Social Behavior, 25,* 350–371.

Aronoff, G. M., & Evans, W. O. (1982). The prediction of treatment outcome at a multidisciplinary pain center. *Pain, 14,* 67–73.

Beck, A., & Steer, R. (1987). *The Beck Depression Inventory manual.* New York: Harcourt Brace Jovanovich.

Bergh, I., Sjöström, B., Odon, A., & Steen, B. (2000). An application of pain rating scales in geriatric patients. *Aging, 12,* 380–387.

Birren, J. E. (2000). Using the gift of long life: Psychological implications of the age revolution. In S. H. Qualls & N. Abeles (Eds.), *Psychology and the aging revolution: How we adapt to longer life* (pp. 11–24). Washington, DC: American Psychological Association.

Blazer, D. G. (1994). Epidemiology of late life depression. In L. S. Schneider, C. F. Reynolds III, B. D. Lebpwotz, & A. J. Friedhoff (Eds.), *Diagnosis and treatment of depression in late life* (pp. 9–19). Washington, DC: American Psychiatric Press.

Blazer, D. G., George, L. K., & Hughes, D. (1991). The epidemiology of anxiety disorders: An age comparison. In C. Salzman & B. D. Lebowitz (Eds.), *Anxiety in the elderly* (pp. 17–30). New York: Springer.

Brattberg, G., Parker, M. G., & Thorslund, M. (1997) A longitudinal study of pain: Reported pain from middle age to old age. *Clinical Journal of Pain, 13,* 144–149.

Bruce, B. K., Rome, J. D., Malec, J. F., Hodgson, J. E., Suda, K. S., Payne, J. E., & Maruta, T. (1992). *Cognitive impairment: A primary reason for the exclusion of the elderly from chronic pain rehabilitation programs?* Paper presented at the meeting of the American Pain Society, San Diego, CA.

Buckelew, S. P., Shutty, M. S., Hewett, J., Landon, T., Morrow, K., & Frank, R. G. (1990). Health locus of control, gender differences and adjustment to persistent pain. *Pain, 42,* 287–294.

Carstensen, L. L. (1992). Social and emotional patterns in adulthood. Support for socioemotional selectivity theory. *Psychology and Aging, 7,* 331–338.

Casten, R. J., Parmelee, P. A., Kleban, M. H., Lawton, M. P., & Katz, I. R. (1995). The relationships among anxiety, depression, and pain in a geriatric institutionalized sample. *Pain, 61,* 271–276.

Center for Substance Abuse Treatment. (1998). *Substance abuse among older adults* (DHHS Pub. No. 1998: 98-3179). Washington, DC: U.S. Government Printing Office.

Charles, S. T., Reynolds, C. A., & Gatz, M. (2001). Age-related differences and change in positive and negative affect over 23 years. *Journal of Personality and Social Psychology, 80,* 136–151.

Cohen, M. E., & Marino, R. J. (2000). The tools of disability outcomes research functional status measures. *Archives of Physical Medicine and Rehabilitation, 81*(12 Suppl. 2), S21–S29.

Cook, A., & Thomas, M. (1994). Pain and the use of health services among the elderly. *Journal of Aging and Health, 6,* 155–172.

Corran, T. M., Gibson, S. J., Farrell, M. J., & Helme, R. D. (1994). Comparison of chronic pain experience between young and elderly patients. In G. F. Gebhart, D. L. Hammond, & T. S. Jensen (Eds.), *Proceedings of the 7th World Congress on Pain, Progress in pain research and management* (Vol. 2, pp. 895–906). Seattle, WA: IASP Press.

Cutler, R. B., Fishbain, D. A., Rosomoff, R. S., & Rosomoff, H. L. (1994). Outcomes in treatment of pain in geriatric and younger age groups. *Archives of Physical Medicine and Rehabilitation, 75,* 457–464.

Cutrona, C. E., & Russell, D. W. (1987). The provision of social relationships and adaptation to stress. *Advances in Personal Relationships, 1,* 37–67.

Deardorff, W. W., Rubin, H. S., & Scott, D. W. (1991). Comprehensive multidisciplinary treatment of chronic pain: A follow-up study of treated and non-treated groups. *Pain, 45,* 35–43.

Dorfman, R. A., Lubben, J. E., Mayer-Oakes, A., Atchison, K., Schweitzer, S. O., DeJong, F. J., & Matthias, R. E. (1995). Screening for depression among a well elderly population. *Social Work, 40,* 295–304.

Douzjian, M., Wilson, C., Shultz, M., Berger, J., Tapino, J., & Blanton, V. (1998). A program to use pain control medication to reduce psychotropic drug use in residents with difficult behavior. *Annals of Long-Term Care, 6,* 174–179.

Eich, E., Reeves, J. L., Jaeger, B., & Graff-Radford, S. B. (1985). Memory for pain: Relation between past and present pain intensity. *Pain, 23,* 375–380.

Erskine, A., Morley, S., & Pearce, S. (1990). Memory for pain: A review. *Pain, 41,* 255–265.

Ferrell, B. A. (1991). Pain management in elderly people. *Journal of the American Geriatrics Society, 39,* 409–414.

Ferrell, B. A., Ferrell, B. R., & Osterweil, D. (1990). Pain in the nursing home. *Journal of the American Geriatrics Society, 38,* 409–414.

Ferrell, B. A., Ferrell, B. R., & Rivera, L. (1995). Pain in cognitively impaired nursing home patients. *Journal of Pain and Symptom Management, 10,* 591–598.

Ferrell, B. A., Stein, W. M., & Beck, J. C. (2000). The Geriatric Pain Measure: Validity, reliability and factor analysis. *Journal of the American Geriatrics Society, 48,* 1669–73.

Ferrell, B. R. (1996). Patient education and nondrug interventions. In B. R. Ferrell & B. A Ferrell (Eds.), *Pain in the elderly* (pp. 35–44). Seattle, WA: IASP Press.

Fingerhood, M. (2000). Substance abuse in older people. *Journal of the American Geriatrics Society, 48,* 985–995.

Fisher, J., & Noll, J. P. (1996). Anxiety disorders. In L. L. Carstensen, B. A. Edelstein, & Dornbrand, L. (Eds.), *The practical handbook of clinical gerontology* (pp. 304–323). Thousand Oaks, CA: Sage.

Fletcher, A. E., Dickenson, E. J., & Philp, I. (1992). Audit measures: Quality of life measures for everyday use with elderly patients. *Age and Ageing, 12,* 142–150.

Flor, H., Fydrich, T., & Turk, D. C. (1992). Efficacy of multidisciplinary pain treatment centers: A meta-analytic review. *Pain, 49,* 221–230.

Floyd, F., Haynes, S., Doll, E., Winemiller, D., & Lemsky, C. (1992). Assessing retirement satisfaction and perceptions of retirement experience. *Psychology and Aging, 7,* 609–621.

Forman, W. B. (1996). Opioid analgesic drugs in the elderly. *Clinics in Geriatric Medicine, 12,* 489–500.

Fry, P. S., & Wong, P. T. P. (1991). Pain management training in the elderly: Matching interventions with subjects' coping styles. *Stress Medicine, 7,* 93–98.

Gallo, J. J., Rabins, P. V., Lyketsos, C. G., Tien, A. Y., & Anthony, J. C. (1997). Depression without sadness: Functional outcomes of nondysphoric depression in later life. *Journal of the American Geriatrics Society, 45,* 570–578

Gatz, M. (2000). Variations on depression in later life. In S. H. Qualls & N. Abeles (Eds.), *Psychology and the aging revolution: How we adapt to longer life* (pp. 173–196). Washington, DC: American Psychological Association.

Gatz, M., & Hurwicz, M. L. (1990). Are old people more depressed? Cross-sectional data on CES-D factors. *Psychology and Aging, 5,* 284–290.

Geerlings, S. W., Beekman, A. T. F., Deeg, D. J. H., & van Tilburg, W. (2000). Physical health and the onset and persistence of depression in older adults: An eight-wave prospective community-based study. *Psychological Medicine, 30,* 369–380.

Gibson, S. J., Farrell, M. J., Katz, B., & Helme, R. D. (1996). Multidisciplinary management of chronic nonmalignant pain in older adults. In B. R. Ferrell & B. A. Ferrell (Eds.), *Pain in the elderly* (pp. 91–99). Seattle, WA: IASP Press.

Gibson, S. J., & Helme, R. D. (1995). Age differences in pain perception and report: A review of physiological psychological, laboratory, and clinical studies. *Pain Reviews, 2,* 111–137.

Gibson, S. J., & Helme, R. D. (2000). Cognitive factors and the experience of pain and suffering in older persons. *Pain, 85,* 375–383.

Gilson, B. S., Gilson, J. S., Bergner, M., Bobbit, R. A., Kressel, S., Pollard, W. E., & Vesselago, M. (1975). The Sickness Impact Profile: Development of an outcome measure of health care. *American Journal of Public Health, 65,* 1304–1310.

Graham, J. R. (1990). *MMPI–2: Assessing personality and psychopathology.* New York: Oxford University Press.

Grayson, D. A., Mackinnon, A., Jorm, A. F., Creasey, H., & Broe, G. A. (2000). Item bias in the Center for Epidemiologic Studies Depression Scale: Effects of physical disorders and disability in an elderly community sample. *Journals of Gerontology Series B: Psychological Sciences Social Sciences, 55B,* P273–P282.

Guccione, A. A., Felson, D. T., Anderson, J. J., Anthony, J. M., Zhang, Y., Wilson, P. W., Kelly-Hayes, M., Wolf. P. A., Kreger, B. E., & Kannel, W. B. (1994). The effects of specific medical conditions on the functional limitations of elders in the Framingham study. *American Journal of Public Health, 84,* 351–358.

Hall-Lord, M. L., Larsson, G., & Steen, B. (1999). Chronic pain and distress in older people: A cluster analysis. *International Journal of Nursing Practice, 5,* 78–85.

Harkins, S. W. (1996). Geriatric pain: Pain perceptions in the old. *Clinics in Geriatric Medicine, 12,* 435–459.

Harkins, S. W., Kwentus, J., & Price, D. D. (1990). Pain and suffering in the elderly. In J. J. Bonica, J. D. Loeser, C. R. Chapman, & W. E. Fordyce (Eds.), *Management of pain* (2nd ed., pp. 552–559). Philadelphia: Lea & Febiger.

Harkins, S. W., & Price, D. D. (1997). Assessment of pain in the elderly. In D. C. Turk & R. Melzack (Eds.), *Handbook of pain assessment* (pp. 325–331). New York: Guilford Press.

Harper, R. G., Kotick-Harper, D., & Kirby, H. (1990). Psychometric assessment of depression in an elderly general medical population: Over- or underassessment? *Journal of Nervous and Mental Disease, 178,* 113–119.

Helme, R., Gibson, S., Bradbeer, M., Farrell, M., Neufeld, M., & Corran, T. (1996). Multidisciplinary pain clinics for older people: Do they have a role? *Clinics in Geriatric Medicine, 12,* 563–582.

Herr, K. A., Mobily, P. R., & Smith, C. (1993). Depression and the experience of chronic back pain: A study of related variables and age differences. *Clinical Journal of Pain, 9*(2), 104–114.

Hinrichsen, G. A. (1997). Interpersonal psychotherapy for depressed older adults. *Journal of Geriatric Psychiatry, 30,* 239–257.

Hopman-Rock, M., Kraaimaat, F. W., Odding, E., & Bijlsma, J. W. J. (1998). Coping with pain in the hip or knee in relation to physical disability in community-living elderly people. *Arthritis Care and Research, 11,* 243–252.

Hybels, C. F., Blazer, D. G., & Pieper, C. F. (2001). Toward a threshold for subthreshold depression: An analysis of correlates of depression by severity of symptoms using data from an elderly community sample. *Gerontologist, 41,* 357–365.

James, I. A., Kendell, K., & Reichelt, F. K. (1999). Conceptualizations of depression in older people: The interaction of positive and negative beliefs. *Behavioural and Cognitive Psychotherapy, 27,* 285–290.

Kaasalainen, S. J., Robinson, L. K., Hartley, J. M., Knezacek, S., & Ife, C. (1998). The assessment of pain in the cognitively impaired elderly: A literature review. *Perspectives, 22,* 2–8.

Kaplan, G. A., Haan, M. N., & Wallace, R. B. (1999). Understanding changing risk factor associations with increasing age in adults. *Annual Review of Public Health, 20,* 89–108.

Kaplan, R., & Kepes, E. (1989). *Pain problems over 70 and under 40 years.* Paper presented at a meeting of the American Pain Society, Phoenix, AZ.

Karel, M. J., & Hinrichsen, G. (2000). Treatment of depression in late life: Psychotherapeutic interventions. *Clinical Psychology Review, 20,* 707–729.

Kee, W. G., Middaugh, S. J., Redpath, S., & Hargadon, R. (1998). Age as a factor in admission to chronic pain rehabilitation. *Clinical Journal of Pain, 14,* 121–128.

Kee, W. G., Middaugh, S. J., & Pawlick, K. L. (1996). Persistent pain in the older patient: Evaluation and treatment. In R. J. Gatchel & D. C. Turk (Eds.), *Psychological approaches to pain management* (pp. 371–402). New York: Guilford Press.

Keefe, F. J., Caldwell, D. S., Baucom, D., Salley, A., Robinson, E., Timmons, K., Beaupre, P., Weisberg, J., & Helms, M. (1999). Spouse-assisted coping skills training in the management of knee pain in osteoarthritis: Long-term followup results. *Arthritis Care and Research, 12,* 101–111.

Keefe, F. J., Caldwell, D. S., Baucom, D., Salley, A., Robinson, E., Timmons, K., Beaupre, P., Weisberg, J., & Helms, M. (1999). Spouse-assisted coping skills training in the management of knee pain in osteoarthritis: Long-term followup results. *Arthritis Care and Research, 12*(2), 101–111.

Keefe, F. J., Lefebvre, J. C., Egert, J. R., Affleck, G., Sullivan, M. J., & Caldwell, D. S. (2000). The relationship of gender to pain, pain behavior, and disability in osteoarthritis patients: The role of catastrophizing. *Pain, 87,* 325–334.

Keefe, F. J., & Williams, D. A. (1990). A comparison of coping strategies in chronic pain patients in different age groups. *Journal of Gerontology, 45*(4), 161–165.

Keller, L. S., & Butcher, J. N. (1991). *Assessment of*

chronic pain patients with the MMPI–2. Minneapolis: University of Minnesota Press.

Kendig, H., Browning, C. J., & Young, A. E. (2000). Impacts of illness and disability on the well-being of older people. *Disability and Rehabilitation: An International Multidisciplinary Journal, 22,* 15–22.

Kerns, R. D., & Rosenberg, R. (1995). Pain-relevant responses from significant others: Development of a significant-other version of the WHYMPI scales. *Pain, 61*(2), 245–249.

Kerns, R. J., Turk, D. C., & Rudy, T. E. (1985). The West Haven–Yale Multidimensional Pain Inventory (WHYMPI). *Pain, 23,* 345–356.

Kramarow, E., Lentzner, H., Rooks, R., Weeks, J., & Saydah, S. (1999). *Health and aging chartbook. Health, United States, 1999.* Hyattsville, MD: National Center for Health Statistics.

Krulewitch, H., London, M. R., Skakel, V. J., Lundstedt, G. J., Thomason, H., & Brummel-Smith, K. (2000). Assessment of pain in cognitively impaired older adults: A comparison of pain assessment tools and their use by nonprofessional caregivers. *Journal of the American Geriatric Society, 48,* 1607–1611.

Lang, F. R., & Carstensen, L. L. (1994). Close emotional relationships in late life: Further support for proactive aging in the social domain. *Psychology and Aging, 9,* 315–324.

Lansbury, G. (2000). Chronic pain management: A qualitative study of elderly people's preferred coping strategies and barriers to management. *Journal of Disability and Rehabilitation, 22,* 2–14.

LaRue, A., Goodman, S., & Spar, J. E. (1992). Risk factors for memory impairment in geriatric depression. *Neuropsychiatry, Neuropsychology, and Behavioral Neurology, 5,* 178–184.

Lavsky-Shulan, M., Wallace, R. B., Kohout, F. J., Lemke, J. H., Morris, M. C., & Smith, I. M. (1985). Prevalence and functional correlates of low back pain in the elderly: The Iowa 65+ rural health study. *Journal of the American Geriatric Society, 33,* 23–28.

Leveille, S. G., Guralnik, J. M., Hochberg, M., Hirsch, R., Ferrucci, L., Langlois, J., Ranatanen, T., & Ling, S. (1999). Low back pain and disability in older women: Independent association with difficulty but not inability to perform daily activities. *Journal of Gerontology: Medical Sciences, 54A,* M487–M493.

Lewinsohn, P. M., Seeley, J. R., Roberts, R. E., & Allen, N. B. (1997). Center for Epidemiologic Studies Depression Scale (CES-D) as a screening instrument for depression among community-dwelling older adults. *Psychology and Aging, 12,* 277–287.

Lipchik, G. L., Milles, K., & Covington, E. C. (1993). The effects of multidisciplinary pain management treatment on locus of control and pain beliefs in chronic non-terminal pain. *Clinical Journal of Pain, 9,* 49–57.

Livingston, G., Watkin, V., Milne, B., Manela, M. V., & Katona, C. (2000). Who becomes depressed? The Islington community study of older people. *Journal of Affective Disorders, 58,* 125–133.

Manton, K. G., & Gu, X. (2001). Changes in the prevalence of chronic disability in the United States black and nonblack population above age 65 from 1982 to 1999. *Proceedings of the National Academy of Sciences of the United States of America, 98,* 6354–6359.

Melding, P. (1991). Is there such a thing as geriatric pain? *Pain, 46,* 119–121.

Mendes de Leon, C. F., Glass, T. A., Beckett, L. A., Seeman, T. E., Evans, D. A., & Berkman, L. F. (1999). Social networks and disability transitions across eight intervals of yearly data in the New Haven EPESE. *Journal of Gerontology: Social Sciences, 54B,* S162–S172.

Mendes de Leon, C. F., Seeman, T. E., Baker, D. I., Richardson, E. D., & Tinetti, M. E. (1997). Black–white differences in risk of becoming disabled and recovering from disability in old age: A longitudinal analysis of two EPESE populations. *American Journal of Epidemiology, 145,* 488–497.

Middaugh, S. J., Kee, W. G., King, S. R., Peters, J. R., & Herman, K. (1992). Physiological response of older and younger pain patients to biofeedback-assisted relaxation training. *Biofeedback and Self-Regulation, 17,* 304–305.

Middaugh, S. J., Levin, R. B., Kee, W. G., Barchiesi, F. D., & Roberts, J. M. (1988). Chronic pain: Its treatment in geriatric and younger patients. *Archives of Physical Medicine and Rehabilitation, 69,* 1021–1026.

Middaugh, S. J., Woods, S. E., Kee, W. G., Harden, R. N., & Peters, J. R. (1991). Biofeedback-assisted relaxation training for chronic pain in the aging. *Biofeedback and Self-Regulation, 16,* 361–377.

Miller, C., & LeLievre, R. B. (1982). Method to reduce chronic pain in elderly nursing home residents. *Gerontologist, 22,* 314–317.

Miller, J., Neelon, V., Dalton, J. NgVandu, N., Bailey, D. Jr., Layman, E., & Hosfeld, A. (1996). The assessment of discomfort in elderly confused patients: A preliminary study. *Journal of Neuroscience Nursing, 28,* 175–182.

Nahit, E. S., Silman, A. J., & MacFarlance, G. J. (1998). Occurrence of falls among patients with new episode of hip pain. *Annals of Rheumatology and Disability, 57,* 166–168.

National Institute of Mental Health. (2001). *Older adults: Depression and suicide facts* (NIH Pub. No. 01-4593). Washington, DC: Author.

Norton, P. J., Asmundson, G., Norton, R., & Craig, K. D. (1999). Growing pain: 10-year research trends in the study of chronic pain and headache. *Pain, 14,* 67–73.

O'Brien Cousins, S. (2000). "My heart couldn't take it": Older women's beliefs about exercise benefits and risks. *Journals of Gerontology Series B: Psychological Sciences and Social Sciences, 55B,* P283–P294.

Okifuji, A., Turk, D. C., & Curran, S. L. (1999).

Anger in chronic pain: Investigation of anger targets and intensity. *Journal of Psychosomatic Research, 61,* 771–780.

Olin, J. T., Schneider, L. S., Eaton, E. M., & Zemansky, M. F. (1992). The Geriatric Depression Scale and the Beck Depression Inventory as screening instruments in an older adult outpatient population. *Psychological Assessment, 4,* 190–192.

Ostir, G. V., Carlson J. E., Black, S. A., Rudkin, L., Goodwin, J. S., & Markides, K. S. (1999). Disability in older adults. Prevalence, causes, and consequences. *Behavioral Medicine, 24,*147–156.

Parmelee, P., Katz, I., & Lawton, M. P. (1992). Depression and mortality among institutionalized aged. *Journal of the American Geriatric Society, 41,* 517–522.

Parmelee, P., Smith, B., & Katz, I. (1993). Pain complaints and cognitive status among elderly institution residents. *Journal of Gerontology: Psychological Sciences, 47,* P3–P10.

Popp, B., & Portenoy, R. K. (1996). Management of chronic pain in the elderly: Pharmacology of opioids and other analgesic drugs. In B. R. Ferrell & B. A. Ferrell (Eds.), *Pain in the elderly* (pp. 21–34). Seattle, WA: IASP Press.

Puder, R. S. (1988). Age analysis of cognitive-behavioral group therapy for chronic pain outpatients. *Psychology and Aging, 3,* 204–207.

Rabins, P. V. (1996). Barriers to diagnosis and treatment of depression in elderly patients. *American Journal of Geriatric Psychiatry, 4,* S79–S83.

Redpath, S., Middaugh, S. J., Kee, W. G., & Levin, R. (1992). *Medication profiles of older versus younger patients evaluated by a chronic pain rehabilitation program.* Paper presented at the meeting of the American Pain Society, San Diego.

Riemsma, R. P., Taal, E., Wiegman, O., Rasker, J. J., Bruyn, G. A., W., & Van Paassen, H. C. (2000). Problematic and positive support in relation to depression in people with rheumatoid arthritis. *Journal of Health Psychology, 5,* 221–230.

Rokke, P., & Scogin, F. (1995). The credibility of treatments for depression among younger and older adults. *Journal of Clinical Geropsychology, 1,* 243–257.

Rosentiel, A., & Keefe, F. J. (1983). The use of coping strategies in chronic low back pain patients: Relationship to patient characteristics and current adjustment. *Pain, 17,* 33–44.

Roy, R., & Thomas, M. (1986). A survey of chronic pain in an elderly population. *Canadian Family Physician, 32,* 513–516.

Roy, R., Thomas, M., & Cook, A. (1996). Social context of elderly chronic pain patients. In B. R. Ferrell & B. A. Ferrell (Eds.), *Pain in the elderly* (pp. 111–117). Seattle, WA: IASP Press.

Rummans, T. A., Davis, L. J., Morse, R. M., & Ivnik, R. J. (1993). Learning and memory impairment in older, detoxified, benzodiazepine-dependent patients. *Mayo Clinic Proceedings, 68,* 731–737.

Ruzicka, S. A. (1998). Pain beliefs: What do elders believe? *Journal of Holistic Nursing, 16,* 369–382.

Ryan, R. M., & La Guardia, J. (2000). What is being optimized?: Self-Determination theory and basic psychological needs. In S. H. Qualls & N. Abeles (Eds.), *Psychology and the aging revolution: How we adapt to longer life* (pp. 145–172). Washington, DC: American Psychological Association.

Sarason, I. G., Levine, H. M., Basham, R. B., & Sarason, B. R. (1983). Assessing social support: The social support questionnaire. *Journal of Personality and Social Psychology, 44,* 127–139.

Satariano, W. A., Haight, T. J., & Tager, I. B. (2000). Reasons given by older people for limitation or avoidance of leisure time physical activity. *Journal of the American Geriatrics Society, 48,* 505–512.

Schaie, K. W. (1993). Ageist language in psychological research. *American Psychologist, 48,* 49–51.

Scudds, R. J., & Robertson, J. M. (2000). Pain factors associated with physical disability in a sample of community-dwelling senior citizens. *Journal of Gerontology: Medical Sciences, 55A,* M393–M399.

Sengstaken, E. A., & King, S. A. (1993). The problems of pain and its detection among geriatric nursing home residents. *Journal of the American Geriatric Society, 41,* 541–544.

Sorkin, B. A., Rudy, T. E., Hanlon, R. B., Turk, D. C., & Stieg, R. L. (1990). Chronic pain in old and young patients: Differences appear less important than similarities. *Journal of Gerontology, 45,* 64–68.

Spencer, W. D., & Raz, N. (1995). Differential effects of aging on memory for content and context: A meta-analysis. *Psychology and Aging, 10,* 527–539.

Stanley, M. A. Novy, D. M., Bourland, S. L., Beck, J. G., & Averill, P. M. (2001). Assessing older adults with generalized anxiety: A replication and extension. *Behaviour Research and Therapy, 39,* 221–235.

Stenager, E. N., Stenager, E., & Jensen, K. (1994). Attempted suicide, depression, and physical diseases: A 1-year follow-up study. *Psychotherapy and Psychosomatics, 61,* 65–73.

Thomas, M. R. (1999). *The changing nature of pain complaints over the lifespan.* New York: Plenum Press.

Thomas, M. R., & Roy, R. (1988). Age and pain: A comparative study of the younger and older elderly. *Journal of Pain Management, 1,* 174–179.

Tibblin, G., Bengtsson, C., Furunes, B., & Lapidus, L. (1990). Symptoms by age and sex. The population studies of men and women in Gothenburg, Sweden. *Scandinavian Journal of Primary Health Care, 8,* 9–17.

Toomey, T. C., Mann, J. D., Abashian, S., & Thompson-Pope, S. (1991). Relationship between perceived self-control of pain, pain description and functioning. *Pain, 45,* 129–133.

Turk, D. C., Kerns, R. D., & Rosenberg, R. (1992). Effects of marital interaction on chronic pain and disability: Examining the down side of social support. *Rehabilitation Psychology, 37,* 259–274.

Turk, D. C., Okifuji, A., & Scharff, L. (1995). Chronic pain and depression: Role of perceived impact and perceived control in different age cohorts. *Pain, 61,* 93–101.

Victor, C. R., Henderson, L. M., & Lamping, D. L. (1999). Evaluating the use of standardized health measures with older people: The example of social support. *Reviews in Clinical Gerontology, 9,* 371–382.

Walker, D. A., & Clarke, M. (2001). Cognitive behavioural psychotherapy: A comparison between younger and older adults in two inner city mental health teams. *Aging and Mental Health, 5,* 197–199.

Weiner, D., Peterson, B., & Keefe, F. (1999). Chronic pain-associated behaviors in the nursing home: Resident versus caregiver perceptions. *Pain, 80,* 577–588.

Weiner, D., Peterson, B., Ladd, K., McConnell, E., & Keefe, F. (1999). Pain in nursing home residents: An exploration of prevalence, staff perspectives, and practical aspects of management. *Clinical Journal of Pain, 15,* 92–101.

Williamson, G. M., & Schulz, R. (1992). Pain, activity, restriction, and symptoms of depression among community-residing elderly adults. *Journal of Gerontology, 47,* 367–372.

Yesavage, J. A., Brink, T. L., Rose, T. L., Lum, O., Huang, V., Adley, M., & Leirer, V. O. (1983). Development and validation of a geriatric depression screening scale: A preliminary report. *Journal of Psychiatric Research, 1,* 37–49.

U.S. Census Bureau. (2000). *Population projections of the United States by age, sex, race, Hispanic origin, and nativity: 1999 to 2100.* Washington, DC: Author.

U.S. Census Bureau. (2001). *The 65 years and over population: 2000.* Washington, DC: Author.

Zarit, S. H., Femia, E. E., Gatz, M., & Johansson, B. (1999). Prevalence, incidence and correlates of depression in the oldest old: The OCTO study. *Aging and Mental Health, 3,* 119–128.

Index

Page numbers followed by *f* indicate figure, *n* indicate note, and *t* indicate table